D0875595

THE ABUSE OF MAN

*An Illustrated History of
Dubious Medical Experimentation*

THE
ABUSE OF
MAN

*An Illustrated History
of Dubious Medical
Experimentation*

WOLFGANG WEYERS, M.D.

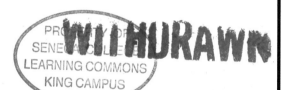

Ardor Scribendi, Ltd.

NEW YORK · 2003

For information, write:

ARDOR SCRIBENDI, LTD.

145 East 32nd Street, 10th Floor, New York, New York 10016
Tel: 212.448.0083   Fax: 212.448.0552

ISBN 1-893357-21-X

Library of Congress Control Number: 2003100021

Printed in the United States of America

ACKNOWLEDGEMENTS
AND APOLOGIES

A book like this cannot be written without help, and I am deeply grateful to the people mentioned below for their considerable contributions. Some helped chiefly by their patience – including my friends and partners at the Center for Dermatopathology in Freiburg, Susanna Borghi and Carlos Díaz, and, especially, my wife, Imke Weyers. Others helped me through their past research and writing about this complex subject that engaged me so thoroughly. Numerous excellent studies concerning the history of experiments carried out on human subjects and the development of regulations to control them provided me with information and inspiration. These ranged from Maurice H. Pappworth's *Human Guinea Pigs* in 1967 and David J. Rothman's *Strangers at the Bedside* in 1991 to Susan E. Lederer's *Subjected to Science* in 1997 and Jonathan D. Moreno's *Undue Risk* in 1999. Human experimentation connected specifically with dermatovenereology also has been the focus of many articles and books. Among the most helpful were Walter B. Shelley's review in 1983 of "Experimental disease in the skin of man" in *Acta Dermatovenereologica*; Elke Tashiro's assessment in 1991 of experiments in venereology in the nineteenth century in *Die Waage der Venus*; James H. Jones' *Bad Blood* of 1993, concerning syphilis experiments at Tuskegee; and the book in 1998 titled *Acres of Skin*, in which Allen M. Hornblum recorded the history of experiments performed on inmates of Holmesburg Prison by dermatologists at the University of Pennsylvania during the third quarter of the twentieth century. The excellent work already done by my colleagues provided a solid foundation on which to build this one.

Many other people helped by providing articles, photographs, and other information. I am grateful to Bernard Cribier (Strasbourg), Allen Hornblum (Philadelphia), Heinz Kutzner (Friedrichshafen), Heinrich Dennhöfer (Cologne), and members of the Institutes of the History of Medicine of the universities of Berlin, Dresden, Frankfurt, Freiburg, Heidelberg, Munich, and Vienna. Of particular assistance were the librarians at the University of Freiburg, where, in a matter of hours, one can obtain almost any needed article or book. I also wish to thank those who helped bring the book to completion, including the chief executive officer of Ardor Scribendi, Ltd., Andrew Zwick, Dee Mosteller and Florence Nygaard who edited the manuscript, Matt Kaukeinen and Zenaida Vega of Ardor Scribendi who integrated everything and readied all of it for printing and publication, and Betsy Peare who oversaw the production of it. Jerry Kelly was responsible for the design and typesetting. And, of course, no one contributed more substantially to this work than my teacher and dear friend, A. Bernard Ackerman, who encouraged me to pursue this study, sent me scores of articles, edited scrupulously the first (very rough) manuscript and at least seven drafts thereafter, and provided countless thoughtful insights. More need not be said. Only Bernie Ackerman can appreciate how truly grateful I am.

In addition to acknowledgements, I also must express apologies. A study of the abuse of man in medical experiments is bound inextricably to moral judgments. Those judgments, although heartfelt, may not always be fair. For example, some people listed as coauthors of articles mentioned in this book about ethically dubious experiments may not have been involved directly themselves in the actual experiments. (If such were the case, however, this author feels that they should not have allowed their name to be associated in any way with those articles.) Also, some of the studies reviewed may have been ethically impeccable, including a responsible weighing of risks and benefits, careful selection of test subjects, and proper process of informed consent of subjects; these facts were not evident in those published reports. If most, or all, of the just mentioned requirements were fulfilled by the researchers, it should have been noted specifically by them in the articles. That no such evidence was given may be attributed to the attitude of the time, which attached little or no importance to the need for justification of the ethics of a study. If, for that or any other reason, a particular study, implicated here as a case of human abuse, actually was sound ethically, then it should not have been included and those who conducted the experiments deserve my apology. An apology also is in order for my selection arbitarily of the studies under review in this volume. A primary criterion for inclusion was inherent defenselessness of the test subjects – e.g., children, the elderly or very ill, and those incarcerated in prisons or other institutions. In many instances, when test subjects were not specified as to their status within society, I felt that they should not be regarded necessarily as victims of abusive behavior by experimenters. For example, some of the experiments described on prisoners actually may have been more ethically sound than countless others that were excluded from this present work because test subjects in them were not identified as being members of a population that was vulnerable. These considerations should be kept in mind by the reader.

More succinctly, I wish to apologize to any individual who has been unjustly, albeit unintentionally, implicated by me in the abuse of man, and to my readers, who have been given a history that despite my best efforts is far from complete.

I also want to take this opportunity to confess my own sins of omission and to apologize to a few of my patients. Over the past

16 years, I, on occasion, have subjected patients whose diseases were particularly interesting to yet another biopsy or diagnostic procedure without telling them that those procedures were more for my benefit than for theirs, that they served primarily to satisfy my curiosity and only secondarily to help with enabling diagnosis and selecting treatment. I do not believe that any of those patients were done any other harm; their right to purely autonomous decisions, however, was neglected. While writing this history of the abuse of man in medical experiments, I have given much thought to my own behavior professionally, and hope that my readers will do the same about theirs.

PREFACE

Self-esteem is essential to a meaningful life, but it is both a blessing and a curse. We acquire self-esteem, in part, through an inner belief that we are better than someone else. No human is completely free of this egoistic conviction. In other words, self-esteem does not derive entirely from within oneself; it comes also from comparing ourselves with others. It is much easier, therefore, to acquire self-esteem through comparison with those who are considered to be weaker, less successful, or less valuable than we are. In short, the feeling of self-esteem, which in itself is commendable, has a dark side, and no small number of atrocities in the history of man – among them suppression and enslavement, war and genocide – are the result of this ugly alter ego.

A lasting, fruitful relationship between society as a whole and individual human beings is possible only when the feelings and claims of superiority are abandoned, and the rights of others are respected. This is not always easy because the concepts of inferiority and superiority are summoned easily by external circumstances, such as differences among nations in military and/or economic might, or disparity among individuals in physical appearance, wealth, knowledge, and social status. They also are evoked by special situations, the most seductive, perhaps, being the relationship between a patient and a physician. The patient often is debilitated by poor physical or emotional health. He or she* is entirely dependent on the physician, who likely has a higher social status; makes more

* For purposes of simplicity – and because most of the physicians referred to in this book are men – patients and doctors who go unnamed will be designated hereafter by masculine pronouns.

– ix –

money; is more knowledgeable (at least about the problems that caused them to meet in that particular setting); is emotionally uninvolved; is, by necessity, "allowed" at times to subject the patient to additional pain; and makes pronouncements of diagnoses and prognoses like sentences in a court of law. Functioning continually in this state of distorted inequality, physicians are prone – sometimes inadvertently – to develop feelings of superiority, to regard patients as inferior beings, and to neglect the right of his or her charges to make their own decisions. For this reason, it is especially important for physicians to be aware of and to moderate such feelings. The only physician who accomplishes his duties optimally, beyond the limits of technical medical precepts, is the one who has respect for his patient; who acts not as dictator but as partner in the challenge, and often the struggle, to achieve well-being of a patient; and who can lend support to that patient emotionally as well as physically.

This demand is, or should be regarded as, the gold standard for the practice of medicine. To fulfill it requires continuous effort and awareness not only of the impact, but also of the signs and symptoms that result from not regarding patients as human beings of equal value. In the daily practice of medicine, this awareness can be communicated by verbal and nonverbal messages from patients to superficial, impersonal, or arrogant behavior – providing the physician is alert to those signals. The dangers associated with a physician's feeling of superiority, however, can be appreciated best by studying incidents in the past that illustrate how horrendous are the consequences of that attitude when it is unbridled. The most striking examples come from medical experiments in which human beings were used as unwitting guinea pigs and suffered temporary or permanent damage to their health without due process of informed consent. Almost invariably, subjects in those experiments were considered by society to be inferior. Most of those experiments would not have been possible without the belief of researchers that the interests of subjects could be disregarded with impunity.

It is undeniable that much that is positive derived from what often were inhumane medical experiments on human beings, including the vast, rapid increase in our knowledge about diseases and how to treat them effectively. In some studies, ethical requirements were observed carefully and test subjects were chosen thoughtfully as authentic volunteers. In many others, however, this was not the case. The focus of this book is on the abuse, rather than the use, of man by medical research. The reason for this is not sensationalism. Most of the experiments have been recorded already in public forums and have been decried. Nor is this intended to praise the superior moral conduct of contemporary researchers by contrast with the behavior of colleagues in times past. The history of questionable experiments on humans continues to the present, and it is not possible to draw a definitive line at which a survey such as this one can be ended logically.

There is no desire here to settle personal scores. Most physicians mentioned in this history are dead. Of those who are still alive, most are unknown personally to me. The reason for revisiting the subject of abuse of man in medical experiments is simply that much can be learned from negative example. Only by awareness of man's inhumanity to man medically, and the assessment of the factors that led to and enabled those abuses to be carried out, is there any possibility that physicians and researchers in the future will shrink from the idea of ever perpetrating them.

Writing a history about dubious human experimentation is an endeavor without end. Too many experiments have been performed at too many times and in too many places, and for too many reasons, to allow analysis of all of them in a single book. For that reason, previous studies have concentrated on certain periods (such as the nineteenth and early twentieth centuries), certain places (such as Germany or the United

States), or certain subjects (such as radiation experiments). Such confinement of subject both sharpens the view and narrows it at the same time. In order to understand factors crucial in the development overall of human experimentation and the concepts that galvanized those experiments, however, the view must not be too narrow. I chose, therefore, to discuss times, places, and subjects in a continuum, and to sharpen the view by emphasizing the particular specialty in medicine that has been the most important in the history of unethical experimentation on human beings, namely, dermatology.

Why dermatology? One reason is that the skin, as the external covering of the body, is easy to observe. Results of experiments can be studied directly and at any time. Moreover, the skin is an extensive organ that allows multiple experiments to be carried out simultaneously. This advantage is used routinely for purposes of diagnosis (e.g., patch tests to contact allergens) and for therapy (e.g., attempts to find the modes most expedient for treatment of a condition externally). The skin also has been utilized widely for purposes of research.

The second reason for the involvement prominently of dermatologists in human experiments is the fact that the development of both modern dermatology and human experimentation began at approximately the same time and in the same geographic region – around the end of the eighteenth and the beginning of the nineteenth centuries, first in England, then in France, and then in Germany and Austria. One of the first nontherapeutic experiments on humans, involving inoculation of a patient with matter from venereal disease, was carried out in the latter part of the 1700s by John Hunter in England. It was there, roughly at the same time, that modern dermatology was established by the English physician, Robert Willan, in his pioneering textbook on cutaneous diseases in which skin diseases were classified according to the morphologic attributes of individual lesions (Fig. 1, 2). During the first decades of the

Preface

nineteenth century, the center of experimental medicine shifted to France. The same was true for dermatology as it was advanced by French physicians like Laurent Theodore Biett (Fig. 3) and Pierre Louis Alphée Cazenave (Fig. 4), who built on Willan's work to expand knowledge of skin diseases. In the latter two thirds of the century, ex-

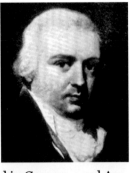

perimental medicine was most advanced in Germany and Austria; at the same time, dermatology in those countries came to the forefront through the influence of Ferdinand Hebra and Moriz Kaposi in Vienna, Heinrich Köbner and Albert Neisser in Breslau, Edmund Lesser in Berlin, and Paul Gerson Unna in Hamburg. Despite its preeminence, however, dermatology was not yet an accepted medical discipline in German-speaking countries; it was not until the end of the nineteenth century that the first chairs for dermatology were established in universities. As a young discipline, dermatology was replete with unresolved problems, and practitioners of it needed quick answers to improve their capability for treatment and to win acceptance among the other, more powerful and respected branches of medicine. For both purposes, using humans as test subjects seemed to be highly expedient.

The third, and per-

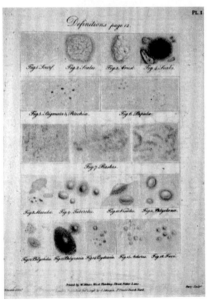

FIG. 2
Definitions of primary lesions of the skin according to Robert Willan (1798).

– xiii –

FIG. 3
*Laurent
Theodor Biett
(1780-1840)*

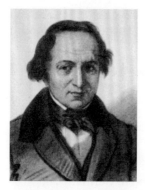

FIG. 4
*Alphée
Cazenave
(1795-1877)*

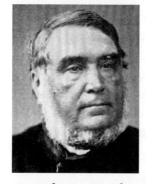

haps the most important, rationale for the connection between dermatology and experimentation in humans is the long association of dermatology with venereology. Since the outbreak of syphilis epidemically in Naples in the late fifteenth century, venereal diseases were perceived as the most terrible threat to health, not only because of their severity, but because of the widely held perception that being infected with such a disease is the penalty for an immoral style of life. Venereal diseases were extremely common, and many carriers were asymptomatic, meaning that their having sexual intercourse with anyone could be lethal to the partner. No definite cure for syphilis existed, and the modes of treatment, such as exposure to hot steam of mercury, were agonizing, as well as mostly ineffectual (Fig. 5). As a result, a diagnosis of syphilis usually was considered to be a death sentence.* Diagnoses of venereal disease at that time were based almost exclusively on findings in the skin, hence the association of dermatology and venereology (Fig. 6). With the advances in dermatology – especially discrimination among eruptions on the basis of minute morphologic changes – the diagnosis of syphilis and its distinction from other cutaneous diseases, such as psoriasis and lichen planus, became much more reliable. Nevertheless, diagnosis of syphilis remained imprecise and largely inaccurate, primarily because it had not been distinguished from other venereal conditions, like gonorrhea and chancroid, that were thought to be manifestations of the same disease. Intense research on venereal

* One can hardly fail to notice the similarities with modern-day AIDS.

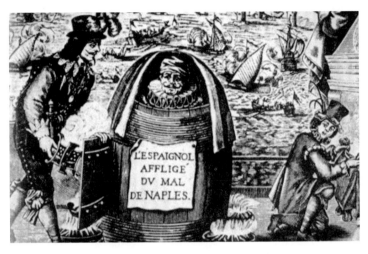

FIG. 5
*Syphilis (or
"Mal de
Naples") being
treated by
exposure to hot
steam of
mercury.*

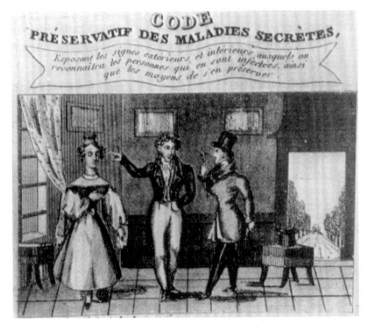

FIG. 6
*"How to
protect oneself
from secret
maladies"
(French poster
of the 19th
century
depicting
cutaneous
signs of
syphilis).*

diseases, therefore, was considered by the medical profession to be mandatory. But this research was compromised by the fact that during that period the pathogenic organisms responsible for venereal diseases could not be grown in cultures or in animals. Although reports about monkeys being infected with syphilis date to the mid-nineteenth century, the findings of these studies were not widely accepted until 1903, when Elias Metchnikoff and Emile Roux succeeded in inducing syphilis in a young chimpanzee. Until that time, the only experiments in the study of venereal diseases were conducted on human beings.

The high prevalence of venereal diseases; their severity in the absence of effective treatments; the multitude of questions about their interrelationships, propagation, and natural course; and the lack of an experimental animal model all contributed to the frequency with which experiments on humans were performed in the discipline of dermatovenereology. Toward the end of the nineteenth century, those experiments elicited wide public discussion, aggravated by anti-Semitic propaganda motivated by the fact of an ever growing number of Jewish physicians who were practicing dermatology in Germany. This led to the world's first governmental decree, issued in Prussia in 1900, concerning experiments on human beings. In the early twentieth century, two experiments in regard to syphilis conducted in the United States by Udo J. Wile and Hideyo Nogushi resulted in heated debates about experiments on humans and induced efforts to include specific rules about this type of testing in the *Code of Ethics* of the American Medical Association. During the Second World War, the skin, by virtue of its accessibility, was utilized for purposes of research that mostly was nonconsensual. For example, the efficacy of sulfonamides was tested by treating experimentally induced infections in inmates of German concentration and extermination camps. Skin diseases, such as scabies, were studied intensely by the Allies, and experiments concerning the effects of poison gas on human skin were part of the war effort of many countries.

Following the war, human experimentation became big business, especially in the United States, where the pharmaceutical, cosmetic, and chemical industries were obligated by the Food and Drug Administration to test all new drugs for possible adverse effects on humans prior to those medications being made available to the public. In the early 1970s, it again was the revelations of an experiment in dermatovenereology – the infamous Tuskegee Syphilis Study – that prompted the U.S. government to enact the Federal Regulations for the Protection of Subjects of Research.

In short, the history of human experimentation and the history of dermatology are linked intimately, integrally, and inextricably. The lessons that can be gleaned from those histories – of what is wrong and what is right, and how to behave – are of more than mere historical interest. They are of inestimable importance for every physician and every patient, not only today, but for all days to come.

TABLE OF CONTENTS

CHAPTER I

INTRODUCTION

There are many ways to acquire knowledge and experience. The most common is the performance of tests on human beings, either on oneself or on others. This is how each of us learns, from the earliest days of our lives, about pain and comfort, and the effects of our behavior on other people. As we use others for enlightenment, so others use us. Experiments on human beings are an essential aspect of learning and as long as they are conducted in the spirit of benevolence, they are acceptable. Confidence in the benevolence of others is the foundation of human experimentation, as it is in any kind of meaningful social intercourse.

During our lives, this confidence in the good will of man is challenged many times. It is necessary, therefore, to reinforce that confidence if positive and gratifying social exchange is to be maintained. This is especially true for situations in which individuals are highly vulnerable, as in the relationship between a patient and a physician. A person in pain who places his entire being in the hands of someone else must be sure that this confidence will not be abused. The special need to reinforce the faith of patients in physicians was recognized early on and propagated in a unique professional code of ethics, the Oath of Hippocrates.

The Hippocratic Oath actually has nothing to do with the Greek physician Hippocrates, just as the *Corpus Hippocraticum,* a collection of roughly 60 manuscripts about various

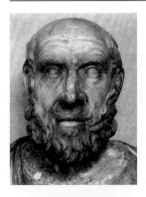

FIG. 7
*Hippocrates
(Roman bust,
2nd century
B.C.)*

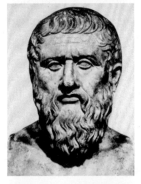

FIG. 8
*Plato (Roman
copy of a Greek
sculpture)*

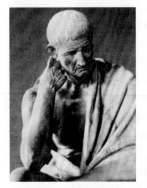

FIG. 9
*Aristotle
(Roman copy
of a Greek
sculpture)*

aspects of Greek medicine, was not written by Hippocrates (Fig. 7) himself. Who Hippocrates of Cos was and what he contributed to medicine is not really known. The first mention of Hippocrates was in Plato's dialogue, Protagoras, in which Hippocrates was said to have the same status among physicians as Phedias held among sculptors and Protagoras among Sophists (Fig. 8). Plato's pupil, Aristotle, described Hippocrates as being small in stature but large as a physician (Fig. 9). The prominence given to Hippocrates in the writings of Plato and Aristotle may have prompted administrators of the famous library at Alexandria to assemble various medical scriptures under the name of Hippocrates. Although the extent to which the "Father of Medicine" contributed to the Hippocratic Collection is controversial, the Oath of Hippocrates surely was written after his lifetime, probably in the fourth century B.C. The Oath was unknown to most Greek physicians and became important only in Christian and Islamic medicine. In the oldest scriptures of the Collection preserved, dating from the tenth century A.D., the Oath was used as a preamble to whatever followed (Fig. 10). As of the sixteenth century, it was sworn by physicians at the outset of their professional lives, and eventually it became the standard credo for the practice of medicine.[1]

I · Introduction

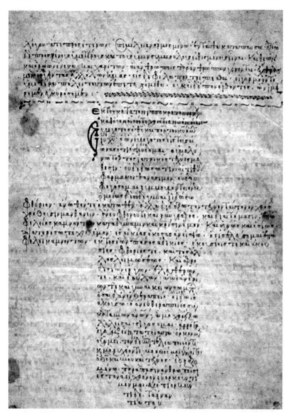

FIG. 10
Oath of Hippocrates (Byzantine manuscript, 12th century)

According to the Hippocratic Oath, practitioners of medicine must respect and support those who taught them medicine; carry out their duties with "purity and piety;" enter the home of others only for the good of a patient, free of any conscious wrong or misdeed; provide medical care only in the best interest of a patient and never in a harmful or unjust way; never give any person a deadly drug, even if asked for; and keep secret anything confidential seen or heard during treatment and during social intercourse outside the practice of medicine. In the course of two and a half millennia, the Oath of Hippocrates has been modified many times and translated into most languages. It no longer is sworn to Apollo and Aesculapius, but to God,

Christ, and Allah, or the medical community. Some directives pertaining specifically to conditions that existed at the time of Hippocrates, for example, to refrain from certain surgical procedures, have been abandoned. Most of the fundamental principles of the Hippocratic Oath, however, have been maintained, that is, to uphold the sanctity of patient confidentiality, to practice medicine free of any conscious wrong, "to help, or at least to do no harm."[2,3]

It was in regard to the rule of *primum non nocere* (above all, do no harm), especially, that interpretation of the Hippocratic Oath changed over centuries and from society to society. The Hippocratic school was exceedingly strict about *non nocere;* treatment was confined mostly to dietary regimens and rules concerning sleep, physical activities, and other aspects of behavior. By those measures little, if any, harm could be done; by employing them almost exclusively, however, Hippocratic physicians eventually were accused of doing nothing but "waiting for death."[4] Most Greek and Roman physicians, including Galen, considered to be the founder of experimental physiology, advocated more active forms of treatment, such as use of phytotherapeutic mixtures. The Hippocratic concept that diseases resulted from disturbances in the equilibrium of the four humors of the body – blood, phlegm, yellow bile, and black bile – became the basis of attempts to extract excess fluids by cupping, scarifying, bloodletting, and inducing emesis. Those regimens were associated inevitably with some harm to patients in the interest of what was thought to be beneficial ultimately.

The Abuse of Man in the Ancient World

The rule never to do harm also was violated in experiments performed on humans for the sole purpose of acquiring knowledge. For example, some physicians experimented with different kinds and concentrations of poisonous plants. Attalus III

I · Introduction

(Philometor) (Fig. 11), who reigned at Pergamum about 137 years before Christ, offered cocktails of them to friends, pretending they were edible herbs, for the insidious purpose of studying their effects.[5] In Alexandria, the greatest anatomist of antiquity, Herophilus of Chalkedon (Fig. 12), who is credited with having identified and named the duodenum, may have acquired his knowledge through vivisection, that is, cutting into living human beings. At a time when disease was thought to result from temporary alterations in the equilibrium of humors, vivisection seemed to be a promising method for unraveling the mysteries of health and disease. According to the Roman encyclopedist, Aulus Cornelius Celsus (Fig. 13), Alexandrian anatomists of the first century used criminals sentenced to death by Ptolemaic kings "for dissection alive, and contemplated, even while they breathed, those parts which nature had before concealed."[6] Celsus also noted that vivisections led to controversial debates about ethical aspects among the different Greek schools of medicine. The Empiricists, who refrained from experiments and philosophical speculations, and emphasized the importance of studying actual signs and symptoms of disease, criticized the cruelty of vivisectionists and the fact

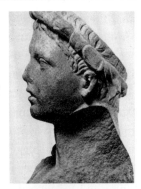

FIG. 11
Attalus III. (Philometor) (2nd cent. B.C.)

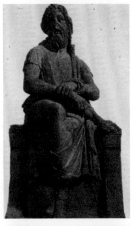

FIG. 12
Herophilus of Chalkedon (3rd cent. B.C.)

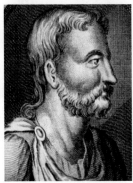

FIG. 13
Cornelius Celsus (detail of a print dated 1765)

"that the art dedicated to the health of man is used not only to bring him to death but even to do this in the most dreadful manner." In contrast, the so-called dogmatists defended vivisection of criminals by pointing out the value for "innocent humans of all times."[7] By the time of Galen (Fig. 14), in the second century, experiments on humans were rejected. Galen acquired new knowledge about anatomy and physiology primarily by cutting into monkeys and pigs (Fig. 15), and the wholesale transfer of his findings to conditions in human beings resulted in misconceptions that were passed on for many centuries.

FIG. 14
Claudius Galenus teaching medicine (miniature in a medieval manuscript, c. 1500)

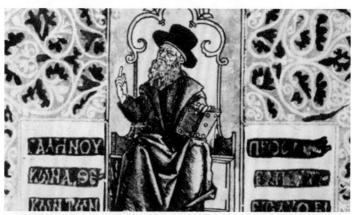

FIG. 15
Picture of dissection of a pig by Galenus.

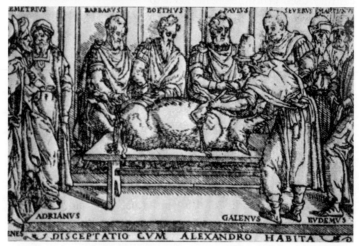

I · Introduction

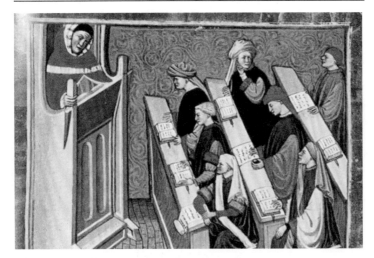

FIG. 16
Teaching at the University of Bologna, early 15th century: Knowledge was sought through reading books, rather than through observation of nature.

Christianity as an Impediment for More Than 1000 Years to New Knowledge in Medicine

With the rise of Christianity, medical experiments of all kinds came to a halt. People no longer were interested in acquiring knowledge about the material world; they wanted to know about God and heaven. The knowledge they sought could be found only in the Bible and other religious texts. Hence, study was devoted almost exclusively to books, and intellectual argument was confined to interpretation of those works whose truthfulness was thought to be beyond doubt.[8] This unshakable trust in religious texts was transferred to volumes on secular issues, including the medical books by Galen. For many centuries, Galen's theories concerning health and disease, and his methods of treatment went unchallenged (Fig. 16). Even when autopsies were performed routinely in the fourteenth century, professors of medicine refused to acknowledge what was in front of their eyes, adhering thereby to incorrect concepts about the human body taught to them through the works of Galen (Fig. 17).[9]

FIG. 17
*Dissection
scene by
Bartolomeus
Anglicus (late
15th century).*

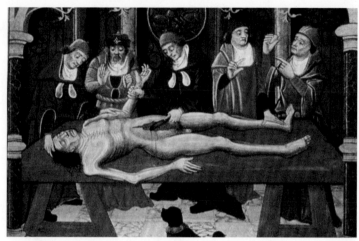

FIG. 18
*Ibn Sina
(Avicenna,
980-1037)*

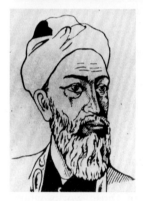

FIG. 19
*Maimonides
(1125-1204)*

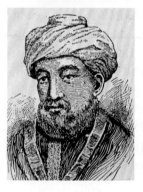

Although only a minimum of medical research was carried out in the Middle Ages, some preeminent physicians acknowledged the need for studying the effects of drugs on human beings. In the eleventh century, the Islamic scientist and philosopher Ibn Sina (Avicenna) (Fig. 18) recommended that a drug be studied in different circumstances in order to assess its effects, and he insisted that "the experimentation must be done with the human body, for testing a drug on a lion or a horse might not prove anything about its effects on man."[10] The practices of research of that time remain obscure, but experiments on humans doubtlessly were performed. In the twelfth century, such experiments motivated the Jewish physician and philosopher, Maimonides (Fig. 19), to counsel colleagues to treat patients always as ends in themselves, not as means for learning new truths. In the thirteenth century, the English philosopher, Roger Bacon (Fig. 20), excused inconsistencies in therapeutic practices among contemporary physicians on the following grounds: "It is exceedingly difficult and dangerous to perform operations on the human body, wherefore it is more difficult to work in that science than in any other . . . The operative and practical sciences which do their work on insensate bodies can multiply their experiments till they get rid of deficiency and errors, but a physician cannot do this because of the nobility of the material in which he works; for that body demands that no error be made in operating upon it, and so experience is so difficult in medicine."[11]

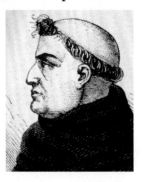

FIG. 20
Roger Bacon
(1214-1294)

Advances in Medicine During the Renaissance

Experiments became much more numerous during the Renaissance when secular, in lieu of religious, issues shifted to the center of interest (Fig. 21, 22). Knowledge from books no longer was deemed to be sacrosanct; nature itself became an object of study. The theoretical foundation of the modern scientific method was laid by Leonardo da Vinci (Fig. 23) in these lines: "I shall test by experiment before I proceed further, because my intention is to consult experience first and then with reasoning show why such experience is bound to operate in such a way. And this is the rule by which those who analyze the effects of nature must proceed, and although Nature begins with the cause and ends with the experience, we must follow the opposite course, namely . . . begin with the experience and by means of it investigate the cause."[12] Like other sciences, medicine detached

FIG. 21
*A human being
counts only as part of
God's universe
(miniature from the
13th century).*

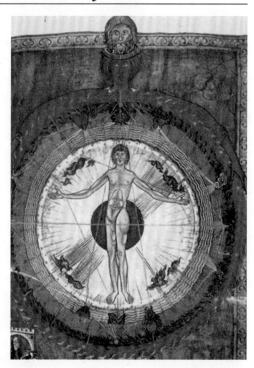

FIG. 22
*Human beings,
and worldly
matters, are in
the foreground,
whereas Christ
is in the
background
("The
Flagellation of
Christ," Piero
della Francesca,
15th century).*

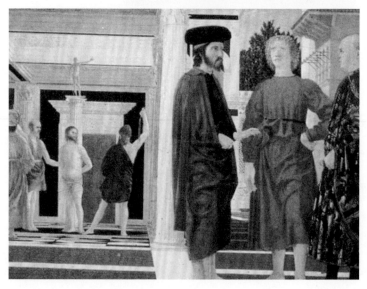

I · Introduction

slowly from ancient dogma. In 1528, one of the proponents of medical empiricism, the German alchemist, Paracelsus (Fig. 24), burned in public the works of Galen and Avicenna in order to demonstrate how great was his opposition to medical orthodoxy then extant. Paracelsus spoke in the language of the common people from whom he collected information about folk medicine. He insisted that "practice should not be based on speculative theory; theory should be derived from practice. Experience is the judge; if a thing stands the test of experience, it should be accepted; if it does not stand the test, it should be rejected."[13]

Within one hundred years, more advances were made in medicine than in the previous one thousand years. As the natural laws of mechanics pertaining to everything material were unraveled, the human body also was found to be governed by mechanical forces. In 1543, the Belgian physician, Andreas Vesalius (Fig. 25), described the body as a 'fabric'; his fundamental treatise, *De Humani Corporis Fabrica*, corrected many mistakes of Galen and became the foundation of modern anatomy (Fig. 26, 27). The discovery of the unidirectional circulation of blood by William Harvey (Fig. 28) in

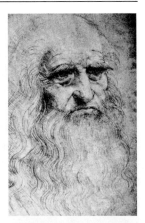

FIG. 23
Leonardo da Vinci (1452-1519)

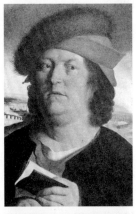

FIG. 24
Theophrastus Bombastus von Hohenheim (Paracelsus) (1493-1541)

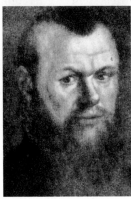

FIG. 25
Andreas Vesalius (1514-1564)

FIG. 26
Andreas Vesalius pictured in "De humani corporis fabrica."

FIG. 27
The "Muscle Man" in "De humani corporis fabria" by Andreas Vesalius.

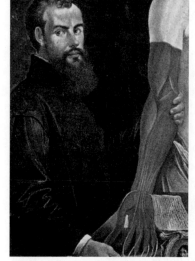

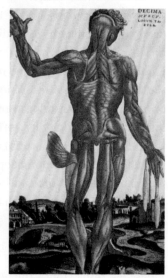

England in 1628 reinforced the notion that the human body works like a machine (Fig. 29, 30). In 1632, French philosopher René Descartes (Fig. 31) wrote a treatise on man titled, *Traité de L'homme*, which went unpublished for 30 years because of fear of persecution by the church. According to Descartes, God created the human body according to the laws of mechanics, which determined its functions in an automatic, perpetual way. Descartes referred to man as a *machine de terre*, compared the urinary tract to a system of intercommunicating pipes, applied laws of optics

FIG. 28
William Harvey (1578-1657)

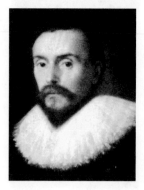

to the function of the eye, and explained nerve reflexes by circulation of a neural spiritus (Fig. 32, 33). The concept of man as an earthly machine implied that the human body, like other mechanical devices, could be manipulated. As a result, an experimental approach came to prevail in medicine and enhanced interest in experiments on humans.[14]

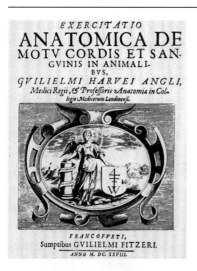

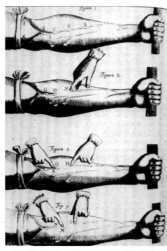

FIG. 29
Title page of
Harvey's
study.

FIG. 30
Experiment
on the
circulation of
blood
(William
Harvey,
1628).

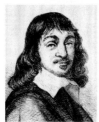

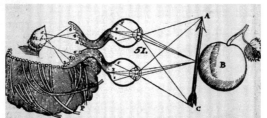

FIG. 31 René
Descartes (1596-1650)

FIG. 32 The mechanism of vision (from Descartes).

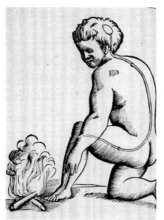

FIG. 33
The mechanism of reflexes
(from Descartes).

The Abuse of Man

The Enlightenment and a New Emphasis on the Rights of Patients

FIG. 34
*Immanuel
Kant (1724-
1804)*

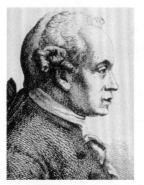

The development of empiricism coincided with increasing awareness of the worth of an individual human being. The eighteenth century was characterized by the Enlightenment, a spiritual current that was defined by Immanuel Kant (Fig. 34) thus: "Enlightenment is man's emergence from his self-incurred immaturity. Immaturity is the inability to use one's own understanding without the guidance of another. This immaturity is self-incurred if its cause is not lack of understanding, but lack of resolution and courage to use it without the guidance of another."[15] In short, the proponents of Enlightenment tried to induce people to use their brain. This educational effort was thought to pave the way for a glorious future; firm was belief in progress and fervent was desire to improve conditions of living according to rational solutions. The hardships borne by common people that for centuries had gone unacknowledged, including the deplorable status of health, became subjects for consideration and concern. Even absolute monarchs began to recognize the importance of the health of their soldiers and farmers. At that time, few physicians possessed an education that might be termed academic and they treated only those persons who moved in the highest circles of society, a service for which they were paid handsomely. Treatment of ordinary people, therefore, was the province of barbers, charlatans, and so-called surgeons who were barbers authorized to perform minor operations, such as bloodletting. To meet the demand for more physicians, surgeons were given full recognition as physicians, academies for surgery were founded, and new hospitals were built.[16]

I · Introduction

In the spirit of enlightenment, basics about diseases and how to avoid them were taught in numerous medical publications designed for laymen. The most popular of these texts, *Avis au Peuple sur Sa Santé* (Advice to the People About Health), begun in 1761 by the Swiss physician Auguste Tissot (Fig. 35), went through 15 editions and was translated into 17 languages (Fig. 36).[17] Some philosophers of the Enlightenment became involved directly in public health; Jean-Jacques Rousseau (Fig. 37), for example, discouraged swaddling of infants and advocated nursing by mothers. The "American Hippocrates," Benjamin Rush (Fig. 38), a committed revolutionary and signer of the American Declaration of Independence, argued that physicians ought to share a rich body of information with their patients in order to enable those supplicants to understand their own medical problems and the measures taken by the physician to rectify them. He anticipated that medical benefits would flow from increased comprehension and reflection by patients, as was the case in other arenas of human life.[18] These prescriptions were in stark contrast with traditional concepts of the relationship between patient and physician. As but some examples, it was felt that the truth about diseases, if

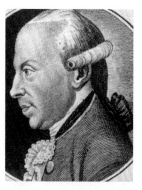

FIG. 35
Simon André (Auguste) Tissot (1728-1787)

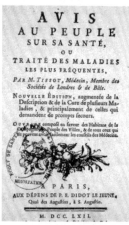

FIG. 36
Avis au Peuple sur sa Santé by Simon Auguste Tissot.

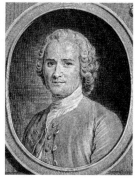

FIG. 37
Jean-Jacques Rousseau (1712-1778)

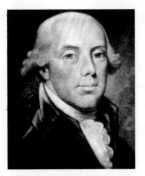

FIG. 38
*Benjamin
Rush
(1745-1813)*

known by the patient, could impede the process of healing; that patients had to pay obedience unconditionally to physicians; and that physicians were entitled to conceal from patients the actual nature of their disease. In the *Corpus Hippocraticum,* physicians had been advised bluntly of the wisdom of "concealing most things from the patient, while you are attending to him . . . turning his attention away from what is being done to him . . . revealing nothing of the patient's future or present condition."[19]

According to the classic ethical rudiments of medicine, as conveyed by the Hippocratic Oath, physicians had a moral duty to act benevolently, that is, to promote health by cure or prevention of disease without allowing interference of any other kind from any other interest. The idea of beneficence overshadowed all other moral principles, such as respect for the autonomy of patients. When interacting with physicians, patients were denied the right to be informed and to make their own decisions; they were obliged to follow the physicians' directives without question. In short, the Hippocratic scriptures imposed duties on physicians, but they did not confer rights on patients. With the call of enlightenment to make use of the power of reason, however, people began to think not only about solutions to practical problems, but also about their own social status, prospects, and rights. The proponents of enlightenment claimed that every individual had rights that were inalienable, rights that no one could take away from them. Among those rights, stated clearly for the first time in 1776 by Thomas Jefferson (Fig. 39) in the American Declaration of Independence, were life, liberty, and the pursuit of happiness.[20] During the French revolution, health, too, was declared to be a right of all citizens.[21]

I · Introduction

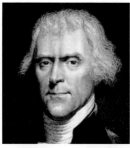

FIG. 39
*Thomas
Jefferson
(1743-1826)*

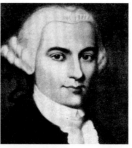

FIG. 40
*Thomas
Percival
(1740-1804)*

The focus on inalienable rights influenced the relationship between physicians and patients. Interest in medical ethics was revived, and Thomas Percival's (Fig. 40) *Code of Ethics,* published in Manchester in 1803, became the model for all later proscriptions (Fig. 41). Recognizing the dependence of patients on physicians, Percival counseled physicians to disregard their egos and to attend strictly to the patients' medical needs. He did not suggest that patients should be involved in the process of decision-making, but he advised that they be informed about their diseases, with the exception of situations that were emergencies, terminal, and/or might be worsened by honesty that was all too candid.[22] To prevent harm was understood to be the most important moral obligation of physicians. Freedom from harm also began to be perceived as a right that could be claimed of physicians by patients. The disparate concepts of respect for the rights of patients and the increasing interest in human experimentation were not easy to integrate, that duality becoming a continuous source of conflict in times that followed.

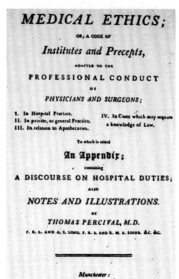

FIG. 41
*Title page of
Thomas
Percival's book
on Medical
Ethics.*

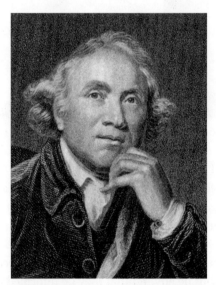

FIG. 42
John Hunter (1728-1793)

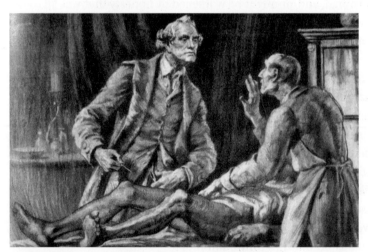

FIG. 43
John Hunter inoculating himself (drawing by Julius Merész).

CHAPTER 2

STUDIES BY INOCULATION

The best interest of individual human beings and the principle of preventing harm were never violated more openly than through experiments that employed inoculation, that is, the deliberate infection of persons with pathogenic organisms for the expressed purpose of producing disease. One of the first inoculation experiments conducted diligently was carried out by John Hunter of London (Fig. 42), who is remembered for his description of the hunterian chancre, to wit, the hard, painless ulcer of primary syphilis. In 1767, Hunter injected pus from a patient with gonorrhea into the penis of a subject referred to simply as "the patient." Some authors later claimed that Hunter had used his own penis for the experiment and praised his heroic inoculation of self, but Hunter's original article provides no evidence for that assumption. As a result of the inoculation, the patient (whoever it was) developed a formidable chancre and signs of indubitable secondary syphilis, namely, a typical syphilitic exanthem and generalized lymphadenopathy.[1, 2] This outcome, apparently caused by infection of the patient with both diseases concurrently, strengthened the erroneous concept of the unity of the "virus" of gonorrhea and syphilis, and established experimentation on humans as standard scientific methodology (Fig. 43).

The Abuse of Man

The Fallacy of Syphilis and Gonorrhea Being the Same Disease

Before long, the procedure employed by Hunter was duplicated by venereologists of different schools and different countries. Some corroborated Hunter's findings and supported his conclusions; his compatriots, Harrison and M'Coy, for example, produced ulcers on the penis of several persons by inoculation of gonorrheal matter.[3] Other authors who failed to produce ulcers in that fashion came to the opposite conclusion, that syphilis and gonorrhea were unrelated. In 1793, Benjamin Bell of Edinburgh described self-inflicted experiments performed by two colleagues who were unable to produce syphilis by inoculation of pus of gonorrhea, although one of those young men developed syphilis following inoculation of pus from a syphilitic chancre.[4] In 1806, the American physician, James Tongue, reported on "Experimental proofs, that the lues venerea and gonorrhea, are two distinct forms of disease." These "proofs" were the results of inoculation experiments in which Tongue infected several healthy individuals with syphilis.[5] In 1812, Jean-François Hernandez of Toulon used 17 prisoners under his care as human guinea pigs. He inoculated their skin with gonorrheal pus but failed to produce lesions of syphilis, which did much to weaken the theory of the unity of the "virus."[6, 7] Nevertheless, the issue remained controversial, especially in France, where the contagiousness of syphilis continued to be denied vehemently. According to the nineteenth century "physiologist" school of François-Joseph-Victor Broussais (Fig. 44), all maladies were caused by an inflammation of tissues. To Broussais, syphilis was nothing but a phlegmon,

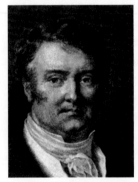

FIG. 44
*François
Joseph Victor
Broussais
(1772-1838)*

and the "venereal virus" either was dismissed as nonexistent or reduced to the level of a mere irritant.[8] Three Parisian medical students who tried to test Broussais' hypotheses by self-inoculation of syphilitic matter developed chancres and buboes, and one was afflicted so severely that he opened his crural artery in an attempt at suicide.[9]

The contagiousness of syphilis and the uniqueness of both syphilis and gonorrhea became generally accepted through the work of Philippe Ricord of Paris (Fig. 45). In his *Traité Pratique des Maladies Véneriénnes* of 1838, Ricord reported on hundreds of negative inoculations with pus of gonorrhea. His method, however, differed from that of Hunter, Tongue, and Hernandez. Ricord inoculated patients with pus taken from their own urethra into their own thigh, rejecting in the process the use of healthy individuals as test subjects. Although he believed that "inoculation is the sole rigorous diagnostic method available in the present state of science," he was "firmly convinced that it is not permissible for a physician to communicate to a healthy man, for any reason whatsoever, a disease the consequences of which it is impossible to predict."[10]

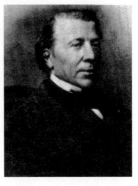

FIG. 45
Philippe Ricord (1800-1889)

The Fallacy of Secondary Syphilis Not Being Contagious

The injection of patients with matter from their own lesions also failed to produce syphilis because, once a patient was infected with that disease, the rapidly ensuing immune response prevented the development of new lesions at the sites of inoculation. Ricord, however, concluded from those "failed" autoinoculations that secondary syphilis was not contagious. The same conclusion was reached by John Hunter and on the same grounds – that the numerous negative responses to inoculation of patients with secondary syphilis via material from their own lesions proved lack of infectiousness of it.[11] The contagiousness of secondary syphilis became a major issue and a battlefield for experimentation on human beings. Among the first to join the battle was William Wallace of Dublin. In a series of articles in *The Lancet* in 1836 (Fig. 46), he told precisely how he had succeeded in inducing classic syphilis by inoculation of material from secondary lesions of the disease. This is what he wrote:

The operation of inoculation I perform in one of three ways; first, by making a puncture with a lancet and applying the matter of either an ulcer or of the condylomata to the wound; secondly, by removing the cuticle with the ointment of cantharides, and applying lint immersed in matter to the denuded surface; or, thirdly, by removing the cuticle from a small extent of surface, with the finger covered by a towel, and by applying the matter to the surface of the cutis thus exposed. The results were similar, whenever the inoculation succeeded, whether the first, or the second, or the third mode was adopted. The part, in general, first healed, and appeared for some time free from disease. But, in the course of two or three weeks after, the seat of the inoculation swelled, and became red and somewhat painful. It then desquamated, or appeared scaly. The tumidity and scaliness increased. The scales then gradually became scabs or crusts, and the spot gradually acquired a fungoid elevation. In a few cases the scaly tubercle soon after its appearance formed an ulcer . . . It seldom, if ever, happened, when inoculation succeeded, that secondary symptoms did not occur.[12]

The precise number of "successful inoculations" performed by Wallace was not provided in *The Lancet,* but obviously they were legion. Following the description of nine cases in which patients had developed syphilis as a result of his inoculations, Wallace remarked as follows: "As time will not permit me to review more . . . experiments . . . I must premise that . . . they are only a small proportion of those made by me during the investigation of those important points."[13] Despite this evidence, the issue of whether secondary syphilis was contagious remained controversial. One reason was that, in those days, knowledge could not be disseminated as it can be today. There were no international medical congresses, and medical journals were devoid of pictures because of the prohibitive cost of reproduction of images. In Wallace's articles on the subject, drawings of the findings in his patients were referred to repeatedly but were not actually shown. As a result, critics of Wallace called into question the accuracy of his observations. Moreover, they argued that Wallace's test subjects could have acquired syphilis by incidental sexual intercourse engaged in concurrently.[14]

To exclude the latter possibility, the ideal guinea pigs for the study of venereal diseases were prepubescent children, who were used for this purpose without restraint. Examples of that abuse are the experiments of Johann Ritter von Waller of the University of Prague. Waller described them in 1851 under the title, *On the Contagiousness of Secondary Syphilis* (Fig. 47). He admitted that, on the basis of clinical observation alone, the contagiousness of secondary syphilis

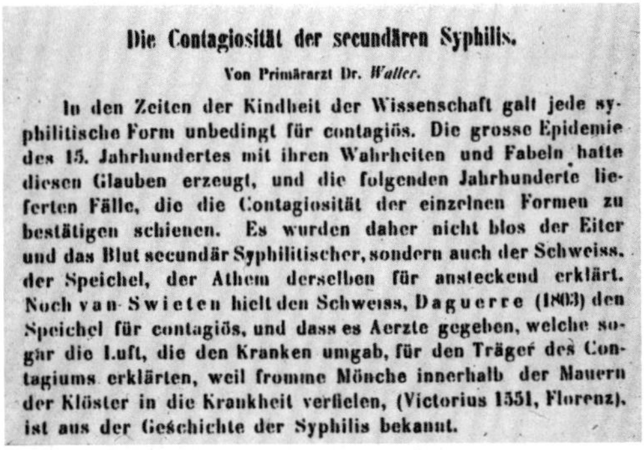

Die Contagiosität der secundären Syphilis.

Von Primärarzt Dr. *Waller.*

In den Zeiten der Kindheit der Wissenschaft galt jede syphilitische Form unbedingt für contagiös. Die grosse Epidemie des 15. Jahrhundertes mit ihren Wahrheiten und Fabeln hatte diesen Glauben erzeugt, und die folgenden Jahrhunderte lieferten Fälle, die die Contagiosität der einzelnen Formen zu bestätigen schienen. Es wurden daher nicht blos der Eiter und das Blut secundär Syphilitischer, sondern auch der Schweiss, der Speichel, der Athem derselben für ansteckend erklärt. Noch van Swieten hielt den Schweiss, Daguerre (1803) den Speichel für contagiös, und dass es Aerzte gegeben, welche sogar die Luft, die den Kranken umgab, für den Träger des Contagiums erklärten, weil fromme Mönche innerhalb der Mauern der Klöster in die Krankheit verfielen, (Victorius 1551, Florenz), ist aus der Geschichte der Syphilis bekannt.

FIG. 47 *Title page of the article by Waller on the contagiousness of secondary syphilis.*

could hardly be doubted. He also described several examples of infection of children through contact with lesions of secondary syphilis in their parents, siblings, or nurses. He was not, however, satisfied with this kind of evidence. "I strived after certainty," he stated, "and thought to be able to reach it only by inoculation ... For this purpose, I chose such individuals who had never suffered of a syphilitic or venereal affection and whom I could observe over a long period of time."[15]

These conditions were fulfilled by two boys, 12 and 15 years of age, who, following inoculation of pus of *condylomata lata* and the blood of patients with secondary syphilis, developed classic syphilitic exanthemas with widespread papules and ulcerated nodules that persisted for several months. When the exanthemas subsided, mucous patches appeared on tonsils and condylomata lata on oral mucous membranes, and one boy developed ulcers on a tonsil and the nasal mucosa. Waller demonstrated his test subjects repeatedly to his colleagues whom he wished to enlist as witnesses to the validity of his diagnoses. Although Waller concluded that "the solution of the controversy has been achieved,"[16] he felt compelled to perform additional inoculations, this time on three boys between the ages of 10 and 14. Because two of these boys were foundlings and blind, they were considered by Waller to be "especially suited for the experiment, as they will spend the entire life in a shelter for the ailing and will always remain under medical observation." Following inoculation of syphilitic blood, one of the boys developed signs of indisputable syphilis, namely, a macular exanthem, ulcerated nodules at the sites of inoculation, mucous patches, and ulcers of the tonsils (Fig. 48, 49, 50, 51).[17] The subsequent fate of the boys never was commented on by Waller, nor was there any indication of an interest in it by him or even of remorse on the part of the physician. In his indifference to the welfare of his test subjects, Waller did not distinguish himself from most of his colleagues who applauded, rather than condemned, his experi-

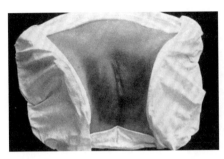

FIG. 48
Primary lesion of syphilis in a prepubescent child.

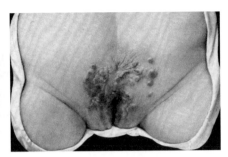

FIG. 49
Condylomata lata in a child.

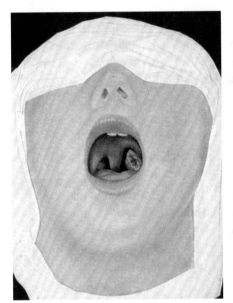

FIG. 50
Ulcer on a tonsil in a child.

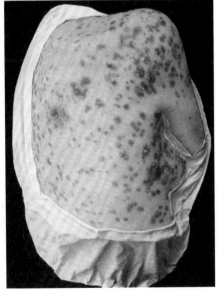

FIG. 51
Severe secondary syphilis.

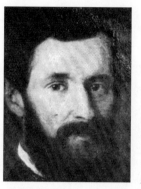

FIG. 52
*Franz
Rinecker
(1811-1883)*

ments. For instance, Franz von Rinecker (Fig. 52), the director of dermatology at the University of Würzburg, had this to say in that regard: "Although not very numerous, Waller's experiments surpass those of Wallace in terms of precision and description of detail, and his inoculation experiments with blood from patients with secondary syphilis are entirely new and their success all the more surprising."[18]

Given this point of view, it is not surprising that Rinecker tried to substantiate Waller's findings. In 1852, he induced syphilis experimentally in two young physicians who had placed themselves "with commendable celerity" at his disposal. Rinecker also experimented on a 12-year-old boy who suffered from Huntington's chorea. Without having obtained the consent of the boy or his parents, Rinecker inoculated him with material from syphilitic lesions, inducing a local reaction. To have corroboration of the accuracy of his observations, Rinecker demonstrated his test subjects, again and again, to Rudolf Virchow and other colleagues at the University of Würzburg (Fig. 53) and noted with approval that "the door is thrown open again for free, uninhibited research."[19]

In the years that followed, the inoculation experiments of Waller and Rinecker employing material from lesions of secondary syphilis were duplicated many times. For example, in 1852 and 1858, Anton Christian August von Hübbenet of the University of Kiev induced syphilis in two young, healthy soldiers in the Russian army and refrained from treating them until he had displayed them "to as many physicians as possible in order to give them the opportunity to convince themselves of the truth of the fact."[20] In 1855, inoculations that took in nine of 14 test subjects were described at a meeting of the Association

2· Studies by Inoculation

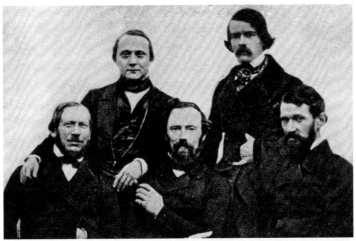

of Physicians of the Palatinate, and it was concluded that "with respect to the experiments described, there seems to be no doubt that secondary syphilis can truly be transmitted by inoculation."[21] Despite these attestations that secondary syphilis was contagious, the French government considered it necessary in 1858 to charge the Medical Academy of Paris with carrying out additional experiments to clarify the issue once and for all. For that purpose, a commission was formed consisting of Alfred Velpeau, Philippe Ricord, Alphonse Devergie, Depaul, and Camille Melchior Gibert, five of the most respected French syphilologists of that time. For purposes of preparing his report to the government, Gibert (Fig. 54) performed four inoculations with pus of condylomata lata, all of which resulted in signs of secondary syphilis. Gibert, who is remembered still for his description of *pityriasis rosea,* also mentioned two "successful" inoculations by his colleague, Joseph-Alexandre Auzias-Turenne.[22, 23] The commission came to the conclusion

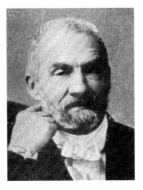

FIG. 54
*Camille
Melchior
Gibert
(1797-1866)*

that "there are secondary or constitutional affections of syphilis that apparently are contagious."[24]

Attempts to Distinguish Syphilis from Chancroid by Inoculation Experiments

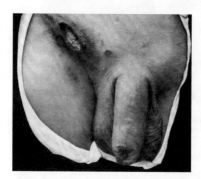

FIG. 55
Lesion of chancroid on the prepuce in conjunction with an ulcerated bubo.

Meanwhile, another question had shifted to the center of interest – whether chancroid was a variant of syphilis or a separate and distinct disease (Fig. 55). The first to distinguish chancroid from syphilis was Ricord's pupil, Léon Bassereau, who, in 1852, noted that only hard chancres were associated with systemic disease (*chancre précursor de la vérole*), whereas soft chancres either remained localized or were followed by a purulent lymphadenitis (*chancre à bubon suppuré*). Bassereau had arrived at that conclusion without experimental evidence, wholly on the basis of epidemiologic studies (the so-called confrontation of patients with one another). Two years later, the term "chancroid" was introduced by another pupil of Ricord, F. F. Clerc of Paris, who observed that chancres developing after inoculation of patients with material from their own lesions always were of soft consistency, never becoming hard. In Clerc's view, chancroid was a variant of the hard chancre of syphilis that developed in patients who were already infected and, therefore, were partially immune.

In subsequent decades, the relationship of hard and soft venereal chancres was debated hotly, evoking scores of inoculation experiments on behalf of resolution of the quandary. The names of the scientists involved read like a *Who's Who* of dermatology. In 1860, Felix von Bärensprung of Berlin (Fig. 56), who is appreciated to this day as the author of the second textbook of dermatopathology and for having elucidated the pathogenesis of zoster, induced generalized syphilis in two young and previously healthy prostitutes by inoculating them with material from a hard hunterian chancre. Using the same subjects, he found that material from the soft ulcer of chancroid did not cause systemic disease.[26] In 1861 and 1862, Ferdinand von Hebra (Fig. 57), the leading dermatologist of the mid nineteenth century, and one of his assistants at the skin clinic of Vienna performed numerous inoculations with material from hard and soft chancres – inducing generalized syphilis in three patients who had consulted the clinic originally because of prurigo and lupus vulgaris.[27] At the same time, Josef Lindwurm of Munich (Fig. 58), the first full professor of dermatology and syphilology in Germany, reported on five examples of experimentally-induced generalized syphilis and several fruitless attempts to induce syphilis through inoculation of material from lesions of chancroid. Lindwurm succeeded, too, in producing mixed chancres in three patients, either by transferring material from chancroid to syphilitic chancres or vice versa.[28] In 1883, Isidor Neumann of Vienna (Fig. 59), the first to describe *pem-*

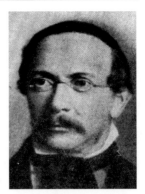

FIG. 56
*Felix von
Bärensprung
(1822-1864)*

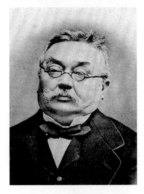

FIG. 57
*Ferdinand von
Hebra
(1816-1880)*

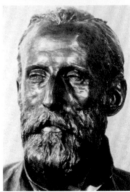

FIG. 58
*Josef
Lindwurm
(1824-1874)*

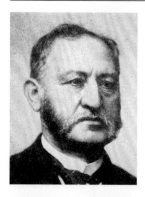

FIG. 59
*Isidor
Neumann
(1832-1906)*

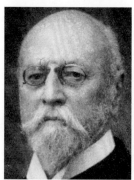

FIG. 60
*Ernst Finger
(1856-1939)*

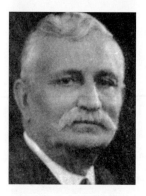

FIG. 61
*Agosto Ducrey
(1860-1940)*

phigus vegetans, recognized that mothers of infants with congenital syphilis were resistant to syphilis themselves, although ulcers could be induced in them by inoculation of material from lesions of chancroid.[29] Two years later, Neumann's successor as chairman of the Second Department of Dermatology of the University of Vienna, Ernst Finger (Fig. 60), demonstrated that soft ulcers of the genitalia were not specific, but could be induced by inoculation of pus of diverse origin, such as impetigo, ecthyma, and acne.[30] When Augosto Ducrey (Fig. 61) determined in 1889 that the bacterium *Haemophilus* was the infectious agent of chancroid, thereby establishing chancroid as a specific disease, he grew the organisms on the skin of human test subjects. Subsequently, other authors confirmed the etiologic role of *Haemophilus Ducreyi* by transferring bacteria over several generations from one patient to another. Among the physicians who performed these experiments were several famous dermatologists, for example, Edvard Welander, William Dubreuilh (Fig. 62), Abraham Buschke (Fig. 63), and Johann Heinrich Rille (Fig. 64).[31]

Experiments also were performed on humans to clarify other issues, such as the contagiousness of coagulated blood of patients with secondary syphilis. Pietro Pellizzari, director of the clinic for venereal diseases in Florence, induced syphilis in a young physician by inoculation of noncoagulated blood, whereas two other physicians who were inoculated with coagulated blood did not develop syphilis. Other matters that lent themselves to experimentation were the contagiousness of breast milk of mothers with syphilis (inoculation of a 16-year-old prostitute by R. Voss of St. Petersburg resulted in syphilis, whereas the inoculation failed to take in two other girls, aged 13 and 15), the contagiousness of sperm of patients with syphilis (French physician, Mireur, reported on inoculation experiments in 1867), and the contagiousness of lymph nodes in secondary syphilis (a previously healthy patient acquired syphilis through inoculation by Ernst Bumm, a student of Franz Rinecker).[32]

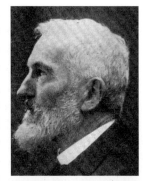

FIG. 62
*William
Dubreuilh
(1857-1926)*

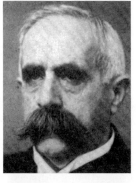

FIG. 63
*Abraham
Buschke
(1868-1943)*

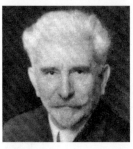

FIG. 64
*Johann
Heinrich Rille
(1864-1956)*

Abuse of Man in Inoculation Experiments on Gonorrhea

Once the gonococcus had been identified by German dermatologist, Albert Neisser, in 1879, inoculation experiments were performed with cultures of those bacteria. In 1880, Arpad Bókai of the University of Budapest reported on the results of inoculations of cultures of micrococci into the urethra of six healthy persons, noting with regret the following: "This small number is caused by the fact that we found only few individuals (mostly students) who offered themselves voluntarily for the infection and were known by us to be reliable men in every respect." Although Bókai succeeded in inducing gonorrhea in three of the test subjects, he concluded that the micrococci used for the inoculations "do not differ, in regard to shape, size, and other qualities, from other micrococci that do not elicit blennorrhea."[33]

In 1882, similar experiments using gonococci were carried out by Leo Leistikow and Friedrich Löffler of Berlin. Leistikow was a student of Paul Gerson Unna, with whom he published a textbook in 1897 on the therapy of skin diseases. Löffler (Fig. 65), a pupil of Robert Koch, is well known to this day for his descriptions of the bacteria of glanders, diphtheria, and erysipeloid. When working with gonococci, Leistikow and Löffler tried to transfer the bacteria to various animals, such as rabbits, rats, guinea pigs, and apes. Those attempts were unsuccessful, and Leistikow concluded that "the inoculations of apes have to be repeated several times, and only if it is confirmed that gonorrhea is a disease specific for humans, one would have to wait for a disciple of science devoted enough to have the inoculation of cultured material performed on himself." Apparently the wait took too long, and Leistikow inoculated his cultures into the urethra of a patient with nongonorrheal urethritis, in-

FIG. 65
*Friedrich
Löffler
(1852-1915)*

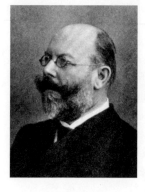

ducing a purulent discharge with abundant gonococci.[34] In 1883, Max Bockhart, a student of Rinecker, reported on the inoculation of cultures of gonococci into the healthy urethra of a human being. Bockhart, who described a superficial form of folliculitis that came to be known as "impetigo of Bockhart," had chosen as his test subject a terminally ill patient who subsequently developed severe urethritis, cystitis, and nephritis, and whose kidneys were found at autopsy to contain abscesses replete with bacteria.[35]

Nevertheless, the causative role of gonococci in gonorrhea continued to be doubted because of reports of negative inoculations with cultures of dubious quality. For example, George Sternberg of Philadelphia (who later became Surgeon General of the United States) inoculated himself and two colleagues in 1885 with cultures of gonococci, but failed to induce gonorrhea. In his article he told of his difficulties in finding volunteers for the experiment and did that in these words: "My friend Dr. Keirle had informed me that several gentlemen connected with the City Dispensary had consented to furnish healthy urethras for the experiments ... I had informed Dr. Keirle that I thought it best to make the experiment upon unmarried men to prevent the possibility of serious secondary consequences ... But the unmarried men failed me at the last moment with the exception of one young gentleman, Mr. W. A. Wegefarth, of Baltimore, a medical student. Contrary to my expectation, Dr. Keirle himself had determined to test the 'gonococcus' on his own urethra, and with this example before me I could do no less than join the experiment, although I confess that I did so with some hesitation, notwithstanding the negative results which I had previously obtained in a similar experiment."[36]

In the same year, the issue of whether gonococci were responsible for gonorrhea was decided by results published in a monograph by Ernst Bumm (Fig. 66).[37] Because Bumm did not wait for volunteers, he was able to conduct a larger series of inoculation experiments. In a culture medium based on human blood, he was able to sustain pure cultures of

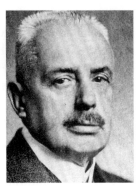

FIG. 66
*Ernst Bumm
(1858-1925)*

gonococci for up to 20 generations, continuing to induce typical gonorrhea by intraurethral inoculations. Subsequently, the culture media for gonococci were improved, and each time the success had to be demonstrated by inoculation experiments. For example, in 1891, an Italian physician, G. Alfuso, induced gonorrhea in a young man by intraurethral inoculation of gonococci cultured in the serous effusion of joints.[38] In 1892, Ernst Wertheim, a gynecologist in Prague, cultured gonococci in Petri dishes containing human serum and transferred them into the urethra of a patient with general paresis. This induced severe gonorrheal urethritis that lasted for at least two months and was associated still with "a rather strong purulent secretion" at the time Wertheim published the results of his experiments.[39] Wertheim's technique for growing gonococci in culture was reexamined by several other physicians, including an assistant at the skin clinic of Breslau by the name of Steinschneider, who infected two volunteers with cultures of gonococci, and Karl Menge, an assistant at the department of gynecology of the University of Leipzig, who transferred cultures of gonococci into the urethra of two patients with cancer.[40]

The question of whether gonococci were confined to the urogenital tract or could infect other tissues, too, stimulated several researchers to perform inoculation experiments. Among them was C. G. Åhmann, an assistant of Edvard Welander at the St. Göran hospital in Stockholm, who cultured gonococci from the blood of a patient with bacteremia and inoculated the organisms into the urethra of a healthy person. The test subject developed severe gonorrheic urethritis, epididymitis, prostatitis, pneumonia, pleuritis, tendovaginitis, myositis, and arthritis. Åhmann cautioned that "the inoculation, unfortunately, worked all too well, and the unlucky course of this case is a sincere warning for anybody who feels inclined to repeat the experiment."[41] His warning, however, went unheeded; two years later, Pio Colombini, an assisant at the skin clinic of the Univer-

sity of Siena, cultured gonococci from
the blood of a patient with gonococcemia and inoculated the bacteria
into the urethra of a 20-year-old man.
The experiment succeeded, resulting
in gonorrheal urethritis that lasted
for many months. Gonococci also
were isolated from the endocardium,
knee joint, and various soft tissues of
that person, and the success of the

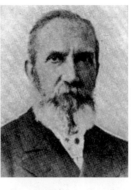

procedure was demonstrated each time through inoculation
experiments.[42]

Numerous experiments on humans concerned the question
of whether gonococci were responsible for ophthalmoblennorrhea. Hubert Sattler of Vienna (Fig. 67) transferred infected
vaginal flux into the eye of a newborn who developed severe
ophthalmoblennorrhea. Eugen Fraenkel of Hamburg (Fig. 68)
used three moribund children in a similar study and succeeded
in inducing ophthalmoblennorrhea in one of them. In Dresden,
gynecologists Leopold and Wessel deliberately refrained from
carrying out Karl Credé's method for prevention of ophthalmoblennorrhea in 18 newborns of
women with and without gonorrhea.
They noted that only one neonate,
whose mother had gonorrhea, developed severely purulent ophthal-
moblenorrhea from which myriad
gonococci could be recovered. Similar
experiments were carried out by several other gynecologists and ophthal-
mologists on newborns and blind
adults.[43]

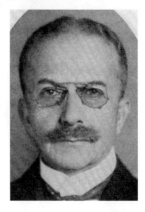

Abuse of Man by Inoculation Experiments
Using a Host of Bacteria, Viruses, and Fungi

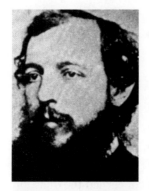

FIG. 69
Daniel
Cornelius
Danielssen
(1815-1894)

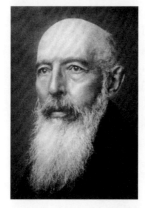

FIG. 70
Gerhard
Henrik
Armauer
Hansen
(1841-1912)

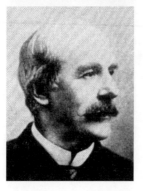

FIG. 71
Émile Vidal
(1825-1893)

Inoculation studies were not confined to venereal diseases. In the 1840s and 1850s, the Norwegian physician, Daniel Cornelius Danielssen (Fig. 69), honored for his delineation of the cutaneous manifestations of leprosy, tried unsuccessfully to induce that disease by inoculation of leprous material into his own skin and that of several other test subjects. After having been the first to identify *Mycobacterium leprae*, Danielssen's younger colleague, Gerhard Henrik Armauer Hansen (Fig. 70), tried to cultivate the bacillus on artificial media and to infect various animals with it. Because his attempts were all in vain, Hansen resorted to an experiment on one of his patients. In 1879, he transferred material from leprous nodules into the conjunctiva of a woman with maculoanaesthetic leprosy, hoping to demonstrate the contagiousness of leprous tissue and the conversion of tuberculoid leprosy to lepromatous leprosy.[44]

In the 1870s, Émile Vidal of Paris (Fig. 71) tried numerous inoculations with material from lesions of impetigo and ecthyma.[45] He also succeeded in reproducing herpes simplex in four

patients by autoinocula-
tion of fluid from vesicles
of the disease.[46] In 1875,
the chair of the pediatric
clinic of the University of
Prague, J. Steiner, reported on the inoculation of
fluid from lesions of varicella in two infants, both
of whom developed the
typical eruption of chickenpox.[47] In 1883, Friedrich Fehleisen, a student
of Franz Rinecker in
Würzburg, inoculated
streptococci from bullae
of erysipelas into human

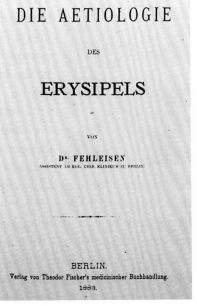

DIE AETIOLOGIE

DES

ERYSIPELS

VON

Dᴿ FEHLEISEN
ASSISTENT AM KGL. CHIR. KLISIKUM ZU BERLIN.

BERLIN.
Verlag von Theodor Fischer's medicinischer Buchhandlung.
1883.

FIG. 72
*Title page of
the booklet, The
Etiology of
Erysipelas, by
Friedrich
Fehleisen.*

skin, inducing severe erysipelas in six of seven test subjects, one
of whom nearly died from the effects of the procedure (Fig.
72).[48] In 1888, Curt Schimmelbusch of the University of Halle
inoculated two patients with cancer, 10 and 18 years of age, with
Staphylococcus aureus in order to elucidate the cause of furuncles. Previous self-inoculations of staphylococci by Carl Garré
(Fig. 73) and Max Bockhart had resulted in impetigo and furuncles. Garré, an assistant at a pri-
vate laboratory in Basel had developed a large carbuncle that was associated with pain, fever, and lymphadenitis. The infection lasted for
three weeks, and, when it subsided,
Garré was left with 17 scars on his
forearm.[49] Nevertheless, Schimmelbusch did not pause (Fig. 74) from
duplicating Garré's technique of inoc-

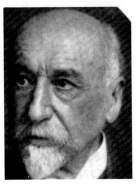

FIG. 73
*Carl Garré
(1857-1928)*

FIG. 74
*Curt
Schimmelbusch
(1860-1895)*

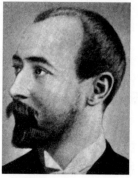

ulation in his own patients. By rubbing pure cultures of staphylococci into the skin for five minutes, he produced scores of pustules, one of which turned into a large furuncle (Fig. 75, 76).[50]

In 1891, Filipp Josef Pick (Fig. 77), the chairman of the department of dermatology of the Charles University of Prague, reported on the results of inoculations of cultures of favus into the skin of 11 children and two adults. All of the test subjects had been admitted to the hospital already because of other skin diseases, and most of them developed fungal disease during the experiments.[51] One year later, Pick published the results of inoculation studies with material from lesions of molluscum contagiosum. The test subjects were two children, aged 9 and 11, who were under his care previously because of unrelated skin diseases. Ten weeks after the inoculations, both children developed papules at the test sites, and Pick stated that he was "very pleased to produce,

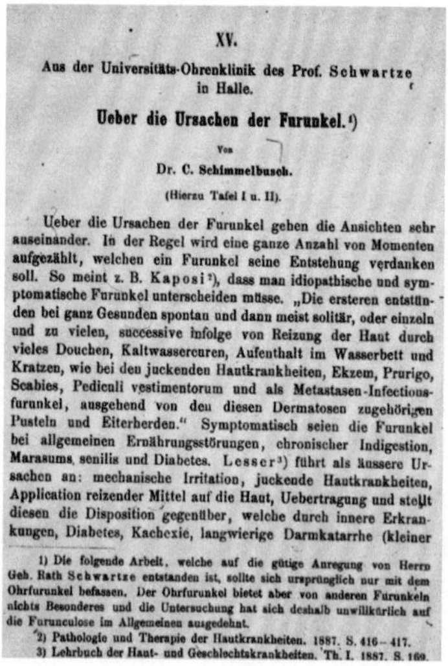

FIG. 75
*Titel page of the
article by
Schimmelbusch.*

XV.

Aus der Universitäts-Ohrenklinik des Prof. Schwartze in Halle.

Ueber die Ursachen der Furunkel.

Von

Dr. C. Schimmelbusch.

(Hierzu Tafel I u. II).

Ueber die Ursachen der Furunkel geben die Ansichten sehr auseinander. In der Regel wird eine ganze Anzahl von Momenten aufgezählt, welchen ein Furunkel seine Entstehung verdanken soll. So meint z. B. Kaposi, dass man idiopathische und symptomatische Furunkel unterscheiden müsse. „Die ersteren entstünden bei ganz Gesunden spontan und dann meist solitär, oder einzeln und zu vielen, successive infolge von Reizung der Haut durch vieles Douchen, Kaltwassercuren, Aufenthalt im Wasserbett und Kratzen, wie bei den juckenden Hautkrankheiten, Ekzem, Prurigo, Scabies, Pediculi vestimentorum und als Metastasen-Infectionsfurunkel, ausgehend von den diesen Dermatosen zugehörigen Pusteln und Eiterherden." Symptomatisch seien die Furunkel bei allgemeinen Ernährungsstörungen, chronischer Indigestion, Marasmus senilis und Diabetes. Lesser führt als äussere Ursachen an: mechanische Irritation, juckende Hautkrankheiten, Application reizender Mittel auf die Haut, Uebertragung und stellt diesen die Disposition gegenüber, welche durch innere Erkrankungen, Diabetes, Kachexie, langwierige Darmkatarrhe (kleiner

1) Die folgende Arbeit, welche auf die gütige Anregung von Herrn Geh. Rath Schwartze entstanden ist, sollte sich ursprünglich nur mit dem Ohrfurunkel befassen. Der Ohrfurunkel bietet aber von anderen Furunkeln nichts Besonderes und die Untersuchung hat sich deshalb unwillkürlich auf die Furunculose im Allgemeinen ausgedehnt.

2) Pathologie und Therapie der Hautkrankheiten. 1887. S. 416—417.
3) Lehrbuch der Haut- und Geschlechtskrankheiten. Th. I. 1887. S. 169.

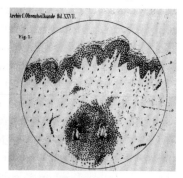

FIG. 76
*Drawing of the histopathology of a
furuncle that was produced by
rubbing pure cultures of
staphylococci into the skin
(from the article by
Schimmelbusch).*

2· Studies by Inoculation

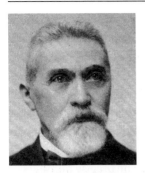

FIG. 77
*Filipp Josef
Pick
(1834-1910)*

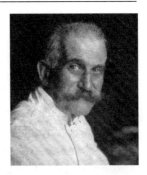

FIG. 78
*Joseph
Jadassohn
(1863-1936)*

under the microscope, clear evidence of molluscum bodies." One of the lesions was excised and the diagnosis of molluscum was confirmed histopathologically.[52]

In 1896, Joseph Jadassohn of Breslau (Fig. 78), who developed the patch test for identifying contact allergens and described for the first time several skin diseases (e.g., pachyonychia congenita and nevus sebaceus), reported on 74 inoculations of material taken from viral warts and given to nine test subjects, six of whom developed warts at some sites of inoculation. Jadassohn performed most of these experiments on himself and on colleagues at his clinic, but he also inoculated three "adult men" and one 3-year-old child. The child was inoculated even after previous experiments had demonstrated convincingly the contagiousness of the material. As a consequence of the experiment, the 3-year-old developed numerous "typically papillomatous and relatively large warts" on both hands.[53]

In 1898, Siegfried Grosz and Rudolf Kraus of the University of Vienna studied non-gonorrheal urethritis by transferring cultures of *Pseudomonas pyocyaneus*, *Escherichia coli*, and *Staphylococcus aureus* to human urethrae. Most of their test subjects "had never had a gonorrheal infection; juvenile individuals (14-18 years of age) were chosen preferentially for the experiment." Grosz and Kraus found that "it is possible to induce a transient purulent urethritis by inoculation of living bacteria (*P. pyocyaneus*, *E. coli*, *S. aureus*)." A transient purulent urethritis also was induced by intraurethral inoculations of dead bacteria, including gonococci. Intracutaneous injections of dead gonococci in 11 patients produced fever and painful local inflammatory reactions.[54]

In brief, following Hunter's first trial with infectious material in 1767, inoculation experiments were carried out by most of the leading dermatovenereologists of the nineteenth century. They also were performed by scores of assistant physicians whose names have long been forgotten. The precise numbers of these experiments and of the patients who had to endure the consequences of scientific endeavor are not known. Many more experiments were conducted than those recorded in the literature, and many more were described than those mentioned specifically in this chapter.

CHAPTER 3

THE CALL OF CONSCIENCE

Although many questionable experiments on humans were described in medical journals and at scientific meetings of the nineteenth century, they aroused hardly a peep of protest from physician colleagues of the investigators. When considered in the context of the ethical code of the medical profession, which mandated that physicians act always in the best interest of their patients, the absence of a vocal response by the medical community is startling. The development of experimental medicine, however, had resulted in a conflict in ethics between the welfare of individual patients and what was perceived to be the welfare of society. In this conflict – which continues even to this day – researchers tended to overlook damage to individuals for the sake of a greater good. For example, Anton von Hübbenet defended the experimental infection of soldiers with syphilis by saying that "If the experiments contribute to the elucidation of truth in such an important matter, the suffering of a few individuals is not too high a price paid by mankind for such a useful and practical result."[1]

Furthermore, the traditional ethical codes of medicine applied only to the relationship between physician and patient, with no consideration being given to the relationship between researcher and test subject. The ethics involved in the introduction of new therapeutic modalities were addressed, however briefly, by some authors. In 1803, Thomas Percival wrote in his *Code of Ethics* thus: "It is for the public good ... that new remedies and new methods of chirurgical treatment should be devised but, in the accomplishment of the salutary purpose, the gentlemen of the faculty should be scrupulously and conscientiously governed by sound reason, just analogy, and well-authenticated facts."[2]

In the best tradition of paternalism in medicine, Percival left to the physician alone the decision about whether a new remedy or new method of treatment surgically should be devised; the patient was not asked to consent in his or her own treatment. Consent of patients was demanded for the first time in 1830 by J. W. Willcock of England, apparently as much for the benefit of the physician legally as for the patient. Willcock strongly advocated medical experiments on humans, emphasizing that he was "not to be understood as speaking of the wild and dangerous practices of rash and ignorant practitioners, which fall properly under the head of want of skill and knowledge; but of deliberate acts of men of considerable knowledge and undoubted talent, differing from those prescribed by the ordinary rules of practice, but which they have good reason, from a knowledge of the human system and of the particular disease ... to believe will be attended with benefit to the patient, although the novelty of the undertaking does not leave the result altogether free of doubt." Willcock continued in these words: "When an experiment of this kind is performed with the consent of the party subjected to it, after he has been informed that it is an experiment, the practitioner is answerable neither in damages to the individual, nor on a criminal proceeding ... But if the practitioner performs his experiment without giving such information to, and obtaining consent of, his patient, he is liable to compensate in damages any injury which may arise from his adopting a new method of treatment."[3]

3 · The Call of Conscience

Three years later, American Army physician William Beaumont (Fig. 79) offered a reasonable set of guidelines for medical experiments in order to provide an ethical framework for nontherapeutic trials conducted by himself. One of his patients, a French Canadian hunter named Alexis St. Martin (Fig. 80), had suffered an accidental gunshot wound to the abdomen that, in healing, left an open fistulous tract. Beaumont utilized this tract to study the physiology of the stomach, justifying his research by defining the conditions under which such experiments on human beings should be performed as follows:

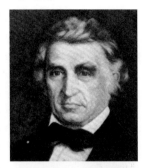

FIG. 79
*William
Beaumont
(1785-1853)*

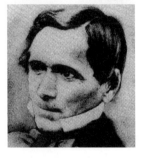

FIG. 80
*Alexis St.
Martin
(1803-1880)*

1. There must be recognition of an area where experimentation in man is needed . . .

2. Some experimental studies in man are justifiable when the information cannot otherwise be obtained.

3. The investigator must be conscientious and responsible . . .

4. Whenever a human subject is used, a well considered, methodological approach is required so that as much information as possible will be obtained. No random studies are to be made.

5. The voluntary consent of the subject is necessary . . .

6. The experiment is to be discontinued when it causes distress to the subject . . .

7. The project must be abandoned when the subject becomes dissatisfied.[4]

This and other ethical codes for experiments on humans were proposed in the early 1830s, a time when systematic medical experiments had just begun. The impact of those proposals, however, was practically nil. The comments of Willcock and Beaumont went largely unnoticed, and even Percival's gentle admonitions in regard to the study of a new surgical remedy or method – conscientiousness, scrupulous care, and sound reason – were violated flagrantly in most inoculation experiments. These experiments aroused neither criticism nor resistance among members of the medical community.

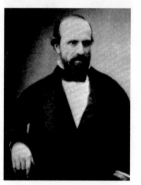

FIG. 81
Paul Diday
(1812-1894)

There were a few exceptions to the rule of no outcry by physicians to cavalier experimentation on humans by colleagues. As one example, the French syphilologist, Paul Diday (Fig. 81), who conducted the first systematic study of congenital syphilis, condemned the inoculation experiments of William Wallace. Diday also performed inoculations but only on animals and on himself. Once, using material from a human chancre, he produced a pustule on the ear of a cat, from which he obtained matter that he inoculated into his own penis. The result was a phagedenic ulcer and a virulent draining bubo that laid him up for months.[5] To use other human beings for this kind of test was unacceptable to Diday. Although in 1858 he referred in his own textbook on syphilis to Wallace's experiments, Diday asked rhetorically whether the "love of wisdom" could ever justify "perpetration of a crime?"[6]

The call of conscience also was heard following the infection of children with syphilis by Johann Ritter von Waller. The editor of the German translation of Ricord's *Letters About Syphilis* asked this question: "Who entitles Mr. Waller to deal in this way with children who have been referred to him for healing? From where does a physician take the right . . . to play fully intentionally such an offhand game with the health and life of a human being?"[7]

3 · The Call of Conscience

In 1853, Georg Gustav Klusemann, a public health physician in Burg, Germany, published a forceful and elaborate condemnation of von Waller's experiments in the *Quarter Annual Journal for Forensic and Public Medicine* (Fig. 82). Klusemann regarded von Waller's study as "an unjustifiable misuse of the power of a physician, a misuse that is even greater and more objectionable in the cases under discussion because the experiments have not been performed in a private practice, but in a hospital." And Klusemann went on to state, heartfeltly and trenchantly, the following: "Whoever knows the class of human beings who turn to hospitals for help against their maladies . . . knows that such people, forced to accept charity and to deal with men who are placed high above them in regard to education and rank in the society, lose very easily all their power of self-determination and submit to the authority of these quasi-superiors in a way that they regard their wishes and suggestions as being orders that have to be obeyed under any condition. If this kind of behavior is very common among adults, how much more frequent must it be with children. And are the latter, and surely also the majority of the former, able to oversee all the consequences of such scientific experiments to their full extent, or even only to appreciate them if explained to the best of one's ability? But is it not a necessary precondition, if

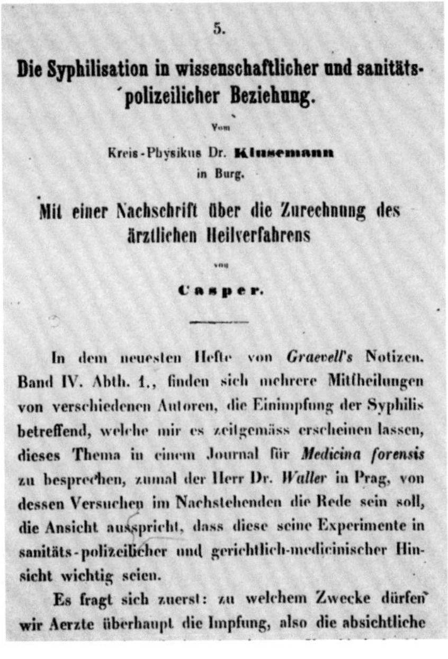

5.

Die Syphilisation in wissenschaftlicher und sanitätspolizeilicher Beziehung.

Von

Kreis-Physikus Dr. **Klusemann**
in Burg.

Mit einer Nachschrift über die Zurechnung des
ärztlichen Heilverfahrens

von

Casper.

In dem neuesten Hefte von *Graevell's* Notizen, Band IV. Abth. 1., finden sich mehrere Mittheilungen von verschiedenen Autoren, die Einimpfung der Syphilis betreffend, welche mir es zeitgemäss erscheinen lassen, dieses Thema in einem Journal für *Medicina forensis* zu besprechen, zumal der Herr Dr. *Waller* in Prag, von dessen Versuchen im Nachstehenden die Rede sein soll, die Ansicht ausspricht, dass diese seine Experimente in sanitäts-polizeilicher und gerichtlich-medicinischer Hinsicht wichtig seien.

Es fragt sich zuerst: zu welchem Zwecke dürfen wir Aerzte überhaupt die Impfung, also die absichtliche

FIG. 82
*Title page of
the article by
Klusemann.*

one wants to perform such experiments with somebody, that this person knows all the consequences a priori? – I am thoroughly convinced that this is absolutely necessary."[8]

In short, although Klusemann considered mandatory disclosure fully and decision with free will for participation of subjects in a test, he doubted whether these conditions were realistic in view of the dependent situation of patients socially. Klusemann wrote with emphasis that "The job of the physician is 'to heal,' but not 'to make ill,' which may not even happen in the interest of science." He insisted that in case of the slightest possibility of permanent damage to a person's health, "it is not compatible with the duties and the profession of the physician to carry out such experiments." On the other hand, he understood that some therapeutic interventions were necessarily of an experimental nature and might be associated with side effects. The intent of such treatment, however, should be to correct a malady. Klusemann concluded that inoculations should be performed only as experiments on oneself, exclusively, "in order to sacrifice oneself, not others, on the high altar of science." In an afterward to the article by Klusemann, the editor of the journal, Johann Ludwig Casper, alerted readers to section 197 of the *Prussian Criminal Code*, which stipulated that intentional application of a poison was punishable by 10 to 20 years' imprisonment.[9]

Legal Actions Against Physicians for Alleged Abuse of Man

Whereas no legal proceedings were instituted against von Waller, other physicians had to defend themselves in court. The most prominent were Franz Rinecker and Armauer Hansen. Rinecker was charged in 1854 for "vaccination with syphilitic poison" of two junior physicians of the University of Würzburg and of a 12-year-old boy. In the name of His Highness the Most

Powerful King of Bavaria, he was sentenced to serve eight days in prison and to pay the expenses of the trial (Fig. 83). This sentence, however, was overturned at a second trial and Rinecker was exonerated. The only penalty for doing harm to a patient was an official rebuke by the Academic Senate of the University, which issued this statement: "Because of careless violation of his profession, commit-

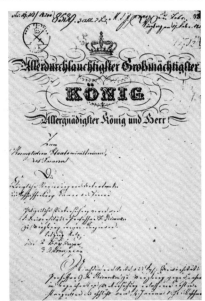

FIG. 83
Document of the sentence imposed on Franz Rinecker and issued by the King of Bavaria.

ted under extenuating circumstances in his function as professor and chairman of the polyclinic through inoculation of the boy Ehrenberg with syphilitic lymph, we give a rebuke to the Royal Full University Professor Dr. Franz Rinecker, by virtue of today's disciplinary resolution, in the sincere expectation that he will henceforth consider to avoid such scientific experiments on non-healthy persons or without legally binding approval by the person."[10, 11]

Armauer Hansen, the medical health officer for leprosy in Norway and resident physician at the Bergen Leprosy Hospital, was charged with having transferred leprous material into the conjunctiva of a patient (Fig. 84). The woman, described by an expert witness as "nervous and hysterical," had refused the procedure, but to no avail. She later claimed that her vision had declined and that she had pain in the eye for several weeks as a result of an experiment she had not sanctioned. In May 1880, Hansen was found guilty by the Law Courts of the City of Bergen. He was sentenced to pay the expenses connected with

FIG. 84
*Armauer
Hansen in his
laboratory.*

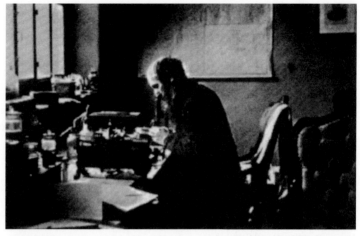

the trial and was relieved of his position as director of the Leprosy Hospital.[12]

Other less renowned physicians also were convicted of negligence. Georg Hübner, a public health officer from Bamberg, Franconia, was charged with infecting numerous patients with syphilis in the process of providing vaccinations against smallpox.[13] In Lyon in 1859, Antoine Gailleton (Fig. 85), who eventually became clinical professor in syphilitic and cutaneous diseases of the University of Lyon and mayor of that city, and his young assistant, Joseph Frédéric Guyenot, were sentenced to pay fines of 100 and 50 francs, respectively, for having infected a 10-year-old boy with syphilis. Whereas the defendants em-

FIG. 85
*Antoine
Gailleton
(1829-1904)*

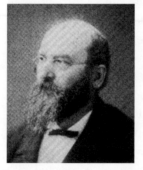

phasized the necessity for freedom in science and the importance of their experiments for public health, the prosecutors argued that physicians, outside the domain of therapy, had to be judged by normal legal standards, according to which this type of experimental inoculation fulfilled the criteria of causing willful bodily harm.[14, 15]

3 · The Call of Conscience

The Defense of Experiments on Humans as Marshaled by Basic Scientists, Chief Among Them, Claude Bernard

The debate about inoculation experiments prompted the famous French physiologist, Claude Bernard (Fig. 86), whose classic experiments illuminated several functions of the liver, the digestive properties of the pancreas, and the control of blood circulation by the nervous system, to address in 1865 the ethical rudiments of experimental medicine in his book

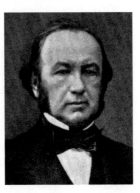

FIG. 86
*Claude
Bernard
(1813-1878)*

Introduction à L'Etude de la Médicine Expérimentale (Introduction to the Study of Experimental Medicine). Bernard defended experiments on living beings in these lines: "We have succeeded in discovering the laws of inorganic matter only by penetrating into inanimate bodies and machines; similarly we shall succeed in learning the laws and properties of living matter only by displacing living organs in order to get into their inner environment. After dissecting cadavers, then, we must necessarily dissect living beings, to uncover the inner or hidden parts of the organism and see them work; to this sort of operation we give the name of vivisection, and without this mode of investigation, neither physiology nor scientific medicine is possible; to learn how man and animals live, we cannot avoid seeing great numbers of them die, because the mechanisms of life can be unveiled and proved only by knowledge of the mechanisms of death."[16]

Like most physicians of the mid nineteenth century, Bernard criticized the interference of the public into what he viewed to be the innate sphere of medicine. This is some of what he wrote in that regard: "The physiologist is not a person of fashion ... he

– 49 –

is a man of science, absorbed by the scientific idea which he pursues: he no longer hears the cry of animals, he no longer sees the blood that flows, he sees only his idea and perceives only organisms concealing problems which he intends to solve. Similarly, no surgeon is stopped by the most moving cries and sobs, because he sees only his idea and the purpose of his operation. Similarly again, no anatomist feels himself in a horrible slaughterhouse; under the influence of a scientific idea, he delightedly follows a nerve filament through stinking livid flesh, which to any other man would be an object of disgust and horror. After what has gone before we shall deem all discussion of vivisection futile or absurd. It is impossible for men, judging facts by such different ideas, ever to agree; and as it is impossible to satisfy everybody, a man of science should attend only to the opinion of men of science who understand him, and should derive rules of conduct only from his own conscience."[17]

In short, Bernard demanded nothing less than to exempt physicians from laws that governed all other members of society. This self-assured demand reflected the growing power of physicians in the nineteenth century. In France, the number of physicians who had been qualified by a university grew from a few hundred at the time of the French Revolution in the late 1700s to about 20,000 in 1890. Many physicians were active in politics; some physicians even became members of the French parliament. Physicians attended at schools and factories for purposes of health control, and they were asked by courts to testify about the cause of death and about the accountability of defendants. The rapid advancement of medical knowledge resulted in unprecedented esteem for physicians, and the revolutionary findings of Louis Pasteur and others were compared to the revolution in physics instigated by the works of Galileo and Sir Isaac Newton.[18]

Whereas the growing power of physicians formed the basis for Bernard's categorical rejection of intrusions from outside the realm of medicine into it, his demand that physicians be guided only by their own conscience reflected what the French Nobel Laureate, Charles Nicolle, later would call "medical individualism."[19] With the increase in knowledge and the refutation of many traditional concepts, it became evident that medical "truths" were relative and likely to be outdated soon. Likewise, yesterday's misconceptions could be tomorrow's innovations. Under such circumstances, the confidence of physicians in their own experiences and their freedom completely in regard to therapeutic decisions were valued highly by them. In their daily practice, physicians were essentially unrestricted, and they were accustomed to disregard taboos by virtue of special rights that were denied others (e.g., the right to maintain patient confidentiality, to dissect corpses, and to injure others purposefully in the course of surgical procedures). The irreverence for taboos that was deemed to be an inalienable right of medicine was claimed, too, by Bernard for medical research. Nevertheless, Bernard acknowledged the existence of ethical limitations and he did that thus: "The principle of medical and surgical morality . . . consists in never performing on man an experiment which might be harmful to him to any extent, even though the result might be highly advantageous to science, i.e., to the health of others."[20]

Unlike Bernard, most physicians of that time did not reflect on the advantages and disadvantages of medical experiments on humans. The sentence imposed by the Lyon court for the experiments of Guyenot and Gailleton met with stern disapproval by the international medical community. In medical journals, "the striking position of French police prosecutors vis-à-vis science" was attacked. Viennese dermatologist, Heinrich Auspitz (Fig. 87), who first described the phenomenon of acantholysis whereby spinous cells of the epidermis come apart from one another, and what came to be known as the Auspitz phenomenon of punctate bleeding that follows immediately on the yanking

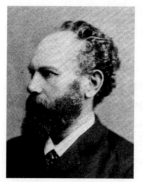

of psoriatic scale, voiced his amazement at the sentence, especially because the boy who had served as test subject seemed to have recovered completely.[21, 22] In 1866, Auspitz published a book titled, *Die Lehren vom syphilitischen Contagium und ihre thatsächliche Begründung* (Concepts of the Syphilitic Contagion and Their True Foundations), in which he summarized all that was known then about inoculation experiments. Not a single word, however, was written by him concerning the dubious ethical aspects of the experiments (Fig. 88).[23]

At last, the views of scientists prevailed and no more legal trials for experiments on humans were instituted until the end of the nineteenth century. The arguments about the propriety of medical experiments highlighted several issues: informed consent given freely of test subjects was mandatory; this condition hardly could be fulfilled, however, if test subjects were under duress, in a dependent position socially, or unable intellectually to realize the consequences of the experiments, especially in regard to ones performed on children; and any serious or permanent damage to health had to be avoided scrupulously. In subsequent years, however, these strictures were paid no heed, and any criticism of free reign of physicians in regard to experimentation on humans was considered to be an assault on freedom of science.

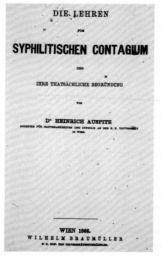

3 · The Call of Conscience

Physician-Experimenters Were Aware That What They Did Was Wrong

Despite all assertions to the contrary, however, it is evident that the scientists themselves were aware that what they had done and were doing was wrong. One piece of evidence on behalf of that thesis is the fact that during that period the largest inoculation study of syphilis was published anonymously. It was presented in 1855 at a meeting in Kaiserslautern in southwestern Germany by someone who claimed to know the author and to be qualified to guarantee the credibility of him scientifically. In this study, material from syphilitic lesions was injected into 11 persons, eight of whom developed severe systemic disease with fever and widespread skin lesions. Pus from those lesions was transferred to three other persons who also contracted syphilis, a fate they shared with six of nine additional subjects in whom infectious blood was smeared on open wounds. The identity of the physician responsible, Julius Bettinger (Fig. 89) of Frankenthal, was not revealed until more than 30 years after his death.[24, 25] Another study, the author of which remained anonymous, was presented at the 12th International Medical Congress in Moscow in 1897. A German-born Viennese neuropsychiatrist, Richard von Krafft-Ebing (Fig. 90), reported on findings of an unnamed "scientifically outstanding and very reliable colleague" who had inoculated patients suffering from general paresis with material from primary lesions of

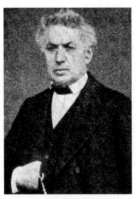

FIG. 89
Julius Bettinger (1802-1887)

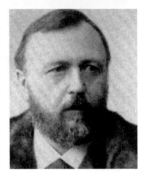

FIG. 90
Richard Krafft-Ebing (1840-1912)

syphilis in an attempt to prove a relationship between the two conditions.[26]

That scientists were aware of questions about the ethical probity of their experiments also can be intuited from the exaggerated assertions by them that "no real harm" was done. Even Bettinger's study of syphilis published anonymously was said to have been done "without violating the laws of humanity and under conscientious observation of the conditions that allow such experiments to be performed."[27] Few authors conceded that they had endangered the health and life of their test subjects. Nearly all ignored the advice of colleagues who called attention to those dangers in unambiguous terms. For example, in regard to syphilis, Anton von Hübbenet alerted fellow investigators to the fact that inoculations "can inflict the most severe, incurable damage to the health of persons serving as test objects."[28] Likewise, C. G. Åhmann of Stockholm described the fate of a patient who developed severe gonococcemia following intraurethral inoculation of gonococci and warned his colleagues not to duplicate the experiment.[29] As to chancroid, Felix von Bärensprung wrote that "I have recently seen very bad cases of patients who had inoculated themselves or had been inoculated by physicians: ulcers of the size of a coin or a palm that did not heal in two, three months and were followed by lymphangitis, phlebitis, and metastatic abscesses"[30](Fig. 91, 92).

In general, the risks associated with inoculations went unmentioned in scientific articles. It was emphasized by the authors, over and over again, how harmless were the experiments. Even in regard to syphilis, many articles concluded with the suggestion that infected test subjects had been healed completely by virtue of the efficacy of a brief course of treatment. This assumption was supported by the natural course of syphilis in which primary and secondary lesions disappear after a few weeks and the patient appears to be healthy again. That the disease was not eradicated and that severe complications,

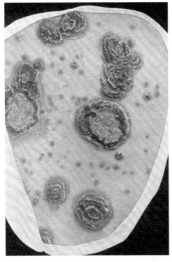

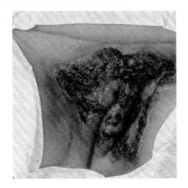

FIG. 92
Severe example of chancroid.

FIG. 91
Severe example of syphilis.

such as general paresis and tabes dorsalis, were late sequelae of syphilis, was not understood in those days. The signs and symptoms induced by inoculations – ulcers, fever, and pain – were minimized consistently in articles about those experiments.

Another sign of awareness of physicians of the dubious aspect of inoculation experiments was the pretext that those experiments served therapeutic purposes primarily. On the basis of that contention, the appearance of a normal, beneficent relationship between patient and doctor – the one seeking and the other providing medical care – could be maintained. From an ethical point of view, therapeutic trials were disassociated from nontherapeutic medical experiments, and those who conducted the former were less subject to criticism. In recognition of this fortuitous circumstance, many authors sought to attach to their studies the pretense of therapeutic consideration.

When Joseph Guyenot was tried by a court in Lyon for having performed a "successful" inoculation of syphilis in a 10-year-old boy, he made an effort to present his "vaccination" as a reasonable method for treating an unrelated infection of the scalp from which the boy suffered.[31] Friedrich Fehleisen, whose inoculation experiments substantiated the role of streptococci in the cause of erysipelas, chose as his test subjects patients suffering from cancer or lupus vulgaris, arguing that the inflammation associated with erysipelas might have a beneficial effect on the underlying disease.[32] Likewise, intraurethral inoculations of cultures of gonococci were performed on patients with latent gonorrhea under the curious assumption that transformation of the disease into a more acute stage might improve the effectiveness of therapeutic measures. This idea was propagated by Ernst Finger especially and enabled him and others to study gonococcal infections experimentally by gaining the permission of patients to perform them. Dermatologist Joseph Jadassohn, for example, transferred gonococci to the urethra of six patients with latent gonorrhea, arguing that he "was justified to carry out such inoculations" because of Finger's assertion "that chronic gonorrhea seems to heal better after inoculation of extraneous gonococci."[33]

Double Standard of Physician-Experimenters Based on Social Class and Economic Status

The fourth, and perhaps most important, indication that physicians were well aware of the reprehensibility of their experiments was the method they employed for selecting test subjects. Those chosen were not private patients from the upper or middle classes of society, but rather the poor and uneducated, the exception being some medical students and junior assistants. In brief, subjects were persons judged to be inferior, whose health and lives were thought by their "superiors" to be unimportant.

In general, test subjects were completely dependent individuals who had no real choice about hardly anything. In the south of the United States, the ideal test subjects were slaves who helped advance the career of their masters by ingesting newly formulated remedies and by enduring painful, sometimes lethal experimental surgical procedures.[34] Natives of the European colonies were used for a variety of medical experiments ranging from studies on the contagiousness of malaria to trials of experimental drugs.[35] Between 1909 and 1914 in the German colonies, for example, hundreds of Africans who were presumed to suffer from sleeping sickness were interned in camps and treated compulsorily with concoctions of arsenic. Those drugs not only were ineffective, but highly toxic; many test subjects lost their lives (Fig. 93).[36]

The bulk of medical research, however, was performed in

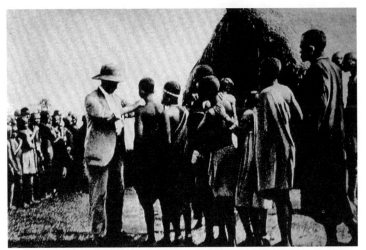

FIG. 93
Experimental treatment in Africa with "Bayer 205," a then newly-developed compound for sleeping sickness (1923).

Europe, especially in Germany, which by the mid nineteenth century had become the Mecca of medicine. At German hospitals, research and management of patients were related closely to one another; when patients could not pay the usual fees, they were expected to participate in scientific studies as compensation for their treatment.[37] According to a survey of articles published between 1880 and 1900 in the *Deutsche Medizinische Wochenschrift*, almost 90 percent of test subjects came from

FIG. 94
*Poor quarter
in Berlin in
1916.*

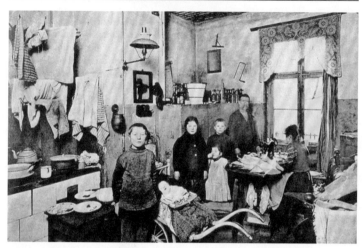

the lower classes (Fig. 94).[38] They were not thought worthy by physicians, and in publications they were referred to not as "persons" or "patients," but as "the infected" or "the material."[39] Treatment of these patients in German hospitals during the late nineteenth century was catalogued in grim detail by a surgeon at the Johns Hopkins Hospital, John M. T. Finney, in these words:

I won't go into the details as to all I saw. I was so disgusted and out-raged by what I did see that I never returned. On that one occasion the patient was a young woman about twenty. She was wheeled into the operating room on a stretcher, then stripped of all her clothing, lifted to the operating table and tied there by the orderlies with bandages binding her legs together and her arms to her sides, with her head pulled back over the end of the table and tied fast there in a most uncomfortable position. Thus she could not move her head, arms, or legs but could only cry. The whole procedure was brutal . . . When the surgeon himself came in, she was crying loud-ly and begging for mercy. He walked over and gave her a resound-ing smack on the cheek and . . . told her to be quiet. He then pro-ceeded to do the operation, a most painful one, without a drop of anesthetic of any kind, believe it or not. The poor girl screamed and cried until she stopped from sheer exhaustion. The details of the operation are too horrible to relate. I waited until after it was over, just long enough to go up and ask the operator – I won't call him a surgeon – why he hadn't given the poor girl an anesthetic. With a shrug of the shoulder he replied, 'It wasn't necessary. We could hold her.' Fortunately, that experience was unique, but I must say that it made me thankful to get out of Germany without having to have a surgical operation done on myself or any of my family.[40]

In her autobiography, the Jewish physician, Käte Frankenthal (Fig. 95), recalled her own experience in Germany in these riveting and poignant remarks: "At that time, patients in public hospitals were treated rather harshly. Not that there was a lack of scientifically founded treatment. We had excellent physicians . . . but they were chiefly scientists, and patients

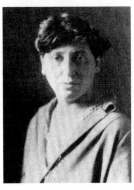

FIG. 95
Käte Frankenthal (1889-1976)

were material. Great advances necessitate great sacrifices . . . I heard this undeniable truth in all tones, especially by very young assistants. Every beginner took a chance on future fame as a scientist and used patients as material. True harm was done only rarely. But how much blood was taken! How many injections done for experimental purposes! How many painful examinations for training purposes! Before the war, the assistant was the unchallenged chief of his unit – this was acknowledged not only by staff, but also by patients. How often did I hear those young physicians shout: 'Do you know what is good for you, or do I? If you do not obey, you can go home . . .'"[41]

In most instances, such intimidation was unnecessary. Because of the long tradition of authoritarianism in Germany and Austria, orders of superiors, including doctors, rarely were challenged. Foreign visitors to German and Austrian departments of medicine were amazed by the stoicism of patients and their deference to authority. Among these was the editor of the *Annales de Dermatologie et de Syphiligraphie*, Adrien Doyon

(Fig. 96), who described his visit in 1883 to Hebra's skin clinic in Vienna as follows:

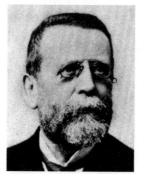

The patients are in their beds when the visit begins, but the moment the professor arrives they get up, put on the blue striped hospital gowns of cotton twill that are issued to everyone, and seat themselves on benches in the center of the room. From there they are summoned one by one to a table at which the professor is seated and on which instruments and dressing materials are laid out. When they appear before the chief of service they undress completely and . . . climb onto a chair where they then turn around and back again, submitting without a word not only to the most minute examinations but even to operative procedures . . .[42]

The Past Presages the Future in Regard to Experimentation on Humans

This attitude of doctors and patients ensured that informed consent given freely to experiments on humans was nothing more than illusion. Moreover, scientists continued to select as test subjects not only patients who could be called "average," but

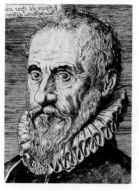

especially persons whom society did not value highly; in fact, they were believed to be inferior. This applied to prison inmates who, since antiquity, had been used for medical experiments. That tradition was much in evidence during the Middle Ages, just as it has been maintained in modern times. For example, Ambroise Paré (Fig. 97), the greatest figure in surgery

during the Renaissance, once suggested that a prisoner be used for testing the claim that a bezoar stone possessed by King Charles IX of France
was an antidote for every ill. To escape
hanging, the prisoner agreed to take
the poison along with the stone, and
he promptly died within a few
hours.[43] In England in 1721, condemned prisoners at Newgate Prison

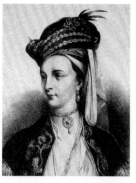

FIG. 98
*Lady Mary
Wortley
Montagu
(1689-1762)*

were offered a pardon by King George I if they would participate in variolation, the experimental injection of matter of
smallpox for the purpose of inducing immunity to the disease.
This program had been initiated by Lady Mary Wortley Montagu (Fig. 98), poet and wife of the British Ambassador to
Turkey. During her stay in Constantinople, Lady Montagu had
noted that "the small pox, so fatal, and so general amongst us, is
here entirely harmless, by the invention of ingrafting, which is
the term they give it here." Her ladyship was so "satisfied of the
safety of this experiment" that she tried it on her own daughter
before proceeding to the larger trial at Newgate Prison. Variolation eventually proved to be an effective way to induce immunity, but it also was the cause of many deaths (not that of the Montagu child) and the source of numerous outbreaks locally of
smallpox. In the 1760s, British physician, Robert Sutton,
recorded 1,200 fatalities among 30,000 persons who were inoculated with matter of variola.[44] The Newgate convicts, however, developed only cutaneous lesions and were sent home,
being spared the hangman's noose.[45]

Between 1772 and 1782, the Bicêtre in Paris, a combination
prison and hospice for the indigent, homeless, aged, orphaned,
infirm, and criminally inclined among the Parisian lower class,
received nearly 50 requests for permission to test in its facilities new drugs and other therapies for venereal disease.[46] In

FIG. 99
*Georg
Friedrich
Hildebrandt
(1764-1816)*

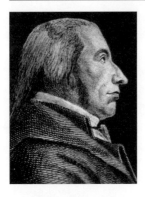

FIG. 99
*Georg
Friedrich
Hildebrandt
(1764-1816)*

FIG. 100
*Casimir
Davaine
(1812-1882)*

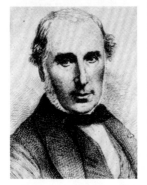

Germany in 1786, Georg Friedrich Hildebrandt (Fig. 99) called for medical experiments to be carried out on prisoners who had been sentenced to death. "It would be desirable for physicians," he theorized in his book *Versuch einer philosophischen Pharmakologie* (Attempt at a Philosophical Pharmacology), "to use the opportunity of conducting experiments on persons destined for death more frequently in order to determine their effects on the bodies of other people ... Other human beings without an interest in the experiments will consent only rarely to experiments whose success is dubious, and to conduct such experiments by use of cunning or force would be irresponsible."[47]

In 1812, Jean-François Hernandez utilized prisoners in Toulon for intracutaneous injections of pus of gonorrhea.[48] Decades later, when the French physiologist, Claude Bernard, demanded that scientists be forbidden to perform "on man an experiment which might be harmful to him to any extent," he excluded specifically prisoners sentenced to death, as long as they were caused no additional suffering.[49] Following Bernard's advice, the French pioneer of bacteriology and helminthology, Casimir-Joseph Davaine (Fig. 100), fed larva-infected sausage to a condemned female prisoner to see whether worms would develop in her intestines after her death.[50]

During a visit to Hawaii, the Hamburg dermatologist, Eduard Arning (Fig. 101), used a prisoner waiting for execution to study the contagiousness of leprosy. The prisoner was rewarded by commutation of his sentence to life imprisonment, but after four years he developed signs of leprosy and his state of health soon became deplorable.[51] After publication of his experiment in Germany, Arning was criticized for having taken advantage of the prisoner's desperate situation.

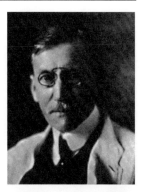

FIG. 101
Eduard Arning
(1855-1936)

Similar objections were heard on other occasions that were analogous. As early as 1827, Karl F. H. Marx of Göttingen had insisted that prisoners, who obviously were vulnerable, should not be exploited to force their participation in medical experiments because "the increasing humaneness of our times precludes . . . experiments on miscreants."[52] In regard to prisoners, though, the call of conscience remained exceptional;

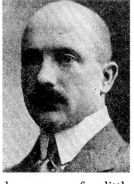

FIG. 102
Ernst
Wertheim
(1864-1920)

convicts generally were considered to be persons of so little worth that experiments on them were conceived to be totally justifiable.

What was true for convicts was true equally for prostitutes. When von Bärensprung performed inoculations on young prostitutes in order to study the contagiousness of secondary syphilis, he argued as follows "I considered myself justified to undertake a series of experiments on persons who, because of their freely selected profession, expose themselves daily to unpunished experiments with gonorrhea and syphilis. I vaccinated several prostitutes who had the undeserved luck of not yet having become syphilitic."[53] Mentally disabled patients provided another source of "suitable" test subjects. The chairman of gynecology at the German University of Prague, Ernst

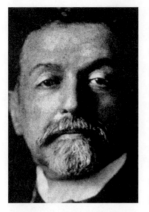

Wertheim (Fig. 102), employed what he called "idiots" and "paralytics" for study of gonorrhea, and did not forget to thank his peer, the chairman of psychiatry (Fig. 103), for providing those patients as test subjects. "I am highly indebted to Professor Arnold Pick," he acknowledged, "for his permission to carry out the inoculation experiments on human beings by use of suitable paralytics of his clinic."[54]

Yet another fertile source of subjects for human experimentation were persons who simply were too ill to object. In those days, mortally ill patients were generally referred to as *corpora vilia* ("cheap" or "worthless" bodies), and they were treated accordingly as raw material for scientific studies (Fig. 104). In publications concerning experiments on humans, the hopeless state of the health of test subjects often was noted as an extenuating circumstance.[55] Among the pitifully few physicians who voiced concern about it, J. A. Gläser of Hamburg wrote in 1898 thus: "We cannot accept as justification for a study . . . that its victim is an 'ailing patient whose end must be anticipated shortly.' The best of physicians and with them the entire profession have acknowledged until now, and will hopefully continue to acknowledge, that the less they are able to bring patients confiding in them to convalescence, the more they are obliged to mitigate their suffering."[56] Instead of lessening their suffering, however, physicians subjected these patients to additional pain. Examples of abuses are legion. Among the most disturbing was the routine use of moribund patients by Viennese dermatologist, Ernst Finger, to study through inoculations the quality of his culture media for gonococci.[57]

3 · The Call of Conscience

Unconscionable Abuse of Orphans and Disadvantaged Minors by Physician-Experimenters

Experiments on persons who could not express their own will were especially rife among those with no relatives who could act on their behalf and interfere. This applied particularly to medical experiments on children, making the orphan an ideal test subject. In the eighteenth and early nineteenth centuries, children in general were regarded poorly; foundlings were bought

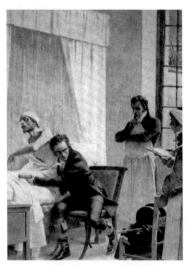

and sold, and child labor was the rule. Against this background it is not surprising that children were among the first subjects to be chosen for experimental medical procedures.[58] In 1703, Dr. Zabdiel Boylston of Boston inoculated children with matter of smallpox, using his son and two of his slaves as the first subjects in testing this theory of prevention, which was derived directly from descendants of the first slaves brought from Africa. In the 1750s, Queen Caroline of England requested that several "charity children" be variolated before the new and frightening procedure was tried on scions of the royal family.[59] Francis Home, a member of the College of Physicians in Edinburgh, in 1759, subjected young children to experimental inoculation with measles.[60] When medical experimentation increased dramatically in the nineteenth century, children continued to be favorite test subjects. In the last two decades of that century, 32 percent of all nontherapeutic experiments on humans in Germany were performed on children.[61]

Johann Ritter von Waller, for instance, used foundlings for inducing experimental infection with syphilis. Another example is an inoculation study on young subjects by Carl Janson of Stockholm utilizing sterilized fluid from lesions of vaccinia. Janson later indicated that he might have erred when he wrote, "I should perhaps first have performed experiments on animals, but the most fit subjects, calves, were difficult to get and maintain because of the high costs, and, therefore – with the friendly permission of the associate professor Medin – I started with experiments on children from the local foundling hospital."[62]

If no orphans were available, it was more difficult to recruit minors as test subjects. In those instances, physicians sought parents who were simple-minded and, therefore, more likely to capitulate to their persuasions about having their children used as fodder for medical experiments. Julius Schreiber of Königsberg, who tried to study the effects of injections of tuberculin on healthy children, later made this admission: "It was difficult to find children, and so I could inject only one boy, casually, for some minor misdemeanor in the clinic. The boy came from a family of workers whose mother had contracted pulmonary tuberculosis. Originally, the parents did not want to permit the injection, but then, as already mentioned, the boy did something wrong, and the father said: 'Well, now you also will be injected. He is going to withstand it, he is healthy.' The boy, however, following injection of 1 milligram, reacted with severe fever that lasted several days . . ."[63]

CHAPTER 4

THE VALUE OF PERFORMING EXPERIMENTS ON HUMANS

T he conviction of physicians that their human subjects for experimentation were inferior – as evidenced by those who were chosen and how they were characterized in articles – served to desensitize the collective medical conscience of the day. The presumption of the importance of experiments on humans for the advancement of medicine and, thereby, of humanity, was another great alleviator of conscience. Franz Rinecker, for instance, defended the deliberate infection of healthy persons with matter of syphilis by arguing that without such experiments there would be no progress.[1] Was Rinecker correct? Were experiments on humans truly requisite for the advancement of medicine?

In 1824, one of the pioneers of experimental medicine, German physiologist Johannes Peter Müller (Fig. 105), made this forthright, but unusual, comment on the value of such experiments:

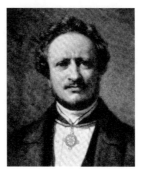

FIG. 105
*Johannes
Müller
(1801-1858)*

Observation is unpretentious, patient, diligent, honest, without prejudice – the experiment is artificial, impatient,

– 67 –

bustling, unsteady, passionate, unreliable ... Nothing is easier than to conduct a bunch of so-called interesting experiments. Whenever one challenges nature violently, she will be forced to give some painful answer ... In anatomic studies, simple observation is much more magnificent than the facile and often enough mendacious physiologic experiment.[2]

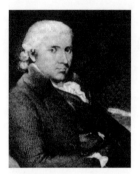

Müller's opinion about experiments was true in general, especially for experiments on humans which, by-and-large, were performed with a sense of haste but without a sense of thoughtful reflection and of unswerving diligence. A sterling example of this shoddiness was the first careless inoculation experiment in 1767 by John Hunter, which gave credence to the erroneous concept of the oneness of syphilis and gonorrhea. One of Hunter's critics was Benjamin Bell of Edinburgh (Fig. 106) who, as recorded in his *Treatise on Gonorrhoea and Lues Venerea* published in 1793, distinguished the two diseases from one another chiefly on the basis of clinical observation, rather than through experimentation. In regard to the inoculation by Hunter, Bell wrote that "it has indeed been said that chancres may be produced by insinuating the matter of Gonorrhoea beneath the skin. But experiments upon this subject are productive of such anxiety and distress, that they never have been, nor ever probably will be, repeated so frequently as the nature of it would require."[3]

Bell was right. The majority of experiments on humans of that time were mere anecdotal exercises rather than controlled, systematic studies. Rarely did those investigations address, let alone resolve, the questions that prompted their having been undertaken in the first place. For example, Danish dermatologist, Erik Pontoppidan, performed many autoinoculations in patients with syphilis for the expressed purpose of clarifying whether excision of a primary lesion early in its course could prevent systemic infection. When Pontoppidan transferred material from a chancre to healthy skin of the same person, he claimed that he was able to induce secondary chancres within the first three days following the experimental infection, whereas a few days later, no secondary chancres developed as a consequence of an ensuing immune response.[4] Viennese dermatologist, Franz Mracek (Fig. 107), noted rightly that Pontoppidan's experiments did not answer the question posed originally. The lack of an immune response in the first three days, Mracek said, could not be interpreted as evidence that syphilis could be healed through excision of the primary lesion early in the course of it.[5] When Daniel Danielssen tried unsuccessfully to induce leprosy by inoculating pleural exudate from lepers into himself and others, Armauer Hansen pointed out that negative results had to be expected because the bacilli of leprosy could not be found in pleural exudate. (Fig. 108). Many

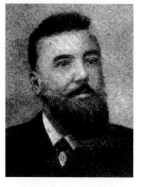

FIG. 107
*Franz Mracek
(1848-1908)*

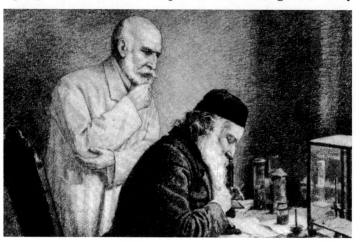

FIG. 108
*Armauer
Hansen (left)
showing
Daniel
Danielssen the
bacillus of
leprosy
(painting by
Karl
Kusnyák).*

other microbes, however, could have been present in that exudate, and Hansen attributed it to simple good luck that none of Danielssen's test subjects had acquired sepsis or pyemia.[6] After the discovery of the causative bacteria of gonorrhea by Albert Neisser in 1879, many investigators rushed to perform inoculations using Neisser's microorganism. The results were diverse and conflicting. In a monograph on gonorrhea in 1885, gynecologist Ernst Bumm criticized most of the reports about the subject as being too imprecise to allow comparisons. He opined that some authors probably even used the wrong types of cocci, that is, ones other than *Neisseria gonorrheae.*[7]

In short, many experiments on humans were futile and, thereby, hampered, rather than advanced, the cause of science. The erroneous concept of the unity of syphilis and gonorrhea could have been corrected much earlier had there not been the misleading evidence provided by Hunter's rash experiment. Likewise, Philippe Ricord's failure at autoinoculation using material from lesions of secondary syphilis led to the mistaken assumption that secondary syphilis was not infectious. Ironically, that sophistic view had not been held before Ricord began his experiments. The inoculations that were performed subsequently to prove the contagiousness of secondary syphilis were completely unnecessary, and that is just how they were perceived by some physicians at the time. In his critique of Waller's experiments with inoculation in the 1850s, Johann Ludwig Casper (Fig. 109) asked this question pointedly: "Can any objective medical critic deny that the manifestations of secondary syphilis are contagious? Is it not true that every older and experienced physician has seen the test of this transferability often enough in daily life, without any help of science, through the companionship and sexual contact of a person with secondary syphilis and a person free of syphilis? Yes, who has ever had any doubt about that before the introduction of syphilis inoculations?"[8]

4· The Value of Experiments

The major breakthroughs of the nineteenth century in dermatology and venereology were achieved by observation of, rather than by experimentation on, humans. Bell's separation of syphilis from gonorrhea, for instance, was based principally on clinical observation. This was true also of Ricord's classification of syphilis into primary, secondary, and tertiary stages. Epidemiologic studies enabled Léon Bassereau to follow the pathways of infection and, as a consequence, to separate syphilis from chancroid.[9] The recognition of the incubation period of syphilis by Joseph Rollet (Fig. 110);[10] the description of late manifestations of congenital syphilis and of the spectrum of cutaneous and noncutaneous changes of

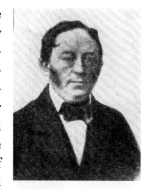

FIG. 109
Johann Ludwig Casper (1796-1864)

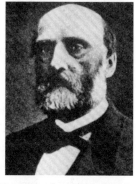

FIG. 110
Joseph Rollet (1824-1894)

syphilis by Sir Jonathan Hutchinson (Fig. 111); the demonstration of *tabes dorsalis* and general paresis as late manifestations of syphilis by Jean Alfred Fournier – all these advances were based on clinical observations and epidemiologic considerations. As such, they did no harm to patients.[11] The same was true for the discovery in 1905 of *Spirochaeta pallida* by the German bacteriologist Fritz Richard Schaudinn and dermatologist Erich Hoffmann.[12] In fact, the claim that experimentation on humans was a prerequisite for the advance of medicine was patently wrong.

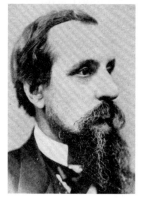

FIG. 111
Jonathan Hutchinson (1828-1913)

The Abuse of Man

The Exaggeration of Worth

Why were experiments on humans so vastly overestimated? The most important reason was the propensity of persons in the late nineteenth century to manipulate, rather than to observe, nature. Anything labeled "experimental" was thought to be vastly superior to traditional ways of acquiring knowledge. At the Third International Congress of Dermatology in London in 1896, Oskar Lassar of Berlin (Fig. 112), a close friend of the dermatologic polymath, Paul Gerson Unna, phrased the credo in these words: "The experiment is the true modern scientific method, whereas case reports in order to support ones own view are basically outdated."[13] Lassar's judgment was as wrong then as it is today; the direct observation of phenomena of nature continues to be an essential aspect of scientific study and is the precondition for planning experiments logically and interpreting the results of them meaningfully.

There are two requisites for any experiment: (1) observation and (2) systematic changes in conditions, in conjunction with scrutiny carefully before, during, and after those changes occur.[14] In many instances, the conditions must be changed by man, especially if experiments concern man-made phenomena, such as assessment of efficacy of new drugs. For other scientific inquiries, it is sufficient, and even preferable, to search for

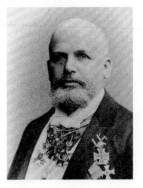

FIG. 112
*Oskar Lassar
(1849-1907)*

changes in conditions that come about naturally, that is, without being caused deliberately by man. In the third quarter of the twentieth century, the anesthesiologist, Henry K. Beecher of Boston, pointed out that "nature presents us with bolder experiments than we would ever dare to perform ourselves."[15] In the realm of dermatovenereology especially, with skin lesions being accessible immediately to the observer, experiments of nature were readily apparent to anyone who chose to observe them and could have been exploited to an extent far greater than they were. In the nineteenth century, however, experimental medicine was entirely new, and enthusiasm for it led to contempt for traditional forms of scientific inquiry and overestimation of the worth of experiments on humans.

Experiments on humans also had the appealing dimension of drama. Although those experiments rarely provided findings that permitted new insights, they did help popularize the findings more than had they been judged by observation alone. For example, the dermatologist, Heinrich Köbner (Fig. 113), who described *epidermolysis bullosa simplex* and the isomorphic phenomenon that today is named for him, behaved like a ham actor when demonstrating the contagiousness of fungi. At a meeting of the Medical Society of Breslau in 1862, Köbner began the theatrics by rolling up one sleeve to show the audience a scutulum on his forearm where he had inoculated himself with scales of favus. Next, he rolled up the other sleeve to display a more advanced lesion of ringworm. For the final act, Köbner opened his shirt to exhibit a fully developed fungal infection on his chest.[16]

Moreover, as noted by Johannes Müller, experiments could be performed quickly and could be carried out relatively simply, in contrast with clinical observation of patients which took time. Whenever physicians became impatient, jumped at conclusions, or wanted to end a debate by proving their own concept conclusively, they tended to deviate from established methods of research and resort to experiments that all too often were imprudent. Even respected scientists were not

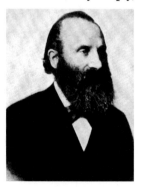

FIG. 113
*Heinrich
Köbner
(1838-1904)*

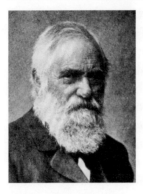

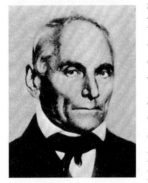

immune to such temptation. In 1892, for instance, the celebrated hygienist, Max Josef von Pettenkoffer of Munich (Fig. 114), who established basic concepts about nutrition and discovered a new amino acid, creatinine, in human urine, decided to challenge Robert Koch's claim that cholera was caused solely by the bacterium, *Vibrio cholerae.* In a dramatic, if less-than-scientific manner, Pettenkoffer swallowed a pure culture of cholera bacilli, after which he suffered only a mild case of diarrhea, allowing him to continue to maintain his thesis that the germ alone did not produce the disease.[17] Among other prominent physicians who risked their lives in self-experimentation was the famous Czech physiologist, Johannes Evangelista Purkinje (Fig. 115), who swallowed enough digitalis to kill nine cats, his purpose being to study the side effects of the drug. Purkinje suffered cardiac pain and irregularity, and vomited for a week afterward, but he survived. French physician, Pierre-Fleurus Tonery, in his zeal to convince the French Academy of Medicine of the extraordinary powers of charcoal to absorb alkaloids, took a dose of strychnine that alone would have been lethal, but wisely mixed it with charcoal as a safeguard.[18]

The Lure and the Risk of Fame

The lure of human experimentation was particularly seductive to younger physicians. In their desire to become famous, they, too, took risks both for themselves and for their patients. The first recorded deliberate experiment that, without question, was of risk to the investigator was performed in 1760 by Anton Störck of Vienna. At the ripe age of 19, Störck ingested increasingly larger quantities of hemlock to assess its safety and/or toxicity.[19] Fortunately for him, he lived. In 1769, 29-year-old William Stark, a student of John Hunter at St. George's Hospital in London, became so intrigued by the relationship between diet and disease that he induced scurvy in himself by living on nothing but bread and water. When hemorrhagic lesions appeared on his gums and skin, Stark consulted his colleague and friend, Sir John James Pringle, for whom is named adenoma sebaceum of tuberous sclerosis (Pringle's disease). Pringle had considerable experience with scurvy, but he had not yet converted to the views expressed by British physician, James Lind, concerning the importance of oranges and lemons in preventing and treating the disease. Pringle's advice to Störk – not uncommon in those days – was to omit salt from his diet. Stark followed that suggestion, continued his dietary experiments, and, in February 1770, the once strapping young doctor died emaciated as a consequence, a mere eight months after having begun his experiment.[20]

In the 1800s, Stubbins Ffirth, a medical student at the University of Pennsylvania, exposed himself to all manner of repulsive material from patients in the last stages of yellow fever. For several nights Ffirth slept on a bed next to an extremely ill patient; he swallowed the patients' vomit, placed drops of it in his conjunctiva, and inhaled its vapors; and he repeatedly cut deep into his skin and subcutaneous tissue in order to deposit black vomit, saliva, sweat, bile, urine, and serum of patients with yellow fever. Apart from inflammation, headaches, and nausea that were temporary, Ffirth suffered no adverse effects and concluded that "the disease cannot be communicated by the secretions or excretions." Although Ffirth's contributions to the elucidation of yellow fever were given no attention by his contemporaries, medical historians later acknowledged that "there are very few pages in the history of medicine which bespeak a heroism comparable to that of Ffirth."[21]

In 1885, another medical student, Daniel Alcides Carrión of

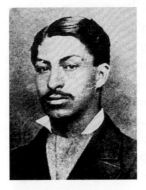

FIG. 116
*Daniel Alcides
Carrión (1858-
1885)*

Peru (Fig. 116, 117), for a variety of reasons, some of them complex psychologically, inoculated himself with material from skin lesions of Oroya fever. Seven weeks later he died of the infection. As a mestizo, Carrión belonged to a class of the population that was considered to be inferior. This circumstance may have enhanced his desire to prove himself through accomplishments, even at risk of death. Although Carrión's self-inoculation was reckless and his death unnecessary, he became a national hero. His portrait, transformed deliberately in such a way that he could not be recognized as a mestizo, is well known in Peru to this day.[22] Likewise, other scientists who performed such experiments on themselves and others were praised enthusiastically. Heinrich Auspitz called Franz Rinecker an "inspired scientist" of "high courage" and "scientific fire," applauding particularly his "famous inoculations with syphilis."[23] In an obituary about Pietro Pellizari of Florence, Filipp Josef Pick pointed out that the Italian venereologist's work concerning the transmission of syphilis was the foundation on which rested his fame.[24] For mediocre scientists, experiments on humans offered a chance to participate in the progress of medicine and to achieve fame by virtue of heroics rather than ingenuity.

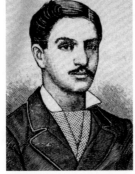

FIG. 117
*Carrión, in his
"official"
portrait that
first appeared
in La Chronica
Medica in
Lima, Peru in
1885; no
longer can he
be recognized
as a mestizo.*

In the days of uncontrolled experimentation on humans at

the end of the nineteenth century, those two words – progress and fame – represented the highest aspirations of man. The entire century was marked by what seemed to be boundless progress. There was an explosion of knowledge, new machines took over men's tasks, industry boomed, and a better age – with better human beings, better societies, better lives – appeared imminent. The enthusiasm for progress was wedded to an obsession for fame. The strongest motivating factor of the day was neither religion, as it had been in previous centuries, nor money, as it would be in the century to follow. What most propelled man was fame. In the 1880s and 1890s, the spectacular advances of bacteriology conferred an abundance of fame on laboratory researchers, whose lives and successes were followed as closely by the public then as those of sports heroes and entertainment superstars

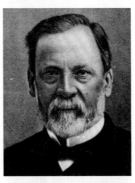

FIG. 118
*Louis Pasteur
(1822-1895)*

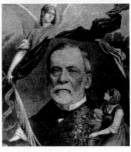

FIG. 119
*Louis Pasteur
pictured as a
Saint.*

today. Robert Koch was such an object of adulation that thousands of handkerchiefs embroidered with his face were sold.[25]

An individual's fame did not belong solely to himself or herself; it extended to an entire nation, enabling the average citizen to feel part of the progress and the fame. At that time, nothing was thought to be more meritorious and satisfying than to bring fame to one's nation, and the front lines of medical research served to bolster strong nationalistic feelings. An example is the competition between what then were the two leading bacteriologists in the world – Louis Pasteur in Paris (Fig. 118, 119) and Robert Koch in Berlin (Fig. 120, 121). Each of Pasteur's advances in germ theory, microbiology, and immunology

FIG. 120
*Robert Koch
(1843-1910)*

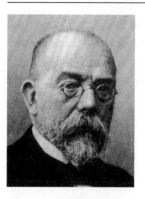

FIG. 121
*Robert Koch
in his
laboratory
(painting by
Max
Pietschmann,
1896).*

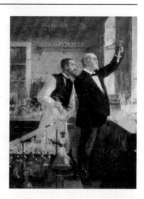

spurred other scientists to look for something new and "bigger." When Koch identified the tubercle bacillus in 1882, it was perceived as a national triumph for Germany and fostered a race for additional discoveries. Like the gold rush in California, where a few major finds induced thousands to go West to try their luck by digging through mountains and streams, Koch's findings induced what was referred to as "bacteriomania." Thousands of physicians throughout the world were digging frantically in search of their own scientific gold mine.[26]

Koch's Postulates

Koch, who lived long enough to be awarded one of the first Nobel Prizes in medicine (Pasteur died too soon to be so honored), set forth guidelines for experimentation in bacteriology. Whenever a finding was made, or a new piece of knowledge was grasped, it had to be tethered securely, which meant it had to fulfill Koch's postulates: (1) the microorganism had to be detected in lesions of the disease; (2) the microorganism had to be isolated and grown in pure culture; (3) inoculation of the culture had to induce a similar disease in susceptible animals; and (4) the microorganism had to be recovered from animals that were inoculated.

In order to turn a discovery into a triumph, it was mandato-

ry that Koch's four conditions be satisfied; any study that fell
short was thought to be defective, regardless of other pieces of
evidence that resulted from it. In the logic of that classic era of
microbiology, even slight alterations of a proven method, for
example, a minor modification of culture media, required fulfillment of Koch's postulates anew.[27] The search for susceptible
animals that might serve to close the circle of reasoning acquired the character of an imperative and was undertaken ob-
sessively. Countless attempts were made to transfer syphilis
and gonorrhea to animals, such as swine, dogs, cats, rabbits,
and guinea pigs. In 1888, Isidor Neumann tried to inoculate the
"virus" of syphilis into three rabbits, a horse, three apes, a hare,
a white rat, a martin, and a domestic cat, all to no avail.[28] Once
Élie Metchnikoff (Fig. 122) and Emile Roux (Fig. 123) had succeeded in 1903 in inducing syphilis in
a chimpanzee (Fig. 124), Albert
Neisser built a monkey house in the
backyard of his villa in Breslau and
stocked it with 200 shrieking simians
for the purpose of compensating,
once and for all, for any lack of experimental animals. When most of the
monkeys succumbed to the bitter
Silesian winter, Neisser changed his
strategy and traveled to Java to carry
out his experiments on long-tailed
primates there. In a more natural setting, he inoculated syphilis in more
than 1,000 monkeys of various types
and studied the responses.[29]

Of course, not everyone could trav-
el to Java, and because of the difficulty
in finding appropriate experimental
animals and the contempt expressed

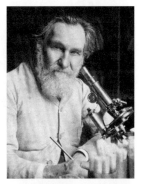

FIG. 122
*Elias
Metchnikoff
(1845-1916)*

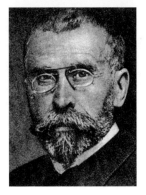

FIG. 123
*Emile Roux
(1853-1933)*

for any work in microbiology that failed to meet Koch's postulates, investigators simply reverted to using the human animal. Nontherapeutic experiments on humans abounded. They were accepted as standard procedures, requiring neither explanation nor apology. Little or no attention was paid to most of those experiments; they were performed perfunctorily and were referred to, if at all, only parenthetically in lectures and textbooks.[30] Although the number of nontherapeutic experiments on humans was great, the value of them scientifically was mostly little. The prodigious harm these experiments caused test subjects went unnoticed and unnoted.

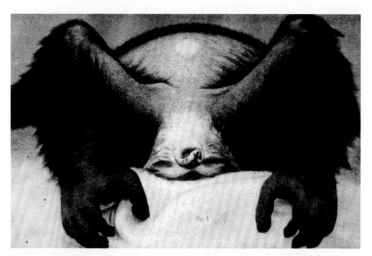

FIG. 124 *Chimpanzee inoculated successfully with material from a chancre of syphilis (from the report by Metchnikoff and Roux in 1903).*

CHAPTER 5

THERAPEUTIC TRIALS

I n principle, any form of medical intervention is an experiment in the sense that the effects of it in an individual patient cannot be foretold. In reality, most therapeutic measures – both medications and technical procedures – are based on vast experience gained through controlled studies or by many years of observation. Only when such experience is lacking may a therapeutic procedure be regarded as truly experimental.

In the nineteenth century, even the most effective modes of treatment lacked thorough grounding in data, and what evidence did exist often was inaccurate and misleading. In recalling medical practice in the Victorian era, Thomas Clifford Allbutt (Fig. 125) mentioned pointedly that although it was customary for physicians at every consultation "to prepare a writing table, pen, and ink for the 'prescription'" and to dispense "a drug for every symptom," hardly any of the drugs administered had been proven effective.[1] With very few exceptions, drug therapy was nothing more than a refined form of charlatanism. This truth was recognized by some important physicians and authors of that time. In an issue

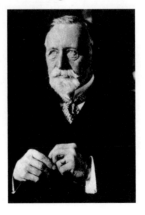

FIG. 125
*Thomas
Clifford Allbutt
(1836-1925)*

of the *Boston Medical and Surgical Journal* for 1861, D.W. Cheever deplored the fact in these words:

Effects are ascribed to drugs which really flow from natural causes, and are but the usual succession of the morbid phenomena; sequences are taken for consequences, and all just conclusions confused. From a want of this knowledge, from defective observation, rash generalizations, and hasty conclusions a priori, have arisen the thousand conflicting theories which have degraded Medicine from its true position as a science, and interfered with its advancement as a practical art.[2]

In the same year, Oliver Wendell Holmes (Fig. 126) gave the students of Harvard Medical School his unvarnished and passionate view of the matter thus:

The disgrace of medicine has been that colossal system of self-deception, in obedience to which mines have been emptied of their cankering minerals, the vegetable kingdom robbed of all its noxious growths, the entrails of animals taxed for their impurities, the poison-bags of reptiles drained of their venom, and all the inconceivable abominations thus obtained thrust down the throats of human beings.

For Holmes, much of the blame for this indiscriminate use of medicinals rested "with the public itself, which insists on being poisoned." He concluded that, "If the whole *materia medica,* as now used, could be sent to the bottom of the sea, it would be all

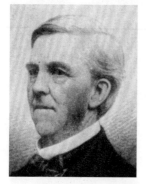

FIG. 126
Oliver Wendell Holmes
(1809-1894)

the better for mankind and all the worse for the fishes."[3]

This type of sloppy therapeutic experimentation had been going on in the name of "good medicine" for centuries, and for that reason there was need urgently for assessing both traditional and innovative forms of treatment in a systematic fashion. In the early nineteenth century, treatment for most conditions still consisted principally of Galen's triad of bloodletting, other methods of fluid extraction, and administration of massive cocktails of vegetable compounds – the more, the better.[4] Any beneficial effects of treatment were chiefly psychological. If an illness were not itself fatal, the natural course of it would lead inevitably to improved health, despite the treatment – unless the cure itself was lethal. Bloodletting, for instance, was debilitating at best, deadly at worst. Patients who had a limited course of this so-called cure would first grow so weak they no longer would care what was happening to them. When the bloodletting stopped, they naturally experienced the pleasant feeling of slowly regaining strength.[5] When repeated excessively, as was the rule in cases believed to be severe, bloodletting contributed to the death of many patients, including such eminences as George Washington. In regard to drugs, Galen had learned that expensive compounds were more effective than cheap ones, and, similarly, generations of physicians that followed him were aided by the effect of placebo.[6] "New" modalities of treatment consisted chiefly of new mixtures of old compounds, and methods that truly were innovative were studied unsystematically and carelessly. For example, the discovery of the circulatory system prompted a host of transfusion experiments by physicians, the first successful transfusion of blood from one animal to another being conducted by British physiologist Richard Lower (Fig. 127). When reports of Lower's experiments reached Paris, the Académie des Sciences appointed Louis XIV's physician, Jean-Baptiste Denis, to carry out his own independent studies of transfusion. In June 1667, after having tried the technique in five dogs, Denis conducted the first transfusion of blood to a human being. The test subject, a

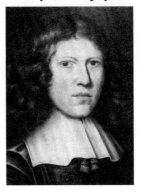

FIG. 127
*Richard Lower
(1631-1691)*

drowsy and feverish young man, was reported to have "rapidly recovered from his lethargy, grew fatter and was an object of surprise and astonishment to all who knew him." Encouraged by this success, Denis repeated transfusion with equally favorable results in another patient. His next two subjects, however, received more than one transfusion, and both died of serum sickness. As a result of this debacle, transfusions were prohibited and were not resumed until the nineteenth century.[7]

Foundations of a Strategy for Testing Therapies

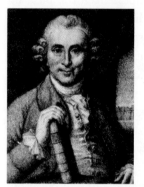

FIG. 128
*James Lind
(1716-1794)*

The foundation of current strategies for the assessment of therapeutic measures was laid in the late eighteenth and early nineteenth centuries. In 1747, the first comparative therapeutic trial in the history of medicine was published under the title, *A Treatise of the Scurvy*. Its author, British naval physician James Lind (Fig. 128), elucidated the cause and advocated treatment of scurvy by experimenting with different kinds of diet among affected members of his ship's crew. "I took twelve patients in the scurvy," he wrote. "Their cases were as similar as I could have them."[8] He fed the sick sailors with various combinations of food, following which he noted substantial improvement only in those who ate oranges and lemons in abundance. None of the test subjects, of course, volunteered for or consented to the experiment. Thus with Lind was born the "therapeutic trial," and, thereafter, experiments regarding therapy were performed by either administering compounds to or withholding them from patients.

Twelve years after Lind's pioneering experiment, Swiss bacteriologist and physiologist, Albrecht von Haller (Fig. 129),

5 · Therapeutic Trials

called attention to the importance of studying treatments systematically. He stressed that "an experiment or a treatment must never be tried only once; truth can never be recognized except by the unchanged success of repeated experience."[9] Subsequently, Anton Störck of Vienna (Fig. 130) advanced experimental pharmacology by first making drugs, then determining the physical and chemical attributes of them, and, last, proving the worth of them in trials clinically. He began with experiments on animals, followed by experiments on himself, and, ultimately, studied those drugs in humans. Although the methods proposed by Störck were sound, his studies of pharmacological compounds were compromised by his own preconceived convictions, which prevented him from rendering any objective judgment.[10] In 1776, Friedrich Gmelin (Fig. 131) recorded in his book, *The History of Poisons* (Geschichte der Gifte), his observation that the reactions of animals to poisons differed from those of human beings. That was the rationale for his concluding there was only one way to study these compounds – by conducting "experiments on the human body itself."[11] Likewise, Georg Friedrich Hildebrandt of Braunschweig warned of pitfalls in applying to humans the results of experiments on animals.[12] In 1799, Johann

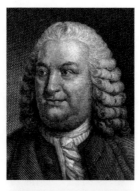

FIG. 129
Albrecht von Haller
(1708-1777)

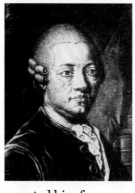

FIG. 130
Anton Störck
(1731-1803)

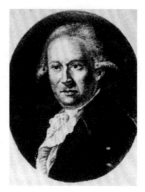

FIG. 131
Johann Friedrich Gmelin
(1748-1804)

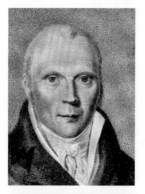

FIG. 132
*Johann
Christian Reil
(1759-1813)*

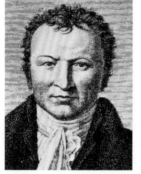

FIG. 133
*Johann
Christian
Gottfried Jörg
(1779-1856)*

Christian Reil, a physician and investigator in Halle (Fig. 132), called for systematic assessment of all drugs given to humans. Reil set forth several requirements for such studies, among them repetition of experiments, standardization of conditions in all experiments, including physical status of test subjects, exclusion of modifying factors, such as concurrent administration of unrelated therapeutic compounds, and assessment of results by observers who were able to think both critically and objectively.[13]

In 1825, Leipzig gynecologist, Johann Christian Gottfried Jörg (Fig. 133), published *Contributions to a Future Pharmacology by Trials of Drugs on Healthy Humans* in which he emphasized that accounts of the effects of drugs predicated on experiments on self were inconclusive. Moreover, he deplored the fallacy of conclusions drawn from a pooling of reports of particular experiments conducted under different conditions and with different dosages and test subjects. To rectify the situation, he founded an "experimenting society" made up of physicians and medical students, the members of which were mandated to try increasing doses of drugs on themselves and to keep detailed records of dates, times, doses, and sensations experienced by them. Jörg's reason for excluding laypersons from participation was not out of respect for the autonomy of patients, but because of his doubts about the ability of patients to provide accurate details and descriptions of the effects of drugs administered to them.[14, 15]

5 · Therapeutic Trials

The Numerical Method

In 1828, Pierre Charles Alexander Louis of Paris (Fig. 134) introduced his "Numerical Method" by which statistics were applied to medical issues. Louis believed that "it is necessary to count" in order to find out "whether a greater number of individuals has been cured by one means than another." He advised that "the different circumstances of age, sex, and temperament, of strength and weakness" had to be taken into consideration, and that, "in order that the calculation may lead to useful or true results, it is not sufficient to take account of the modifying powers of the individual; it is also necessary to know with precision at what period of the disease the treatment has commenced; and especially we ought to know the natural progress of the disease, in all its degrees, when it is abandoned to itself, and whether the subjects have or have not committed errors of regimen."

Louis admitted that the Numerical Method posed "real difficulties in its execution," but insisted that it was the only way to assess accurately the efficacy of treatment. For him it was "because hitherto this method has been not at all, or rarely employed, that the science of therapeutics is still so uncertain."[16]

One motive for the introduction of the Numerical Method was Louis' skepticism about the worth of established forms of treatment. In a study titled, "Recherches sur les Effets de la Saignée dans Quelques Maladies Inflammatoires" (Research on the Effects of Bloodletting in Some Inflammatory Diseases), Louis compared a group of patients treated by the time-honored method of bloodletting with another group of patients in which no treatment had been given. There were no significant differences in results.

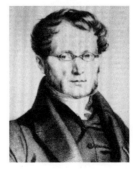

FIG. 134
Pierre-Charles-Alexandre Louis (1787-1872)

Within a short time, a number of similar studies was initiated. For example, Joseph de Larroque, one of Louis' students, planned a study about typhus in which a cohort of 100 patients was to be treated with either purgatives or bloodletting, and another 100 were to be left untreated to serve as controls.[17]

These experiments were criticized harshly by contemporary physicians who clung to traditional modalities of treatment based on concepts of pathogenesis and adjusted to the needs of individual patients. In contrast, the Numerical Method disregarded completely concepts about pathogenesis of that time. In spite of Louis' admonition to give due weight to the "natural progress of the diseases" being studied and to the stage of the disease at which treatment was administered, many studies employing the Numerical Method did not even consider the matter of diagnosis, the consequence of that being the data derived from them had little or no validity. Moreover, the population of patients studied usually was too small to eliminate the possibility of chance being the reason for the differences in results obtained. There also were ethical objections to the Numerical Method. Critics of it claimed that the method represented a violation of the Hippocratic Oath because patients were not regarded as individual human beings, but rather as numbers, and were viewed as mere variables for statistical studies. Observers at the time concluded that "Human life is

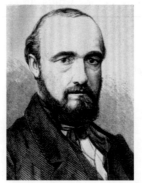

FIG. 135
Carl August Wunderlich (1815-1877)

not esteemed of much value in the hospitals of Paris – an experiment is worth a dozen lives." Others described patients in hospitals as "laboratory animals."[18] The German physician, Carl Reinhold August Wunderlich (Fig. 135), wrote a scathing condemnation of the experiments that then were being carried out on unwitting patients, and he did it in these words:

I cannot raise myself to the position that the doctor's degree or the professorship entitles somebody to make experiments at will with human beings. When I see that a French physician subdivides his patients suffering from typhus into three classes and treats one by bloodletting, the other one by laxatives, and the third not at all, explicitly without any selection, with iron consequence until death, then I have to admit that our times are more barbaric that those in which criminals sentenced to death have been used for surgery and physiologic experiments. It is true that the premier task of medicine is the study of nature, but for the physician, his objects should be more sacred than for the entomologist who pierces his beetles without mercy.[19]

Despite this criticism, the value of comparative therapeutic studies came to be acknowledged. In the European centers of medicine – Paris and Vienna especially – newly built hospitals provided an opportunity to study in this manner large numbers of patients. Most of the early studies about therapy were dictated by skepticism, which was just as well. Patients who were left untreated often did better than those who were treated, providing the additional benefit of allowing physicians to study the natural course of the disease. Because of the limited effectiveness of therapies of the time, the emphasis of physicians was on recognition, rather than treatment, of diseases, reinforcing the perception that patients were simply fodder for study, rather than individuals in need of medical care. Josef Dietl (Fig. 136), an exponent of the Second Viennese School of Medicine, spoke about this subject in 1845 as follows: "Our tendency is a purely scientific one . . . One cannot blame medicine for not being able to heal one disease or the other, but one has to blame it rightly for not having examined diseases properly. The physician has to be judged by the sum of his knowledge, not by the suc-

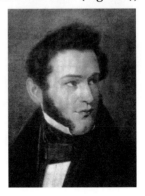

FIG. 136
*Josef Dietl
(1804-1878)*

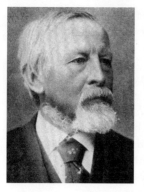

FIG. 137
*Adolf
Kussmaul
(1822-1902)*

cess of his treatment. In the physician, one has to esteem the student of nature, not the artist of healing."[20] In the early twentieth century, a famous German clinician, Adolph Kussmaul (Fig. 137), criticized the therapeutic nihilism of the Second Viennese School of Medicine when he said this: "Teachers and pupils forgot the real task of medicine: healing. This failure resulted in a decline of the most worthy of all human arts, and, in the end, some young physicians were more interested in the confirmation of their anatomic diagnosis than in the success of their courses of treatment."[21]

Prescription for Pharmacology Practiced Systematically

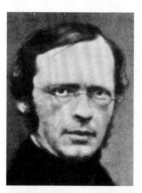

FIG. 138
*Rudolf
Buchheim
(1820-1879)*

With the burgeoning of the chemical industry, the spectrum of effective modalities of treatment began to widen dramatically in the mid nineteenth century. The ability increasingly to produce pure molecules and to modify them by acetylation and other processes resulted in a wave of new drugs waiting to be tested experimentally. Pioneers of modern pharmacology, such as Rudolf Buchheim (Fig. 138), founder of the first institute of pharmacology, and his student, Oswald Schmiedeberg, studied new compounds chiefly through experiments that employed chemical and physical techniques, followed by trials of those compounds in animals. For the ultimate test in human beings, Buchheim considered the observation of effects of a

5 · Therapeutic Trials

drug at the bedside to be insufficient. He advocated clinical trials based on some of the principles set forth by Louis, including large groups of test subjects with approximately the same manifestations of a disease, establishment of control groups whose members were to be left untreated, comparison of different trials, and statistical assessment of results. In 1905, pharmacologist Hugo Paul Friedrich Schulz of Greifswald (Fig. 139) proposed that test subjects be left unaware of the anticipated effects of a compound in order to prevent any influence of suggestion. Schulz also was the first to emphasize that subjects of therapeutic trials must be volunteers.[22]

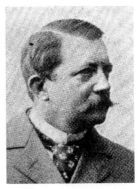

FIG. 139
Hugo Paul
Friedrich
Schulz
(1853-1932)

The development of standards for therapeutic trials, however, was slow and, in general, failed to transform practices of research. With so many diseases lacking effective treatment and so many new compounds becoming available, it is not surprising that many physicians of the late nineteenth century conducted trials that were conceived poorly and conducted hastily, and that failed to meet acceptable standards of the time. The perception that patients were simply grist for research led to uninhibited trials of all types of therapeutic compounds. The burgeoning pharmaceutical industry had no problem with testing its products on human beings, even in the earliest phase of assessment of them. For example, when the hypnotic, Somnal, was first given to patients in 1890, it had been tested only on six rabbits.[23] Even when severe side effects of some drugs were encountered, those medications continued to be administered in clinical studies without further testing in animals. One antipyretic, acetylphenylhydrazine, was found soon after its introduction in 1888 to cause nephritis, hemolysis, severe anemia, and apathy in up to 20 percent of patients. Although these side effects were known, therapeutic trials went on nonetheless, and new indications and uses were promulgated for the drug, among them application topically for psoriasis. J. Oestreicher, an assistant in the private skin clinic of Oskar Lassar in Berlin, found that topical treatment of psoriasis with a 20% ointment of acetylphenylhydrazine resulted in anemia and even in liver disease, the latter evidenced by the development of icterus. German physician, Wilhelm His, Jr. (Fig. 140), stated trenchantly in 1898 that "such compounds should really never be studied in human beings" and stressed deliberately the need for painstaking pharmacologic and toxicologic experiments on animals before clinical trials on humans ever were contemplated.[24]

The desire to study new therapeutic compounds was so strong that it even pushed some physicians beyond the boundary of ethics to the point where they were willing to induce infectious diseases, then to be treated, in healthy persons. In 1898, Edvard Welander (Fig. 141), director of dermatology at St. Göran hospital in Stockholm, inoculated gonococci into the urethra of 15 healthy persons in order to study the efficacy of Protargol, a newly developed antiseptic agent, for prevention of gonorrhea. As a result, one of his test subjects came down with severe gonorrheal urethritis. In the same year, Ernst Frank of Berlin described his experiences with Protargol at the 6th Congress of the German Dermatological Society in Strasbourg.

FIG. 140
*Wilhelm His,
Jr. (1863-
1934)*

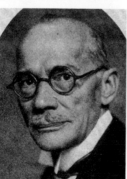

FIG. 141
*Edvard
Welander
(1846-1917)*

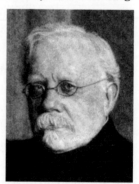

5 · Therapeutic Trials

Frank had performed six "double experiments," to wit, intra-urethral inoculations of gonococci in subjects in whom Protargol had and had not been given concurrently. The test subjects who had received Protargol remained free of disease, but the control group contracted gonorrhea. In order to complete the experiment, the Protargol group was reinfected without having first received the antiseptic, and this time the members of it acquired "regular gonorrhea."[25] In 1906, Élie Metchnikoff of Paris propounded an ointment containing calomen for prophylaxis of syphilis, wagering his honor on the efficacy of it. To prove its potential for effectiveness in humans, Metchnikoff persuaded a resident physician to inoculate himself with syphilis and then to write his doctoral thesis about the treatment of syphilis with Metchnikoff's ointment. At the time of the defense of his thesis, the resident was free of syphilis; a few weeks later, however, he developed signs of the disease.[26]

The Trials of Immunization

Despite the development of many new chemical compounds, the most intriguing therapeutic trials of the nineteenth century involved immunization against infectious agents. The impetus to conduct such trials had been Edward Jenner's (Fig. 142) success in 1798 at vaccination against smallpox. This triumph, in the midst of a therapeutic drought, was breath-

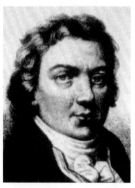

FIG. 142
*Edward Jenner
(1749-1823)*

taking. Having observed that milkmaids who contracted the pox from swine or cows seemed to be immune to the more virulent smallpox, Jenner first inoculated his own son with swinepox, but failed to induce immunity. Next, he "selected a healthy boy, about eight years old, for the purpose of inoculation for the cow-pox. The matter . . . was inserted . . . into the arm of the boy by means of two incisions." Whether the boy, James Phipps, was a willing subject, whether his parents had been informed about risks associated with the procedure, and whether the parents had consented to have their son "selected" for the experiment is not known. James, however, lived in Jenner's neighborhood, and it may be supposed that some degree of trust must have existed between the researcher and his subject (Fig. 143, 144).[27]

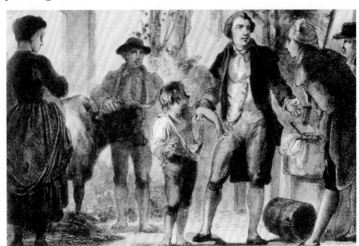

FIG. 143
The first vaccination against smallpox by Edward Jenner (color litograph, 1865).

FIG. 144
Different stages of a lesion of vaccinia (from the French translation of Jenner's report, "Traité de l'inoculation vaccine," 1800).

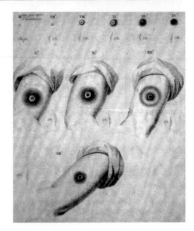

5 · Therapeutic Trials

Jenner's original account cited 14 persons who previously had cowpox and did not develop smallpox when inoculated subsequently with infectious material of it. A further 10 patients were infected artificially with cowpox, and after having been inoculated, four of them did not develop smallpox. Several similar trials followed. A few months after Jenner's report, George Pearson of London published the results of his own experiments in which five people – of whom three had cowpox and two had not – were inoculated with smallpox. The first physician to use the method in America, Benjamin Waterhouse, vaccinated 19 boys with cowpox. Afterward, he inoculated 12 of the boys with smallpox, along with two others who had not been vaccinated. Only the two unvaccinated children developed smallpox. Consent of test subjects was not a matter for consideration.[28]

Pasteur's Spectacular Immunization

In July 1885, almost 100 years after Jenner's report on vaccination against smallpox, Louis Pasteur (Fig. 145) staged the most spectacular immunization of the nineteenth century. He was consulted by the family of a nine-year-old boy who had been bitten by a dog that presumably was rabid. The boy had no symptoms, but

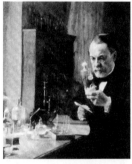

FIG. 145
Louis Pasteur in his laboratory (painting by Albert Edelfelt, 1885).

his family feared for his life and asked the great doctor to save him (Fig. 146). Pasteur accepted the challenge and treated the boy with a series of injections that began with highly attenuated, nonlethal strains of the rabies virus and progressed, step-by-step, to increasingly more lethal strains. The boy survived, Pasteur was celebrated as a hero, and his method of immunization proved to be effective in subsequent trials. Nevertheless,

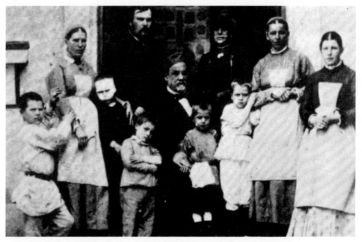

Pasteur's attitude toward the experimental introduction into a human of a potentially life-threatening agent was cavalier and violated his very own principles of conduct. Pasteur himself had emphasized that rabies vaccine should not be introduced into humans without having been studied extensively first in animals, the reason being "experimentation, permitted on animals, is criminal on man." He also wrote that "proofs must be multiplied ad infinitum on diverse animal species before human therapeutics should dare to try this mode of prophylaxis on man himself."[29]

None of his own conditions had been met before Pasteur tried his vaccine on the boy. Although he later testified that he had "succeeded in immunizing fifty dogs of all ages and breeds to rabies without having had a single failure," none of those experiments had been brought to completion prior to the experiment on the boy. Moreover, Pasteur had used a strategy diametric to that for immunization of infected animals, the latter starting with lethal strains of the virus and moving gradually to more attenuated strains. It also should be noted that rabies, although fatal once symptoms of it become manifest, develops in only a small minority of those bitten by an infected animal. In all likelihood, the boy would have survived even without Pasteur's interventions. The explanation of Pasteur that he had "resolved, though not without great anxiety, to try the method which had proved consistently successful on the dogs" because "the death of the child appeared inevitable," was neither sound nor convincing.[30] The ethical implications of Pasteur's experiment were recognized by many of his contemporaries, and he was criticized severely at meetings in 1887 of the Académie de Médicine in Paris. The subsequent success of his vaccine and the fears of destroying a medical icon of France eventually silenced his critics.[31]

In his pioneering work that led to the development of vaccines against chicken cholera in 1880, anthrax in 1881, and rabies in 1885, Pasteur was influenced greatly by the ideas of the syphilologist, Joseph-Alexandre Auzias-Turenne (Fig. 147). When he first embarked on his studies, Pasteur was given a volume of the complete works of Auzias-Turenne, who proposed that the virus of rabies be used "in a therapeutic role." Pasteur also discussed practical aspects of immunization with some of Auzias-Turenne's former colleagues who earlier had worked with the French scientist on experiments with bovine pleuropneumonia and rabies.[32]

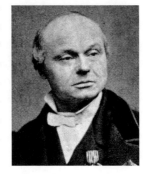

FIG. 147
Joseph-Alexandre Auzias-Turenne (1813-1870)

The Rise of Syphilization

Auzias-Turenne had derived most of his ideas about the induction of immunity from his studies of syphilis. In the 1840s, he had introduced the concept of "syphilization," which he defined as "the condition of an organism in which the organism is no longer able to express the manifestations of syphilis, as a result of a kind of syphilitic saturation." The "saturation" was achieved through repeated inoculation of material from a chancre of the disease. Auzias-Turenne noticed that after several of these inoculations, lesions at the site of inoculation became less acute and subjects did not develop any signs of secondary syphilis. Auzias-Turenne originally studied syphilization in monkeys, but his claim to have syphilized those animals met with disbelief. One of his critics, Adrien-Auguste Cullerier, chief surgeon at the hospital of Lourcine in Paris, asserted in 1844 that the only way to prove those claims would be to inoculate a human being with matter from sores of one of the monkeys. No scientist with a conscience would try that.[33] Philippe Ricord challenged Auzias-Turenne, saying that "One ought to have the courage of one's convictions; it is necessary to know how to die for science just as one dies for one's country. Monsieur Auzias ought to inoculate himself, therefore, with pus from the ulcerations of his monkeys and wait for the manifestation of the symptoms."[34]

This was merely the opening salvo in an unremitting attack for 20 years on Auzias-Turenne, during which his critics derided him primarily for lacking the courage to experiment on himself. As a matter of fact, Auzias-Turenne *had* undergone syphilization, but he chose to keep it to himself. Every time he was taunted, he simply told his heckler that it was none of that person's business as to whether he had experimented on himself. In his diary, this is how he explained his reasons for discretion in that regard:

Suppose one of two things. (1) I have syphilized myself and I will not say so: (a) because if I were to develop bad health, people would not hesitate to attribute it to syphilization; (b) because if I were to proclaim my observation, people would be capable of anything against me – speculations, calumnies, scrutinization of public and private life, etc. (as has well been shown already). (2) I have not syphilized myself: (a) because I lack courage; (b) because I did not have syphilis; (c) because I reserved myself for other occasions, wishing to perform other experiments on myself. And so – what does all that do to syphilization? Is syphilization right or not? True or false? That is the whole question. The rest does not matter.[35]

5 · Therapeutic Trials

Whether syphilization was right or wrong was difficult to decide. The decrease in size and severity of skin lesions at sites of inoculation indicated that an immune reaction had occurred; most subjects on whom syphilization was performed did not ever show signs of "constitutional syphilis." The reasons for the absence of any signs of secondary syphilis following syphilization were that: (a) the material used for syphilization often came from lesions of chancroid, rather than from chancres of syphilis; (b) many subjects had acquired syphilis previously, resulting in immunity that prevented onset of systemic manifestations of the disease; (c) the development of an immune response was accelerated by the saturation; and (d) syphilis, following the appearance of a chancre, may remain otherwise inapparent clinically for many years. The consequences of deliberate induction of syphilis, therefore, were likely to go undetected until long after the experiments were completed and the authors were honored for their "successes."

Syphilization actually resulted in considerable morbidity and even death. Among the earliest victims of the procedure was an enthusiastic follower of Auzias-Turenne, a 27-year-old German physician named Lindemann, who offered himself as a test subject and received dozens of inoculations in 1850 and 1851. In September 1851, Lindemann developed a chancre accompanied by lymphadenopathy and lesions on the tonsils. Following the appearance of these signs of indubitable syphilis, treatment by syphilization was accelerated in a desperate attempt to halt the progress of the disease. Despite expectations to the contrary, however, the inoculations continued to produce ever more extreme chancres. In an editorial in the journal, *L'Union Médicale*, Lindemann was described as "A young man who makes a remarkably fine and intelligent impression but whose arms and legs are eroded by phagedenic chancres and his entire body impregnated with syphilitic virus . . . [he] resists all entreaties for therapy . . . [and] wants to push the experiment to its conclusion . . . ' But you could die of it,' one tells him – ' So much the better,' he responds. 'My death will prove that the doctrine of syphilization is but a terrible error and will prevent other such misfortunes.'"[36]

The fate of the heroic Lindemann did, in fact, do much to discredit syphilization, which was rejected in 1852 as both a preventive and curative procedure by the Paris Academy of Medicine. Auzias-Turenne, however, remained undeterred. He insisted that in Lindemann's case his own instructions regarding the procedure of syphilization had not been followed precisely. He later admitted to experimenting, beginning in November 1850, on 300 human subjects, and affirmed that 17 of the 300 had been completely syphilized, that is, inoculation no longer produced chancres. Similar claims were made by Casimiro Sperino, director of the Hospital for Venereal Women in Turin, Italy, who practiced syphilization on 52 women under his care "with happy consequences." Although the consequences were not quite as happy for many of the women – syphilization required several months in a hospital and was associated with painful ulcers that left patients studded with scars – no severe complications were recorded by Sperino and immunity did appear to have been achieved. The chancres produced by inoculation were said to have become less painful and to have healed faster than usual.[37]

Encouraged by the ostensible induction of immunity against syphilis, Auzias-Turenne touted syphilization not only as a prophylactic measure, but as a treatment for secondary syphilis. When skin lesions disappeared as a result of the natural course of the disease, Auzias-Turenne attributed the improvement to his treatment. Despite rejection of the procedure in France, where it had been developed, syphilization remained popular for several decades in other countries, especially in Norway where it was advocated by the prestigious chairman of dermatology in Christiania, Carl Wilhelm Boeck (Fig. 148), and by his colleague, Daniel Cornelius

5 · Therapeutic Trials

Danielssen. Boeck and Danielssen even used syphilization for the treatment of other cutaneous diseases, such as leprosy. In general, little harm was done by the inoculations; when, however, material from a true syphilitic chancre, rather than from a lesion of chancroid, was used, syphilis with potentially fatal consequences was the result.[38]

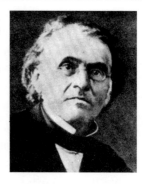

Koch's Tuberculin

Mechanisms of immunity were not even understood vaguely in those days. When Robert Koch introduced tuberculin as a new therapeutic agent against tuberculosis, he thought that its effect was related to its capability to enhance necrosis within tuberculous tissue. Koch gave the first account of tuberculin at the Tenth International Medical Congress in Berlin on August 4, 1890, announcing the availability of a substance "that is able to terminate the growth of tubercle bacilli not only in the test-tube, but also in animals."[39] Three months later, Koch described results of his first trials in human beings, saying "that the diseased tissue becomes necrotic already after a single injection and is later discharged as a dead mass" (Fig. 149).[40] Because of the enormous morbidity and mortality resulting from tuberculosis at that time, Koch's re-

FIG. 149
The preliminary report of Robert Koch about experimental treatment of tuberculosis in humans with tuberculin was considered to be so sensational that the Deutsche Medizinische Wochenschrift published it in a special edition ("Extra-Ausgabe") on November 13, 1890.

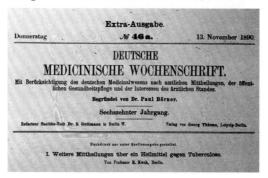

port was welcomed enthusiastically by both physicians and the laity, and was given extensive play in the press. Within a matter of weeks, patients with tuberculosis flocked to hospitals, demanding the new treatment. Physicians from all over the world scrambled to obtain samples of tuberculin. In the closing months of 1890, 24 articles on tuberculin were published in the *Deutsche Medizinische Wochenschrift* alone.[41]

Koch advocated use of tuberculin for lupus vulgaris especially and for an early stage of pulmonary tuberculosis, and he asserted that by virtue of the efficacy of it tuberculosis could be "improved and almost healed," even in advanced stages. As a result, the drug was used freely for indications that never had been studied in experiments on animals. Although most of the so-called trials had a therapeutic dimension, many were purely experimental. Tuberculin was given not only to moribund patients suffering from tuberculosis or from other diseases, but also to healthy individuals for the purpose of studying its effects on them. For example, Ludwig Lichtheim of Königsberg treated a tuberculous child "in an absolutely hopeless condition in the final stage of meningitis" with tuberculin in order to determine "whether the latter caused any damage."[42] Not all physicians were as intemperate in their experiments with tuberculin. Pediatrician Eduard Henoch of Berlin (Fig. 150), who characterized what now is known as Henoch-Schönlein purpura, re-

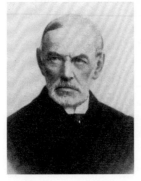

FIG. 150
*Eduard
Henoch
(1820-1910)*

frained from administering tuberculin to children with tuberculous meningitis because of fear of the danger of intracranial edema. When a child was in the last stage of the disease, however, he decided "to put it [tuberculin] to the test." At autopsy, he found his apprehensions verified and was forced to this conclusion: "From the standpoint of a physician, one cannot administer a drug whose effect, because of increased intracranial pressure, holds out the indubitable prospect of shortening life."[43] According to the chairman of dermatology of the University of Breslau, Albert Neisser, some injections of tuberculin were performed for reasons other than therapeutic ones, that is, "in order to study the effects of the compound at the autopsy of those patients who, anyhow, were prone to die."[44]

Although Koch had provided no additional information about the nature of tuberculin – trying as he was to keep it under wraps in anticipation of an enormous financial windfall – he was showered with honors and praised as a benefactor of mankind. Within a few months, however, it became apparent that the efficacy of tuberculin therapeutically was very limited, and that treatment with it was associated with severe side effects, including heightened inflammation followed by ulceration of lesions, pain, fever, anemia, icterus, and diarrhea. Some patients even died from the treatment itself. By the middle of 1891, three deaths and a few close calls had been recorded after tuberculin had been administered to patients with lupus vulgaris, and clinicians who had conducted those trials were shaken badly by the experience. The chairman of dermatology at Hôpital Saint-Louis in Paris, Ernest Besnier (Fig. 151), expressed this opinion ardently about a trial of tuberculin as follows: "I do not consider myself justified to continue an experiment of which I have accepted full responsibility of its demonstration. But today my conviction is established. I do not believe that any physician is justified in inoculating men with the extracts of the toxins of tuberculosis and I shall not again practice the inoculations."[45]

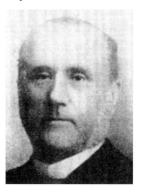

FIG. 151
*Ernest Besnier
(1831-1909)*

FIG. 152
*Emil von
Bering
(1854-1917)*

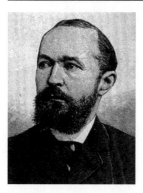

FIG. 153
*Shibasaburo
Kitasato
(1856-1931)*

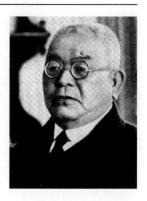

Immunization Against Diphtheria and Tetanus

Only a few weeks after the introduction of tuberculin, the first experiences with immune sera against diphtheria and tetanus were described by Koch's students of bacteriology, Emil von Behring of Germany (Fig. 152) and Shibasaburo Kitasato of Japan (Fig. 153). Twelve years later, Behring would be awarded the first Nobel Prize for Physiology or Medicine in recognition of his demonstration of immunization against the two diseases. Behring's attitude was much more reserved than that of Koch, and the title of his article, "About the development of immunity against diphtheria and tetanus in animals," communicates clearly that the treatment for him was still wholly experimental (Fig. 154). Behring cautioned against the simple transfer of data derived from experiments on animals to conditions in humans. He insisted that further experiments on animals be performed before therapeutic trials in humans were undertaken. His reluctance was criticized by clinicians who claimed it was unethical to withhold from patients a therapy that was far more effective than any other available. Following the great success of Behring's immunizations during epidemics of diphtheria in 1893 and 1894, the antiserum was put to use prophylactically. At that time, allergic phenomena were unknown and the development of anaphylactic reactions to antisera, which were ex-

5 · Therapeutic Trials

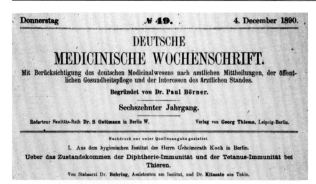

Donnerstag   № **49.**   4. December 1890.

DEUTSCHE
MEDICINISCHE WOCHENSCHRIFT.

Mit Berücksichtigung des deutschen Medicinalwesens nach amtlichen Mittheilungen, der öffentlichen Gesundheitspflege und der Interessen des ärztlichen Standes.

Begründet von Dr. Paul Börner.

Sechszehnter Jahrgang.

Redacteur Sanitäts-Rath Dr. S Guttmann in Berlin W.   Verlag von Georg Thieme, Leipzig-Berlin.

Nachdruck nur unter Quellenangabe gestattet.

I. Aus dem hygienischen Institut des Herrn Geheimerath Koch in Berlin.

Ueber das Zustandekommen der Diphtherie-Immunität und der Tetanus-Immunität bei Thieren.

Von Stabsarzt Dr. Behring, Assistenten am Institut, und Dr. Kitasato aus Tokio.

FIG. 154
Title page of the article in which Bering and Kitasato in 1890 described the sera against diphtheria and tetanus.

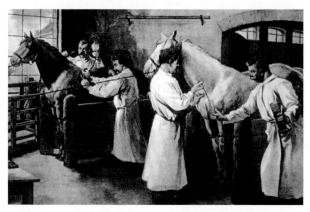

FIG. 155
Serum against diphtheria collected from horses (aquarelle by Fritz Gehrke, 1906).

tracted from horses, could not be anticipated (Fig. 155).[46] In 1896, administration prophylactically of serum against diphtheria resulted in the death of a 2-year-old boy. The death was highly publicized because the youngster was the son of a renowned Berlin pathologist, Robert Langerhans (Fig. 156), whose even more famous brother, Paul, discovered the islets in the pancreas and the dendritic antigen-presenting cells in the epidermis named for him. Robert Langerhans had given the lethal injection himself, and he described his son's sudden death and the

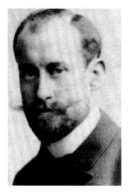

FIG. 156
Robert Langerhans (1859-1904)

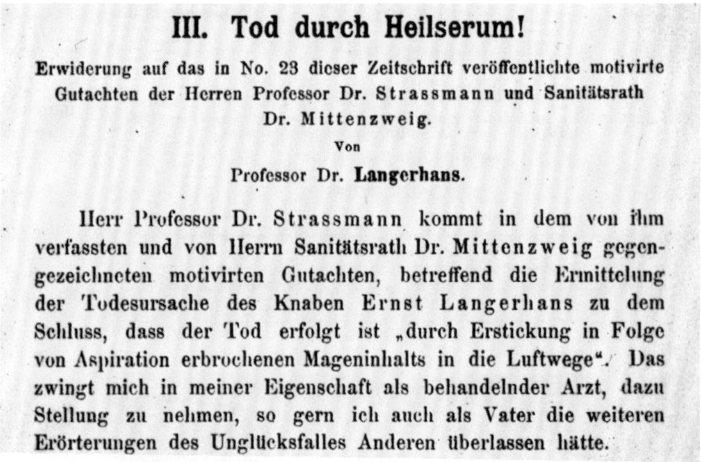

FIG. 157
*Title page of
the article
titled "Death
through
therapeutic
serum" by
Robert
Langerhans.*

III. Tod durch Heilserum!

Erwiderung auf das in No. 23 dieser Zeitschrift veröffentlichte motivirte
Gutachten der Herren Professor Dr. Strassmann und Sanitätsrath
Dr. Mittenzweig.

Von

Professor Dr. **Langerhans.**

Herr Professor Dr. Strassmann kommt in dem von ihm
verfassten und von Herrn Sanitätsrath Dr. Mittenzweig gegen-
gezeichneten motivirten Gutachten, betreffend die Ermittelung
der Todesursache des Knaben Ernst Langerhans zu dem
Schluss, dass der Tod erfolgt ist „durch Erstickung in Folge
von Aspiration erbrochenen Mageninhalts in die Luftwege". Das
zwingt mich in meiner Eigenschaft als behandelnder Arzt, dazu
Stellung zu nehmen, so gern ich auch als Vater die weiteren
Erörterungen des Unglücksfalles Anderen überlassen hätte.

post-mortem findings, meticulously and dispassionately, in
an article in the *Berliner Klinische Wochenschrift* titled,
"Death through therapeutic serum" (Fig. 157).[47] In the same
year, an analysis of 2,228 persons to whom the serum had
been administered revealed evidence of resultant serum sickness in 519 (23.3%) and a "deadly collapse" in nine patients.[48]
Although examination of Behring's antiserum prior to use of
it therapeutically had been more intensive and extensive than
for any other compound until that time, assessment of a large
series of patients who had received it led to the conclusion
that preliminary analysis of it had been insufficient and that
accusations in this regard were justified.

Behring's antisera for diphtheria and tetanus were still great
advances and prompted other physicians to initiate studies
similar to those of Behring. Within a few years, more than 60
investigators had carried out trials with sera from various animals, some of which had been inoculated with syphilitic material and with sera of humans who suffered from secondary or tertiary syphilis. In 1892, Albert Neisser, chairman of dermatology
at the University of Breslau, tried to induce immunity against
syphilis in healthy persons by infusion intravenously of serum

from patients suffering from overt syphilis. At that time, the question of whether cell-free serum from syphilitics was contagious was still in debate. Moriz Kaposi, chairman of dermatology at the University in Vienna, believed that infection through cell-free serum was possible and, in a review of the subject in 1892, he cited several published examples as verification of his position. Neisser, however, remained convinced that serum was noncontagious and that reports of infections resulting from injection of it had to be attributed to contamination of sera with red corpuscles in the blood. In 1898, Neisser published the results of experiments he had carried out with syphilitic serum free of cells in eight female patients who had come to his clinic because of a variety of dermatologic problems, all of which were unrelated to syphilis. Four of those patients – aged 10, 14, 16, and 24 years – remained free of syphilis. The other four subjects, all of whom were prostitutes, acquired syphilis within one-half year, two years, three years, and four years, respectively, after receipt of the infusions. Neisser concluded "that immunity has not been achieved by the infusions." He also conceded that the syphilis could have been caused by his treatment, but dismissed that possibility as highly unlikely. "I am completely convinced," he wrote, "that the prostitutes have been infected in another 'normal' way."[49]

Introduction of Chemotherapeutic Components

The most important therapeutic advance in the history of venereal diseases was the introduction of the first chemotherapeutic compound, Salvarsan, by Nobelist Paul Ehrlich (Fig. 158) in 1910 (Fig. 159, 160). Three years earlier, in a lecture to the Berlin Medical Society, Ehrlich had outlined his objectives in this way: "What we want is a *chemotherapia specifica*, i.e., we are looking for chemical agents which, on the one hand, are taken up by certain parasites and are able to kill them and, on

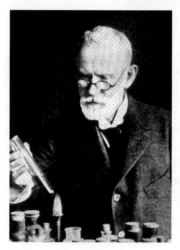

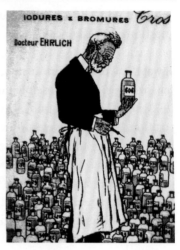

FIG. 158
Paul Ehrlich (1854-1915)

FIG. 159
French postcard showing Ehrlich
engaged in countless attempts to
produce Salvarsan (E606).

the other hand, in the quantities necessary for this lethal action,
are tolerated by the organism without too great damage."[50]

Ehrlich recognized that effective chemotherapeutic agents
were associated inevitably with injury to a patient, and he emphasized that side effects had to be accepted for a greater good.
"It is often maintained," he wrote in 1910 in his seminal monograph called *The Experimental Chemotherapy of Spirilloses*,
"that for the treatment of human beings, and especially in the
case of syphilis, only absolutely harmless substances should be
used. If this restriction is accepted, any progress in chemotherapy becomes impossible."[51] In view of undesired side effects,
Ehrlich considered it essential to inform patients about the
risk-benefit ratio of treatment prior to administering it. Just as
a surgeon weighs the threat of a particular pathological process
left to its own devices against the risk of a particular operation,
Ehrlich maintained that a chemotherapeutist must "tell his patient what possibilities of risk exist and how frequent they are."
Ehrlich acknowledged that it was impossible to provide accu-

rate information until a sufficiently large base of data from clinical trials was available. In the initial trials, he cautioned, unexpected side effects could never be anticipated fully or excluded entirely.[52]

Because of these considerations, the introduction of Salvarsan differed in several ways from that of earlier compounds that emerged from therapeutic trials. The toxicity of the compound had been studied exhaustively in experiments on animals prior to use of it in hu-

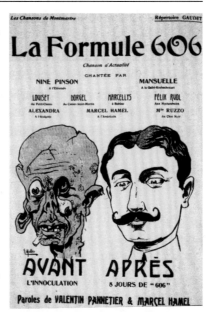

FIG. 160 *"La Formule 606" and expectations for it by the public (before and after treatment).*

mans, and all clinical trials had been supervised closely by Ehrlich himself. Some 60,000 packages of Salvarsan were released to select directors of skin clinics who had agreed to place their entire records of the patients at Ehrlich's disposal. In this way, Ehrlich was able to monitor unexpected side effects, control the quality of different batches of the compound, and check the effects of minor modifications in the application of it, such as the use of different solvents. Despite these safety measures, some patients experienced untoward side effects, including fever, colic, diarrhea, icterus, convulsions, and paresis; some even succumbed to the treatment.[53]

CHAPTER 6

WARRIORS AGAINST DISEASE

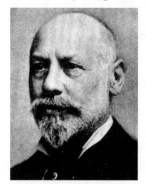

FIG. 161
Moriz Kaposi
(1837-1902)

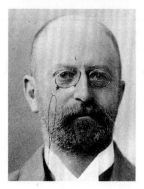

FIG. 162
Edmund
Lesser
(1852-1918)

C uriously, following the denouncements of the experiments of Waller and Rinecker in Austria and in Germany, respectively, Guyenot and Gailleton in France, and Hansen in Norway, practically no notice was given to ethical issues regarding experimentation in humans. In contrast to the situation prior to 1885, no attempts were made in the medical literature to justify experiments on humans; there was no need for that because those considerations were thought to be superfluous and, therefore, inappropriate for scientific articles.[1] In lectures at universities by such personages as Ernst Finger, Maximilian von Zeissl, and Moriz Kaposi in Vienna (Fig. 161), inoculation experiments were mentioned only elliptically, as though they were standard medical procedures.[2] In discussions of experiments on humans at medical meetings, ethical concerns played no role at all. Leading dermatologists like Albert Neisser, Oskar Lassar, Paul Gerson Unna, and Edmund Lesser (Fig. 162) criticized some of the conclusions drawn from experiments done on humans, but the necessity for such experiments was not questioned at all and the matter of obtaining the consent of persons about to be tested never was addressed.[3] Over the years, experiments on humans had slowly, but surely, become a tradition that was passed from one generation of physicians in medical centers to the next – from Isidor Neumann to Ernst Finger, from Filipp Josef Pick to Ernst Wertheim, from Franz Rinecker to Max Bockhart, Ernst Bumm, and Friedrich Fehleisen, and so on.[4] By the end of the nineteenth century, most physicians, from the time they were in medical school, were familiar with the phenomenon of human experimentation and they performed those experiments, reflexively, whenever expedient.

This was the case especially in Wilhelmine Germany (1871–1918) as a consequence, in part, of the high value Germans placed on the rights of the state versus the rights of individual human beings. In contrast to other European countries like France and the United Kingdom, Germany for centuries had been fragmented into dozens of tiny states, a situation that hampered development politically, culturally, and economically. Throughout the nineteenth century, unification of the nation was the highest political goal of most Germans, and when this goal at last was achieved in 1871, it was hoped that the new unified state would be strong and sovereign in its relationship to other nations, as well as to its own citizens. At that time, education in Germany was influenced mightily by the philosophy of Georg Wilhelm Friedrich Hegel (Fig. 163). According to that last great philosopher of idealism, the state held a high-

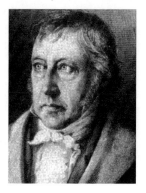

FIG. 163
*Georg Wilhelm
Friedrich Hegel
(1770-1831)*

er position than the individual; serving the state was the highest honor an individual could attain. Based on the belief that the fundamental reality, or Absolute, is spiritual rather than physical, Hegel taught that the progress of history consisted of bringing uncontrolled natural will into harmony with a universal principle, a higher reality. In Hegel's view, the state (especially in the form that existed in Prussia) was the worldly organization that most closely approximated reality, and individual citizens could come close to reality only through participation in the state.

The supreme importance attached to the state was fostered further by new findings in biology in regard to cells. Following the description of cell division by Robert Remak in 1852, Rudolf Virchow, who was both a pathologist and a statesman, confirmed the theory that all cells grow from preexisting cells. In 1861, he introduced the concept of a "cell state," comparing individual cells to citizens and the body to a state. For Virchow, one of the founders and most prominent representatives of the German Liberal party, liberal principles applied perfectly to both biology and politics. He emphasized the individuality of both cells and citizens, and was opposed to hierarchical concepts of control of either of them. In contrast, other biologists, such as Ernst Haeckel (Fig. 164), a philosopher and the first German scientist to advocate Darwin's theory of evolution, contended that the more differentiated an organism was, the more

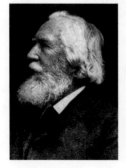

FIG. 164
Ernst Haeckel
(1834-1919)

necessary it was to control it. Just as "higher" organisms required a more developed brain, more highly developed societies needed more control by the state. This view superseded liberal concepts of biology and of state, and gave legitimacy to authoritarian structures. The development of bacteriology – accompanied by the discovery that hoards of alien parasites invade the "cell state," which resists them with complex mechanisms of defense – reinforced the analogy of body and state, and the belief that if the nation itself were to be healthy, central control was requisite to insure the health of individual citizens.[5]

Public Health: More Care, More Control

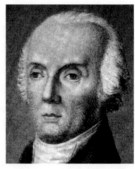

FIG. 165
Johann Peter Frank
(1745-1821)

Control of the health of individual citizens for their own benefit had been advocated since the late eighteenth century. One of the earliest and most prominent proponents of a system of public health was the German physician Johann Peter Frank (Fig. 165). In his *System einer vollständigen medicinischen Policey* (System for Complete Medical Control), published in six volumes between 1779 and 1827, Frank suggested that private and public life – including aspects as disparate as marriage, nutrition, clothing, housing, and public safety – be reorganized according to the requirements of health.[6] The Utopian concept of a healthy state had far-reaching implications, ranging from compulsory enrollment of citizens in public health insurance to improvement of public hygiene. In the nineteenth century, creation of a modern supply of clean water, construction of sewers, organization of disposal of garbage, and plans for development of cities based on cleanliness and avoidance of overcrowding were responses of the government to the findings and proposals of hygienists like Max von Pettenkofer.

Other physicians emphasized the misery of the working class as an important factor in the pathogenesis of disease and urged social reforms. Frank, again, was among the earliest to call for reform in ownership of land as a means of improving public health. Virchow, in 1848, analyzed an epidemic of typhus in Upper Silesia and concluded that the extreme poverty of the population there was the chief reason for the ease with which the disease became disseminated. According to the founder of social hygiene, Alfred Grotjahn, "the objective of public health care is not the health of a few privileged persons, but the generalization of physical care for all classes of our people. It also aims at coming generations, and its ultimate goal is nothing more or less than the eternal youth of our people."[7] Inherent in this lofty aspiration was the implication that persons with incurable hereditary diseases had to be prevented from propagation, even if that meant killing them. One of the first to consider this method as a viable option was Ernst Haeckel, who, in 1904, referred to the killing of crippled newborns as a "useful measure."[8] Although the time to translate these concepts into practical policy had not yet come, the soil for it was cultivated amply. Eradication of diseases was thought to be a duty owed not only by the state to its citizens, but also by citizens to the state. In order to fulfill those duties, individual citizens were expected to subordinate themselves to those who were responsible for the maintenance and improvement of public health.

Focus on the Microbe

These concepts of care for health were given a boost by triumphs in bacteriology. By the last quarter of the nineteenth century, bacteriology had succeeded cellular pathology as the frontier of science. German and German-trained bacteriologists were world leaders in this field and were responsible for the vast majority of microorganisms being identified. Among these were the bacteria of relapsing fever, anthrax, gonorrhea, tuberculosis, glanders, cholera, diphtheria, typhus, and tetanus.[9] The shift of emphasis in medicine from pathology to bacteriology was accompanied by a new philosophy regarding patients and disease. Virchow had stressed the importance of both the individual cell and the individual patient, pleading for democracy and social reform as means of improving public health. In contrast, bacteriologists focused on what they perceived to be more advanced mechanisms – such as the induction of immunity – and on the life of the microbe rather than of the man. Emil von Behring criticized Virchow's famous report about the Silesian typhus epidemics, calling it a "political pamphlet" rather than a serious medical study. "In our century," he wrote in 1893, "the beginning of the social era has manifested itself by attributing diseases to social misery." Behring contrasted those "social/political considerations" with the methods of bacteriologists who, "undeterred by the current of the time and not influenced by religious, philosophical, and mystical speculations, focus on diseases themselves as objects of scientific study and seek to prevent and heal diseases on the basis of that study."[10]

The type of public health care that Behring had in mind was based primarily on compulsory vaccination against infectious diseases. The first such measure was compulsory vaccination against smallpox, which was established by law in 1874, and was contrary to the wishes of many citizens who resented the increasing intrusion of the state into their private lives. In the

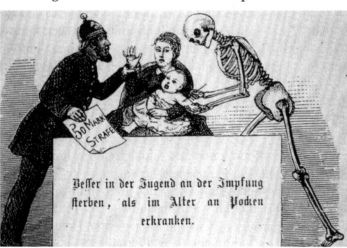

FIG. 166
Propaganda poster against compulsory vaccination (1881). The text reads: "Rather die from vaccination in one's youth than acquire small pox at an old age." The paper held by the policeman proclaims "Fine, 50 Marks."

Beſſer in der Jugend an der Impfung
ſterben, als im Alter an Pocken
erkranken.

year following the enactment of the law, 30,000 signatures were collected in support of having it repealed, all to no avail (Fig. 166).[11] This was Wilhelmine Germany, where health was perceived to be a national issue that could be resolved only by technocratic means. In order to secure the future of the nation, health was to be imposed on citizens who were obliged to endure whatever physicians regarded as being necessary. The authoritarian attitude was fostered by a military education of many physicians and favorable disposition of them subsequently to a military mentality. In fact, most Prussian bacteriologists appointed to university chairs between 1887 and 1900 had a military background. For example, Friedrich Löffler had military training and his father was a leading army doctor; Behring had been proposed by the army to work in Koch's laboratory.[12] In that era, a comparison with soldiers in battle helped glamorize bacteriologists, who began to see themselves as "warriors against disease" (Fig. 167).

The importance of the battle against infectious diseases was underscored by increasing awareness of the wickedness of the "enemy" – in this case, venereal diseases. Syphilis had always terrified people, but in times past it had been deemed curable ultimately. In the last decades of the nineteenth century, Parisian dermatologist Jean Alfred Fournier debunked that illusion by demonstrating that even though the infection might seem to disappear, manifestations of it

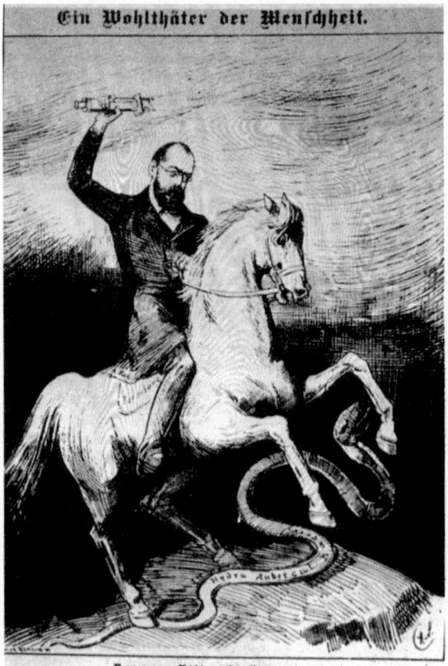

FIG. 167
Caricature of Robert Koch of November 18, 1890, shortly after the introduction of tuberculin. Koch, referred to as "a benefactor of mankind," is pictured as a new St. George, trampling the hydra of tuberculosis, the tube of a microscope being his only weapon.

Ein Wohlthäter der Menschheit.

Der neue Ritter St. Georg.

such as *tabes dorsalis* and general paresis, could appear late in the course of the process.[13] With better recognition of the clinical spectrum of syphilis, the prevalence of it could be appreciated more accurately. Fournier pointed this out in 1900 when he wrote as follows: "Syphilis . . . is flourishing in our days. It is found in abundance in our clinics, polyclinics, and consulting rooms. It fills not only specialized hospitals, which have already become too small, but has spread widely across general hospitals . . . and I would bet that there is not a single department today in which one cannot find some interesting specific affection of the brain, spinal cord, heart, liver, kidneys, etc . . . On the other hand, it is not a secret for anyone that syphilis populates . . . asylums for lunatics, invalids, and so forth."[14]

The terror that syphilis evoked was described graphically in 1907 by the Austrian physician and writer, Fritz Wittels, in these lines:

The nightmare of syphilis always seemed to be dreadful enough. It hid behind every kiss and affected the entire surface of the body with boils and abscesses. The nose, the extremities, the intestines dissolve. Mercury displaces the nightmare, but it comes back, and who is healed remains fearful for years, when going to bed in the evening, that a new eruption may be present the next morning. . . . Even more dreadful than syphilis is tertiary syphilis. When the pain of the disease, like a feverish dream, has long been forgotten, it suddenly whistles in the air, and back it flies, and grasps your brain with claws until that organ fades away. These prospects poison all zest for living.[15]

As a result, suicide was not uncommon following a diagnosis of syphilis. In 1903, Fournier reported on 18 such patients, noting that "the number of suicides that come to our knowledge is probably much lower than their real number, because many families conceal such catastrophes." A well-known Austrian writer, Stefan Zweig (Fig. 168), recalled in his autobiography that "many young people took a gun immediately after having

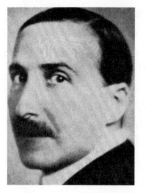

been informed of the diagnosis [of syphilis] because they found it intolerable to live suspecting, as did they and their families, that they are incurable."[16]

The impact of gonorrhea on health had long been minimized compared with that of syphilis. Toward the end of the nineteenth century, however, serious conditions, such as salpingitis, peritonitis, arthritis, and sepsis, were recognized as common complications of gonorrhea, and the importance of asymptomatic carriers of the disease was acknowledged. According to estimates of the 1890s, 80 to 90 percent of the entire population was infected with gonorrhea. Because the disease so often resulted in sterility, it represented a major obstacle to goals of national policy in regard to population, such as the adequate supply of workers for industry and soldiers for the army.[17] In this sense, the fight against venereal disease was regarded as a national effort that had to be engaged without restraint. The warriors against disease were in charge. They had to fulfill their duty, and the animals and human beings used in their experiments were at best their soldiers and at worst their victims.

FIG. 169
Fedor Krause
(1857-1937)

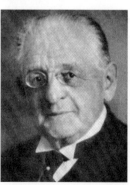

FIG. 170
August von
Wassermann
(1866-1925)

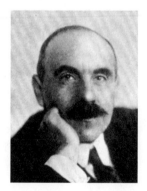

Exceptions to this attitude on the part of physicians were so rare they deserve to be mentioned specifically. In 1882, surgeon Fedor Victor Krause (Fig. 169) of the Charité Hospital in Berlin reported on unsuccessful attempts to transfer cultured gonococci to the eyes of cats, pigeons, mice, and rabbits. Krause, who introduced the surgical techniques of free skin transplants and extirpation of the gasserian ganglion for treatment of trigeminal neuralgia, concluded that although humans seemed to be the only subjects susceptible, "naturally, this experiment could not be carried out."[18] August von Wassermann (Fig. 170), who with Albert Neisser and Carl Bruck developed the first serologic test for syphilis in 1906, advanced the same point of view. After a lecture delivered in 1897 about toxins of gonococci, he was asked whether he had tested the toxins in humans. Wassermann acknowledged that although it was tempting, it was taboo. This is what he said: "It is natural that I am reluctant and consider it to be inadmissible to carry out such experiments with patients entrusted to us by the Charité."[19] J.A. Gläser of Hamburg made this withering criticism:

With the expansion of experimental medical research and with the great successes of surgical techniques, some physicians have come to believe that they are unrestricted masters of the patients under their care and that they can command them at will "for the greater fame of science."[20]

In general, however, the morality of human experimentation was discussed only rarely, and when it was, the experiments themselves were felt to be justified. When it came to medical research, concerns about ethical conduct were abandoned. Like officers in battle, the warriors against disease argued that their activities must be placed above ethical codes

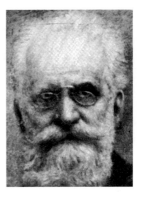

FIG. 171
*Eduard Láng
(1841-1916)*

characteristic of civilian life.[21] In that spirit of *noblesse oblige*, Viennese dermatologist, Eduard Láng (Fig. 171), wrote these lines in 1904:

At first blush, the question may arise whether the aims of research are high enough to justify the approach to human beings as the most noble field for experimentation. The nobility of the aim cannot be doubted; one may even say boldly, and without calling forth opposition, that we aspire to one of the greatest goals when working on the eradication of such a wicked disease as syphilis. From every single member of the army, we expect to meet death coldbloodedly when spiritual ideals or material goods of the fatherland are at stake; almost daily we witness that work in mines and caissons, in tunnels and on railways, in industrial plants and other enterprises causes casualties for the mere generation of material goods; why then should not the initiation of progress for the sake of salvation of suffering mankind justify the recruitment of a relatively small number of individuals for a great idea. The soldier feels ennobled and elevated when his soul is inflamed for the patriotic fight. Surely, man also is amenable to enthusiasm when it comes to sacrifices on the altar of science that serve the welfare of entire mankind.[22]

CHAPTER 7

THE MERGER OF ANTIVIVISECTIONISM AND ANTI-SEMITISM

For most of the nineteenth century, discussions about the morality of medical experiments were restricted to medical circles; the public in general took little notice of such things. This attitude stemmed from an unquestioning belief in authority that protected physicians from indictment for misdemeanors, and was abetted by the absence of any journalistic press with a mass circulation. Concern for ethical aspects of medical experiments became manifest in England in the early 1800s, but there the interest was mostly in animals, rather than humans.

The Royal Society for the Prevention of Cruelty to Animals, the first organization of its kind, was founded in London in 1824.[1] In the 1860s, that Society began to direct its attention to scientific experiments on animals and to do that by searching the medical literature for abominable examples of grievous injury to them, the purpose being to denounce those acts of villainy in articles, posters, and leaflets. The search reaped a bounty of incidents marked by cruelty. A particularly heinous example was an experiment by the Viennese dermatologist, Gustav Wertheim (Fig. 172), who painted 25 dogs with turpentine and then proceeded to set them on fire in order to study the effect of

FIG. 172
*Gustav
Wertheim
(1822-1888)*

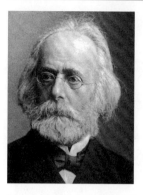

FIG. 173
*Paolo
Mantegazza
(1831-1910)*

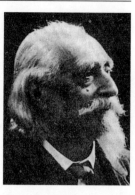

burns.[2] Italian physiologist, Paolo Mantegazza (Fig. 173), tortured rats with needles and tongs in order to assess the influence of severe pain on respiration. French physiologist, François Magendie (Fig. 174), whose experiments on animals helped establish halogens, strychnine, emetine, quinine, morphine, and other drugs as beneficial therapeutic agents, delivered a nonanesthetized pregnant dog of its puppies through a lethal abdominal section with the aim of studying motherly love at the moment of death. His colleague, Claude Bernard (Fig. 175), three-time winner of the Grand Prize in physiology from the Académie des Sciences, constructed an oven to monitor the effects of heat on live rabbits and dogs. Bernard announced dispassionately that "the animals always show the

FIG. 174
*Francois
Magendie
(1783-1855)*

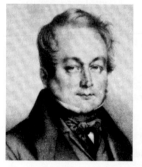

same sequence of characteristic symptoms. At first, the creature is slightly excited, soon the respiration and blood circulation are accelerated. The animal opens its mouth and breathes heavily, and soon it is impossible to count its heartbeats; at last it falls into convulsions and usually dies with a cry"[3] (Fig. 176).

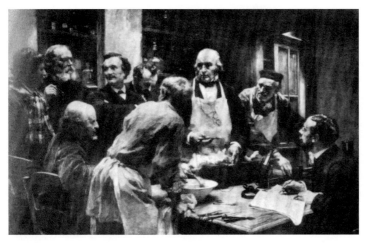

FIG. 175
Claude Bernard (third from right) performing a vivisection (painting by Louis Lermitte, 1889).

FIG. 176
Apparatus of Claude Bernard for study of the effects of heat on animals (1876).

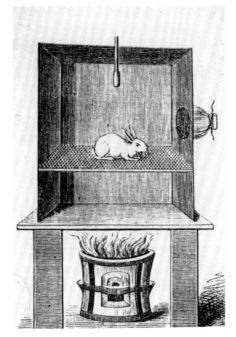

A Good Thing Goes Bad

Unfortunately for them, the opponents of animal experimentation went too far. In their zeal for uncovering examples of cruelty, they began to exaggerate and falsify reports of medical experiments, and persecute scientists by way of inaccurate and unfair accusations. The first and most prominent example of such harassment was a campaign against a German-Jewish physiologist, Moritz Schiff (Fig. 177), who at the time was a member of the faculty of the University of Florence. Schiff, whose work in neurophysiology was pioneering, was accused falsely of slaughtering thousands of dogs in his experiments. With extraordinary support from their English counterparts, Italian protectors of animals reviled Schiff, insulted his family, and tried to take control of his laboratory. Those assaults drove Schiff from Florence in 1876, whereupon he accepted a position at the University of Geneva.[4] The ten-

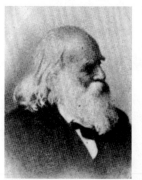

FIG. 177
Moritz Schiff
(1823-1896)

dency to exaggeration and falsification also is reflected in the contrasting and confusing epithets that the protectors of animals gave to their opponents and to themselves. They called their enemies "vivisectionists" – "vivisection" meaning the "dissection of living bodies" – whereas they dubbed themselves "antivivisectionists." The connotation of vivisectionist was negative and conveyed a sense for denigration of experiments of all kinds on animals.[5]

Employing propaganda of this type, antivivisectionists induced the British government to propose a bill, termed the Cruelty to Animals Act, that came before parliament in 1876. The bill was endorsed by leading persons in public life, including members of the aristocracy and clergy, among them luminaries such as Lord Ashley, 7th Earl of Shaftesbury; William Thomson, Archbishop of York; and Cardinal Henry Edward Manning, a former Anglican who had become the head of the British Roman Catholic Church. The churches sympathized with antivivisectionists not only because of their desire to promote the rights of living creatures, but of their contempt for physiology, which impeded the role of metaphysics and hindered practice of organized religion. So wild were the attacks against vivisectionists from English pulpits that Carl Ludwig of the University of Leipzig (Fig. 178) – not only one of the world's leading physiologists, but also a pioneer of the German movement for the protection of animals – likened them to the days when witches were persecuted.[6] Although many

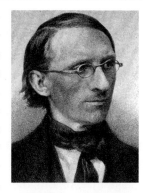

FIG. 178
Carl Ludwig
(1816-1895)

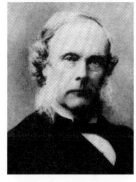

FIG. 179
Joseph Lister
(1827-1912)

respected scientists, like Joseph Lister (Fig. 179), Sir James Paget (Fig. 180), and Charles Darwin (Fig. 181), certified experiments on animals as being indispensable for the advance of medicine, the Cruelty to Animals Act was passed with a small

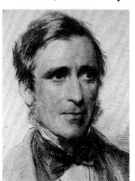

FIG. 180
James Paget
(1814-1899)

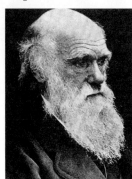

FIG. 181
Charles
Darwin
(1809-1882)

majority. Henceforth, all experiments on animals in England were subject to approval by the state.[7]

With logistic and financial support from England, the anti-vivisectionist movement spread across Europe, taking hold firmly in Germany especially. In 1879, the most important anti-vivisectionist pamphlet in the German language, *Die Folterkammern der Wissenschaft* (The Torture Chambers of Science) by Ernst von Weber, galvanized a national campaign against experiments on animals. So vituperative was the language that, in a matter of months, it became one of the most hotly debated political issues of the day (Fig. 182). Like his models among the English, von Weber quoted extensively, but one-sidedly and out of context, from the medical literature, describing in vivid detail cruel experiments that had been performed in the distant past but that he connected indiscriminately to current practices in experimental medicine.[8] This highly emotional brochure communicated the distinct impression that physicians, in general, and physiologists, in particular, were "brutal murderers," "juggernauts," and "monsters of hell."[9] Within a short time, these very terms were adopted by von Weber's followers, including Richard Knoche, a Catholic military priest in Hannover, who condemned, while conducting a worship service, the abyss

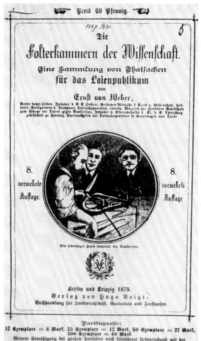

FIG. 182
Title page of The Torture Chambers of Science, 1879.

into which science falls when it becomes detached from Christian belief and morality. Another acolyte was Friedrich Zöllner, an astrophysicist at the University of Leipzig, who prophesied gloomily that the next attempt at assassination of the German Kaiser would be by a vivisectionist. Paul Förster, a schoolteacher and ardent anti-Semite, whose brother, Bernhard, was married to Friedrich Nietzsche's sister, proposed that vivisectionists should dissect one another. Even composer Richard Wagner got into the act by characterizing physiologists as "pitiless human beings."[10]

In the early 1880s, the parliaments of the German Reich and of its member states were bombarded with petitions demanding a general prohibition of vivisection. In the Reichstag, the German imperial parliament, Rudolf Virchow stressed emphatically how important were experiments in animals to the progress of medicine and to the health, and even survival, of countless human beings. He noted that since the Cruelty to Animals Act had been passed, not a single significant article about physiology had come from England. As a consequence, the proposals of the antivivisectionists were dismissed by parliament, at least temporarily, in 1880 and 1882.[11] Following a new petition to the Prussian parliament in 1883, however, a majority of conservative and nationalist parliamentarians supported the antivivisectionists' motion and charged the government with responsibility for the preparation of legislative measures in that regard.[12] The result, in 1885, was a very moderate edict by the Prussian Minister of Culture, Gustav von Gossler, in which baseline rules for experiments on animals were established. These, of course, were the same old rules that had been standard in Prussian universities for years, and they were worded carefully so as not to curtail any possibility of research in physiology.[13] The antivivisectionists, discontent with this result, continued their propaganda, but their petitions no longer had any impact because of the new regulations that had been adopted.[14]

Revival of Anti-Semitism

At this same time, Germany was confronted with another powerful movement – a new wave of anti-Semitism. Contempt for Jews was a longstanding tradition throughout Europe, a consequence largely of the centuries-long control of the spiritual life of the masses by the Roman Catholic Church. Among all the peoples of Europe, Jews had been the only ones to refuse to be converted, which was perceived as an affront to Christianity. Tensions between Christianity and Judaism were aggravated by the fact that both religions shared the same foundation – the Old Testament of the Christian Bible was the Hebrew Scriptures for Jews. The interpretation of those scriptures was a source of constant conflict, and the mere existence of a different view of the meaning of the Bible was considered a challenge to the authority of the Church of Rome. The refusal of Jews to be baptized, despite their profound knowledge of the Bible, was said to be proof of their perfidy. This image of the "evil" Jew was nurtured by the Church, particularly on Good Friday and Easter Sunday, and was transmitted, unquestioned, from generation to generation, being integrated into common parlance, surfacing in jokes and seemingly innocuous phrases, and imparted through art in the form of derogation in novels, poems, paintings, and sculptures. Eventually, contempt for Jews became so much a part of European culture that it was absorbed, naturally and inevitably, in the process of elementary education.[15]

Anti-Semitism was more prevalent in Germany and Austria than in other European countries, such as France and England, the reasons for that being several. The religious tolerance of the Enlightenment arrived in Germany later than in countries that neighbored it to the west, and there were many more Jews living in Germany and Austria than in most other countries. In the process of emancipation that culminated in establishment of full equality of rights in the constitution of the unified Ger-

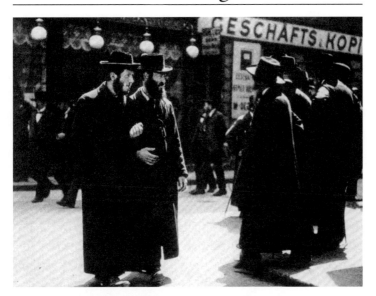

FIG. 183
*Orthodox Jews
in a street of
Vienna.*

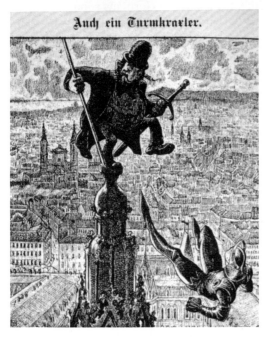

FIG. 184
*The Jew on top of the
city hall of Vienna
replacing the old
"Man of City Hall."*

man Reich of 1871, German Jews became highly successful in the arts, sciences, and economy. More visible than ever, they now generated increasing public interest, as well as envy. There was resurgence of traditional anti-Semitism that had lain relatively dormant for most of the nineteenth century. It was in 1873 that the term anti-Semitism was coined by Wilhelm Marr, a failed journalist who predicted the "victory of Jewry over Germandom." Within the next decade, the first anti-Semitic political parties were founded. A worldwide economic depression in the 1870s was blamed on Jewish capitalists, whom the anti-Semites claimed had engaged in financial manipulations to undermine the country. The situation was aggravated by the immigration from Eastern Europe of orthodox Jews whose foreignness was strikingly apparent in their flowing black caftans, black hats, and long side curls. The perception of orthodox Jews as being overtly different from real Germans soon was transferred to the entire Jewish community. Jews no longer were perceived to be simply adherents of a different religion, but members of a different race that was incompatible biologically with Germans. The preeminence of Jews in public life was said to be a manifestation of the domination of Germans by aliens[16] (Fig. 183, 184).

The Merging of the Antis

Like the antivivisectionists, anti-Semites tried to exert pressure on the government by means of petition. When that petition was presented to German chancellor Otto von Bismarck, in April 1881, it had 225,000 signatories who demanded the prevention, or at least the restriction, of immigration of Jews from other countries and the barring of Jews from positions in the German government, in schools, and in universities. The rationale was the need for "the emancipation of the German people from a form of alien domination which it cannot endure for any length of time." Among the men who initiated the petition was Bernhard Förster, leader of a small anti-Semitic party and brother of the antivivisectionist and anti-Semite, Paul Förster.[17] The antivivisectionists and the anti-Semites were fast becoming not only allies, but one and the same. This was true of many leaders and prominent supporters of the antivivi-

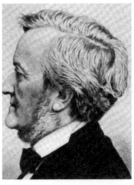

FIG. 185
*Richard
Wagner
(1813-1883)*

sectionist movement, including Ernst von Weber, Friedrich Zöllner, and Richard Wagner. It was Wagner who said, "I am perhaps the last German who knows how to hold himself upright in the face of Judaism which already rules everything"[18] (Fig. 185). It was not only the proponents of antivivisectionism and anti-Semitism who were merging, but also their opponents. Rudolf Virchow (Fig. 186), for example, attacked the petition of the anti-Semites, promoted a counterpetition, and deplored in public assemblies the fact that this kind of religious intolerance was still possible in Germany. Virchow said this: "... the concurrence of Jewish elements in the life of the city as well as the state has taken place in a national sense, supportive truly of the state. The friendship to Jews is a special peculiarity of Berlin ... I really want to know if there is another city in the world where Jews have accomplished so much."[19]

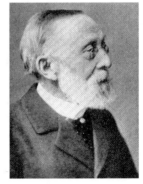

FIG. 186
*Rudolf
Virchow
(1821-1902)*

Personal ties, mutual opponents, and similar strategies wedded antivivisectionism and anti-Semitism. The most important ingredient of this incongruous mixture, however, was fanaticism. The antivivisectionists' criticism of experiments on animals, as justified as it was in many instances, was greatly exaggerated, especially when one considers that antivivisectionists ignored other painful infringements on the rights of animals, such as dog fights, hunting, and castration.[20] Moreover, antivivisectionists themselves were not always delicate when it came to the treatment of fellow human beings. Ernst von Weber, for instance, in a book about the German colonies abroad, suggested that rhinoceros whips should be used to punish Negroes, even though a few strokes of these sadistic devices were sufficient to kill a man.[21] In 1882, Bernhard Förster wrote in Richard Wagner's anti-Semitic journal, *Bayreuther Blätter,* these provocative words: "If you, Mr. Physiologists, really are devoted so deeply and wholly to the knowledge of animal vital functions and wish to bring sacrifices for science – why don't you sacrifice one from your own midst? You call the case of your science high and holy – so, for God's sake, serve it with your lives!"[22] His brother, Paul, advised as appropriate treatment of vivisectionists that they be "squashed and pierced with nails."[23] He also insisted that all experiments on animals be substituted for by experiments of physiologists on themselves. His antipathy to physiologists was expressed thus: "We would not consider it a disaster if some of these by-products of human society would kick the bucket; they are absolutely dispensable."[24]

The reckless call to torture and kill vivisectionists had its counterpart in the demands of anti-Semites for "proper treatment" of Jews, namely, expulsion or eradication of them. For example, the influential Austrian politician, Georg von Schönerer, spoke of the duty of the Nordic race "to eradicate parasitic races, as one has to eradicate venomous snakes and wild beasts of prey."[25] Karl Lueger, mayor of Vienna, declared in a public forum that he did not care "whether Jews are hanged or decapitated."[26] Austrian publisher, Lanz von Liebenfels, advocated the use of the "castration knife" as a means to solve the "Jewish problem,"[27] and French writer, Pierre-Joseph Proudhon, warned that "the Jew is the born enemy of the human race. One must send this race back to Asia or exterminate it . . . by fire or fusion or by expulsion. The Jew must disappear."[28] Despite these harsh sentiments, antivivisectionists and anti-Semites presented themselves consistently as humanitarians. To this end, an excellent opportunity for both groups became possible with the debate about experiments on humans now being conducted within the province of dermatovenereology.

CHAPTER 8

ANTI-SEMITISM AS A VEHICLE TO MORALITY

At the outset of the antivivisectionist movement, experiments on humans hardly had been a matter for consideration. Every now and then, antivivisectionists had remarked, with a sense of relief, that cruel experiments on human beings were prevented by law, and they surmised that it was legal consequences only that held back physiologists from subjecting human beings to the same dreadful experiences as they inflicted on animals.[1] In an open letter in 1880 to Ernst von Weber, Richard Wagner had expressed his suspicion that physicians did not give succor to the "poor worker," but actually took advantage of him by performing "interesting experiments for the evaluation of physiologic problems."[2] Two years later, the priest, Richard Knoche, claimed "that patients in hospitals sometimes only serve as experimental objects for the attending physicians who use them to study scientific problems."[3] At first, the antivivisectionist movement was rooted entirely in protection of animals and it took a decade before its interest shifted to experiments on humans.

For antivivisectionists, experiments on humans became ever more important when all attempts by them to introduce new regulations concerning experiments on animals were blocked and interest of the public in the subject declined. The denouncement of experiments on human beings was designed to inject new life into a flagging movement and to win support from different parts of the population, especially the working class, which previously had shown no enthusiasm for the cause of antivivisectionism.

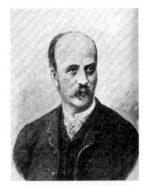

The first time that an experiment on humans induced wide public debate was in 1891 when heated discussion followed a presentation at a meeting of the Medical Academy of Paris by the French physician, André-Victor Cornil (Fig. 187). Cornil told in detail how a "foreign surgeon" had transplanted tissue of mammary carcinoma onto the opposite healthy breast in order to study the question of whether cancer cells could be transferred successfully by way of a surgical procedure. Two patients were involved in this study and both of them developed nodular malignant neoplasms. Although Cornil explained that he had not performed the grafts of cancer himself, but had only analyzed the data, his article about the growth of cancer in previously healthy tissue caused dismay in colleagues and in laypersons alike.[4] The French journal, *Progrès Médical,*

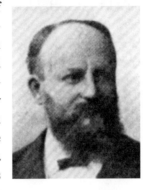

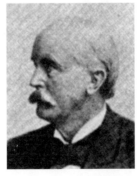

was quick to disclose that the "sad priority" in this experiment belonged to a German physician, Eugen Hahn (Fig. 188), the director of surgery at a municipal hospital in Berlin.[5] As a consequence, the discussion about experiments on humans moved to Germany and was nurtured by reports about other experiments that recently had been carried out there. The famous professor of internal medicine, Hugo von Ziemssen of Munich (Fig. 189), took advantage of the circumstance of the chest wall of a patient with cancer having already been resected and used it to perform electrophysiologic studies on the heart,[6] and the pediatrician, Alois Epstein of Prague, studied the contagiousness of roundworms by "feeding" them to children.[7] In 1892, these and other examples of dubious experiments on humans were collected by the physician, B. Koch, and published in a booklet titled *Ärztliche Versuche an lebenden Menschen* (Experiments of Doctors on Living Human Beings).[8] Three years later, the priest, Philipp Horbach of Marburg, authored another booklet on the subject under the title *Menschen als Versuchsthiere* (Human Beings as Experimental Animals).[9] In both brochures, descriptions of experiments on humans were exaggerated, taken out of context, falsified often, and were replete with nationalistic exhortations and anti-Semitic undertones.

Ever Closer Merger of Antivivisectionists and Anti-Semites

Experiments on humans were grist for the mill of anti-Semites for several reasons. One was that most anti-Semites were high-

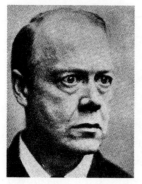

FIG. 190
*Houston
Stewart
Chamberlain
(1855-1927)*

ly conservative and had nothing but contempt for modern science. For example, the philosopher, Houston Stewart Chamberlain (Fig. 190), an exponent of anti-Semitism and racism, began his book, *Foundations of the Nineteenth Century*, by declaring proudly that he was an "unlearned man" and by praising dilettantism as a "reaction against the narrow slavery of science."[10] In regard to medicine, this attitude meant that anti-Semites tended to adhere to traditional proscriptions for a healthy, natural life and to non-invasive forms of treatment. In contrast, recent advances in medicine, based chiefly on experimental data, were met with suspicion. Like many other aspects of modern life, such as industrialization, and pollution of water and air, experimental medicine came to be identified with Jews and was said by anti-Semites to be a manifestation of the typical materialistic attitude of Jews. The link between experimental medicine and Jews was tightened further by the fact that Jews, in comparison to the percentage of them in the general population, were over-represented in medicine. Yet another factor was that Jews in medicine were stifled in pursuit of an academic career. Instead of becoming full professors, most Jewish medical scientists did not advance beyond the status of university lecturers. Because they remained in a subservient, dependent position, they had to prove themselves continuously by noteworthy accomplishments scientifically. In addition, the chance of Jews having a career in the more respected fields of medicine was much worse than in newly established ones, such as pharmacology, physiology, immunology, and dermatovenereology, in all of which experimental studies were more popular. For these various reasons, Jews were involved prominently in experimental medicine and the constellation of negative factors just mentioned attracted the attention of anti-Semites.[11]

That attention was increased further by questionable experiments on humans that meshed with traditional prejudices against Jews, for example, that Jews poisoned wells and conducted ritual murder of children. The ritual murder charge, a medieval relic of European anti-Jewish propaganda that Jews employed the blood of a Christian child in preparing matzo and wine for Passover, continued to be raised in court, e.g., in 1891 in Xanten on the Rhine, in 1899 in Polna, Bohemia, and in 1900 in Konitz, Prussia.[12] It was tempting for anti-Semites to couple

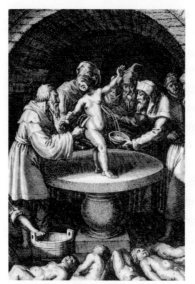

those myths with the infection of children in medical experiments (Fig. 191). Another fable about Jews claimed that the Talmud forbade Jewish physicians to heal Christians and, on the contrary, permitted them to test the toxicity of drugs on Christians. This tale dated to 1700 in accusations by the protestant theologian, Johann Eisenmenger, and was revived in connection with trials about therapeutics. The prejudice that Jews were dirty and vermin-ridden found an analogue in the experimental infestation of human test subjects with microorganisms. The widely held belief that Jews were over-active sexually seemed to be supported by their involvement in experiments on humans that concerned sexually transmitted diseases.[13]

The prominent role of dermatovenereologists in experimentation on humans was especially riveting for anti-Semites because there were more Jews in dermatovenereology in Germany and Austria than in any other field of medicine. In the nineteenth century, dermatovenereology was still a young specialty and esteem for it was low. Most physicians avoided the study of skin diseases because it meant exposure constantly to "ugly" lesions, unaesthetic and smelly forms of treatment, and contact with patients who had contracted diseases sexually and who, thereby, were considered to be inferior socially. The disgust for dermatology of most physicians offered opportunities to Jews for a career when few others were available to them. At the University of Vienna, for instance, the director of dermatology, Ferdinand

Hebra, could recruit only Jewish assistants, many of whom eventually acquired worldwide fame, e.g., Heinrich Auspitz, Isidor Neumann, Filip Josef Pick, and Moriz Kaposi. The leading dermatologists in the German Reich also were Jewish; among them were the first director of dermatology at the University of Breslau, Heinrich Köbner; his successor, Albert Neisser; Edmund Lesser, who founded the famous Berlin school of dermatology; and Paul Gerson Unna, the Nestor of external pharmacotherapy and maestro of dermatopathology. Because of relative lack of competition, Jewish dermatologists could even become a professor and chairman of a university department, and that position allowed them to accept Jewish assistants to a degree that their non-Jewish colleagues never would. Eventually, the public identified Jews so closely with the practice of dermatology that all dermatologists were regarded as Jews and often were referred to as "Felljuden," a derogatory term meaning "fur Jews," which was a play on words: that Jews traditionally traded in furs and now traded in human skin.[14] The fact that these "fur Jews" were involved prominently in human experimentation became the springboard for a political campaign that was supported avidly by both antivivisectionists and anti-Semites.

The campaign was initiated inadvertently in October 1898 by a series of articles in the liberal Munich newspaper, *Münchener Freie Presse,* under the title, "Poor people in hospitals" (*Arme Leute in Krankenhäusern*) (Fig. 192). The authors summarized descriptions of unconscionable experiments on humans that had been extracted by them from the brochures of Koch and Horbach. Ironically, the main author of the series was Ludwig

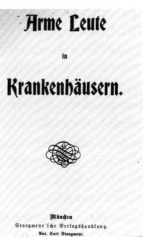

FIG. 192
Title page of the booklet,
Poor People in Hospitals.

Quidde, a liberal journalist who was married to a Jew, and whose first publication had been an attack on anti-Semitic agitation at German universities. Quidde was aware of the potential misuse of his articles for anti-Semitic propaganda, but he considered his message to be too important to be withheld by such considerations.[15] "To be pulled down into the dirt of anti-Semitic baiting," he wrote, "is an ill fate to which even the best cause is susceptible."[16] Following a recounting of numerous inoculation studies, the articles concluded with this challenge: "These experiments are a blood toll, extracted from poverty forcefully by perfidy and betrayal, a mockery of charity and a social attitude about which our time brags so much. And, therefore, in the face of the flaccidity of those who are in power, we call upon public opinion for the protection of poor people in hospitals."[17]

The articles generated an outcry. In numerous letters to the editor, human experiments, some of which had been abstracted from anti-Semitic writings, were cited passionately. Conservative and anti-Semitic newspapers quoted from the *Münchener Freie Presse,* and, in the process, changed the emphasis of the articles: the main focus no longer was that heinous experiments had been performed on humans, but that those experiments had been performed by Jews.[18] This was the case, for instance, with Ernst Finger's experiments 20 years before on transfer of exudate from lesions of congenital syphilis in infants to skin of their mother in order to determine whether those women were immune to the "virus." Finger's experiments, which had been performed without consent of patients, certainly were objectionable. For anti-Semites, however, the experiments were not quite objectionable enough. They made it sound much better – or worse – by claiming, incorrectly, that "most of those who were inoculated with the poison of syphilis were children and women in childbed."[19]

Another letter to the editor concerned a series of injections of bacteria into the urethra of young, healthy men, those injections having been given at the skin clinic of the *Rudolphstiftung* in Vienna, which was directed by Franz Mracek, the editor of a renowned three-volume textbook of dermatology, and in the serotherapeutic institute there, which was directed by Richard Paltauf, who first described "lymphogranulomatosis maligna," one of the manifestations of

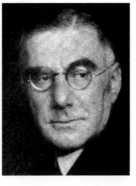

FIG. 193
*Siegfried Grosz
(1869-1922)*

Hodgkin's disease. The experimenters, Siegfried Grosz (Fig. 193) and Rudolf Kraus, published their results in 1898, and later that year had to defend themselves in court.[20] (Fig. 194) Although both physicians were acquitted because no serious harm had been done to any patient, the abuse of patients in medical experiments without the consent of them having been obtained was criticized by the court. The anti-Semites jumped on this immediately and distorted the facts immensely. Grosz and Kraus were accused falsely of infecting their test subjects with gonococci and the experiments were presented as an example of the typical Jewish materialistic attitude that leads to dangerous medical practices – even though one of the authors was not Jewish.[21]

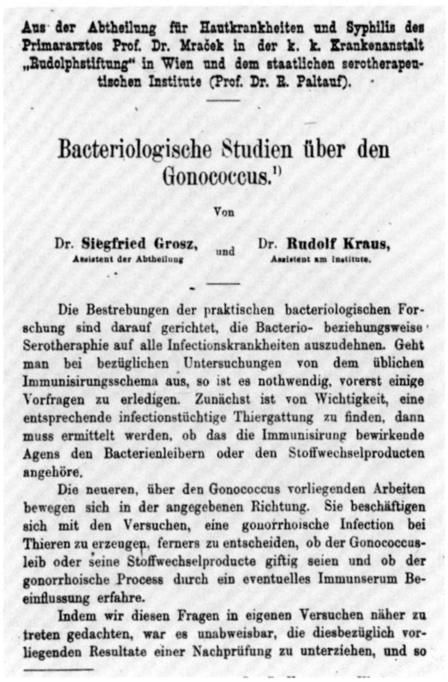

There did not have to be a Jew involved in dubious medical experiments in order for the anti-Semites to blame Jews in general

FIG. 194
Title page of the article by Grosz and Kraus about gonorrhea, 1898.

Aus der Abtheilung für Hautkrankheiten und Syphilis des Primararztes Prof. Dr. Mraček in der k. k. Krankenanstalt „Rudolphstiftung" in Wien und dem staatlichen serotherapeutischen Institute (Prof. Dr. R. Paltauf).

Bacteriologische Studien über den Gonococcus.[1)]

Von

Dr. **Siegfried Grosz,** und Dr. **Rudolf Kraus,**
Assistent der Abtheilung   Assistent am Institute.

Die Bestrebungen der praktischen bacteriologischen Forschung sind darauf gerichtet, die Bacterio- beziehungsweise Serotheraphie auf alle Infectionskrankheiten auszudehnen. Geht man bei bezüglichen Untersuchungen von dem üblichen Immunisirungsschema aus, so ist es nothwendig, vorerst einige Vorfragen zu erledigen. Zunächst ist von Wichtigkeit, eine entsprechende infectionstüchtige Thiergattung zu finden, dann muss ermittelt werden, ob das die Immunisirung bewirkende Agens den Bacterienleibern oder den Stoffwechselproducten angehöre.

Die neueren, über den Gonococcus vorliegenden Arbeiten bewegen sich in der angegebenen Richtung. Sie beschäftigen sich mit den Versuchen, eine gonorrhoische Infection bei Thieren zu erzeugen, ferners zu entscheiden, ob der Gonococcusleib oder seine Stoffwechselproducte giftig seien und ob der gonorrhoische Process durch ein eventuelles Immunserum beeinflussung erfahre.

Indem wir diesen Fragen in eigenen Versuchen näher zu treten gedachten, war es unabweisbar, die diesbezüglich vorliegenden Resultate einer Nachprüfung zu unterziehen, und so

for these practices. To induce in readers the desired conclusion, anti-Semites simply added an exclamation mark in parenthesis (!) after any Jewish-sounding name. The bearers of those names, however, often were Christian. The name of Curt Schimmelbusch, a Berlin surgeon who conducted experiments in humans to clarify the pathogenesis of furuncles and whose Christianity was carefully concealed, became an impetus to anti-Semitic baiting. In connection with Schimmelbusch's experiments, the Vienna-based *Deutsches Volksblatt* blared indignantly that "patients in hospitals are not research material for our Jewish physicians," and commented thus about experiments on humans: "This very common abuse seems to be caused partially by the inundation of the medical profession by non-Aryan members."[22]

Virulence in Vienna

Anti-Semitism was especially virulent in Vienna, a consequence of that city's status as capital of the Austro-Hungarian Monarchy, which was afflicted by severe rifts among its different national groups, Germans, Czechs, Poles, and Croatians among them (Fig. 195). Each of these groups blamed the others

FIG. 195
Cartoon depicting the fear of Germans in Austria (right) of being outnumbered by Czechs (left) and Jews (middle) (from the paper Kikeriki, *1910).*

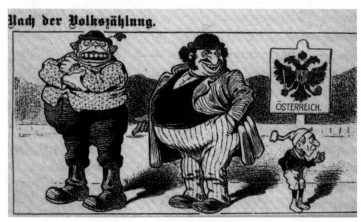

8 · Anti-Semitism

for its troubles and felt that its own rights were being denied constantly. Even though many citizens from the peripheral states of the empire moved to Vienna, the powerful mayor, Karl Lueger (Fig. 196), insisted that the capital was a German city and prohibited all non-German activities in it, such as having special schools or street signs in languages other than German.[23] In this tense nationalistic atmosphere, Jews remained outcasts. Because most of them spoke German or Yiddish (a language derived from German but written in Hebrew characters), they were reckoned by Czechs, Poles, Croatians, and others to be German. The Germans, however, perceived Jews to be aliens who were trying to take over their space.[24]

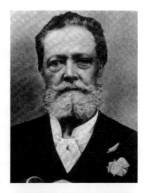

FIG. 196
Karl Lueger
(1844-1910)

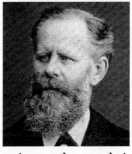

FIG. 197
Hermann
Nothnagel
(1841-1905)

At the University of Vienna, anti-Semitism flourished to such a degree that several professors founded the League for Repulsion of Anti-Semitism. The chairman of this league, the famous clinician and pathologist, Wilhelm Hermann Nothnagel (Fig. 197), soon became the target of virulent attacks by antivivisectionists and anti-Semites. For example, the *Deutscher Volksbote*, an anti-Semitic newspaper based in Mannheim, spewed the following: "What Virchow is in Berlin, Nothnagel is in Vienna. Presumptuous, arrogant, 'liberal,' almost bursting with nothing but 'science,' this Mr. Professor, of course, is also a protector of Jews and, in this capacity, has even risen to the rank of chairman of the League for Repulsion of anti-Semitism. Together with several Jewish (!) physicians, this gentleman now spends the time in his clinic by torturing poor animals in the worst way. They vaccinate guinea pigs with plague bacilli so that the creatures die with the most terrible pain."[25] The article was published following an accident at the Institute of Pathology of the University of Vienna in which an orderly, a nurse, and a physician, all of whom worked under Nothnagel, had contracted plague from experimental animals and had died soon thereafter. The fact that the deceased physician was an assistant of the "protector of Jews," and that a Jewish physician had been involved in the treatment of the victims was reason enough for anti-Semites to conjure up a vision of mankind being destroyed by an epidemic of plague introduced by the Jews. This vision led to fierce public discussion and to heated debate in the Austrian parliament.[26]

The Neisser Case

In the German Reich, the experiment on humans that aroused the greatest public attention was Albert Neisser's (Fig. 198) attempt to induce immunity to syphilis in eight female subjects by infusions of cell-free serum of syphilitics. None of the test subjects had been informed about the nature and intent of the study, and four of them (all prostitutes) eventually contracted syphilis, although the interval of time was such that the infection likely came by way of another more natural route.[27] Short-

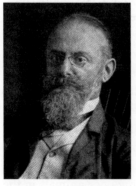

FIG. 198
Albert Neisser
(1855-1916)

ly after publication of the work in 1898 in the major German dermatology journal, *Archiv für Dermatologie und Syphilis* (Fig. 199), Neisser's study was included by the *Münchener Freie Presse* in its series on questionable experiments on humans, the work being presented in a deliberately false manner that qualified as caricature. The authors stated that "the intravenous infusion . . . is per se associated with mortal danger; the slightest entrance of air into the puncture wound can result in sudden death."[28] They also claimed that it was "by far more probable" that syphilis in the test subjects had been caused by the infusions than by a later infection during sexual intercourse.[29] The "Neisser case" was picked

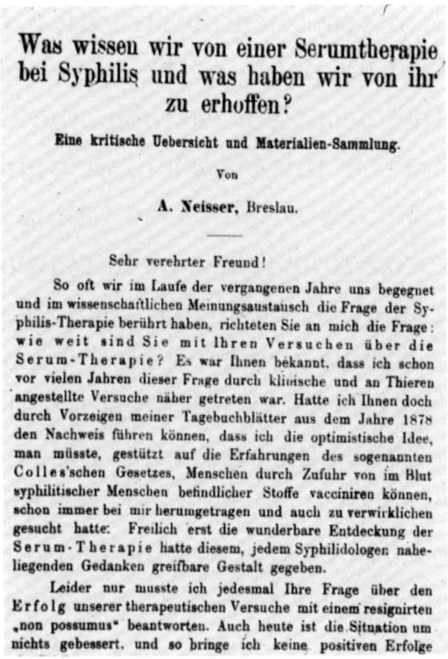

Was wissen wir von einer Serumtherapie bei Syphilis und was haben wir von ihr zu erhoffen?

Eine kritische Uebersicht und Materialien-Sammlung.

Von

A. Neisser, Breslau.

Sehr verehrter Freund!

So oft wir im Laufe der vergangenen Jahre uns begegnet und im wissenschaftlichen Meinungsaustausch die Frage der Syphilis-Therapie berührt haben, richteten Sie an mich die Frage: wie weit sind Sie mit Ihren Versuchen über die Serum-Therapie? Es war Ihnen bekannt, dass ich schon vor vielen Jahren dieser Frage durch klinische und an Thieren angestellte Versuche näher getreten war. Hatte ich Ihnen doch durch Vorzeigen meiner Tagebuchblätter aus dem Jahre 1878 den Nachweis führen können, dass ich die optimistische Idee, man müsste, gestützt auf die Erfahrungen des sogenannten Colles'schen Gesetzes, Menschen durch Zufuhr von im Blut syphilitischer Menschen befindlicher Stoffe vacciniren können, schon immer bei mir herumgetragen und auch zu verwirklichen gesucht hatte: Freilich erst die wunderbare Entdeckung der Serum-Therapie hatte diesem, jedem Syphilidologen naheliegenden Gedanken greifbare Gestalt gegeben.

Leider nur musste ich jedesmal Ihre Frage über den Erfolg unserer therapeutischen Versuche mit einem resignirten „non possumus" beantworten. Auch heute ist die Situation um nichts gebessert, und so bringe ich keine positiven Erfolge

FIG. 199
Title page of the article by Albert Neisser about serum therapy in syphilis, 1898.

up enthusiastically by anti-Semitic newspapers, exaggerated dramatically, and, in March 1899, was broached in the Prussian parliament in Berlin by the conservative, von Pappenheim. Although Neisser's test subjects had been three children and five young prostitutes, Pappenheim averred "that he [Neisser] has conducted trials in eight innocent children which we would even disapprove of were they vivisections in animals."[30] Supported loudly by other parliamentarians, Pappenheim demanded rigorous disciplinary measures against the persons responsible in order to restore the honor of German science.[31]

Neisser himself had already alerted the government about the article in the *Münchener Freie Presse*,[32] and the Prussian Minister of Culture had initiated an examination of the case. When challenged in parliament, the minister declared that should the accusations be substantiated he would "interfere without regard for the person."[33] Additional pressure on the government came from the press, especially from the *Münchener Freie Presse* and from conservative papers with anti-Semitic inclinations.[34] The articles referred to "The Syphilis Serum of Privy Councillor Neisser,"[35] criticized Neisser's experiments as "scientific atrocities" and "criminal science,"[36] and advised the public of the existence of experiments on humans by other Jews. For example, the *Deutsche Tageszeitung* reported that "On this occasion, we want to remind of the fact that another Jewish physician [Alois Epstein] has cultivated roundworms from feces and has given this brew in a candied form to orphans of one to four years of age."[37]

A trial against Neisser brought by the Royal Disciplinary Court received wide and rapt attention by the public. In December 1900, the case ended with an official rebuke of Neisser and a fine of 300 marks. That, plus the expenses of the trial, added up to 1,545 marks, roughly two-thirds of Neisser's annual salary.[38] For Neisser, however, this, the most unpleasant incident of his professional career, was not yet over. Until his death, Neisser continued to be attacked in anti-Semitic publications that claimed he had been guided by the alleged Talmudic principle to use non-Jewish patients for scientific experiments.[39] Ironically, Neisser had converted to Christianity many years before.

Greed: A Favorite Theme

One of the chief prejudices against Jews – that they were usurers obsessed by thirst for money – could not be related so easily to experimentation on humans. Anti-Semites who wanted to play this favorite chord on their instrument of agitation could do little more than refer to it in a vague manner. For example, in reference to accidental cases of plague at the University of Vienna in 1898, the local *Deutsches Volksblatt* had this to say: "As in the Middle Ages, in the time of darkest superstition, when magicians tried with strangest experiments to find the philosopher's stone that would enable them to produce large quantities of gold, a number of physicians have assembled in a kind of secret conspiracy in order to turn themselves, through experiments with pathogens of the most diverse diseases, into scientific capabilities and then, like the 'magicians,' to transform this advertisement for themselves into gold." The newspaper, of course, left no doubt that it was referring to the avarice of Jewish physicians[40] (Fig. 200).

The first opportunity for anti-Semites to demonstrate a relationship between Jewish usury and experimentation on humans came in 1910 after the release by Paul Ehrlich of Salvarsan for treatment of syphilis. That Jewish Nobel laureate was aware of potential side effects of the drug and had taken exceedingly careful note of the experiences of other scientists who were too hasty in their

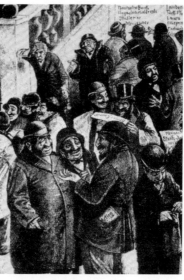

FIG. 200
Anti-Semitic cartoon depicting "Jewish haggling."

propagation of newly developed compounds. Examples of that prematurity were deaths following administration of Koch's tuberculin and of Behring's serum against diphteria. Ehrlich also had his own unhappy experiences with precursors of Salvarsan that had been assessed in small clinical trials, occasionally with serious side effects, such as amaurosis that occurred in two of 120 patients who had been treated by the dermatologist, Eduard Arning of Hamburg. Before releasing Salvarsan commercially, Ehrlich had given free samples to colleagues whom he considered reliable enough to provide him with thorough analysis clinically beforehand. In the course of the earliest clinical studies, significant side effects, including deaths of some patients, had been duly noted, and the dosage and modes of application were modified. Nevertheless, because of the relative effectiveness of Salvarsan, physicians who could obtain the

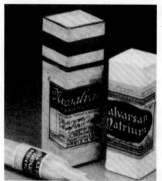

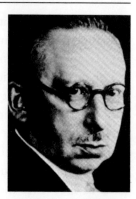

drug were flooded with patients and some of them made a fortune from employing the treatment, to the great dismay of other dermatologists who had not received samples and therefore were suspicious of a conspiracy. Another angry and loud group was the faith healers and charlatans, who, because of the efficacy of Salvarsan, no longer were sought after, who were prohibited from treating patients with syphilis now that there was effective treatment for it, and who thus were deprived of income. When Salvarsan was made available commercially, its price was criticized as being unduly high, and opponents spoke of a "Salvarsan syndicate" that profited by propounding an extremely dangerous drug and suppressing all negative reports that might jeopardize financial success[41] (Fig. 201).

These accusations were disseminated enthusiastically by a physician of little renown, Richard Dreuw, who was loosely connected with the Berlin police, being involved part-time in the health control of prostitutes, and who called himself a "police doctor." Furious about Dreuw's attacks, Felix Pinkus (Fig. 202), a nephew of Paul Ehrlich and a brilliant embryologist, anatomist, and dermatopathologist who was the first to characterize *lichen nitidus,* the hair disc, and the mantle of the follicle, induced the Berlin Police Department to terminate its contract with Dreuw. Dreuw's attacks, however, only became more vitriolic and were supported by anti-Semitic newspapers like the *Deutsches Volks-*

blatt, which referred to Dreuw as an "undaunted fighter" against the powerful Salvarsan syndicate and bemoaned the fact that "Jewish scientists especially are involved in the financially very lucrative field of luetic diseases."[42]

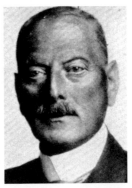

The editor of the journal, *Der Freigeist* (The Free Spirit), Karl Wassmann, proclaimed in 1913 that the Jewish director of the skin clinic in Frankfurt, Karl Herxheimer (Fig. 203), had treated prostitutes with Salvarsan against their will, and had "mutilated" and even killed them in that process. According to Wassmann, "Professor Herxheimer and his associate are nothing but agents of profit-seeking industrialists to whom nothing is sacred. The profit-seeking of certain people even includes premeditated murder." Herxheimer, who 20 years later would die in the concentration camp at Theresienstadt, was among the most respected dermatologists in Germany, having been responsible for calling attention to the filamentous structure of epithelial cells, the existence of an authentic basement membrane between epidermis and dermis, the Jarisch-Herxheimer reaction, a hypersensitivity reaction in the treatment of syphilis, and acrodermatitis chronica atrophicans, a disease now appreciated to be a late manifestation of an infection by *Borrelia.* Against the advise of Paul Ehrlich, he filed suit against Wassmann, whose slanderous assertions were disproven and who was sentenced to one-year imprisonment.[43]

In March 1914, the issue of a Salvarsan syndicate was even debated in the Reichstag, in which supporters of Dreuw spoke inaccurately of more than 275 casualties secondary to treatment with Salvarsan.[44] Refutation of these figures did not put an end to public attacks on Ehrlich and to the fiction of a Salvarsan syndicate run by Jews. Ten years after the debate in the Reichstag, Adolf Hitler, in his book, *Mein Kampf,* referred to Salvarsan as "the crafty application of a question-able drug."[45]

In summary, ethical problems associated with experimentation on human beings began to be acknowledged widely and discussed publicly in the 1890s. Because the most objectionable experiments had been performed by dermatovenereologists, among whom there were more Jews than in any other field of medicine, anti-Semites saw a chance for gaining a propaganda advantage and condemned Jewish scientists at the same time that they presented themselves as fighters for higher moral standards. Paradoxically, morality became a vehicle to anti-Semitism. Nevertheless, the public debate had some advantages: it alerted to ethical problems in medicine and galvanized efforts to overcome them. The converse also was true: anti-Semitism became a vehicle to morality.

CHAPTER 9

THE DAWN OF
INFORMED CONSENT

Throughout the history of medicine – well into recent times – physicians have dealt with patients as objects rather than as subjects, expecting them to be docile, obedient, and acquiescent in enduring, without question and surely without challenge, measures imposed on them. In early times, a patient was given no information whatever about his disease. The rationale for this was that telling the truth to a patient about diagnosis and prognosis would cause despair and resignation, thereby hampering recovery. Prescriptions were written in Latin, in large measure in order to keep their contents secret from persons they were designed to benefit. Because the fundamental ethical principle of medicine was reputed to be "beneficence," any deception by a physician was believed to be justified in order to prevent a patient from becoming anxious, agitated, or sorrowful, with effects ultimately that would be deleterious. In Hippocratic writings, the physician was portrayed as one who decides and commands, the patient as one who accedes to those commands.[1]

This attitude of paternalism and authoritarianism on the part of physicians was heightened in the Middle Ages by the influence of religion, the Roman Catholic Church in particular demanding of its members obedience absolutely. An example in the early fourteenth century of that prevailing attitude was

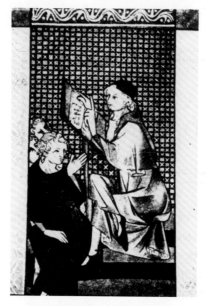

FIG. 204
*Henri de
Mondeville
(1280-1325)*

the admonition to his colleagues of the French surgeon and teacher of anatomy, Henri de Mondeville (Fig. 204), to "... promise a cure to every patient, but ... tell the parents or the friends if there is any danger." At the same time, he counseled that patients should be required to "obey their surgeons implicitly in everything pertaining to their cure." Mondeville advised that physicians "ought to comply with lawful requests insofar as they do not interfere with the treatment." When it came to matters of importance, however, a patient was denied the right of codetermination. Physicians were free to compel obedience by monitoring, withholding, or exaggerating information selectively, and to refuse to deliver any medical care in the "unfortunate" event that a patient was defiant.[2]

Change in Attitude of Physicians During the Enlightenment

With the Enlightenment in the eighteenth century came a change; honesty, rather than deception, was established as a rule for defining the relationship between a doctor and his patient. In his *Lectures on the Duties and Qualifications of a Physician*, John Gregory of Edinburgh, a teacher of Benjamin Rush, suggested that even in a circumstance in which prognosis was grim, physicians should "give a hint to the patient of his real danger" because the patient might have "made no settlement of his affairs, and yet perhaps the future happiness of his family may depend on his making such a settlement." At the same time, Gregory acknowledged that "a deviation from truth sometimes is . . . both justifiable and necessary." Never did he imply that the physician should seek the consent of a patient to therapeutic measures or involve a patient actively in the process of making decisions.[3] With minor modifications, Gregory's ideas concerning the relationship between physicians and patients were promulgated by other authors of that time, including Thomas Percival, whose *Code of Ethics* had a profound effect on the way physicians came to view themselves.[4]

For most of the nineteenth century, the consent of patients to therapeutic measures and to participation as subjects in experiments was not viewed as a matter of importance, although there were exceptions. In 1830, J. W. Willcock insisted that a medical experiment be performed only "with the consent of the party subjected to it, after he has been informed that it is an experiment . . . "[5] William Beaumont referred to "the voluntary consent of the subject" as a precondition for medical experiments on human beings.[6] On other occasions, after flagrant violations by physicians of the most basic rules of decency and common sense had become known, the relevance of consent was acknowledged publicly. This was in connection mostly with inoculation experiments in dermatovenereology. Franz Rinecker's experiment in 1852 in which syphilis was inoculated in a 12-year-old boy resulted in a rebuke by the Academic Senate of the University of Würzburg. Rinecker was instructed "to avoid such scientific experiments . . . without legally binding approval by the person."[7] In 1853, Georg Gustav Klusemann condemned studies on syphilis by Johann Ritter von Waller, declaring that consent in a test was insufficient if the subject of it was not "able to oversee all the consequences to their full extent of such scientific experiments."[8] For Klusemann, neither consent alone nor consent that followed on information having been provided about the experimental nature of a procedure was sufficient. In his judgment, for consent to be valid, subjects of tests had to be made aware of all possible consequences of them. This was the first time that informed consent in its modern sense was demanded explicitly. Unfortunately, these thoughts, expressed in the mid nineteenth century, remained mere sentiment, failed to evoke discussion widely, and had no impact on the actual management of patients and on research of the day.

The Will of the Patient Becomes Official

The situation changed at the end of the nineteenth century when the issue of human experimentation moved outside medical circles. In 1891, following the reports of serious side effects after administration of tuberculin, the Prussian Ministry of the Interior instructed physicians at state prisons to employ tuberculin with extreme caution and "only in fresh or otherwise suitable cases and not against the will of the patient." At long last, the will of the patient was given recognition in an official document.[9] Neither did the decree go unnoticed by the international community of physicians. In the *British Medical Journal* and the *Journal of the American Medical Association* (*JAMA*) it was reported that according to the Official Regulations in Germany,

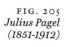

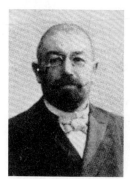

"the remedy must in no case be used against the patient's will."[10] Seven years later, the Neisser case led to the first governmental decree concerning human experimentation and, specifically, about informed consent.

In the wake of the heated debates engendered by the Neisser case, many physicians continued to defend experiments on humans and to condemn any curtailment of the "freedom of science." This opinion was stated by the renowned medical historian, Julius Pagel of Berlin (Fig. 205), in these lines:

For physicians, the question whether or not Neisser was justified in carrying out his experiments does not exist. For them, the Neisser case only leads to the necessity to close ranks in order to defend those scientists in their midst who keep the flag of science flying from unjustified attacks intra et extra muros, so that the dignified striving of our profession, that at all times has been responsible for its fame, will not wane, namely, to prevent diseases and to help suffering mankind. This is for us the ethics of the Neisser case.[11]

The German physician, Karl Ernst von Baer, attacked Prussian parliamentarian von Pappenheim and Minister of Culture Studt, in these words: "If the will of these gentlemen was fulfilled, medicine would still be in the state of Hippocrates, and natural healers, homeopaths, and charlatans, instead of physicians, would be responsible for the art of healing."[12]

In general, however, the need to reconsider the practices of human experimentation was now being acknowledged openly. Ernst von Düring (Fig. 206), a student of Paul Gerson Unna and chairman of dermatology at the University of Istanbul, wrote of the matter in the *Münchener Medizinische Wochenschrift* in 1899 thus:

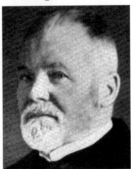

FIG. 206
Ernst von Düring (1858-1944)

"All experimental inoculations of gonorrhea, syphilis, cancer . . . can only be called crimes and must be condemned. That physicians do not denounce to public prosecutors all such cases that come to their knowledge . . . can be explained by their rejection of everything that looks like showing-off; however, one should not believe that we do not condemn, with deep ethical concern, activities that harm our fellow human beings and that can only hamper, but never support, true progress in science and humanity."[13]

Von Düring's words illustrate clearly the difficulty physicians had in declaring experiments on humans reprehensible, particularly when public discussion of that subject could be injurious to their own professional reputation. Von Düring saw this predicament in terms of being a challenge to the traditional self

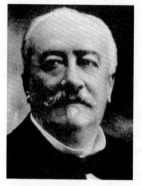

FIG. 207
Alfred
Fournier
(1832-1914)

image of physicians as benefactors. Patients still were considered mere objects that had to be protected from abuse, rather than subjects with the right to determine what was in their own best interest. In like manner, the world's leading syphilologist of the time, Alfred Fournier (Fig. 207), had this to say in his textbook, *Traité de la Syphilis,* published in 1898:

The experiment with healthy human beings is a procedure for which, out of respect for the dignity of our art, I cannot accept the name 'method' and which, cynically, consists of inoculating the product of a lesion of syphilis into a healthy person in order to see whether or not the product contains the infectious matter of syphilis . . . If I had to judge the morality of such conduct, I would declare resolutely what I think of it and what every physician who is a decent human being with respect for his art has to think of it.

The next year, the reminder of morality in medicine stated bitingly by Fournier was quoted in the *Münchener Freie Presse,*[14] which publication went even further than he, criticizing not only the violation of medical ethics, but the existence of medical ethics as a legitimate concept. The newspaper argued that "to speak about ethics of a specific profession results from the same terminological confusion in the field of morality that has brought forth the experiments under consideration and attempts to justify them. These gentlemen always seem to forget that there is only a single, general ethics, and not so and so many ethics in specific professions."[15] The substance of the article in the *Münchener Freie Presse* differed from most commentaries by physicians in that it emphasized unflinchingly the rights of patients. It questioned whether physicians had "the legal right to treat poor patients as research material, as elements without rights who cannot claim free disposition of their own body."[16] Experimental modalities of treatment were said to be justified only if they served to benefit patients. The newspaper, however, made it clear that "such an experiment with a new compound or a new surgical procedure, if associated with any risk at all, can only be made with the explicit and free approval by the patient. Gratuitous treatment must not be used as a lever to obtain the consent of poor patients that would be denied in the case of a decision given freely, and even less can a dangerous experiment be performed without the approval of the patient."[17]

The Issue of Consent Being Valid

Whereas physicians who criticized experiments on humans, like von Düring and Fournier, concentrated on violations of the ethical code of medicine, and newspapers, like the *Münchener Freie Presse*, stressed the right of patients to autonomy and free choice, the concept of "informed consent" had not yet been articulated unambiguously. When Albert Neisser was interrogated by the Royal Disciplinary Court in January 1900, he contended that he had abstained from asking his patients for their consent to experiments "because, exactly from the moral point of view, I have not attached any importance to such consent, and I never will. If I had aspired to being protected formally, I surely would have procured consent because nothing is easier than to induce incompetent people, through friendly persuasion, to give any consent sought, especially when dealing with such harmless, routine matters as an injection."[18]

Neisser's assistants in carrying out the experiments saw

things differently. Friedrich Westberg stated that the patients of Neisser had not been informed about the nature of the injection because they would have "articulated their rejection of such a therapeutic measure . . . clearly enough."[19] Another assistant,

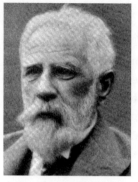

FIG. 208
*Max Rubner
(1854-1932)*

Otto Lasch, testified that " . . . we never carried out bloodletting or injections in patients who rejected them explicitly. Moreover, the defendant had instructed us to refrain from any measures against persons who were resistant, but I believe that he knew perfectly well that we never would have achieved our aim had we told them the full truth."[20]

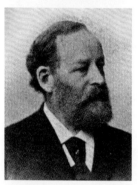

FIG. 209
*Robert
Michaelis
Olshausen
(1835-1915)*

Following the debate about the Neisser case in the Prussian parliament, the Minister of Culture asked a committee of experts on public health for its opinion about the matter. Among the members of the committee were pathologist Rudolf Virchow, hygienicist Max Rubner (Fig. 208), gynecologist Robert M. Olshausen (Fig. 209), and two former pupils of Franz Rinecker, the renowned professor of internal medicine, Carl Gerhardt (Fig. 210), and psychiatrist Friedrich Jolly (Fig. 211). In its report, the committee made clear that consent of patients was requisite and that patients had to be informed about all risks of medical procedures before they were performed. The communication stated further that "From

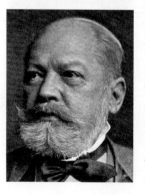

FIG. 210
*Carl Gerhardt
(1833-1902)*

Neisser's report, it does not become clear whether the test subjects have been informed about possible risks to their health and whether they consented to the experiment nevertheless. Both requirements must be preconditions of the experiment."[21]

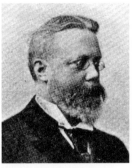

FIG. 211
Friedrich Jolly
(1844-1904)

Other expert testimony was given by lawyers, who also emphasized the importance of consent by patients. Ludwig von Bar of Göttingen averred that in the absence of consent, nontherapeutic experiments fulfilled the criteria of "willful bodily harm," and that their scientific purpose in such an instance could not be regarded as an "extenuating circumstance." Even if test subjects gave consent, however, any nontherapeutic experiment that resulted in severe harm or death was deemed an offense that would subject the perpetrator to a trial in court. In the view of Bar, test subjects could revoke their consent at any time, and minors were not elegible for experiments because neither they nor their parents could give legally binding consent to an experiment on them.[22] Bar also warned experimenters that it was necessary to present all appropriate information to test subjects prior to requesting their consent. "Of course," he said, "a precondition of legally relevant consent is that the consenting person is not uninformed about the consequences of the physical procedure he may choose to undergo, although strictly scientific insight, with consideration of all vaguely possible and highly improbable results, cannot be required."[23] Another lawyer, by name Leydig, argued that the responsibility exclusively of the director of a clinic was to prevent assistants and medical students from performing experiments on humans at will. Moreover, Leydig demanded that test subjects must be informed in writing about the purpose, course, and possible consequences of experiments, and that consent, too, must be given in writing.[24]

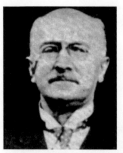

In November 1899, Berlin psychiatrist Albert Moll (Fig. 212) told of other questionable experiments performed on humans, and reflected on the circumstances that made them possible. This is some of what he wrote:

The main duty of the physician is treatment of ill individuals. But he also has to prevent healthy persons from disease, judge diseases in court, teach medicine, and expand his science. All these activities are often performed by the same person. The scientist, for example, is at the same time the managing physician. This situation is of special interest because both activities, on occasion, may come into conflict with one another. If the physician serves exclusively the patient who is entrusted to him, it is impossible that this specific case be used for purposes of scientific research; if, however, he also serves the elucidation of a scientific problem, then he may be tempted to neglect the welfare of the individual under his care.[25]

In connection with the Neisser case, Moll was asked by the Prussian government to turn over his documents concerning experiments on humans, but he refused to do that without a guarantee that no legal proceedings would be instituted against the scientists responsible. The guarantee was not given and Moll kept his documents.[26] Nevertheless, his message was heard. Moll considered experiments on humans to be justifiable only if subjects of tests were able to comprehend possible dangers posed by the tests to the same extent as could the experimenters. This was a condition that, in Moll's view, could never be fulfilled when dealing with children, the mentally disabled, persons who were unconscious, and the mortally ill.[27]

The Prussian Decree

During the debate about the Neisser case, a number of principles pertaining to human experimentation came to be formulated. Some of these had been discussed briefly in the 1850s, but now they became the basis of an official decree issued by the Prussian Minister of Culture on December 29, 1900. This is what was set forth in the document:

I. I wish to point out to the directors of clinics, polyclinics, and similar establishments that medical interventions for purposes other than diagnosis, therapy, and immunization are absolutely prohibited, even though all other legal and ethical requirements for performing such interventions are fulfilled, if:

1. The person in question is a minor or is not fully competent on other grounds.

2. The person concerned has not declared unequivocally that he consents to the intervention.

3. The declaration has not been made on the basis of an appropriate explanation of adverse consequences that may result from the intervention.

II. In addition, I prescribed that:

1. Interventions of this nature may be performed only by the director of the institution himself or with his special authorization.

2. In every intervention of this nature, an entry must be made in the medical case-record book certifying that the requirements laid down in Items 1–3 of Section I and Item 1 of Section II have been fulfilled, specifying details of the case.[28]

As a consequence of this decree, discussion of the public about dubious experiments on humans dwindled, which was precisely what the Prussian government intended when it issued the order. The decree yanked the teeth of the antivivisectionists (and anti-Semites), even though experimentation on humans continued to be a subject of debate in medical circles, albeit on a much smaller scale. In 1902, Moll published a comprehensive monograph titled, *Ärztliche Ethik* (Medical Ethics) (Fig. 213), in which he criticized the edict of the Prussian government on various grounds. For example, he bemoaned the

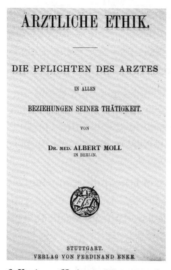

ÁRZTLICHE ETHIK.

———

DIE PFLICHTEN DES ARZTES

IN ALLEN

BEZIEHUNGEN SEINER THÄTIGKEIT.

VON

Dr. med. ALBERT MOLL
IN BERLIN.

STUTTGART.
VERLAG VON FERDINAND ENKE

fact that the decree was not fortified by the power of law. It imposed onerous limits for mundane, nonharmful procedures on minors – literally banning "the cutting off of a hair in a 20-year old" – while being too lax about more serious matters, such as disregarding completely experiments that were carried out in private institutions. Moreover, Moll rallied to the cause of simple informed consent by test subjects being woefully insufficient. He questioned the accuracy and adequacy of information that would be given by scientists to future test subjects and speculated that some patients would consent to experiments "only out of fear that they might otherwise be regarded as unfriendly and be treated accordingly." Rather than leaving decisions about experimentation on humans strictly to the scientists, Moll proposed that advisory boards consisting of "scientists, physicians, lawyers, and other learned men" be formed to review and approve all such experiments.[29]

Moll's book was not welcomed warmly by the German medical community. It received scathing reviews and went out of print after only one edition. Most physicians insisted that physicians alone retain control of medical experiments and rejected any curtailment of research by the government. In 1904, Julius Pagel protested simplistically that "The fact that at all times the best physicians have considered it to be their right and their professional duty to assess, on occasion, questions of biology and pathology through experiments on their patients favors the principle justification of these experiments."[30]

The mentality of Pagel was widespread among physicians.

9 · The Dawn of Informed Consent

It is not surprising, therefore, that questionable experiments on humans continued to be conducted. In 1904, Walther Scholtz of Jena (Fig. 214), who later became chairman of dermatology at the University of Königsberg (now Kaliningrad, Russia), reported on inoculations of secretions of non-gonorrheal urethritis into the urethra of healthy persons. There was no mention of consent of subjects.[31] In 1905, Benjamin Lipschütz (Fig. 215), an assistant in the department of dermatology in Vienna of Ernst Finger, reported on autoinoculations in 70 subjects of material from lesions of chancroid, the result being induction of lesions that became ulcerated. Lipschütz, who is remembered still for his original descriptions of *erythema chronicum migrans* and of intranuclear inclusion bodies in herpes simplex, assured readers that "none of the inoculated persons suffered any harm, either through a complicating swelling of lymph nodes or through a significantly elongated healing time." He concluded that "in our view, the inoculation may still be used as a diagnostic procedure in cases in which the diagnosis is uncertain and in scientific studies, especially of bubos, where it has proved to be superior to examinations by culture."[32] One year later, the Prussian regulations concerning experimentation in humans were adopted by the Austrian government, too.[33]

In 1913, dermatologist Egon Tomaszewski of the Charité hospital in Berlin, along with neurologist, Edmund Forster, performed brain biopsies on live patients with general paresis

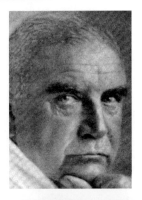

FIG. 214
Walter Scholtz
(1871-1947)

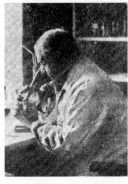

FIG. 215
Benjamin
Lipschütz
(1878-1931)

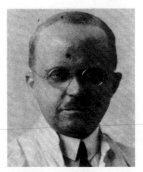

FIG. 216
Rudolf Habermann (1884-1941)

for the purpose of demonstrating spirochetes.[34] In fact, it already had been established beyond doubt through autopsies that general paresis was a specific manifestation of syphilis and that spirochetes were present in the brain of paretic patients.[35] Tomasczewski and Forster, however, trumpeted that they were the first "to sample fresh material from living paretics and to demonstrate living spirochetes in the first two cases."[36] In 1914, dermatologist Rudolf Habermann of Bonn (Fig. 216) reported on a trial in which vaccine against gonorrhea was given to two patients who had gonorrhea and to healthy control subjects. The patients with gonorrhea developed fever, whereas the controls did not. Consent of test subjects was not a consideration.[37]

Positive Effects of the Decree

Nevertheless, the Prussian decree concerning experimentation in humans left its mark. Although experiments on humans continued to be performed, authors of articles about them now tended to offer justifications for their studies, as Benjamin Lipschütz did for his inoculations of material from lesions of chancroid. Such attempt at justification was almost unheard of only a few years earlier. Furthermore, scientists resorted increasingly to experiments on themselves in order to avoid criticism and legal trouble. In 1903, for example, Tomasczewski wrote of cutaneous inoculations of cultures of *Haemophilus ducreyi*, and emphasized that "I have carried out the vaccination experiments exclusively on myself."[38] In 1905, Max Juliusberg, a dermatologist at the University of Bern, induced *molluscum contagiosum* by inoculation of an ultrafiltrate of material from a lesion for the purpose of demonstrating the viral nature of the transmissible agent. The test subjects for the experiment were Juliusberg himself and "two colleagues who have kindly placed themselves at my disposal."[39] Interestingly, authors of that time tended to "clean up" some of the unconscionable experiments of the past, calling them, in scientific articles, euphemistically, but incorrectly, "experiments on self." In an article about "Prophylaxis and therapy of gonorrhea" in 1900, W. Stekel of Vienna referred specifically to the "self-experiments" of Edvard Welander, who had inoculated 15 healthy persons with the gonococcus, infecting one of them in his attempt to elucidate the efficacy of compounds thought to be prophylactic against gonorrhea. Physicians who had performed scores of experiments on humans and had built their scientific reputation on the integument of unsuspecting victims, suddenly dismissed such experiments as being superfluous. For example, when gynecologist Ernst Wertheim was asked at a medical congress in September 1899 (at a time when the Neisser case was still pending) whether he had checked the results of a venereological study by performing inoculations, he replied that he did not consider inoculations on human beings to be necessary.[40]

The changing attitude about human experimentation that followed the decree of the Prussian government is illustrated best by the research on syphilis that was carried out in the ensuing years. One of the first experimental studies undertaken after the issuing of the decree was conducted by two physicians in the skin clinic of the University of Breslau, Ernst Baermann and Viktor Klingmüller (Fig. 217), the latter eventually becoming chairman of dermatology in Kiel. In 1904, Baermann and Klingmüller inoculated themselves with a filtrated discharge from lesions of syphilis, failed to de-

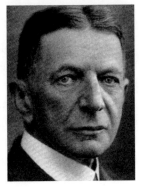

FIG. 217
Viktor
Klingmüller
(1870-1942)

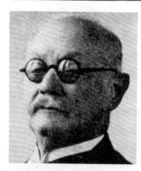

FIG. 218
Louis Török

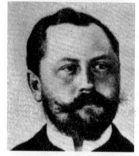

FIG. 219
*Fritz
Schaudinn
(1871-1906)*

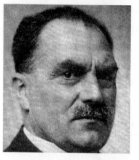

FIG. 220
*Erich
Hoffmann
(1868-1959)*

velop syphilis, and concluded, therefore, that the causative microorganism was not filterable.[41] A year earlier, Metchnikoff and Roux had succeeded in infecting a chimpanzee with syphilis, thereby establishing an animal model for the disease. In 1907, Hungarian dermatologist Louis Török (Fig. 218) condemned, unequivocally, the continued performance of human experiments in regard to syphilis thus: "Syphilis vaccinations on human beings, including syphilitics, are inadmissible ... One can use apes for experimental purposes. Who does not have apes available should wait patiently for others to perform the studies."[42]

By 1905, at least 25 authors had claimed to have discovered the causative organism of syphilis; all of them were proven wrong subsequently. Nevertheless, when Fritz Schaudinn (Fig. 219), with the help of Erich Hoffmann (Fig. 220), identified *Spirochaeta pallida* by microscopy and established that agent as being responsible for the disease, his claim was accepted almost immediately. The reason was that other students of the subject could employ successfully the very same method used by Schaudinn and Hoffmann for examining the discharge of lesions of syphilis and substantiate, thereby, the findings. Fulfillment of Koch's postulates for demonstrating the causative role of an organism no longer was thought to be mandatory, a mentality that would have been unthinkable just a few years before[43] (Fig. 221).

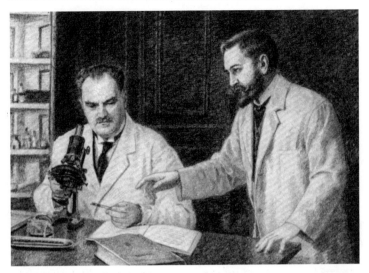

FIG. 221
Erich Hoffmann (left) and Fritz Schaudinn (painting by Karl Krusnyák).

CHAPTER 10

THE AMERICAN APPROACH TO EXPERIMENTATION ON HUMANS

The concept of informed consent and the first official decree about experimentation in humans emanated from Prussian Germany around 1900. It was a consequence of public concern about a common practice of the medical field that violated flagrantly accepted rules of moral conduct and impaired the confidence of the population in the nation's system of health care. In other countries, where human experimentation was not as prolific as in Germany, the situation was less dramatic. There was less concern of the public and fewer reasons for governments to issue specific regulations that pertained to experimentation on humans. Nevertheless, questionable experiments in humans were not confined to Germany. Science is not the exclusive endeavor or domain of one nation, and the global character of science was becoming increasingly apparent as the world grew smaller by virtue of advances in communication and transportation. Numerous medical journals established in the second half of the nineteenth century ensured dissemination worldwide of information about the most recent findings and concepts. Among the most notable in the realm of dermatology were the *Annales de Dermatologie et de Syphiligraphie,* founded

10 · The American Approach

by Adrien Doyon in 1868, the *Archiv für Dermatologie und Syphilis* by Filipp Josef Pick and Heinrich Auspitz in 1869, and the *British Journal of Dermatology* by Malcolm Morris and Henry Ambrose Grundy Brooke in 1888.[1] In the last two decades of the century, scientists began to convene regularly at international meetings to exchange information and compare techniques. For example, the first International Congress of Dermatology was held in Paris in 1889, the second in Vienna in 1892, and the third in London in 1896.[2] Young physicians came from all over the world to institutes of dermatology in England, France, and Germany for the purpose of completing their training, and when they returned to their native countries, they took home not only knowledge of diagnosis and treatment, but also of methods of research. In the process they acquired some habits that led to abuses in experimentation on humans.

In 1874, for example, Robert Bartholow (Fig. 222) of Cincinnati, Ohio, used a feeble-minded woman with a rodent ulcer of basalcell carcinoma of the scalp as a test subject to study the reaction of the brain to electrical stimuli. The stimuli were delivered by needle electrodes inserted into the exposed substance of the brain (Fig. 223). The retarded patient apparently was asked if she would consent to the study and she was said to have given "a cheerful assent to the proposed experiments." With increasing intensities of electrical current, however, the woman's good cheer vanished. Bartholow noted that "her countenance exhibited great distress, and she began to cry . . . the arm presently was agitated

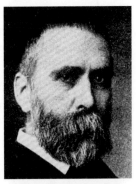

FIG. 222
*Robert
Bartholow
(1831-1904)*

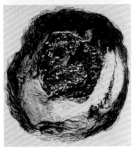

FIG. 223
*Woodcut of an
ulcer on the scalp
of Bartholow's
experimental
subject showing
what seems to be
a large basal-cell
carcinoma
("rodent ulcer").*

with clonic spasm; her eyes became fixed, with pupils widely dilated; lips were blue and she frothed at the mouth; her breathing became stertorous; she lost consciousness, and was violently convulsed on the left side. The convulsions lasted five minutes, and were succeeded by coma. She returned to consciousness in twenty minutes from the beginning of the attack, and complained of some weakness and vertigo." When the patient died a few days later, Bartholow performed an autopsy and found "extensive thrombus formation in the longitudinal sinus."[3] Ironically, Bartholow conducted this awful experiment at the Good Samaritan Hospital!

Among the most notorious examples of dubious experimentation in humans was a study in 1896 by a physician at Harvard Medical School, Arthur H. Wentworth, in which more than 45 lumbar punctures were performed on sick infants. Many of the babies died shortly after the puncture, seemingly from the effects of their underlying illness. At that time, the safety of lumbar puncture, a new procedure, had not been established. Wentworth's punctures were wholly experimental in nature and his attitude toward his test subjects was cavalier. In an article about the experiments, Wentworth stated simply that "after several months' consideration, I resolved to try some control experiments on normal cases in order to determine whether or not the operation was a dangerous one."[4]

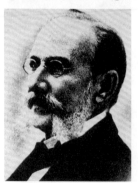

FIG. 224
*Carlos Juan
Finlay
(1833-1915)*

In the 1880s, Carlos Finlay, a Cuban physician (Fig. 224), was the first to identify the mosquito that carries the virus of yellow fever. Attempting to produce yellow fever in healthy individuals to prove his point, he allowed mosquitoes to feed for two to four days on a patient who had symptoms of yellow fever. He then let the same mosquitoes bite uninfected persons. Finlay failed to produce yellow fever because he was not aware that at least 12 days must elapse before the infected mosquito is infectious to another person. As a consequence, the cause of yellow fever escaped him.[5] In his follow-up article about the study, Finlay made no mention of obtaining permission from his more than 100 potential victims.

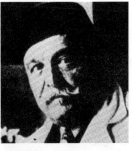

FIG. 225
Guiseppe Sanarelli (1864-1940)

Another scientist who tried to resolve the mystery of yellow fever was Giuseppe Sanarelli (Fig. 225), Director of the Institute for Experimental Hygiene at the University of Montevideo. In 1897, Sanarelli claimed to have found the causative bacillus of yellow fever by fulfilling Koch's postulates; he isolated it, cultured it, and transmitted it to laboratory animals and to five human subjects, three of whom died of the infection.[6] Sanarelli's description of one of these experiments on a human subject reads like a script for a horror movie:

> The subject received an intravenous injection of 10 cc of a filtered culture. This was followed within fifteen minutes by nausea and vomiting, general agitation, and pain in the lumbar region. Gradually the abdominal region became painful and the slightest pressure with the hands over the abdomen or in the lumbar region caused severe pain . . . The patient complained of severe headache during the night and continued to vomit . . . Delirium interrupted by brief periods of coma continued during the second day, after which the patient's condition improved . . . On the second day an explorative puncture of the liver and kidney was made and some juice was obtained through the aspirating needle. Under the microscope this was found to contain, from the liver, hepatic cells in a profound state of fatty degeneration and, from the kidney, epithelial cells in a state of intense tumefaction and granular degeneration . . . The fever, congestions, haemorrhages, vomiting, steatosis of the liver, cephalgia, rachialgia, nephritis, anuria, uraemia, icterus, delirium, collapse . . . constitute the indivisible basis of the diagnosis of yellow fever.[7]

The Abuse of Man

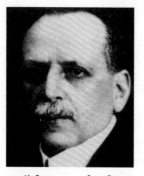

Although the results of Sanarelli's experiments were impressive, his conclusion was not. The disease he produced in these patients had nothing to do with yellow fever. The organism inoculated by Sanarelli was later found to be the bacillus of hog cholera.[8]

In the same year (1897), dermatologist Leopold Freund of Vienna (Fig. 226) became the first to report on the use of radiation for the purpose of treatment. Freund wrote in the *Wiener Medizinische Wochenschrift* that "the experimental object was a girl with a widespread *nevus pigmentosus piliferus.*" Having read about hair loss incidental to sites of radiation, Freund applied X-rays in varying intensities to different parts of the girl's nevus and

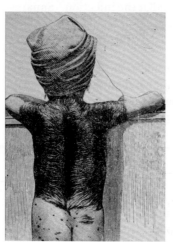

FIG.227
Five-year-old girl with a large congenital melanocytic nevus on the back who served as "experimental object" in the first therapeutic trial of radiation by Leopold Freund of Vienna in 1897.

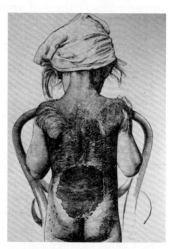

FIG.228
Consequences of irradiation in the girl: hair was removed from the nevus, but a large zone of necrosis progressed to become a huge ulcer that, in time, eventuates in radiation sclerosis, a fertile field for development of maligment neoplasms.

succeeded in removing hair from it.[9] The girl, however, developed severe radiation dermatitis. The skin on the lower part of her back, where X-rays had been applied for 42 hours, became necrotic and covered with stinking debris. The girl suffered from severe pain and developed a high fever. Freund concluded that "the unexpected development of necrosis urges caution in experiments with X-rays and moderation in the application of them." Nevertheless, he later recommended X-rays for "epilation treatment on a trial basis"[10] (Fig. 227, 228).

In 1899, Italian physician, Amico Bignami, tried to demonstrate that malaria could be transmitted by mosquitoes of the Culex genus by exposing a healthy person to bites of parasite-carrying mosquitoes.[11] Four years later, another Italian physician was prosecuted by the civil authorities in Rome for inoculating an elderly man with malaria and received a reprimand for "exceeding the boundaries of acceptable research."[12] In Russia, a physician studying the transferability of typhus through inoculation succeeded in infecting several test subjects with typhus.[13]

In Norway, the chairman of dermatology at the University of Christiania (now Oslo), Caesar Boeck (Fig. 229), honored as the first to characterize sarcoidosis, performed an extensive study on the natural course of syphilis by withholding treatment from almost 2,000 infected patients. His speculation that withdrawal of drugs of demonstrably limited value, such as potassium iodide and mercury, might enhance natural resistance against the organism was not proven; his test patients fared worse than others who were treated. When Boeck's successor as head of dermatology, Edvin Bruusgaard, analyzed Boeck's data in 1929, he noted that "exanthems in those pa-

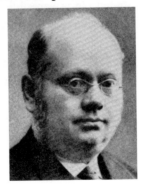

FIG. 229
Caesar Boeck
(1845-1917)

tients were invariably more pronounced, often very persistent; in many patients remnants of the exanthem were still present at release from hospital – furthermore, recurrences were common. We noted early on that in many of those cases there were mild meningitides as a result of the dissemination of the infectious agents in the organism."[14]

Respect for the Individual Lowers Tolerance for Medical Experimentation in America

In brief, experiments in humans were carried out in many countries; many of them were of questionable merit, and many met with justifiable criticism. Nowhere, however, was criticism of human experimentation as vociferous as in the United States. This was not because there were more or worse experiments on humans in the United States than in other developed countries, but because respect for the autonomy of an individual human being was at the core of the American Constitution and of American society. As early as 1833, an American surgeon, William Beaumont, called for the procurement of "free consent" of patients prior to having any medical experiment performed on them.[15] In 1886, Charles Francis Withington of Boston contended that whenever research involved discomfort or risk to patients without the promise of benefit therapeutically, physicians were obligated to inform patients fully of that and obtain their consent before experimentation was begun.[16] Two years later, gynecologist James W. Etheridge advised his colleagues that the consent of patients "obtained without direct or indirect coercion" was mandatory in trials of such risky modes of treatment as caesarean section, which, at that time, was considered to be "the most difficult, dangerous and formidable procedure in operative obstetrics."[17]

The profound respect for the rights of individuals inherent in the Constitution of the United States of America lowered the

threshold of tolerance for unconscionable treatment of patients.
American physicians who had studied in the medical schools of Paris in
the first part of the nineteenth century were aghast at how little human life
was valued in French hospitals, where
patients were "mostly looked upon as
good subjects for the dissecting
knife." In the second half of the centu-

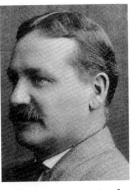

FIG. 230
*John Miller
Turpin Finney
(1863-1942)*

ry, American physicians pursuing postgraduate training in the
hospitals of Berlin and Vienna expressed their distaste for the
attitude displayed by German and Austrian physicians toward
their patients. "They would attempt things that in most other
countries would be considered unjustifiable," commented Baltimore surgeon John M.T. Finney (Fig. 230). He went on to say
that "though the results were fairly satisfactory, the human element was largely lacking. The patient was something to work
on, interesting experimental material, but little more."[18]
Charles Francis Withington noted that "In the older European
countries, where the life and happiness of the so-called lower
classes are perhaps held more cheaply than with us, enthusiastic devotees of science are very apt to encroach upon the rights
of the individual patient in a manner which cannot be justified.
In this country we are less likely to fall in this error."[19]

When two English physicians, William Murrell and Sydney
Ringer (for whom the common irrigation solution is named),
tested a purified form of sodium nitrate in unsuspecting patients, with resultant severe side effects, Withington wrote that
"If the experimenters wished to investigate the physiological
action of the drug they should have called for volunteers; they
had no right to make any man the unwilling victim of such an
experiment."[20] When Giuseppe Sanarelli's claim to have discovered the bacillus of yellow fever was referred to as "simply

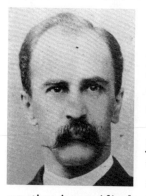

ridiculous" at a medical congress in 1898, the prestigious chairman of the Department of Medicine at Johns Hopkins University School of Medicine, William Osler (Fig. 231), declared that the claim actually was far worse than that. "To deliberately inject a poison of known high degree of virulency into a human being," he said, "unless you obtain that man's sanction, is not ridiculous, it is criminal."[21] The Canadian-born Osler, who had become a titan of American medicine, linked eponymically to conditions such as Osler's nodes in subacute bacterial endocarditis and Osler-Weber-Rendu disease, recognized in Sanarelli's experiments a trend that was a threat to the profession of medicine. In the 1898 edition of his text, *The Principles and Practice of Medicine*, Osler called for regulations concerning experimentation on humans. This is what he wrote:

The work of Sanarelli has been marred by a series of unjustifiable experiments upon men which should receive the unqualified condemnation of the profession. The limitations of deliberate experimentation upon human beings should be clearly defined. Voluntarily, if with full knowledge, a fellow-creature may submit to certain tests, just as a physician may experiment upon himself. Drugs, the value of which has been carefully tested in animals and are found harmless may be tried on patients, since in this way alone may progress be made, but deliberate experiments such as Sanarelli carried on with cultures of known and tested virulence, and which were followed by nearly fatal illnesses, are simply criminal.[22]

The harsh reactions of the American medical community were not reserved exclusively for dubious experiments on humans in Europe. American perpetrators of unethical experiments on humans also were identified and vilified. For example, the lumbar punctures performed in 1896 by Wentworth on infants at the Boston Children's Hospital were condemned in several lay publications and at least one medical journal.[23] Bartholow's experiment in 1874 with electrical stimulation of the brain was criticized as a reckless use of a living human being. The American Medical Association (AMA) passed an official resolution that criticized soundly Bartholow's experiments, characterizing them as "so in conflict with the spirit of our profession, and opposed to our feelings of humanity, that we cannot allow them to pass unnoticed."[24] This stern response to his experiment prompted Bartholow to offer the following apology: "Notwithstanding my sanguine expectations . . . that small insulated needle electrodes could be introduced without injury into the cerebral substance, I now know that I was mistaken. To repeat such experiments with the knowledge we now have that injury will be done by them – although they did not cause the fatal result in my own case – would be in the highest degree criminal. I can only now express my regret that the facts which I hoped would further, in some slight degree, the progress of knowledge, were obtained at the expense of some injury to the patient."[25] Bartholow's response was direct and, for this reason, meritorious.

The assessment by American physicians of unauthorized, potentially dangerous experiments as being criminal was verified by the American legal system. Patients in the United States were far more willing than their counterparts in Europe to file a suit for damages sustained from involuntary experimentation; any departure from standard, proven practices of medicine placed the burden of a favorable result on the physician. In the case of *Carpenter v. Blake* in 1871, a physician was put on trial for having used an innovative, but unorthodox, technique to correct a dislocated shoulder. The court ruled that any deviation from standard practice that lacked the approval of respectable practitioners was not acceptable if it did not benefit the patient.[26] The prospect of lawsuits resulting from experiments on humans constrained American physician-scientists, some of whom were envious of the less restrictive climate in German medicine. When tuberculin became available for the treatment of tuberculosis in 1891, an article appeared in the *JAMA* claiming that "It is fortunate that the 'lymph' is being tested among Germans on German patients, for certainly America would never allow this amount of experimentation involving death in some instances, without what might become troublesome investigations."[27]

In the late nineteenth and early twentieth centuries, the growing number of lawsuits concerning unauthorized surgical procedures prompted surgeons and hospital administrators to introduce forms for written consent. In 1913, the authors of a guide to hospital management cautioned that "It is becoming a common practice of some people, especially the poor and more ignorant classes, to hold surgeons to an unreasonable accountability for their conduct in their cases." Obtaining written consent prior to surgical procedures offered some protection for surgeons when a case ended badly and "some venal lawyer looking for a fee happens to gain the ear of the family of the patients."[28] The importance attached to formal consent by American courts is illustrated well by the case in 1914 of *Schloendorff v. Society of New York Hospitals.* It involved a woman who consented to an exploratory abdominal operation but insisted that no surgical removal be performed. After her surgeon removed a fibroid tumor discovered during the course of the operation, she brought suit against the hospital. Although the procedure actually had benefited the patient, Supreme Court Justice Benjamin Cardozo ruled that "Every human being of adult years and sound mind has a right to determine what shall be done with his own body; a surgeon who performs an operation without his patient's consent commits an assault, for which he is liable in damages."[29]

10 · The American Approach

Antivivisectionism in America

Low tolerance for experimentation in humans was not confined to physicians and lawyers, but was present in the American population at large. The American antivivisectionist movement had millions of followers, organized in several hundred national and local societies across the country. These included the American Society for the Prevention of Cruelty to Animals (ASPCA), founded in 1866; the American Humane Association (AHA) in 1874; and the American Antivivisection Society in 1883. [30] These societies all aspired to be protectors of animals, including the restriction or prohibition of medical experiments on animals; they also were involved in protection of children and in resistance to experiments on humans. Like their European counterparts, American antivivisectionists deplored experiments in animals not only because they caused suffering to fellow creatures, but because they were likely to have a hyposensitizing effect on suffering in general that would erode the quality of medical care by physicians. For example, Elizabeth Blackwell (Fig. 232), the first female graduate of an American medical school, cautioned her colleagues that the reckless sacrifice of animal life "tends to make us less scrupulous in our treatment of the sick and helpless poor. It increases that disposition to regard the poor as 'clinical material,' which has become, alas! not without reason, a widespread approach to many of the young members of our most honourable and merciful profession"[31] (Fig. 233, 234).

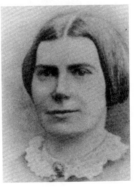

FIG. 232
Elizabeth
Blackwell
(1821-1910)

At the twenty-first annual convention of the AHA in 1897, physician Albert Tracy Leffingwell (Fig. 235) referred to Sanarelli's study about yellow fever as "the Assassination of

FIG. 233
"The little boy who never grew up" (antivivisectionist depiction of vivisectors as being heartless, Life, 1911).

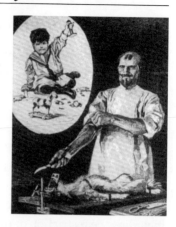

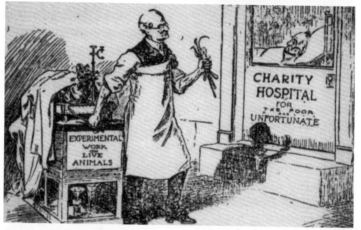

FIG. 234
"Only a Step" (antivivisectionist cartoon emphasizing the relationship between experimentation in animals and in humans, New York Herald, 1914).

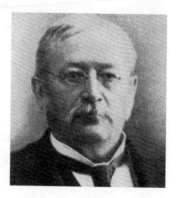

FIG. 235
Albert Tracy Leffingwell (1845-1916)

Human Beings as a Means of Scientific Research." That pronouncement seemed to imply that the grim prophecies of antivivisectionists had been fulfilled. John G. Shortall, the president of the AHA observed that "Having read the accounts of the horrid and cruel destruction of life which has been inflicted upon millions of animals, I have been expecting every year to hear of the experimenter reaching man."[32] Leffingwell was appointed to an AHA committee to study the practice of human experimentation and, within a short time, he compiled a pamphlet that gave alarming examples of such experiments, most of them having been extracted from the European literature. The pamphlet created wide public concern, evoked more articles about the issue, and reinforced feelings of insecurity and fear on the part of the population in regard to modern medicine. Tales of "night doctors" kidnapping negroes for experimentation and dissection flourished in the African-American community. According to an article in 1900 in the magazine *Outlook*, the distrust of hospitals by both the rich and the poor would continue to grow until the public was assured that "the hospital is for man, not vice-versa, for the benefit of patients, not data."[33]

Strategies of Science for Survival in America

How did American scientists get around the widespread rejection of and barriers to their research endeavors? They resorted to four basic strategies that often were employed concurrently: 1) conducting experiments on themselves, 2) recruiting test subjects by offers of money, 3) falsely obtaining consent of subjects by giving incomplete or misleading information about experiments, and 4) using vulnerable populations that had no advocates to aid them in preserving their rights.

Testing a new drug or an untried procedure on oneself before applying it to patients was an accepted attribute of medical research in the nineteenth century. The introduction of anesthet-

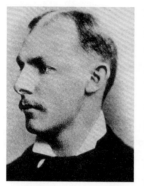

ics, for example, fostered considerable self-experimentation with ether and chloroform prior to physicians having administered these agents to patients. When the anesthetic properties of cocaine were reported on in 1884, many physicians proceeded to try the drug on themselves and their students. Among the best known of these was surgeon William Stewart Halsted of New York City (Fig. 236), who found that cocaine injected into the trunk of a sensory nerve anesthetized the entire region supplied by that nerve. Unfortunately, Halsted, his co-worker Richard J. Hall, and two other assistants who participated in the experiments became addicted to cocaine. The latter three, after living miserable lives, succumbed to their addiction. Halsted himself recovered in large measure, although not completely, after months of hospitalization. Subsequently, he enjoyed a brilliant career, albeit compromised by his lingering addiction, as professor of surgery at Johns Hopkins, where he introduced the use of rubber gloves into surgery. Sadly, Halsted continued to struggle with addiction to opiates for the rest of his life.[34]

Experiments on self were carried out for a variety of reasons. One was convenience; one's own body always was at hand and could be used without the need to ask anyone else. Another reason was the opportunity for researchers to have experiences first-hand that could not be obtained otherwise. That opportunity prompted physiologist Johannes Evangelista Purkinje to swallow digitalis, turpentine, camphor, and numerous other substances for the purpose of studying the effects of them on his body,[35] surgeon August Bier to subject himself to lumbar anesthesia in order "to reach a valid conclusion" about postoperative side effects,[36] and surgeons William S. Halsted and Richard J.

Hall to inject themselves with cocaine in an effort to assess the anesthetizing properties of it. The reason given most commonly for experiments on self by researchers in the United States, however, was the conviction that it was unethical to ask others to be the first to volunteer.

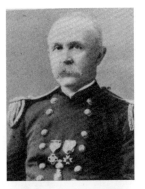

FIG. 237
George Miller Sternberg (1838-1915)

The most famous example of an attitude of offering one's own body first was provided by the American Yellow Fever Commision investigating the transmission of yellow fever by mosquitoes. The commission was formed in 1900 by Surgeon General George Miller Sternberg (Fig. 237), who was concerned about the threat of yellow fever to American troops occupying Cuba at the end of the Spanish-American War. Because no animal model for yellow fever existed, deliberate infection of healthy human beings was considered unavoidable. To their credit, the members of the Yellow Fever Commission, Walter Reed, James Carroll (Fig. 238), Jesse Lazear (Fig. 239), and Aristides Agramonte, gave more consideration to the ethical aspects of experiments on humans

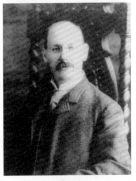

FIG. 238
James Carroll (1854-1907)

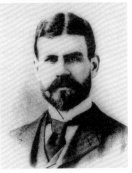

FIG. 239
Jesse W. Lazear (1866-1900)

than did most other physicians of that time. In one of his articles that detailed early meetings of the group, Carroll wrote that "the moral responsibility was . . . considered, and . . . it was agreed that the members of the Board would themselves be bitten and subject themselves to the risk that necessity compelled them to impose on others."[37] Because of previous exposure to yellow fever, Agramonte was considered to be ineligible for the experiment. The three other scientists were not immune; only Carroll and Lazear, however, intentionally applied infected mosquitos to their own skin. Both developed a severe attack of yellow fever. Carroll recovered, but Lazear died of the disease, leaving behind a wife and two children, one of whom was only one month old. Following Lazear's death, the story was spread that he had been bitten accidentally, probably because of fear that his life insurance would be forfeited if it became known that he had infected himself deliberately. Walter Reed (Fig. 240), whose name later became a symbol for heroic self-sacrifice of physician-scientists, left Havana for Washington immediately after having agreed to engage in the self-experiment. The reasons for his hasty departure are not known; according to Carroll, Reed left the morning after the pledge to self-experiment "without a word of explanation." Shortly before Lazear died, Reed wrote a letter in which he rejected the pledge wholesale: "I certainly shall not, with the facts that we now have, allow a 'loaded' mosquito to bite me! That would be fool-hardy in the extreme."[38] Reed's refusal to take the risk himself, however, did not prevent him from permitting American soldiers and Spanish immigrants to expose themselves to the mosquitoes.

In fact, self-experiments were not always what they were

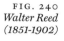

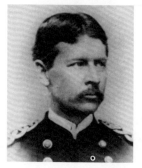

FIG. 240
Walter Reed
(1851-1902)

purported to be and the issue of whether such an experiment on one's own person justifies performing it on someone else was barely mentioned. In the eyes of the public, as well as the judiciary, self-experiments exempted insulated physicians from charges of reckless experimentation on humans (Fig. 241, 242).

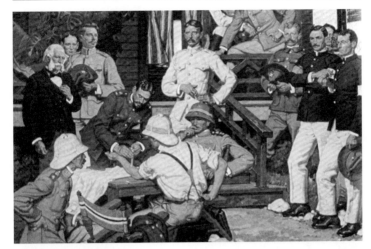

FIG. 241
Experiments in Cuba on yellow fever (painting by Dean Dornwell showing Major Walter Reed placing a mosquito on the arm of James Carroll.

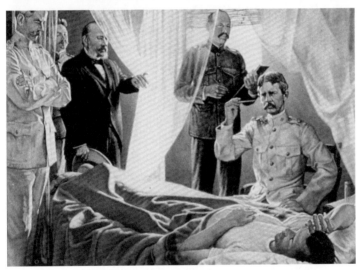

FIG. 242
Experiments in Cuba on yellow fever (from left to right: W.C. Gorgas, A. Agramonte, C. Finlay, J. Carroll, W. Reed).

Recruiting Volunteers for Pay

Because of legal obstacles associated with experiments conducted on nonconsenting patients, American scientists looked for volunteers; the most effective way of finding them was with offers of money. This strategy had been employed successfully in the early nineteenth century by army surgeon William Beaumont. Unable to close a gunshot wound in the stomach of a French-Canadien trapper, Alexis St. Martin, Beaumont, in 1820, decided to take advantage of this unique opportunity to study the digestive process in a human. He paid a small stipend to induce a reluctant St. Martin "to return and submit to the necessary examinations and experiments upon his stomach and its fluids."[39] The indentured research subject, while compliant, was not entirely content with his lot, and he ran away several times.[40] Prior to the Civil War, physicians from the South purchased slaves who were afflicted with medical conditions the scientists wanted to study.[41] In the 1890s, newspapers in New York City carried advertisements offering financial compensation for individuals who were willing to become subjects of medical experiments.[42] Financial compensation also was proffered to newly arrived Spanish immigrants in order to induce them to take part in experiments by the American Yellow Fever Commission in Cuba. Every test participant in that study received $100 in gold for his participation, with a cash bonus of $100 if he developed the disease. For a potentially fatal disease like yellow fever, $200 hardly was appropriate compensation, but scores of impoverished immigrants were attracted to the bait. And, in fact, they received much more than the usual payment to volunteers for medical experiments.[43]

Having recognized the importance attached to consent by colleagues, judges, and the laity, many physicians resorted to sins of omission to get "volunteers" to consent to experiments. They gave incomplete and misleading information, or none at all. Not infrequently, patients who consented to one procedure had an additional procedure performed on them without their knowledge. In one study on hookworm infection, a potentially fatal disease, Claude Smith, a physician in the South of the

United States, placed soil containing larva of the parasite on the foreskin of a patient who was waiting to be circumcised. As Smith explained in *JAMA* in 1904, "the patient seemed to have an idea that it was some medicine preparatory to the operation as nothing was said to him about it." After four minutes, the patient remarked that his prepuce "felt as if a fly was crawling over it, and a minute or so later said that he felt as if needles were sticking in it."[44] Smith seemed totally oblivious to both his own deceit and his patient's suffering consequent to having been infected experimentally.

The study on yellow fever by Walter Reed and his coworkers in 1900 often has been referred to as a model for experimentation in humans because self-experiments by physicians preceded testing in other humans and because "informed written consent" was obtained from their subjects. The decision to use written contracts probably was influenced by Surgeon General Sternberg who, in a letter to Aristides Agramonte in May 1900, advised that experiments on humans "should not be made upon any individual without his full knowledge and consent."[45] Although the Yellow Fever Commission followed that advice, the information given to test subjects was misleading, downplaying as it did the mortal danger associated with contraction of yellow fever and exaggerating the probability that the men working in Cuba would become infected naturally anyway. The waiver that "volunteers" had to sign as part of the consent form was a classic example of obfuscation and the content of the statement to be signed tells why:

"The undersigned understands perfectly that in the case of the development of yellow fever in him, that he endangers his life to a certain extent, but it being entirely impossible to him to avoid the infection during his stay in this island, he prefers to take the chance of contracting it intentionally in the belief that he will receive from the Reed Commission the greatest care and the most skillful medical service."[46]

The Abuse of Man

Resort to Vulnerable Populations

In spite of the highly visible self-experiments, the upbeat, misleading information, and the offers of monetary rewards, volunteers for medical experiments did not come forward readily. Moreover, some experiments required participation of test subjects who could not give legally binding consent. Testing of new vaccines, for example, most often had to be performed in children, they being the only ones who had not been exposed to some of the common infectious diseases. These problems, and the evident intolerance of Americans in regard to experiments on humans, led scientists to utilize the most vulnerable populations – those who lacked advocacy and whose abuse by medical experimentation likely would go unnoticed. Experiments in prisons, orphanages, and lunatic asylums were more common in the United States than in Europe. In 1895, for example, New York pediatrician Henry Heiman reported on successful inoculations with gonococci of two mentally disabled boys, a 16-year-old "idiot" and a 4-year-old "idiot with chronic epilepsy."[47] In the same year, George Miller Sternberg and Walter Reed tested the efficacy of a preparation that "might immunize against" smallpox by running experiments on unvaccinated children in some of the asylums for orphans in Brooklyn.[48] In 1909, Frank Crozer Knowles (Fig. 243), who later became president of the American Dermatological Association (ADA), inoculated matter of mollus-

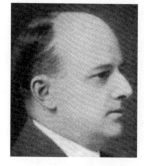

cum contagiosum into the skin of two orphans at St. Vincent's Home in Philadelphia – a boy and a girl, each four years old – to determine the incubation period of the disease.[49] Joseph Stokes, Jr., of the Department of Pediatrics at the University of Pennsylvania School of Medicine, analyzed the effects of "intramuscular vaccination of human beings . . . with active virus of influenza" by experimenting on residents of two large state institutions for the retarded.⁵⁰

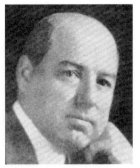

In the early 1900s, the American director of the Biological Laboratory of the Philippine Bureau of Science, Richard Pearson Strong (Fig. 244), used inmates of Bilibid Prison in Manila for experimental vaccinations against cholera and plague (Fig. 245). The number of test subjects was not stated in most of his publications, but the total reached 200 in one report. On November 16, 1906, Strong inoculated 24 prisoners with an experimental cholera vaccine that had been contaminated accidentally with serum of plague. As a result, 13 prisoners died. An investigative general committe instituted by Philippine Governor Smith found that Strong had issued an Executive Order that effectively made the vaccinations compulsory. Strong had "ordered all the prisoners there to form in line . . . without telling them what he was going to do, nor consulting their wishes in the matter." The committee came to the conclusion that "it is not lawful to subject a person, however unfortunate that person's social position may appear, to a dangerous or at least painful experiment, against his will, without his consent clearly and freely given." According to the committee, Strong had for-

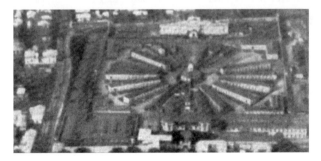

FIG. 245
*Aerial view of
Bilibid Prison,
Manila. At the
top center is the
large white
prison hospital.*

gotten "the respect due every human being in not having asked the consent of persons inoculated." Moreover, the committee suggested that even in the presence of consent, prisoners should not be used as test subjects because "on account of their lack of freedom to resist or protest," they could voice no more than a "humble objection or gentle lamentation."[51]

Although the committee charged Strong with criminal negligence, Governor Smith exonerated him and allowed medical experiments on inmates of Bilibid to continue. Six years after the plague disaster, Bilibid prisoners were used by American physicians, Ernest L. Walker and Andrew Watson Sellards, for a study concerning amebiasis. This time, prisoners were informed about the experiment "in their native language," asked for written consent without any "financial inducements" or "promise of immunity to prison discipline or commutation of sentence," and then asked to swallow gelatin capsules containing the pathogenic organisms.[52] Despite their written consent, participation of prisoners surely was a result of coercion because either of fear of future punishment or hope for better treatment. An independent decision about participation of these subjects in the study was difficult, if not impossible, as a consequence of their being incarcerated.

Dietary Horrors Behind Bars

In 1912, another study carried out at Bilibid Prison involved beriberi, a severe disease caused by a deficiency of thiamine (vitamin B1) and characterized by polyneuritis, cardiac failure, and widespread edema. Prior to this study, for most of the nineteenth century, beriberi had been attributed to an infectious or toxic cause. The first person to show conclusively that it was related to nutrition was the Japanese naval surgeon, Takaki Kanechiro, who almost eradicated beriberi from his navy by changing the daily rations of the personnel. Takaki's findings,

however, were published in 1885 only
in a Japanese journal and one whose
circulation was limited mostly to his
country. In the 1890s, Dutch medical
officer Christiaan Eijkman (Fig. 246)
showed that a paralytic condition resembling beriberi could be produced
in chickens by feeding them a diet consisting solely of polished rice. A study
conducted at different Malay prisons

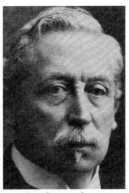

FIG. 246
*Christiaan
Eijkman
(1858-1930)*

confirmed the importance of dietary factors in the pathogenesis of beriberi – the incidence of the disease being much greater
where polished, rather than brown, rice was fed to prisoners.
Eijkman thought, incorrectly, that beriberi was caused by some
toxic chemical produced in response to digestion of polished
rice, rather than by absence of an essential nutrient. Nonetheless, in 1929, one year before his death, he received the Nobel
Prize for Medicine for his experiments on beriberi.[53] By 1912,
evidence in abundance had been accumulated in favor of a nutritional, rather than an infectious, cause of beriberi. Despite
this, a controlled study concerning the effects of various diets
on beriberi was conducted at Bilibid Prison by none other than
Richard P. Strong himself. According to the principal investigator, the prisoners "were told that the experiments were for the
purpose of testing the comparative value of different kinds of
rice as a food; the articles of food comprising the diet that
would be given to them were enumerated, and they were also
told that perhaps they might contract beriberi. The proposition
was stated to them clearly. In addition, they were to be allowed
an abundance of cigarettes of any kind that they wished and
also cigars if they desired them." The offer of cigarettes and cigars cinched the deal, inducing 29 prisoners to participate in the
study. One of the test subjects died as a consequence of the experiment, but Strong was able to confirm that beriberi was the

result of a nutritional deficiency. One year later he was appointed professor and head of the new Department of Tropical Medicine at the Harvard Medical School.[54]

Dietary regimens and their effects on health also were studied behind iron bars within the borders of the United States. To learn whether sulfuric acid, which is used in making molasses, might be injurious, the Louisiana State Board of Health, in 1907, put "Negro prisoners on a steady diet of molasses for five weeks." According to the Board, the inmates did not "object to submitting themselves to the test, because it would not do any good if they did."[55] In 1915, U.S. Public Health Service investigator Joseph Goldberger (Fig. 247) asked Mississippi Governor Earl Brewer for permission to use inmates of a state prison farm for a study on pellagra, a disease caused by a deficiency of niacin and characterized by severe dermatitis in sun-exposed areas, inflammation of mucous membranes, diarrhea, and psychiatric disturbances. As in the case of beriberi, the question of whether pellagra was caused by an infectious agent or a dietary deficiency still was in debate, although evidence in favor of a dietary cause already was overwhelming. As early as 1866, Théophile Roussel of France had noted that in regard to treatment of pellagra, "without dietary measures all remedies fail."[56] In 1914, Casimir Funk, a Polish-born biochemist working in England and who introduced the term "vitamin," had attributed, correctly, pellagra to a vitamin deficiency brought on by consump-

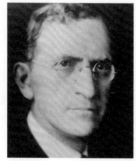

FIG. 247
*Joseph
Goldberger
(1874-1929)*

tion of overmilled corn.[57] Goldberger, himself, had conducted studies at two orphanages and one mental asylum in which pellagra was highly prevalent, and had nearly eliminated the disease by adding animal proteins and legumes to the inmates' diet. Nevertheless, Goldberger considered it important to close the chain of reasoning

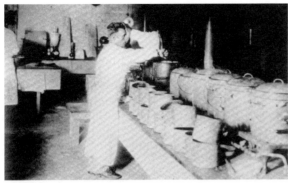

FIG. 248
In Goldberger's laboratory devoted to pellagra, varying deficiency diets were prepared and fed to test subjects.

by inducing pellagra artificially in a population that previously was free of the disease. He found that condition fulfilled at a farm in the Mississippi State Penitentiary system.[58] Because pellagra represented a serious problem in the southern part of the United States, Governor Brewer granted permission to put prisoners on a diet of meat, meal, and molasses for six months, and guaranteed pardons for those who volunteered to be test subjects. It was a successful inducement to which 12 prisoners gave consent. Soon the prisoners developed pellagra. They suffered terribly, and many of them begged to be freed of the "hellish experiment," even if it meant returning to the general population of prisoners. But Goldberger would not allow them to "quit."[59] After successful completion of the study, the test subjects were released and offered free medical care during their period of recovery. As Goldberger noted, however, "they all went off like a lot of scared rabbits"[60] (Fig. 248).

In summary, in the late nineteenth century, American medicine caught up to the standards – both good and bad – of the most advanced countries in Europe. The desire of scientists to perform experiments on humans was hampered in the United States by the high regard its citizens had for the autonomy of the individual. Nevertheless, scientists found ways to circumvent limitations. In the early twentieth century, human experimentation was more common in the United States than in Europe.

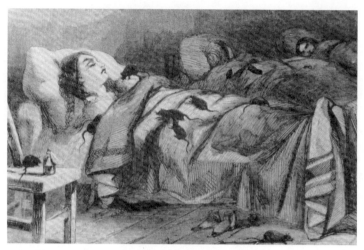

FIG.249
The Bellevue Hospital, New York City: a flagrant example of catastrophic conditions at American hospitals in the mid 19th Century (Engraving from Harper's Weekly, 1860).

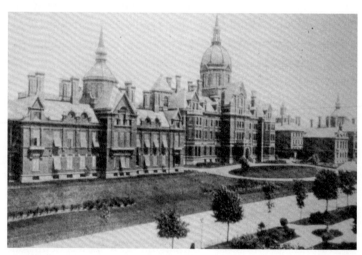

FIG. 250
The Johns Hopkins Hospital in 1889.

CHAPTER II

LEGAL INITIATIVES IN THE UNITED STATES

odern medicine in the United States may be said to have begun in the last quarter of the nineteenth century and gained momentum rapidly. Following the example of Europe, hospitals were built throughout the country, the number of them increasing from 178 with less than 50,000 beds in 1873 (including institutions for the mentally ill) to 4,359 with more than 420,000 beds in 1909 (excluding institutions for the mentally ill) (Fig. 249).[1] As more beds became available, management of patients could be combined with research. In 1889, with the opening of the Johns Hopkins University School of Medicine in Baltimore, standards for education in medicine were raised substantially and dramatically (Fig. 250). For the first time in the United States, students received extensive laboratory instruction in the basic sciences, in addition to training in clinical medicine[2] (Fig. 251, 252). Three years later, the dean of the Hopkins medical school, William Henry Welch, founded the *Journal of Experimental Medicine* for the purpose of publishing articles about original American research. Although he feared initially that it would be difficult to obtain enough manuscripts of sufficient quality for publication, he soon was inundated with usable articles.[3] The Rockefeller Institute for Medical Research inaugurated its laboratories in 1904, and its sixty-bed hospital was opened in New York City in

1910, the first institution of its kind devoted entirely to clinical research[4] (Fig. 253, 254).

These activities resulted both in marked improvement in the quality of medical care and in the reputation of the American medical profession. At the same time, they attracted the attention and induced resentment of the strong antivivisectionist

FIG. 251
Advertisement for "Medical Instruction in the Johns Hopkins Hospital" in 1889.

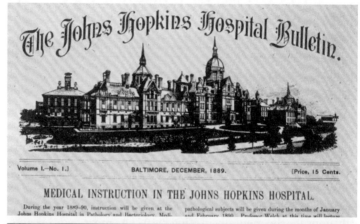

FIG. 252
Members of the first clinical faculty of Johns Hopkins University School of Medicine, Baltimore, Maryland (painting by John Singer Sargant, 1905). From left to right: William Henry Welch, William Stewart Halsted, William Osler, and Howard Attwood Kelly.

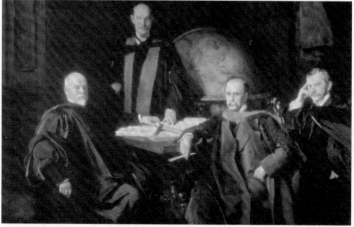

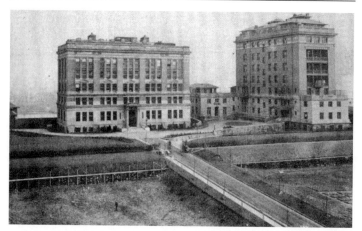

FIG. 253
The Rockefeller Institute and Hospital, New York City, 1910.

movement which was opposed fervently to medical experiments (Fig. 255, 256). In 1896, American antivivisectionists made the first attempt to restrict, at the federal level, experiments on animals. Passage of a bill that would ensure protection of animals given to research in the District of Columbia and in federal institutions was viewed by antivivisectionists as a first step toward the enactment of similar laws at state and local levels. The "Cruelty to Animals Bill," introduced by Senator James MacMillan of Michigan, was similar to the British model of 1876, not only in name, but also in its provisions. These included requirements for the licensing of any person intending to experiment on animals, prohibition of any experiment that

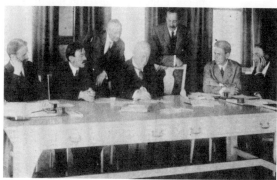

FIG. 254
The original Board of Scientific Directors of the Rockefeller Institute. From left to right: Theobald Smith, Hermann M. Biggs, Simon Flexner, William Henry Welch, T. Mitchell Prudden, L. Emmett Holt, Christian A. Herter.

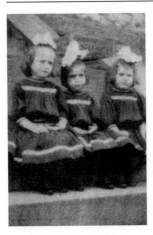

FIG. 255
"Experimental material" (*from an exposé on the use of orphans from St. Vincent's home for medical experiments, Philadelphia, Cosmopolitan, 1910*).

FIG. 256
"Would you like to have your baby inoculated?" (*Pamphlet by the New York Anti-Vivisection Society, 1915*).

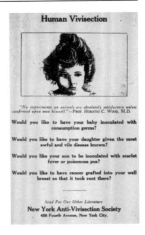

did not have as its intent the expansion of medical knowledge, and proscription of any experiment that was not deemed "useful for saving or prolonging life or alleviating suffering."[5]

The bill was endorsed by prominent public figures, including several members of the U.S. Supreme Court and eminent Protestant and Catholic leaders who considered it to be a compromise that would be acceptable to the medical profession. But this was not the case. American scientists had been forewarned by British colleagues that were such legislation to pass, they could anticipate increased costs and delays in research. On the other hand, the legislation was vague in several crucial re-

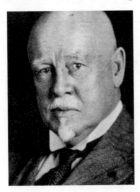

FIG. 257
William Henry Welch (1850-1934)

spects. For example, it did not provide criteria for determining whether an experiment would lead to "useful knowledge" or even what, exactly, was meant by "useful knowledge." The bill, as written, also outlawed experiments on animals for the purpose of confirming findings of other investigators or of honing surgical skills. The tremendous support given the bill as it was proposed in the first public hearings of the Senate Committee of the District of Columbia so alarmed leaders of organized medicine that Welch (Fig. 257) volunteered to lead a fight against the antivivisectionists. A former pupil of Robert Koch and one of the strongest advocates of laboratory science in the United States, Welch called on respected physicians in every state to start a letter-writing campaign "to deluge the Senate with protests" against the bill.[6]

Human Experimentation on Trial

The vote on the bill was postponed because of the Spanish-American War in 1898, but the following year legislation similar to it was proposed "For the Further Prevention of Cruelty to Animals in the District of Columbia." This time, representatives of medicine were better prepared and, at the public hearing on February 21, 1900, they fielded an impressive array of eminent medical authorities who were opposed zealously to bureaucratic restrictions on experiments in animals. Among these were Welch, William Osler, and William Williams Keen, a pioneer in brain surgery and president of the American Medical Association. Opponents of the bill from various medical and scientific societies presented testimonials to the value of vivisection and letters of support from such distinguished British scientists as Michael Foster and Joseph Lister. These ringing endorsements, coupled with concern of the Senate Committee about ambiguities in the proposal, combined to quash the bill.[7]

Among the Senate documents concerning the proposed legislation were reports on several nontherapeutic experiments on humans, including Sanarelli's study on yellow fever and statements from articles by three American investigators. One of those, Henry J. Berkley, an associate in neuropathology at Johns Hopkins, had used moribund patients in 1897 for determining the toxicity of extracts of the thyroid gland. By administering these extracts in gradually increasing doses, he had produced in his test subjects weight loss, disturbances of the circulation of the blood, digestive upset, irritability, and mental excitement so great that it reached "a state of frenzy."[8, 9] Another example in August 1896 pertained to "the vivisection of children in Boston," which consisted of lumbar puncture experiments by Arthur Wentworth, an assistant in diseases of children at Harvard Medical School. Wentworth had tapped the subarachnoid space of the spinal cord of sick infants and children at a time when lumbar puncture still was a new, risky, and unproven procedure.[10, 11] The third example dealt with an enigma in dermatovenereology, namely, whether leprosy and syphilis were separate and distinct entities or manifestations of the same disease. In 1883, George L. Fitch, resident physician to the leper colony on Molokai Island in Hawaii, had inoculated six leprous girls with the "virus of syphilis." The failure of these children to develop signs of syphilis lent credence, Fitch claimed, to the theory of the unity of syphilis and leprosy.[12, 13] Fitch was wrong and he was lucky that none of his vulnerable young charges actually acquired syphilis.

During the hearing of the Senate Committee in February 1900, Jacob H. Gallinger (Fig. 258), senior Republican senator from New Hampshire, questioned physician witnesses about the aforementioned exploitations of vulnerable human beings

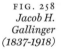

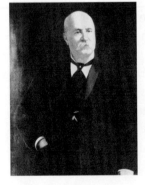

FIG. 258
Jacob H. Gallinger (1837-1918)

carried out in the name of science. The most forthright response came from Osler, who condemned without equivocation those experiments, but declared that very few physicians used patients for experimental purposes. Keen (Fig. 259) informed Gallinger that he disapproved strongly of the experiments under discussion, but he attacked antivivisectionists sharply

11· Legal Initiatives in the United States

for a series of vague references and garbled, inaccurate accounts that, in his view, were "scarcely less culpable" than the experiments themselves. Keen's attempt to avoid discussion of the ethics of experimentation in humans and to shift the focus to antivivisectionists, with their "gross ignorance or wilful disregard of the truth," prompted rancorous exchanges between him and the president of the American Humane Association (AHA), James M. Brown, an argument that went on for months and filled the pages of antivivisectionist magazines and medical journals.[14]

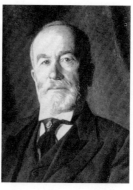

FIG. 259
*William
Williams Keen
(1837-1932)*

Less than two weeks after the public hearing on the bill regarding cruelty to animals, Senator Gallinger introduced a proposal for the regulation of experiments on humans in the District of Columbia. Senate Bill 3424 required prior disclosure of "the objects and methods of the proposed experiment" to commissioners of the District, who could then issue a specific license for performance of the experiment. The application for the license had to include written permission of test subjects "signed in the presence of two witnesses and duly acknowledged before a public notary under seal." A test subject had to be "not less than twenty years of age and in full and complete possession of all his or her reasoning faculties." Experiments in children and in women during and for one year after pregnancy were forbidden; experiments "upon any aged, infirm, epileptic, insane, or feeble-minded person" were prohibited. Moreover, consent obtained from test subjects had to be informed – that is, those subjects had to be "fully aware of the nature of the proposed experiment." The bill did not apply to "any experiments whatsoever made by medical students, physicians, surgeons, physiologists, or pathologists upon one another."[15]

The proposed legislation was rejected out of hand, and harshly, by the medical profession and stimulated Keen, in a private letter to Senator Gallinger, to concede that "unjustifiable experimentation" had occurred, but to warn of the hardships that the legislation would impose on physicians in the District of Columbia. "You know how unreasonable patients are," he said, conspiratorially, "especially if the result is not all that they anticipated. If the Bill 3424 becomes a law, it will inevitably give rise to a large number of suits on the ground of experiment." According to Keen, experiments in humans were so rare that a special act of Congress was not needed to control them. He wrote that "the moral sense of the profession may well be relied upon to prevent any extension of such an objectionable method without any law to restrain it."[16]

Gallinger's bill was defeated, as was a new version of it that he introduced in 1902. Several other legislative proposals for the regulation of experiments in humans also were unsuccessful. In 1905 and 1907, the Chicago-based Vivisection Reform Society urged passage of a bill in the Illinois state legislature "to prohibit such terrible experiments on children, insane persons and certain women as have been performed in late years" and to ensure "that no experiments should be performed on any other human being without his intelligent written consent." In 1913, the American Antivivisection Society supported the introduction of a bill before the Pennsylvania legislature that was meant to regulate experiments in humans. One or more bills restricting experimentation in animals appeared on legislative dockets each year from 1907 through 1923.[17]

The AMA Reacts

The various attempts aimed at restricting medical experiments galvanized leaders of the AMA in 1908 to form a special Council on the Defense of Medical Research. This committee included pathologist Simon Flexner of the Rockefeller Institute, who led the team that identified the polio virus (Fig. 260); Harvey Williams Cushing, formerly of the Johns Hopkins Medical School, who characterized what now is known as Cushing's disease and whose biography of William Osler won a Pulitzer Prize in 1927 (Fig. 261); and pharmacologist David Linn Edsall of the University of Pennsylvania. The committee was headed by physician / physiologist Walter Bradford Cannon of Harvard Medical School (Fig. 262), a pioneer of studies of X-rays and of the function of the autonomic nervous system. For the next 18 years, Cannon coordinated the response of organized medicine to antivivisectionists.[18] In 1909, in an effort to prevent legislative measures, he circulated a set of rules among all American laboratories and medical schools that had acknowledged using animals in research. In what was to be an early application of the "spin factor," these rules were not written in order to change the way animals were being handled and cared for in the best institutions, but to demonstrate

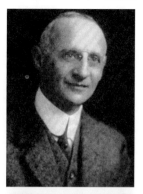

FIG. 260
Simon Flexner
(1863-1946)

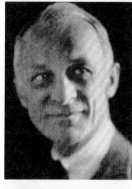

FIG. 261
Harvey
Cushing
(1869-1939)

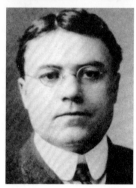

FIG. 262
Walter B.
Cannon
(1871-1945)

to the public "the intent of investigators and the precautions which they take against suffering."[19] In 1910, Cannon could report that 37 medical schools and research institutes had agreed to adopt and enforce the rules. In a letter to Governor Charles E.

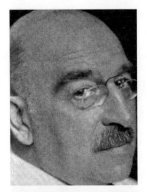

FIG. 263
Ernst Moro
(1874-1951)

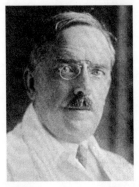

FIG. 264
Clemens von
Pirquet
(1874-1929)

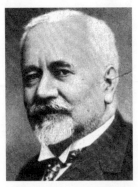

FIG. 265
Albert Léon
Charles
Calmette
(1863-1933)

Hughes of New York, where an anti-vivisectionist proposal was pending in the state legislature, Cannon predicted that before the end of the year, the regulations would "probably be enforced in all the medical laboratories in the United States."[20]

In the second decade of the twentieth century, Cannon was confronted with charges that had reference chiefly to vivisection in humans. Several new examples were ammunition for American antivivisectionists, among these being studies on the use of tuberculin as a diagnostic test for tuberculosis. Three methods had been proposed for that purpose, namely, intramuscular injection by German pediatrician Ernst Moro (Fig. 263); intracutaneous injection by Austrian pediatrician, Clemens Freiherr von Pirquet (Fig. 264), who coined the word "allergy," and intraocular application, by French bacteriologist Albert Léon Charles Calmette (Fig. 265), who, with Camille Guérin, later developed an avirulent strain of *Mycobacterium bovis* or bacillus Calmette-Guérin (BCG) that still is used today for vaccination against tuberculosis. Intracutaneous testing eventually was found to be superior to the other methods. In order to come to that realization, however, the three methods first had to be compared with one another. The ideal test subjects, of course, were children and

11 · Legal Initiatives in the United States

the best sources, that is, the easiest and safest, were orphanages, like the St. Vincent's Home in Philadelphia where tuberculin was tested on roughly 150 children. That some of the young subjects suffered from "serious inflammation of the eye" secondary to intraocular application of tuberculin outraged antivivisectionists. Other experiments in children, such as the inoculation of children with ringworm, fanned the fires of indignation of the public.[21, 22]

Venereologic Experiments Under Fire

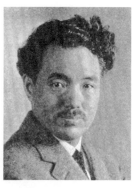

FIG. 266
*Hideyo
Noguchi
(1876-1928)*

The most hotly debated cases, however, were two that involved venereologic experiments. The first was a clinical trial in 1911 of luetin, a serum derived from pure cultures of *Treponema pallidum* that had been developed by Hideyo Noguchi (Fig. 266), a Japanese-born bacteriologist working at the Rockefeller Institute. In analogy with tuberculin in testing for tuberculosis, Noguchi hoped that intracutaneous injections of luetin would prove useful as a diagnostic test for syphilis. The safety of luetin was verified by four failures: to detect live spirochetes by microscopy, cultivate spirochetes from serum, infect rabbits by inoculation of serum, and produce infections during experiments on themselves by Noguchi and some of his colleagues. At that point, William Henry Welch suggested to Noguchi that he test luetin in a more comprehensive trial in human beings. Following Welch's advice, Noguchi contacted dispensaries and hospitals in the New York metropolitan area and obtained 400 test subjects thanks to the "courtesy" of 15 attending physicians. More than half of the subjects were known to have contracted syphilis previously; the others who were free of the disease served as controls. The control group consisted of 100 adults and children with various non-syphilitic diseases and of 46 healthy children between the ages of two and eighteen. None of the test subjects was asked to consent to the procedure. Although the tests caused no serious harm, the mere fact that healthy children and ailing adults had been exposed to material of "one of the most loathsome diseases known to humanity," and this without their knowledge and consent, alarmed the public (Fig. 267). Noguchi, the Rockefeller Institute, and the "courteous" New York physicians who had provided the test subjects were attacked, and rightly so, for having violated the personal rights of human beings under their care.[23, 24]

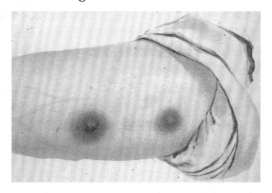

FIG. 267
Pustules following injection of luetin (from Noguchi's article on "luetin").

Even harsher protests were evoked by a study published in 1916 in the *Journal of Experimental Medicine.* Its author was Udo Julius Wile (Fig. 268), founder and chairman of the department of dermatology at the University of Michigan Medical School in Ann Arbor. Wile reported on the successful inoculation of rabbits with spirochetes of syphilis obtained by puncturing the brain of six patients with general paresis (Fig. 269). The very same experiment had been performed three years earlier at the Charité hospital in Berlin by Edmund Forster and Egon Tomasczewski. Several other investigators also had isolated spirochetes in brains at autopsy and cultivated those spirochetes in the testes and scrotal skin of rabbits. Wile repeated these experiments with material recovered from the brain of living patients, hoping to prove the existence of a neurotropic strain of *Treponema pallidum* that might be treated by direct administration into the brain of antisyphilitic drugs. His method for discovering an unknown strain of spirochetes was, at best, question-

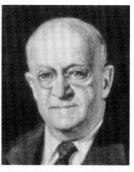

FIG. 268
*Udo Julius Wile
(1882-1965)*

able. To increase his chances of cultivating bacteria, Wile "inoculated the brain substance of several cases into a single rabbit." The rabbit developed lesions, exceptionally rapidly, of syphilis, probably as a consequence of the high number of spirochetes inoculated. That circumstance prompted Wile to postulate, incorrectly, the existence of a distinct neurotropic type of *Treponema pallidum,* namely, "a virulent strain with a shorter period of incubation for the rabbit than exists with other strains." In brief, Wile's study was totally unnecessary and mere repetition of experiments that already had been performed. Moreover, it was flawed scientifically. Even more significant, however, were its flaws ethically. In his article, Wile told that "for my series of experiments six cases were chosen from a large number of patients." He did not mention a word about consent of

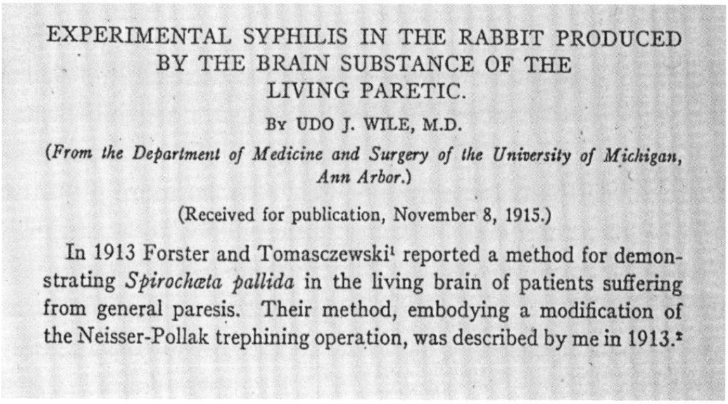

FIG. 269
Title page of the article about Wile's "dental drill" experiments.

EXPERIMENTAL SYPHILIS IN THE RABBIT PRODUCED BY THE BRAIN SUBSTANCE OF THE LIVING PARETIC.

By UDO J. WILE, M.D.

(From the Department of Medicine and Surgery of the University of Michigan, Ann Arbor.)

(Received for publication, November 8, 1915.)

In 1913 Forster and Tomasczewski[1] reported a method for demonstrating *Spirochæta pallida* in the living brain of patients suffering from general paresis. Their method, embodying a modification of the Neisser-Pollak trephining operation, was described by me in 1913.[2]

patients or of their legal guardians. He then described precisely how he pierced the skin and skull above the frontal convolution of the brain with a dental drill and aspirated a small cylinder of brain substance with a long, thin trocar needle.[25] When anti-vivisectionists heard about this blatant "use of patients in our hospitals for purely experimental purposes," accounts severely critical of Wile's "dental drill experiments" appeared in newspapers across the country.[26]

Wile himself remained indifferent to the criticism. "You may quote me as having absolutely no interest in the matter," he informed a reporter, "whatever people may wish to think regarding the experiment."[27] This casual attitude was reminiscent of Claude Bernard's patronizing exhortation in 1865 that "a man of science should attend only to the opinion of men of science who understand him."[28] Representatives of American medicine, however, knew full well that times had changed and that indifference to ethical concerns of the public was bound to result in curtailment of research. In a private letter to Wile, Cannon told the syphilologist pointedly that "no one man has any reason whatever to be disregardful of the conviction, which mankind cherishes, that the right of the individual to determine the uses to which his body shall be put is a sacred right which no investigator is justified in violating."[29] Without identifying Wile by name, Cannon also addressed the issue of experiments in humans in an editorial for *JAMA*. Having acknowledged that the honest desire to advance medical knowledge tempted researchers on occasion to perform procedures without careful consideration of the rights of individual patients, Cannon made this observation: "There is no more primitive and fundamental right which any individual possesses than that of controlling the uses to which his own body is put. Mankind has struggled for centuries for the recognition of this right. Civilized society is based on the recognition of it. The lay public is perfectly clear about it." Physicians who countenanced such abuses, Cannon warned, would suffer hostility and legal action. Cannon concluded with these words:

The medical profession is certainly not called on, in any sense, to support the physician who transgresses the elementary principles of ethics. Especially are the reputation and esteem of medical men endangered by any failure on their part to stand firmly for the fundamental right of the individual with respect for his own person. . . . The sick commit themselves to the care of the physician and surgeon helplessly and with the implicit trust that their welfare alone will be considered. Any practitioner or investigator, no matter how laudable his motives, who fails in scrupulous regard for this trust is liable to do incalculable harm by rousing suspicions, fears, and disrespect as to the character of medical service.[30]

Wile's "dental drill experiments" spurred Cannon further to propose, in 1916, that the AMA adopt a formal resolution in which the conditions for acceptable experimentation – including formal prior consent of patients – would be spelled out. Although many of his colleagues conceded that an official stand on the subject was necessary, they worried about where to draw the line between unjustifiable experiments and harmless studies, such as the collection of blood and urine that, even though unrelated to a patient's treatment, was important for clinical research. They also worried that the obligation to secure informed consent for all these procedures would delay and complicate research significantly.[31] Cannon's colleague at Harvard, Francis Peabody, who wrote a poignant essay on the management of patients, was particularly uneasy with the idea of a patient having to give consent. Although necessary in risky experiments, he felt that that agreement could detract from a physician's responsibility to act always in the best interest of a patient. Peabody asserted that the character of the person doing the research was the principal issue, and that those who pursued a career in scientific medicine were generally "among the more high minded of the profession."[32] Because of these concerns and others, such as implications of the war in Europe for American medicine that at the time were considered to be more important, Cannon's proposal was not entertained in 1916 by the House of Delegates of the American Medical Association.[33]

The Ravages of War Overshadow the Horrors of Experimentation

Cannon's initiative in restricting experimentation on humans was the last of its kind for many years. With thousands of soldiers dying on the battlefields of World War I, medical experiments on animals and human beings seemed to be an issue of relatively little consequence. When antivivisectionists tried to block animal experiments for study of diseases such as trench fever, they were criticized roundly for placing the welfare of animals above the needs of American soldiers, and they lost many of their followers.[34] As a result, experiments that would have aroused vehemence before the war went unchallenged during and after it. For example, between 1920 and 1922, transplants of testes were performed on hundreds of prisoners in California in order to determine whether loss of potency in aged and ill men could be restored. Some prisoners received implants from humans, whereas others were given "the testicles of goats, rams, boars, and deer." The investigator, Dr. L.L. Stanley, noted that it was "fortunate that this work could be carried out in a prison, for in such a place all men are treated alike, and live under the same conditions of food, work and general surroundings. A good opportunity was given for observing the results, because the patients could be under daily observation, and the 'follow-up' conditions were ideal."[35] The dream of an investigator had come true.

In 1926, J.A. McIntosh of Memphis, Tennessee reported on the first "instance of successful experimental transmission of

11 · Legal Initiatives in the United States

granuloma inguinale from one individual to another." The test subject was an African-American male "not previously exposed in any way to the possibility of spontaneously contracting this disease."[36] In the same year, Andrew Sellards of Harvard Medical School told about how he and two coworkers at the Bureau of Science in Manila had "produced yaws experimentally in a group of six volunteers in

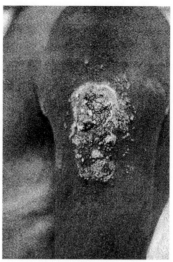

FIG. 270
Lesions of
experimentally
induced yaws
six weeks after
inoculation
(from the
article by
Sellards et al.).

order that we might know the exact time of inoculation and the first appearance of clinical symptoms." The authors did not state whether they had informed the "volunteers" about possible complications, such as ulcerated cutaneous lesions, osteitis, periostitis, and destruction of the central part of the face (Fig. 270).[37] In 1934, two Colorado prisoners were injected with tubercle bacilli at National Jewish Hospital in Denver, in return for which they were pardoned by Governor Edwin C. Johnson. When these experiments became known publicly, they were criticized by citizens who protested that there was "no excuse for releasing upon the community two life-term fellows because they didn't get tuberculosis when inoculated with a preparation of microscopic bugs. "[38] The dubious ethical quality of the experiment went unnoticed.

During this era, even if the ethics of a particular experiment did attract the attention of the public, it created nothing more than a mild stir. In 1921, for instance, *The Nation* criticized a study by three New York pediatricians – Alfred F. Hess of the Hebrew Infant Asylum, and his colleagues, Mildred Fish and Lester Unger – who induced scurvy in orphans by withholding orange juice from their diet for the purpose of developing a diagnostic test for the disease.[39] Although the publication stated that "no devotion to science . . . can for an instant justify the experimenting on helpless infants," it also expressed its admiration for modern medicine and rejected explicitly "antivivisection fanatics and the various freaks and cranks" hostile to medical progress. The editors of the journal, *American Medicine*, exonerated Hess and his colleagues of misconduct and pointed out, defensively, that their research had enabled the orphans to "make a large return to the community for the care devoted to them."[40]

The decline of the antivivisectionist movement was furthered by changes in the editorial style of medical publications. Having learned their lesson, the leaders of experimental medicine saw to it that the most objectionable passages of articles involving human test subjects were deleted. Nobelist Francis Peyton Rous (Fig. 271), editor of the *Journal of Experimental Medicine*, made "judicial" editorial changes such as those routinely. For example, the word "infant" was eliminated from the title of an article on vaccination against colds. The phrase "lice fed on man" in an article on inoculations with a strain of typhus was changed subtly to "lice fed on human volunteers."[41] The fact that test subjects were "volunteers" was emphasized in most articles, although it was far from clear what this really meant because recruitment came chiefly from populations, such as infants,

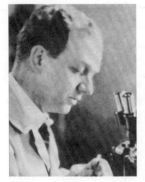

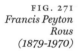

who were vulnerable by virtue of not being able to exercise free will. One pediatrician, William C. Black, infected infants with herpes simplex in order to help clarify the cause of acute infectious gingivostomatitis.[42] His article on the subject was rejected by Rous, who informed the author that infection of a 12-month-old infant with herpesvirus "was an abuse of power, an infringement on the rights of the individual, and not excusable because the illness which followed had implications for science. The statement that the child 'was offered as a 'volunteer' – whatever that may mean – does not palliate the action."[43] Black's article was published subsequently in the *Journal of Pediatrics* and went largely unnoticed by antivivisectionists.

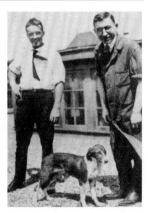

FIG. 272
Frederick Banting and Charles Best with a dog used for experiments at the Institute of Physiology in Toronto, where those co-workers isolated insulin for the first time and used it for therapy of diabetes (1922).

The most important reason for the declining influence of antivivisectionists in America was remarkably impressive results that came from medical research. One such triumph was the discovery of insulin through research on dogs, thereby enabling treatment successfully of diabetic patients in coma or on the verge of it (Fig. 272). Consequently, the American medical profession enjoyed unprecedented popular esteem and the word "experiment" lost its negative connotation. Physicians who in the course of their work acquired an infectious disease were considered heroes, likened to soldiers wounded on a battlefield.[44] They were praised in articles about "martyrs of science" and in books, such as Sinclair Lewis' 1925 Pulitzer Prize-winning novel, *Arrowsmith,* in which was detailed an imaginary test of a newly developed serum on a plague-infested island in the West Indies.[45] Bacteriologist Paul de Kruif's *Microbe Hunters,* published in 1926, recounted dramatic stories of medical scientists "who blazed a path through the darkness of ignorance."[46] One chapter of de Kruif's book was devoted to the experiments by Walter Reed on yellow fever and became the basis of a Broadway play, produced in 1934, called *Yellow Jack,* followed in 1938 by a successful Hollywood film of the same name. In 1931, *Arrowsmith,* too, was turned into a movie that was well received. Other popular films, such as *Men in White* (1934) and

The White Parade (1934), helped enhance respect for experimental medicine.[47] Patients no longer were suspicious of research activities in hospitals; in fact, they welcomed them because those activities seemed to convey that the most advanced methods of diagnosis and treatment were being employed in their very own hospitals. Some people even tried to "give meaning to their lives" by offering their bodies, wholesale, for any experiment that might advance the cause of science.[48]

The American medical community undertook great efforts in the first two decades of the twentieth century to block legal initiatives aimed at the restriction of experiments on humans. Those efforts were successful and in subsequent decades they no longer were necessary.

CHAPTER 12

EXPERIMENTS ON HUMANS IN A TURBULENT TIME

Horrors of the first World War superseded anxiety about medical research involving human beings. In the face of the slaughter of millions of people, experiments involving relatively small groups of humans ceased to be an issue of public interest, not only in the United States, but also in Europe, especially in those countries that had lost the war. Germany and Austria, in particular, were in desperate political and economic shape. The Austro-Hungarian Empire was in a state of complete dissolution and the German-speaking part of it had lost vast territory, including Bohemia and Moravia, which became part of Czechoslavakia; southern Styria, which melded into Yugoslavia; and Southern Tyrol, which became Italian. In the Treaty of St. Germain, the victorious Allied powers imposed onerous reparations on the newly formed Austrian republic and denied its wish to become a province of the German Reich, that rejection contributing to years of political instability.

In Germany, the situation was similar. Following the abdication of the Kaiser in 1918, the country was convulsed by a bloody revolution with fighting raging among opposing political groups. Eventually, a new democratic government was established, its first duty being to the sign the Treaty of Versailles. The treaty imposed severe penalties on Germany, including the loss of one-seventh of its territory and one-tenth of its population, confiscation of industrial equipment, and enormous reparations. As a result, the Democrats who had signed the treaty were defamed as traitors; nationalistic and antidemocratic tendencies were kindled; the economy collapsed; astronomical inflation led to pauperization of much of the population, which was accompanied by unemployment, hunger, and hopelessness.

In this situation, questionable experiments on humans went largely unnoticed and unchecked. In the early 1920s, numerous studies involving the dubious use of human test subjects were published in the German medical literature. For example, Wilhelm Grüter of Marburg induced *herpes corneae* in several blind persons, and noted the following: ". . . inoculation of the material in the normal conjunctiva of animal or man did not result in inflammation of the cornea, not even if the cornea was traumatized. In order to secure success . . . the material must be inoculated directly by cutting the cornea with a lancet."[1] Viennese dermatologist Benjamin Lipschütz, in an attempt to establish the contagiousness of *herpes genitalis*, "considered it to be necessary not to restrict the scope of examinations to microscopy and animal experiments, but to go a step further and to confirm the correctness of the hypothesis by experimental inoculation of human beings." Lipschütz inoculated 31 persons with fluid from vesicles of *herpes genitalis* and succeeded in "inducing typical herpes in the skin of the test subjects following an incubation period of three weeks."[2] In collaboration with Lipschütz, pediatrician Karl Kundralitz of Vienna probed the relationship between zoster (shingles) and varicella (chickenpox) by inoculating children with fluid from vesicles of zoster. Most of the subjects who were less than five years of age developed chickenpox, providing evidence that the virus in both conditions was identical. Lipschütz confirmed the diagnosis clinically by examination histopathologically of sections of biopsy specimens taken from the children. One infant with widespread skin lesions died of pneumonia a few days after the onset of the eruption. Whether or not this was related to the infection induced experimentally cannot be determined from reading Kundralitz's report.[3]

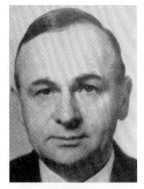

FIG. 273
Walther
Schönfeld
(1888-1977)

Walther Schönfeld (Fig. 273), who later became chairman of the departments of dermatology at the universities of Greifswald and Heidelberg, studied the passage of various dyes from the blood into the spinal fluid of 53 test subjects, some of whom had syphilis and others of whom did not. Schönfeld performed a total of 75 lumbar punctures and found that the passage of dyes into the spinous fluid was enhanced in patients with syphilis, especially in those suffering from paralysis.[4] Hans Martenstein (Fig. 274), an assistant at the department of dermatology of the University of Breslau who later became director of the skin clinic in Dresden-Friedrichstadt, investigated the sensitivity of patients with *xeroderma pigmentosum* and *hydroa vacciniforme* to rays of different spectra. Subjects were exposed to α-, β-, and γ-rays, X-rays, ultraviolet rays, and visible light; skin reactions included erythema, scaling, urtica, vesicles, and bullae.[5, 6] Another Breslau dermatologist, Hans Biberstein (Fig. 275), who later joined

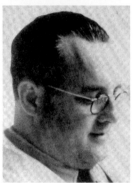

FIG. 274
Hans
Martenstein
(1892-1945)

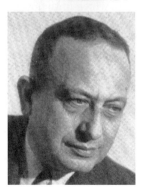

FIG. 275
Hans
Biberstein
(1889-1965)

the voluntary faculty of The Skin and Cancer Clinic of New York University School of Medicine, studied reactions induced by experimental sensitization of patients to potent allergens.[7] In the published reports of all these studies, not a single mention was made of information being provided to patients about possible implications and risks of the experiments and not a single word was written of acknowledgement of their consent.

In the era that followed World War I, experiments on humans again were performed as they had been in the late nineteenth century – uninhibitedly and without heed to the interests and rights of test subjects. The Prussian guidelines of 1900 concerning medical experiments in humans were neglected completely. Performing such experiments at will, with one's conscience as the only guide, continued to be regarded by many physicians as their right professionally. Paul Gerson Unna of Hamburg (Fig. 276), a leading pioneer in dermatotherapy and dermatopathology, articulated his vision of experiments in humans thus:

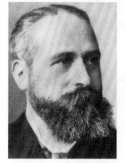

FIG. 276
*Paul Gerson
Unna
(1850-1929)*

The large surface of human skin, so easily accessible for observation, will in the future be of the same, and possibly even higher, value for experimental therapy and pharmacology than the animal body, which until now has been used almost exclusively. I can only call upon qualified pharmacologists to use the dermato-therapeutic experiment more commonly for their studies. Nowhere can controlled examinations be performed so easily and simply, is the method so humane, and the result so directly usable for the therapy of human beings.[8]

That some patients might object to being used for therapeutic experiments did not occur to Unna and he did not take that possibility into account.

A Shift in Direction of Experiments

Although the attitude of physicians concerning the matter of human experimentation essentially was unchanged, a gradual shift did occur in the objectives and methods of research. The great days of classic bacteriology were over, the cause of the most important infectious diseases having been elucidated. Inoculation experiments, therefore, were performed episodically only. Among these experiments was the study concerning the contagiousness of genital herpes by Lipschütz;[9] the experimental induction of trachomata by transfer of genital discharge to the conjunctiva by ophthalmologist Moritz Wolfrum of the University of Leipzig;[10] and the transfer of the filtrated gargle of persons with acute scarlet fever to the tonsils of susceptible children by Deicher of Berlin, who tried to demonstrate that the disease was caused by non-infectious toxins of streptococci, rather than by the bacteria themselves.[11]

In contrast to the waning of inoculation experiments, research on matters immunologic and therapeutic became increasingly important, with some of the most objectionable studies being carried out on children. In 1927, Düsseldorf pediatrician Arno Nohlen used 20 moribund children as test subjects to assess the side effects of intravenous injections of soot. The study was performed under the specious assumption that artificial anthracosis induced by these injections might prove beneficial for patients suffering from thrombemboli to the lung.[12] In the same year, Dr. H. Vollmer of Berlin reported on a trial of the vitamin D compound, Vigantol, for the treatment of rickets, using as subjects "approximately 100 rats and 20 children." In order to rule out other factors that might explain an improvement of rickets, Vollmer kept "test children under unfavorable conditions in regard to diet and light exposure." The results of experiments in animals already had indicated the effectiveness of Vigantol, and none of Vollmer's test subjects ex-

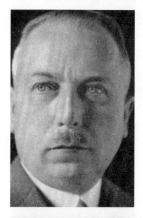

perienced adverse effects. Consent of the parents of the children, however, was not obtained.[13, 14] The chairman of the department of pediatrics of the University of Leipzig, Georg Bessau (Fig. 277), studied different types of diets in infants. Four of 14 infants given a diet that consisted only of powdered milk and rice gruel died, whereas all 20 of the infants who had vegetables added to their diet survived.[15] The

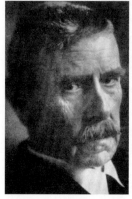

purpose of the study was to confirm the importance of carbohydrates (in a gruel of rice) and vitamins (in vegetables) for ensuring that infants thrived. In order to demonstrate that proposition in a scientifically convincing way, Bessau needed a control group which would receive a diet that he, himself, believed to be inferior. No mention was made of parental consent or of ethical considerations.

The mentally disabled and others with little control physically over their bodies continued to be favorite test subjects. In 1918, psychiatrist/neurologist, Julius Wagner-Jauregg of Vienna (Fig. 278) demonstrated that general paresis of tertiary syphilis could be improved by inducing high fever through injection of blood taken from persons infected with malaria. Although this treatment was associated with terrible side effects – about three percent of the patients died during attacks of fever and even more than that in subsequent weeks – it was the only therapy for dementia paralytica then available. In 1927, Wagner-Jauregg was awarded the Nobel Prize for having introduced "malaria therapy." The availability of patients with malaria in psychiatric sanitariums offered an unexpected, but welcome, opportunity for the German pharmaceutical industry to assess newly synthesized drugs for efficacy against malaria and for toxic side effects. The paralyzed patients could not give their own consent, and their relatives were not asked for it either. The side effects of the various experimental drugs often were dramatic, ranging from severe cyanosis to paresis. When, however, some of the drugs were tried on patients with syphilis who were competent mentally, their blood-curdling screams of protest forced the chief investigator, Peter Mühlens of the Institute for Tropical Medicine in Hamburg, to terminate the trials.[16]

Human Experimentation Becomes a Political Weapon – Again

In the early 1920s, a public debate about questionable experiments in humans was prevented because of political turbulence, such as two failed attempts to overthrow the German government (one by Wolfgang Kapp in 1920 and the other by Adolf Hitler in 1923). In the mid 1920s, however, it was the turbulent political situation that prompted the public to focus its attention again on experiments on humans. Medical research involving humans was rediscovered as a vehicle to political ends, albeit with some associated serious ethical concerns. Among those who utilized this issue for purposes of propaganda were so-called natural healers, a group that presented itself as an alternative to conventional allopathic medicine through emphasis on the importance to health of sun, fresh air, and other gifts of nature. In actuality, the "natural healers" were mostly charlatans with only rudimentary knowledge of basic principles of pathology and pathophysiology. Nevertheless, they consistently attacked conventional medicine with its specialized and often impersonal forms of treatment. Rather than considering individual mechanisms of disease or disturbances of particular organs, they aspired to a unifying "holistic" medicine that treated the whole person by restoring him or her to a balanced, natural life. Natural healers were activists in an anti-vaccination movement, vilifying vaccination on the basis of possible side effects and arguing that "the immunity of children should be strengthened by raising them in fresh air, by skin care, and a diet rich in vitamins and minerals. This alone brings about effective protection."[17]

In Germany, thousands of natural healers created their own schools and edited their own journals. The Reich's Committee of Non-Profit Associations for Life-and Health-Reform (*Reichsausschuss der Gemeinnützigen Verbände für Lebens- und Heilreform*), founded in 1926, had support from approximately five million citizens. According to estimates of 1924, one-seventh of the entire German population preferred the services of natural healers to those of physicians.[18] Natural healers, however, lacked official recognition and benefits, such as coverage of their fees by health insurance programs. In an effort to overcome this handicap, the healers seized any opportunity to bring to the attention of the laity the mistakes and misdemeanors of physicians, including objectionable experiments on humans. Only when representatives of "official" medicine acknowledged wrongdoing on the part of colleagues and entered into serious discussion about the matter, did the natural healers become conciliatory, referring to unethical experiments as deplorable, but rare, exceptions. When there was no serious response to their accusations, however, the healers tended to exaggerate and falsify reports about experiments, implying that those cases were merely the tip of a huge and dangerous iceberg.[19]

Uncivil War Erupts in the Medical Community

Questionable experiments on humans also were used as projectiles in conflicts within the medical profession itself, and there were many such quarrels that stemmed from the particularly stressful economic situation of the time. With the burdens of reparations, inflation, a severely impaired industry, and high unemployment, very little money was available for health care. With the healthcare business drying up, a large excess of physicians became inevitable, many being left unemployed, and those who continued to work in their profession could barely earn a living. In 1926, nearly half of all physicians in Germany earned a salary only slightly higher than that of the average industrial worker. In 1929, 48 percent of German doctors earned less than the official minimum wage for survival, and, in the wake of the world economic crisis, this number escalated to 72 percent.[20] The result was a "civil war" among various factions of physicians, each of which tried to hold its ground against the others. General practitioners vied with specialists, and physicians in private practice opposed those employed in hospitals. Under these circumstances of fierce competition, the publication of dubious experiments on humans came to be regarded as an economic threat or even a weapon that could be used by one faction to damage the reputation of another. For example, Friedrich von Müller (Fig. 279), professor of internal medicine at the University of Munich, accused physicians in private practice of employing reports of onerous experiments in order to diminish the public's confidence in hospitals and to direct patients to themselves.[21]

The most serious conflict within the medical profession was one with a long history, to wit, between physicians in private practice and those who worked in "ambulatories," or polyclinics, operated by public health insurance groups. Through a decree in 1883, all German citizens with low income had to be enrolled in public

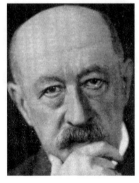

FIG. 279
*Friedrich von Müller
(1858-1941)*

health insurance programs. Only those earning higher wages could be insured privately. Because the limit of income for compulsory enrollment in public health insurance was raised steadily, the portion of the population that was insured publicly increased from 10 percent in 1885 to about 50 percent in 1914.[22] As a result, physicians became more and more dependent on public health insurance payments and, by contract, had to accept much lower fees than those paid by private patients. The financial resources of the public health insurances were exhausted because of the war. To prevent the breakdown of the public health insurance system, the scope was widened further in 1918 to include even more citizens with higher incomes, depriving physicians further of more lucrative private patients. The problem escalated during the astronomic inflation of the early 1920s. By the time a physician received payment, at last, from the public insurance program, the fee had lost much of its original value. On top of this came a federal decree in October 1923 that granted public health insurance the right to issue guidelines for treatment and to control physicians who worked under its auspices. In answer to this growing dilemma, the most powerful organization of physicians in Germany, the Leipzig Association (Leipziger Verband, which became the Hartmannbund), called for a strike by physicians. In December 1923, publicly insured patients, except for emergencies, were treated only on the condition that they agreed to pay their bills immediately. The health insurance groups, having an obligation to provide medical care, responded by opening their own polyclinics and employing their own physicians to run them.[23]

These "ambulatories" were viewed by the Leipzig Association as a major threat, not only because they weakened the position of physicians vis-à-vis public health insurance, but because they seemed to represent a first step toward the "socialization of medicine." Most German physicians were conservative, had strong feelings against socialists and communists, valued their independence professionally, and feared that being reduced to the status of employees would diminish both their income and their respect by laypersons. A minority of physicians, however, welcomed the trend toward socialized medicine with health care being controlled by the state, and being provided freely and equally to everyone. In this conflict of ideas about health care, ambulatories became a symbol of socialized medicine, and they were both attacked and defended vehemently. For example, some branches of the major organizations of physicians tried to exclude doctors who worked in ambulatories from membership and accused them of violating the best interests of the profession.[24]

The Specter of Socialized Medicine

Because physicians with socialist leanings found themselves poorly represented by the established professional organizations, they founded their own unified groups, among them the Association of Socialist Physicians (*Verein Sozialistischer Ärzte*) and the German Panel Fund Physicians Union (*Reichsverband der deutschen Kassenärzte*). The latter league published its own journal called *The Panel Fund Physician* (Der Kassenarzt), edited by Julius Moses (Fig. 280), a physician of Jewish descent, a member of the executive committee of the Social Democratic Party and, from 1920 to 1932, a parliamentarian in the German Reichstag. Moses, in criticizing official medicine for not paying enough heed to social and economic causes of disease, such as poor diet and housing, appeared to adopt, in part, the position of the natural healers. He rallied against the strike of physicians in December 1923, imply-

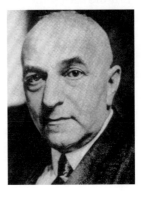

FIG. 281
*Karl
Haedenkamp
(1889-1955)*

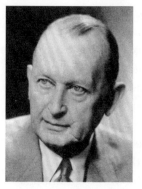

ing strongly that the motivation of these physicians was undue material gain. Through these statements, Moses came to be regarded by many physicians as their worst enemy. The general secretary of the Leipzig Association, Karl Haedenkamp (Fig. 281), referred to him as the "symbol of the undermining spirit" and a "despiser of all concepts of medical honor."[25]

In his broadside against traditional structures and attitudes in medicine, Moses also called attention to dubious experiments on humans. In numerous articles in 1928, he decried Vollmer's study on treatment of rickets, Nohlen's soot injections, and medical experiments of other kinds. Moses took these studies out of context, exaggerated the risks associated with them, attributed them to "raw cynicism" and widespread "experimental mania," and heaped calumny on those "elements in the medical profession who unscrupulously disregard life and health of patients under their care in order to perform questionable experiments on them."[26] In the eyes of most physicians, Moses' "smear-campaign" was both inappropriate and dangerous, and was intended to undermine the confidence of patients in the medical profession as a whole. In an open letter in 1928 to a journal dedicated to the protection of animals *(Tierrecht und Tierschutz)*, a physician in Koblenz wrote that "Dr. Moses, who, together with some other physicians, stands entirely outside the medical profession, probably thought he had found a good opportunity to pick holes in the profession, to prejudice the public against physicians, and, thereby, to work for the ultimate cause of social democrats, namely, the complete socialization of medicine."[27]

Human Experimentation as a Tool of Party Politics

The issue of human experimentation was utilized not only in conflicts between physicians and natural healers and among different groups within the medical profession, but also as a tool of propaganda for party politics. Julius Moses was involved prominently in this as well. In the official journal of the Social Democratic Party, he emphasized that children who were used for medical experiments came from proletarian families without the power to resist.[28] This happened to be true, the authors of some scientific articles having made it abundantly clear how important social background was for recruitment of test subjects. For example, when in 1928 pediatricians Friedrich Kruse and Arthur Stern studied the relationship between elimination of organic acids in the urine and various diets in infants, they pointed out that the subjects "were submitted precisely for that purpose by parents who, because of social misery, wanted to leave their children in the clinic for a while."[29] Moses contended, rightly, that the utilization of social misery for purposes of research was unacceptable and advised that the proletariat needed to be protected from the "crimes of class medicine."[30]

Moses' claims were rejected as pure demagogy. Physician Richard Wolf warned his colleagues against Moses in the blackest terms: "One incautious word delivers you into the hands of the most dangerous fellow human being, the homo politicus . . . We are dealing with men striving for power who take up material for their daily work of agitation wherever they find it."[31] Wilhelm His, Jr. of Berlin emphasized that dangerous experiments performed on humans were exceptional in the extreme and that "the news that reached the public was almost always more or less distorted."[32] In a meeting of the Berlin Chamber of Physicians in June 1928, the celebrated surgeon, August Bier (Fig. 282), reminded his colleagues of examples of self-experi-

FIG. 282
August Bier
(1861-1949)

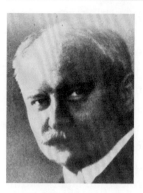

FIG. 283
Ignaz Zadek
(1858-1931)

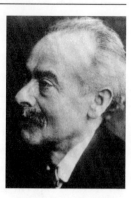

mentation for the purpose of disproving the accusation that only "members of public health insurances and of poorer classes of society" were used as medical test subjects.[33] Bier had performed experiments on himself when he developed the technique of lumbar anesthesia. On the other hand, even the German Minister of Sciences, Arts, and People's Education, Grimme, acknowledged that he did not know "of a single case in which such experiments have been performed in private clinics or sanitariums devoted to the treatment of wealthy patients."[34]

Ignaz Zadek (Fig. 283), chairman and a founding member of the Association of Socialist Physicians, acknowledged that Moses' criticism of experiments on humans was one-sided. He emphasized, however, that proletarians, being the first to be subjected to new forms of treatment, contributed thereby to the safety of modalities that eventually profited members of the bourgeoisie.[35] In a resolution proposed by Socialist and Communist physicians of Berlin, medical experiments on members of the working class were said to result from competition within the giant pharmaceutical industry.[36] A member of the municipal council of Dresden wrote this about the matter: "If those heroes of official medicine consider experiments or trials of chemical compounds to be necessary, they should try them on themselves or on the owners, directors, members of the supervisory boards, and stockholders of those chemical companies that produce the compounds in order to make big money."[37]

Propaganda in connection with the struggle of classes turned human experimentation into an issue of general appeal politically, qualifying it as the subject of repeated debates in the German parliament. In the new General German Penal Code, enacted in 1929, medical interventions were addressed specifically, and a distinction was made between therapeutic and non-therapeutic experiments. Section 263 of the code provided that "interventions and treatments that are carried out only for the purpose of healing and that are consonant with the practice of a conscientious physician and in accordance with the standards of medical care are not injuries physically in the sense of this law."[38] Only if therapeutic interventions were carried out against the explicit will of the patient – and the patient lodged a complaint against the physician – would a penalty of up to three years imprisonment be possible. In contrast, section 264 provided that nontherapeutic experiments were exempt from punishment only if they were carried out with the consent of the test subject and if they did not result in severe physical injury. Critics of the Penal Code complained that it continued to be biased in favor of the physician, based as it was on concepts such as the "practice of a conscientious physician" and on the testimony of expert witnesses who were not likely to testify against a fellow physician in court, thereby making it very difficult to convict a physician of negligence.[39]

The new Penal Code did not end the debate about experiments on human beings. On the contrary, the debate was fueled further by tragic incidents that occurred in the city of Lübeck in 1929 and 1930. On the initiative of the municipal office for public health, the director of the Lübeck General Hospital, Georg Deycke, performed vaccinations against tuberculosis in 251 newborns using Calmette's method. Parents were required to give written consent to the procedure, but the information leaflet distributed to them did not use the word "vaccination" and no mention was made of possible risks. Deycke produced the vaccine himself and accidentally contaminated it with a virulent strain of the tubercle bacillus. As a result, at least 68 infants died of tuberculosis.[40]

The "Lübeck Vaccination Scandal" was interpreted differently by different commentators. The authorities responsible spoke of it as a tragic accident, contending that the vaccinations had been necessary because of the high prevalence of tuberculosis in the region. They emphasized that the tuberculosis vaccination itself had been proven safe in more than 300,000 newborns. On the other hand, some critics referred to the vaccinations in Lübeck as a "gigantic" experiment on humans,[41] an argument that carried legitimacy because the Calmette method still was controversial. In fact, a year before the Lübeck vaccinations, the Reich's Health Council had issued a warning not to perform the Calmette vaccination until more data were available. Eminent pediatricians, such as Clemens von Pirquet of the University of Vienna, rejected the procedure on the basis of its having been assessed insufficiently;[42] others demonstrated flaws in the statistical analysis of Calmette's original data.[43, 44] Even those who initiated the vaccinations in Lübeck had acknowledged the experimental character of them when they asked parents for written consent, a practice that was not employed in those days for routine medical procedures.[45]

Julius Moses attributed the decision of authorities in Lübeck to initiate a vaccination program against tuberculosis to "local medical patriotism" and chronicled the tragic events in a polemic titled *The Death Dance of Lübeck* (Fig. 284). In his view, the only way to counter the "experimental rage" of physicians was through strict control by politicians. An alternative and self-serving solution was suggested by natural healers, namely, that they, rather than physicians, be hired solely in offices for public health. Everyone agreed that the events of

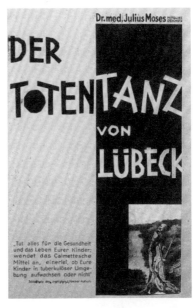

FIG. 284
Title page of the book by Julius Moses published in 1930 and titled "The Death Dance of Lübeck."

Lübeck were likely to undermine the confidence of the public in the system of health care, but representatives of official medicine ascribed this chiefly to the destructive criticism of Julius Moses, who, in turn, joined natural healers in blaming it on the mania for experimentation of practitioners of conventional medicine.[46]

The Convocation of the Reich's Health Council

As a direct reaction to the Lübeck Vaccination Scandal, the Prussian parliament passed a resolution on October 21, 1930 that called on the Reich's government to set forth more effective legal measures to restrict potentially dangerous experiments on humans.[47] The Reich's Health Council, an expert committee that advised the government on matters of health care, was commissioned to draft a decree for governing human experimentation at the federal level. Because the Council was composed of representatives of different groups within the medical

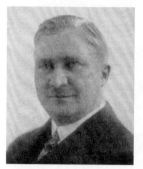

profession, the opinions about what measures were needed differed substantially. For example, Alfons Stauder (Fig. 285), the new president of the two largest German organizations of physicians – the Hartmannbund and the Ärztevereinsbund – argued that the practice of a physician had to be guided by two basic rules: 1) to do no harm, and 2) to heal. In the case of a conflict between those two demands, the decision had to be left entirely to the conscience of the responsible physician, even in experiments that were potentially dangerous. Stauder pointed out that any medical intervention could have adverse effects, depending on the circumstances and the individual patient, and, therefore, could be conceived of as experiment. Nonetheless, a physician was justified in carrying out these interventions, and the same principle had to be applied to other experiments, including nontherapeutic procedures involving persons who were not fully competent. In regard to consent of test subjects, Stauder deemed it sufficient to inform those subjects "about the extent and danger of an intervention within the limits drawn by psychological considerations." He concluded that, "No law and not even the strictest control can prevent experiments on human beings, but only the awareness of physicians about their mission and their good example."[48]

Not surprisingly, Moses expressed a different point of view and called for stricter regulation of experiments on humans. He did, however, concede the necessity of such experiments and dropped the demagogy that had characterized his previous speeches and writings. Moses also stated that a precise ethical code might be more effective than penalties imposed by law. From his vantage, experiments on humans were acceptable if they served "general medical progress and public welfare," if all other methods of research had been exhausted, and if test subjects consented to the experiment after being informed of the possible consequences in a manner that took into account their "perceptive faculties and educational level."

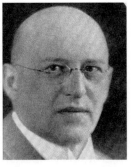

FIG. 286
Arthur Schlossmann (1867-1932)

Arthur Schlossmann (Fig. 286), chairman of the department of pediatrics at the University of Düsseldorf, stressed that scientific data should be published in a manner that did not create the impression that any unkindness had been done to test subjects. He also suggested that experiments should be admissible only under the condition "that they will, under any circumstances, be more beneficial than harmful to a patient," an unrealistic provision that hardly could be realized in practice. Friedrich von Müller, chairman of internal medicine at the University of Munich, proposed several principles for guiding human experiments, including consent of patients, weighing of consequences, careful planning, and investigation carried out in competent and responsible fashion. He concluded that a physician should perform only those experiments "that he would, after conscientious consideration, also perform on himself and his relatives, if necessary." Müller criticized suggestions by the Berlin Chamber of Physicians to create an official regulatory body to control hospitals and to approve any planned medical experiment. "I want to warn of such a measure," Müller wrote, "because such control of leading physicians of hospitals by representatives of professional organizations, the state, or local authorities would result in severe conflicts, not in the least because the definition of the term experiment, and therefore of any intervention, is extremely vague. Such a measure would paralyze the activities of physicians in hospitals and would handicap scientific work at German hospitals in comparison to other countries."[49]

Despite these differences of opinion, all members of the Reich's Health Council agreed that measures had to be taken to protect test subjects from harm medically and the medical profession itself from the consequences of unethical or questionable experiments. In an article that appeared in the *Münchener Medizinische Wochenschrift*, even Stauder, a fierce adversary of Moses, characterized some medical experiments in exaggerated, polemic phrases like these: "Naked cynicism; placing the lives of small children on the same level as those of experimental animals (rats); dubious experiments having no therapeutic purpose; science sailing under false colors; crimes against the health of defenseless children; lack of sensibility; mental and physical torture; martyrization of children in hospitals; the worst forms of charlatanism; disgustingly shameful abominations in the name of science run mad; horrors of the darkest middle ages, outstripping the infamous deeds of the inquisition and the hangman; social injustice; discrimination between the rich and the poor."[50]

The Reich's Circular Sets the Rules

Following discussion of brief presentations by Moses, Müller, Schlossmann, and Stauder at a meeting on March 14, 1930, the Reich's Health Council formulated guidelines for human experimentation. After revision by the Reich's Ministry of Justice, the guidelines were circulated by the Ministry of the Interior on February 28, 1931. In comparison with the Prussian guidelines of 1900, the *Reich's Circular* of 1931 was much more precise. It forbade specifically "exploitation of social hardship in order to undertake innovative therapy" and provided that "publications of results of innovative therapy must respect the patient's dignity and the commandments of humanity." Moreover, the *Circular* was the first document to distinguish between therapeutic and nontherapeutic research. Therapeutic research was defined as "modes of treatment of humans which serve the process of healing, i.e., pursuing in specific individual cases the recognition, healing or prevention of an illness or suffering, or the removal of a bodily defect, even though the effects and consequences of the therapy cannot yet be adequately determined on the basis of available knowledge." Nontherapeutic research was defined as "operations and modes of treatment on humans carried out for research purposes without serving a therapeutic purpose in an individual case, and whose effects and consequences cannot be adequately determined on the basis of available knowledge."

Nontherapeutic research was restricted by four provisions that exceeded the burdens placed on therapeutic research:

(a) Without consent, non-therapeutic research is under no circumstances permissible.

(b) Any human experimentation which could as well be carried out in animal experimentation is not permissible. Only after all basic information has been obtained should human experimentation begin. This information should first be obtained by means of scientific biological or laboratory research and animal experimentation for reasons of clarification and safety. Given these presuppositions, unfounded or random human experimentation is impermissible.

(c) Experimentation with children or minors is impermissible if it endangers the child or minor in the slightest degree.

(d) Experimentation with dying persons conflicts with the principles of medical ethics and therefore is impermissible.[51, 52]

In contrast with the guidelines of 1900, the Reich's Circular did not exclude completely experiments on children and adolescents. Its provisions regarding informed consent were vague; whereas "an appropriate explanation of the adverse consequences that may result from the intervention" had been demanded in the Prussian guidelines as the basis for informed consent, the Circular of 1931 left it "an expedient instruction provided in advance."[53, 54] Moreover, the distinction between therapeutic and nontherapeutic research that was adopted in many subsequent codes is problematic. In principle, experimental inquiry and therapeutic care are opposing concepts. The purpose of an experiment is the acquisition of knowledge and not the betterment of a particular test subject. If an experiment happens to be beneficial to a patient, that is welcome; it is not essential. By calling an experiment "therapeutic" a priori, an outcome that has not yet been demonstrated is presupposed. The distinction between therapeutic and nontherapeutic research was introduced to offer special protection to vulnerable groups of persons that previously were used indiscriminately for all kinds of medical experiments. Although that purpose was achieved, the distinction between therapeutic and nontherapeutic research in the Reich's Circular, and in many codes subsequently, eventually came to be used as an excuse for decreasing requirements for consent whenever researchers could claim some adjunctive therapeutic benefit.[55]

Despite these weaknesses, the *Reich's Circular* provided a much higher degree of protection for human subjects than ever before, including a risk-benefit analysis, requirement for written justification of any deviation from standard protocols, requirement for written justification for the study of particularly

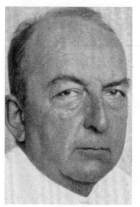

vulnerable populations, and the need to maintain written records. In many ways, the *Circular* was more comprehensive than both the subsequent Nuremberg Code in 1947 and the Declaration of Helsinki in 1964.[56, 57]

On the suggestion of council member Leopold Ritter von Zumbusch (Fig. 287), chairman of dermatology of the University of Munich, the *Circular* included a paragraph requiring that "all physicians in open or closed health care institutions should sign a commitment to these guidelines when entering their employment."[58, 59] The guidelines also were circulated to physicians working in prisons and penitentiaries, and on May 2, 1931, the Prussian Minister of Justice prohibited scientific experiments to be conducted on inmates of Prussian prisons, even if informed consent was given.[60]

The *Circular* issued in Germany by the Reich's Ministry of the Interior in 1931 was not enforceable by law. Nevertheless, it provided precise instructions for experiments on humans and, in conjunction with the General Penal Code of 1929, it gave Germany the most advanced rules in the world, by far, concerning experimentation on human beings.

CHAPTER 13

FROM THE BEST
TO THE WORST

S hortly after the promulgation of the German guidelines of 1931, French bacteriologist and Nobel laureate, Charles-Jean-Henri Nicolle (Fig. 288), criticized not only non-therapeutic experiments in humans, but also the regulations designed to control them. He argued that in regard to dubious experimentation, "once the first step is accepted, there will be no border, there can be no border on the march forward."[1]

Considering what happened in Germany in the ensuing years, Nicolle's remarks were prescient. But was there, as Nicolle seemed to suggest, truly a causal relationship between the best ethical code and the worst atrocities in the history of experimentation on humans? Of course not! The outrageous experiments performed by Nazi physicians in German concentration and extermination camps were conducted in spite of, not because of, the guidelines of 1931, which, parenthetically, remained in effect throughout the entire period of Nazi reign. The only relationship between the guidelines and the subsequent atrocities was that both were consequences of a general tendency in medicine to disregard the health of individual patients either for the sake of progress in science or for the advancement of an individual career. That tendency was most pronounced in the country with the most advanced medical system, namely, the German Reich. The guidelines of 1931 were like a dam built to withstand the force of these tendencies. When the dam could no longer contain them, it burst and the most terrible experiments ensued.

The Superiority of Genes

What were the factors that caused the dam to burst? There were many. First and foremost was the unhesitating belief in the superiority of certain human beings and the inferiority of others. This sentiment, as old as mankind, was heightened by the colonialism and imperialism of the late nineteenth century and acquired now a distinctly racial thrust. At the same time, Darwinism was fomenting, albeit somewhat innocently, the belief in differences in the value of human beings. Black Africans, for example, were thought to be much more closely related to apes than were Caucasians, a view supported by claims of anatomical differences among the races by serious scientists. When the anatomist Paul Schiefferdecker of the University of Bonn (Fig. 289) identified apocrine glands for the first time, he insisted that they occurred in decreasing density in animals, Negroes, and Caucasians, in that order. He attributed this phenomenon to a more advanced state of biological development of Caucasians, implying that Blacks had less value than Whites.[2] Differences in value, however, also were recognized among the various groups of Caucasians, and the idea was advanced that the quality of a race could be enhanced by restricting the birth

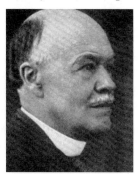

FIG. 288
*Charles Nicolle
(1866-1936)*

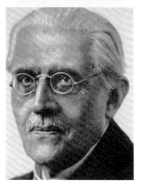

FIG. 289
*Paul
Schiefferdecker
(1849-1931)*

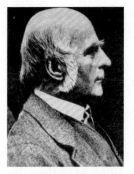

FIG. 290
Francis Galton
(1822-1911)

rate of the "unfit" and increasing reproduction of the "fit." These ideas, first proposed by Sir Francis Galton (Fig. 290), an English scientist and a cousin of Charles Darwin, were promulgated under terms such as "eugenics" and "racial hygiene," designations that soon became popular in many countries.[3]

"Fit" and "unfit" did not refer only to diseases of established genetic character, but to attributes of individuals as well. For example, a high level of education meant "fit," and poor education, low economic status, criminality, alcoholism, and prostitution meant "unfit." Each of these characteristics was thought to spring directly from the genetic make-up of a person. The relatively low birth rate among the upper classes compared with that of the lower classes was perceived, therefore, as a major threat to society and to all mankind. German dermatologist Hermann Werner Siemens (Fig. 291), remembered to this day for his characterization of one type of *epidermolysis bullosa dystrophica*, was one of many representatives of medicine who warned that "the best of human heredity will be swamped with a mess of inferior types" unless the ever rising tide of human beings of poor quality was stemmed.[4]

No developed nation was exempt from those fears. For example, American president Theodore Roosevelt (Fig. 292) referred to the reproduction of persons of "good blood" as the "warfare of the cradle."[5] In America, concerns about the declining quality of the population were aggravated by continuous immigration from other countries. Traditionally, the United States had thought of itself as a "melting pot" of peoples, and

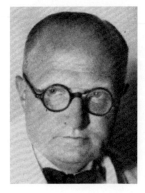

FIG. 291
Hermann Werner Siemens
(1891-1969)

13 · From the Best to the Worst

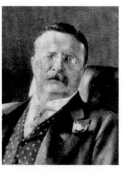

in the Broadway play of 1908, *The Melting Pot* by an English playwright and
ardent Zionist, Israel Zangwill, "the
real American" as portrayed by one of
the characters, was to be "the fusion of
all races, the coming Superman."[6] The
concept of a melting pot, however, applied only to the "German and French-
man, the Irishman and Englishman,
Jews and Russians"[7] – that is, to white Europeans. Asians and
Africans were not welcome in the pot. In 1916, Madison Grant,
a well known racist, in his bestseller, *The Passing of the Great
Race*, argued that America, through unrestricted immigration,
had nearly "succeeded in destroying the privileges of birth; that
is, the intellectual and moral advantages a man of good stock
brings into the world with him." Grant further warned that because the virtues of the "higher races" were "highly unstable"
they were certain to disappear altogether "when mixed with
generalized or primitive characters."[8] The first World War exacerbated these xenophobic tendencies. In the 1920s, a quota system for immigration to the United States was enacted, capping
entry from any one country to two percent of persons born
there, banning all Asians, and favoring northern and western
Europeans at the expense of Slavs and persons from Mediter-
ranean countries.[9]

Eradication of Genetic Flaws and the Rise of Nazism

Restriction on immigration was not the only measure taken to
secure "good blood" for the American people. Another was the
sterilization of citizens deemed to be inferior. This assault on
the rights of an individual was justified by the audacious claim
of the American Breeders Association that "society must look

upon germ plasm as belonging to society and not solely to the individual who carries it." Sterilization of "inferior types" was touted as being cost-effective, not associated with serious medical sequelae, and efficacious in reducing by half, within three or four generations, the number of mentally defective persons in a community.[10] In 1907, the state of Indiana was the first to pass a law allowing compulsory sterilization of the mentally ill and the criminally insane. By the late 1920s, 28 states of the United States and one province in Canada had enacted legislation that, before the year 1930 arrived, resulted in sterilization of some 15,000 men and women. North America's laws served as models for the National Socialist government that took power in Germany in 1933, and the Nazis often quoted those laws in support of their own policies.[11]

Under the Nazi regime, enforced sterilization acquired another dimension, qualitatively and quantitatively. Qualitatively, sterilization was performed more arbitrarily and ruthlessly. The least deviation of a person from the norms of society could result in sterilization, and the threat of enforced sterilization was used commonly to coerce cooperative behavior. Decisions about sterilizations were made by special genetic health courts in hearings that took place outside the scrutiny of the public and that lasted, on average, five minutes. The persons to be sterilized often had to be dragged to those hearings by the police, and, beginning in 1936, they were denied the right to lodge a protest or complaint against a sentence. Only about 10 percent of requests for sterilization were rejected, the reason being that the accuser and the judge often were one and the same person. Consequently, enforced sterilization in Germany reached enormous dimensions, with about 200,000 sterilizations having been carried out between 1934 and 1936. Representatives of racial hygiene estimated that about 10 percent of the German population would need to be sterilized because of "genetic flaws"[12] (Fig. 293).

13 · From the Best to the Worst

The belief that genetic flaws had to be eradicated from humankind was another factor that contributed to large-scale human experimentation under the Nazis. A patient with a genetic disease no longer was considered an individual; only the population at large was of concern to eugenicists. This shift in ethics affected medicine in its entirety and corresponded precisely with the

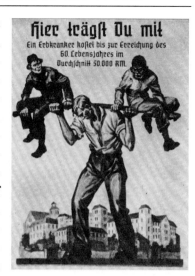

advent of National Socialism. In the view of the Nazis, an individual was not in the least important; all that mattered was the community of the people, which had to be kept pure, sound, and healthy, even if that meant eradication of some of its own members. To this end, enforced sterilization came to be seen as insufficient. With the beginning of World War II, the Nazis established a killing program, referred to euphemistically as "euthanasia." Any person who had been ill for five years or more and was unable to work had to be reported to the government. Decisions about who was to be killed were based entirely on questionnaires that included such items as name, race, marital status, nationality, frequency of visitors and who the visitors were. These questionnaires were assessed by physicians who never actually saw the patients themselves. The condemned patients were carried off to killing centers to be gassed and their corpses burned under the supervision of physicians. Between September 1939 and August 1941, more than 70,000 patients were eliminated in this manner. It was calculated that removal of these unfit specimens from the wards saved not only the master race, but also the hospitals about "245,955.50 Reichmarks per day" or "88,543,980.00 Reichmarks per year." From the vantage of the Nazis, these numbers justified the killings; to them, the euthanasia program was the equivalent of a successful surgical procedure that restored health to the community of the people by eradicating worthless, wholly parasitic elements.[13, 14]

In the eyes of the Nazis, however, there were even more dangerous parasites dwelling in the flesh of the German race, namely, the Jews. According to Hitler, Jews were "bacilli," ever ready to "poison the blood of the national body." Leonardo Conti, the Reich's Health Leader, contended that Jews could only survive "parasitically inside the people." Rudolf Ramm, a medical officer on Conti's staff, wrote that Jews put the German people at risk through "the contagion of poisonous ideas and the destruction of germinating life." Being Jewish, in itself, was thought to be a disease and, therefore, the wholesale killing of Jews qualified as "euthanasia" (Fig. 294). It was carried out by the same personnel who directed the killing of mentally disabled patients and with the same rationale. One of the Auschwitz killer physicians, Fritz Klein, explained to a female inmate (also a physician) that because he himself was a medical

FIG. 294
Nazi cartoon comparing Jews to infectious organisms. The text reads: "With his poison, the Jew undermines the sluggish blood of weak peoples so that a disease arises that causes deterioration rapidly. With us, however, the diagnosis is different: The blood is pure. We are healthy!"

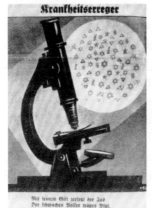

man, he wanted "to preserve life." It was "out of the respect for human life" that he would "remove a gangrenous appendix from a diseased body. The Jew is the gangrenous appendix in the body of mankind."[15] Without the belief that it was justifiable, or even virtuous, to eradicate human beings deemed to be inferior, the outright slaughter and ruthless medical experiments in German concentration camps would have been unthinkable.

13 · From the Best to the Worst

Atrocities for the "Greater Good"

Another important factor in the mindset of the Nazis, including physicians, was the belief that any action was justifiable as long as it served a "greater good." For the Nazis, the greater good was power – power for themselves and for the great nation they aspired to build. In order to acquire, maintain, and enhance power, any deception or cruelty was permissible. Eventually, this included the arrest and murder of former allies, such as Ernst Röhm, founder and commander of Hitler's "Brown Shirts," and other leading officers of the storm troops. In the name of the greater good, a never-ending series of blatant lies and shameless violations of contracts was propagated (Fig. 295).

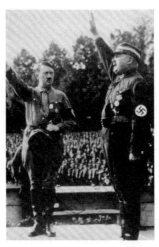

FIG. 295
In 1934, Adolf Hitler (left) ordered the murder of high-ranking members of the stormtroops, including their leader Ernst Röhm (right), one of his oldest companions.

The unconditional striving for power at the expense of such traditional concepts of morality as honesty and decency had a firm intellectual foundation. Many Germans, and other nationalities as well, were influenced by the writings of philosopher Friedrich Wilhelm Nietzsche (Fig. 296), who idealized power. "What is good?" he asked in his book *The Anti-Christ*, to which he answered thus: "All that heightens the feeling of power, the will to power, power itself in man. What is bad? – All that proceeds from weakness. What is happiness? – The feeling that power increases – that a resistance is overcome."[16] Words such as these

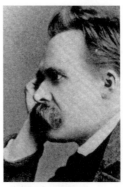

FIG. 296
Friedrich Nietzsche (1844-1890)

served as excuses for violations of principles of morality. The Nazis differed from their political opponents in their utter disgust for weakness and in their ruthless exercise of strength. Nietzsche reasoned that "to require of strength that it should *not* express itself as strength, that it should *not* be a desire to conquer, a desire to subdue, a desire to become master, a thirst for enemies and resistances and triumphs, is just as absurd as to require from weakness that it should express itself as strength."[17] The desire to use strength to acquire power, said Nietzsche, could only be "carried through at the expense of smaller powers. The magnitude of an 'advance' is even to be measured by the mass of things that had to be sacrificed to it; mankind in the mass sacrificed to the prosperity of a single stronger species of man – that would be an advance."[18]

That was exactly the kind of advance to which the Nazis aspired, and for which they were ready to sacrifice mankind *en masse*. Just as the writings of Darwin had unwittingly prepared the ground for fanatics of racial hygiene, the writings of Nietzsche provided rich soil for the uninhibited exercise of strength. With this background, the strength and unscrupulousness of the Nazis impressed, rather than repelled, a large part of the German people, many physicians among them. For example, medical historian Georg Sticker of Würzburg (Fig. 297), who described and named *erythema infectiosum*, wrote

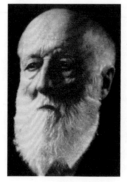

FIG. 297
*Georg Sticker
(1860-1960)*

with unbridled enthusiasm in the prestigious *Münchener Medizinische Wochenschrift* that "A Führer has arisen who has a strong will and speaks out about what we have to want and ought to do, unconcerned with the whimpering of a false, hypocritical humanity. If the German people, says Adolf Hitler, want to recover and continue to live, it . . . must not have ears for the weaklings who cry and bemoan interferences in the holy rights of men."[19]

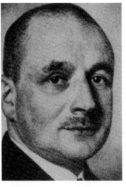

FIG. 298
*Walther
Schultze
(1893-1970)*

In all arenas of life, drastic and unreasonable measures that would have been inconceivable in the days of the Republic were taken by the Nazis on behalf of the greater good. As an example, Walther Schultze (Fig. 298), head of dermatology at the University of Giessen, established a labor camp for "anti-social venereal disease patients." These patients were confined compulsorily, subjected to what Schultze called "the therapy of work," and released only after they had shown signs of "good conduct." "By manual work," Schultze wrote, "the incarcerated subjects shall contribute to reduce the burden of the public to a minimum. By severe physical strain, we want to put those with an aversion to work on another track, to discipline them, and also to achieve a deterrent effect on others."[20] When Schultze reported on this new "mode of treatment" in 1936 in the respected journal, *Dermatologische Wochenschrift (Dermatologic Weekly)*, he offered the following rationale for his novel mode of therapy: "Physicians must no longer content themselves with treating venereal disease patients more or less successfully, but have to attack the evil actively at its roots. Many say that this is impossible, so why engage oneself? That is not National Socialist thinking. We recognize the enemy and attack him, wherever we find him."[21] For Schultze, the greater good was the eradication of venereal diseases, and the measures he initiated to that end – incarceration of patients in a labor camp – would have been thought to be impossible a few years earlier. During the period of the war soon to ensue, the greater good for medical researchers consisted of medical progress and the maintenance of the health of German soldiers. The measures taken to ensure that these two goals were achieved also would have been considered "impossible" a few years earlier, among those measures being large-scale human experimentation that led directly to the deaths of many test subjects.

Rewards for Physicians

Another factor that induced physicians to embrace the Nazi cause was rewards offered for both individuals and the profession as a whole. As a group, physicians profited immensely from the new government. Although the Nazis were sympathetic to natural healers and advocates of a "new German healing" based on exposure to sun, wind, and the gifts of the German soil, and although they derided "official medicine" with its emphasis on mechanisms of disease and disturbances of particular organs as "Jewified medicine," the Nazi government established physicians as the only recognized source for all things truly medical. A powerful new association, the Reich's Chamber of Physicians, was created to organize medical education and supervise medical services; membership in it was compulsory for every practicing physician in Germany. Another new organization, the German Panel Fund Physicians' Union (Kassenärztliche Vereinigung Deutschlands, or KVD), furthered the interests of physicians in private practice by taking over negotiations with public health insurance payers. The ambulatories that had been brought forth by the Weimar Republic were closed; the days of "socialized medicine" were over.[22]

In fact, most of the hopes of the old professional medical organizations were realized. Although these organizations were merged into the National Socialist Physicians' League, their onetime leaders supported the Nazis. On March 22, 1933, Alfons Stauder, president of the Hartmannbund and Deutscher Ärztevereinsbund, telegraphed Hitler that "the principal professional organizations in Germany gladly welcome the firm determination of the Government of National Renewal to build

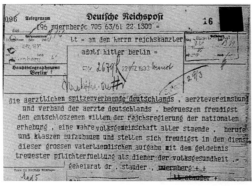

FIG. 299
Telegram of Adolf Stauder to Adolf Hitler proclaiming to him the loyalty of German physicians, dated March 22, 1933.

a true community of all ranks, professions, and classes, and they gladly place themselves at the service of this great patriotic task"[23] (Fig. 299). The former executive director of the Hartmannbund, Karl Haedenkamp, boldly proclaimed that "to serve this state must be the sole objective of the medical profession. We are aware of the duties that we have to fulfill on its behalf. Insofar as we carry them out, we shall earn the right to have our work respected."[24]

A condition for earning the "respect" of the new government – which translated into good will in regard to one's own personal aspirations – was complete subordination to the objectives of the government. Haedenkamp was ready to accept that condition, both as a leading representative of physicians and as a man. Privately, he continued his career in the Reich's Cham-

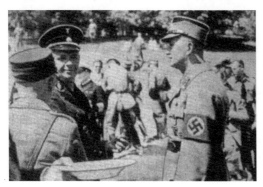

FIG. 300
Karl Haedenkamp (middle) at the inauguration of the "school for leaders of German medicine" (Führerschule der Deutschen Ärzteschaft) in 1935.

ber of Physicians and was instrumental in ousting many Jewish doctors from the practice of medicine (Fig. 300). Following World War II and the fall of the Third Reich, Haedenkamp – a masterful politician – became president of the new German Chamber of Physicians. In contrast, his old adversary, Julius Moses, a socialist and a Jew, was deprived first of the right to work as a physician, then of most of his personal belongings, and finally of his life. In 1942, at the age of 74, Moses was taken to the concentration camp at Theresienstadt, where he soon died of starvation[25] (Fig. 301).

The ridding of Jews from the medical profession was referred to by Haedenkamp as an "employment enhancing strategy."[26] In fact, the strategy led to the creation of thousands of vacant positions that the government dangled as rewards for cooperative behavior. Unemployed physicians who had joined the storm troops before Hitler's ascent to power learned to their delight that they were eligible for immediate placement on insurance-fund panels (Fig. 302). At many universities, contracts were renewed only for members of the Nazi party, and appointments to department chairs were almost impossible to obtain without evidences of active participation in the National Socialist movement.[27] Unemployment among physicians no longer existed (except for Jews and political opponents of the Nazis), and the income of physicians rapidly reached levels higher than ever before (Fig. 303).

FIG. 301
Letter to Dr. Julius Moses on November 18, 1941, informing him of the expropriation of his "furniture, other household belongings, textile fabrics, shoes, bicycles."

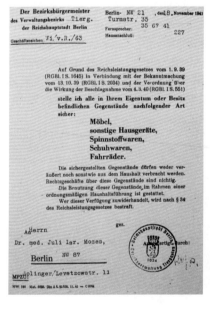

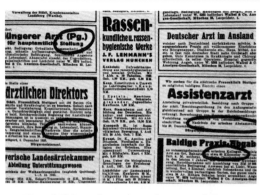

FIG. 302
Advertisement for physicians in a German newspaper following the ousting of their Jewish colleagues. A precondition for even applying for a position was proof of Aryan descent and sometimes membership in the Nazi party (Pg.=Parteigenosse).

The shifting fortunes of most of those in the medical field was accompanied by a swift economic recovery of the German Reich and an equally rapid regaining of its political and military power. Most Germans felt that their country had been humiliated greatly and treated unfairly by the victorious powers of the First World War. The refusal of the Nazis to pay any more reparations or to comply with the restrictions on armaments imposed on Germany by the Treaty of Versailles symbolized resurrection of the nation. Investments in the armed forces helped decrease the unemployment rate from more than six million people in 1933 to fewer than one million by the end of 1937.[28] Popular measures instituted by the Nazis included construction of highways, dispensing of radios *gratis*, provision of inexpensive vacations for workers, and, as one of the first legal

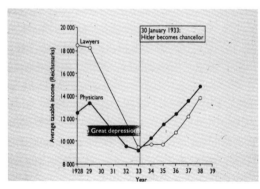

FIG. 303
Graph of income of German physicians compared to that of German lawyers.

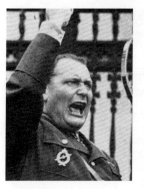

FIG. 304
Hermann
Göring
(1882-1946)

initiatives, promulgation of new regulations concerning experiments on animals. Protection of animals was said to be "a measuring stick for the culture of a nation." When, on August 16, 1933, Prussian Prime Minister Hermann Göring (Fig. 304) forbade "vivisection of animals of all kinds," he earned enthusiastic thanks from animal protectionists. The regulations subsequently were relaxed somewhat, but the Reich's Law for Animal Protection, published on November 24, 1933, insured that approval be obtained from the Reich's Ministry of the Interior for all experiments on animals and that "the animal species used, and the purpose, methods, and results of the experiments" be documented precisely.[29]

Physicians for Hitler

Many factors were instrumental in the wide support enjoyed by the Nazis among the general population and, even more so, among physicians. No other profession was affiliated as closely with National Socialism as was medicine. Nearly half of all German physicians were members of the Nazi party: 26 percent of male physicians belonged to the storm troops (the SA or "Brown Shirts") and seven percent were in the "defense corps" (the SS or "Black Shirts").[30] The active participation of so many physicians in the Nazi movement explains why cruel medical experiments could be carried out on inmates of concentration and extermination camps without their being challenged, and why those experiments could be reported on in respected medical journals and presented at medical congresses with impunity.

A stunning example of unethical medical experimentation run amok was a series of studies concerning the efficacy of sulfonamides in treating deliberately infected inmates of the Ravensbrück camp, a project that was described in vivid detail in May 1943 at a meeting of the Academy for Military Medicine (Militärärztliche Akademie) in Berlin. Most of the elite of German medicine registered for that meeting, including the well known surgeon, Ferdinand Sauerbruch (Fig. 305); pharmacologists Wolfgang Heubner (Fig. 306) and Ferdinand Flury; psychiatrists Max de Crinis and Otto Wuth; and dermatologists Karl Zieler (Fig. 307), Heinrich Löhe, Heinrich Adolf Gottron (Fig. 308), Alois Memmesheimer (Fig. 309), Walter Frieboes (Fig. 310), and Josef Vonkennel.[31] In a brief introduction, the leading clinician of the SS and a childhood friend of Himmler, Karl Gebhardt, informed the audience that he accepted "the full human, surgical, and political responsibility for these experiments." Following presentation of the sulfonamide study by Gebhardt's assistant, Fritz Ernst Fischer (Fig. 311), its results were discussed by participants.[32] No one voiced any ethical concerns, although Fischer had left no doubt that the experiments had been carried out nonvoluntarily in people incarcerated in a concentration camp, and that several of them had died as a consequence of the experiments.[33]

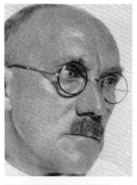

FIG. 305
*Ferdinand
Sauerbruch
(1875-1951)*

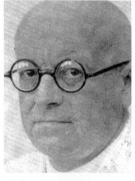

FIG. 306
*Wolfgang
Heubner
(1877-1957)*

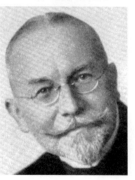

FIG. 307
*Karl Zieler
(1874-1945)*

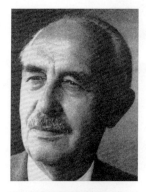

FIG. 308
*Heinrich Adolf
Gottron
(1890-1974)*

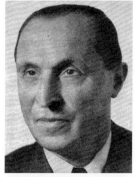

FIG. 309
*Alois
Memmesheimer
(1894-1973)*

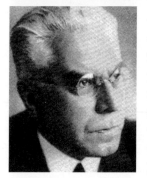

FIG. 310
*Walter
Frieboes
(1880-1945)*

This account does not necessarily indicate that all members of the audience approved of the experiments. Some may have been bothered by them, but one thing is certain – no one had the courage to speak out against them. Lack of moral courage and strict obedience to authority were qualities shared by most German physicians, virtually all of whom had been exposed to authoritarian strictures their entire lives and had come to succeed, in large part, by adapting to them. Raised mostly by highly conservative parents, indoctrinated with nationalism and militarism during their school years, and completely dependent on their department chairs for work as medical assistants, most German physicians had never developed the habit of expressing their own convictions or challenging their superiors.[34] Moreover, they knew that protesting against experiments in humans would be of no avail, the only effect being negative consequences for themselves. The leader of the SS and the Reich's Minister of the Interior, Heinrich Himmler, had stated explicitly that he would regard anybody who challenged the right to conduct experiments on humans at a time when German soldiers were losing their lives as being "guilty of high treason."[35] Failure to oppose dubious experiments in humans resulted from fear that was well founded. Even supporters of the Nazi government knew, full well, that they were not living in a state founded on a constitution and that severe penalties were likely in the case of any perceived misconduct or disloyalty to Hitler.

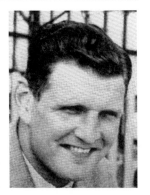

FIG. 311
*Fritz Ernst
Fischer
(born 1912)*

Physicians who, in private, rejected experiments on humans, acquiesced in public. Instead of following their conscience, they tried to soothe it by turning a blind eye to what was going on and repressing what they knew. They resorted to selective, euphemistic, and inaccurate modes of perception. These psychological props were ubiquitous in Nazi Germany, where the killing of chronically ill patients was termed "euthanasia," the transportation of Jews to concentration and extermination camps was referred to as "resettlement," and the wholesale annihilation of the Jewish people was called the "final solution."[36] In like manner, prisoners used for medical studies were designated "patients," and when they died, it was not because of their having been murdered brutally as a consequence of the experiments, but because of "weakness of the heart and circulation." Persons that the SS provided as test subjects for medical experiments were referred to as "criminals sentenced to death," even though many of them were innocent children.[37] Desperate prisoners who offered themselves for experiments in order to get more food and avoid dying of inanition were said to be "willing volunteers."[38] In medical journals, many experiments on humans were passed off as experiments on animals.[39] Even when the use of humans as subjects of research was acknowledged, it was excused by invoking the pressing need of experiments for the progress of science and the welfare of all mankind. Some articles included hypocritical and pious remarks about ethical aspects of experiments in humans. For example, in 1943, geneticists Hans Nachtsheim and Gerhard Ruhenstroth-Bauer, both members of the prestigious Kaiser Wilhelm Institute in Berlin, exposed epileptic children to low pressures of oxygen that were potentially lethal. In their article on *The Role of Oxygen Deficiency in Producing Epileptic Attacks*, their ethical shield read as follows: "For the physician working experimentally with patients, the methodical possibilities are always limited; he has to consider the welfare of the patient. Only exceptionally, in the interest of future patients, a researcher may dare to subject a patient to an experiment whose outcome cannot be foretold with certainty."[40]

In summary, the belief that some human beings are inferior, that eradication of these humans is justifiable or even virtuous, and that the uninhibited exercise of power is acceptable if it serves a greater good, contributed to the collapse of the dam that had been built by the architects of the Weimar Republic to contain the rush of unethical experimentation on humans. So, too, did other factors, such as professional and personal rewards offered by the Nazis, fear of disrupting the established chain of order and obedience, and effective disguise of the nature of the atrocities committed in the name of science. The most important reason for large-scale experiments in human beings by German physicians during the war, however, was the current itself, that is, the curiosity of physicians and their desire to test their ideas, to build their careers, and to add their names to the list of medical pioneers. When these tendencies no longer were held in check, the country that had propounded the most advanced regulations concerning human experimentation became the testing ground of some of the worst atrocities in the history of medical research.

CHAPTER 14

MEDICAL RESEARCH UNDER THE NAZIS

T housands of experiments of both pitiless nature and questionable value were performed in humans prior to the regime of Nazism in Germany. But it is the body of research carried out in the name of the Third Reich that is linked inextricably to such words as "barbaric," "sadism," and "atrocity." What made the experiments in humans under the Nazis so heinous and abominable? First, they were carried out on a scale of proportions so enormous that they defy belief. Second, many of them were of cruelty unparalleled in the annals of history. And third, the circumstances under which they were conducted were horrendous to actualization of the worst nightmares of hell. Test subjects were deprived of any remnant of human dignity and reduced to repositories that could be used at will and then discarded. Whether or not test subjects survived the experiments, their fate had been sealed; they had been sentenced to death for the crime of mere existence. Their only claim on life was their utility: inmates of Nazi concentration and extermination camps were allowed to survive briefly if they could be exploited for work or for medical research (Fig. 312).

Those inmates who did not meet those criteria were killed without delay. Rudolf Höss (Fig. 313), commander of the Auschwitz concentration camp, described the process of determining life or death in these matter-of-fact words:

FIG. 312
Corpses of Jews
in an extermi-
nation camp.

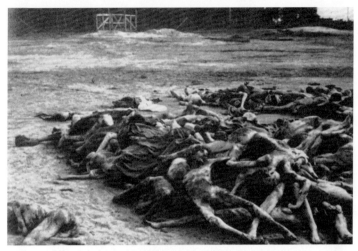

FIG. 312
Corpses of Jews
in an extermi-
nation camp.

Men and women are separated from one another first. Both columns are standing on the ramp. Now the SS physician begins to separate those able to work from those whom he considers unable to work. Those good for work were sent into the camp. Others were sent to the extermination facilities immediately. Children of tender age were exterminated without exception because, on account of their youth, they were unable to work.[1]

Only about 10 percent of the arrivals at Auschwitz were sent to the work camp or pulled aside for medical experiments. The remainder were instructed to undress, remove their jewelry, and tie their shoes together (in order to ensure that pairs could

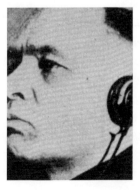

FIG. 313
Rudolf Höss
(1900-1947)

be matched easily for use later). They then were hurried past lines of auxiliary police to the gas chambers, which were camouflaged as shower rooms. Packed in, one person per square foot, they were gassed until all were dead. The corpses were tossed out and burned immediately to make room for the next trainload of arrivals, which was not far behind[2] (Fig. 314).

14 · Medical Research Under the Nazis

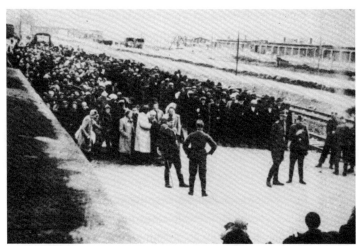

FIG. 314
*Jews being
lined up,
women and
girls on the left
and men and
boys on the
right, for "selec-
tion" at the
railway sta-
tion of the ex-
termination
camp at
Auschwitz.*

It was a "privilege" to be selected a worker or a test subject, that boon consisting of being housed in crowded, filthy barracks shared with lice and fleas beyond number, given rations so meager that everyone suffered severe emaciation, forced to stand naked in the cold and rain for hours, beaten and whipped, denied sleep, and made to perform brutally hard manual labor for 15 to 18 hours a day (Fig. 315, 316). As if this were not enough, prisoners were entirely dependent on the mood of their guards, be they officers of the SS, block leaders, or members of various lower ranks. The latter included the auxiliary police, made up of former Ukrainian prisoners-of-war and other prisoners who had been chosen to enforce obedience and maintain order among their fellow inmates, and to assist in the organization of labor, research, and killing. Invested with tremendous power, these men and women of all ranks often gave way readily to sadistic tendencies. Prisoners were used as personal slaves to wash their masters' feet, clean their boots, laugh at their jokes, and tolerate silently all kinds of physical abuse and psychological denigration.[3] In order to counter boredom, guards often forced prisoners to perform exhausting or humiliating acts, such as senseless physical exercises, or used them as targets for practice in shooting exercises that were judged to be successful only if prisoners were wounded or killed.[4]

Not all human experimentation was carried out on prisoners of concentration and extermination camps. The army, for example, resorted often to using inmates of psychiatric hospitals and prisoners-of-war as test subjects because research in the camps required the approval of the SS. An atmosphere of terror, how-

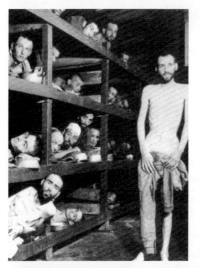

FIG. 315
Barracks of the concentration camp at Buchenwald.

ever, shrouded all experiments, no matter where they were performed. If subjects were not cooperative, they were informed bluntly that they would be killed on the spot.[5]

Experimentation differed not only in regard to the branches of the German forces who conducted them and to the test subjects recruited for them, but also in regard to the

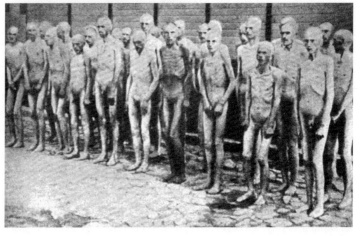

FIG. 316
Prisoners being forced to stand naked in the cold for hours.

subject matter and scientific value of it. In general, the research conducted by the SS was of the lowest quality and had the least value, in part because SS physicians simply were not as good as those affiliated with the army and the air force (Luftwaffe). Only the latter organizations could recruit physicians at will from the universities, whereas in at least the first years of the war the SS was made up entirely of volunteers. For a medical career in the SS, political, rather than academic, merit was most important. In addition, the SS had a virtually limitless supply of test subjects, and, as a result, experiments tended to be performed hurriedly, chiefly to make use of the opportunity available, rather than as steps in a carefully planned study.

The consequences, of course, were severe flaws in the conduct and interpretation of experiments by the SS. In some instances, test subjects were used for several experiments concurrently, thereby muddying the results. One person, for example, might be used at the same time for experimental infections with malaria and tests of liver function.[6] The pathetic physical state of test subjects often precluded meaningful interpretation of data. Such was the case with results from studies about treatment of malaria induced in patients who suffered from active, naturally acquired tuberculosis.[7] Experiments in humans often were not part of a controlled study but were performed simply to satisfy the curiosity of a single physician. For example, Johann Paul Kremer, director of the Institute of Anatomy of the University of Münster, had written his thesis for habilitation about "changes of muscle tissue secondary to starvation." When he was assigned for two and a half months to the extermination camp at Auschwitz as a substitute for a camp physician, he used his time there to add proof to his theories. Emaciated prisoners had to inform him about their original weight, and they then were killed by injections into the heart of phenol so that Kremer could collect and study their muscles.[8] Even physicians who themselves were prisoners and were forced to assist in research

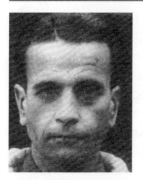

and killing sometimes could not withstand the lure of experimenting on human subjects. The Polish psychiatrist Zenon Drohocki, for example, while incarcerated at Auschwitz, constructed a device for electroshock in order to study its effects in his fellow prisoners.[9]

Poor standardization of methods and insufficient numbers of appropriate experiments invalidated statistical analyses of the research. Waldemar Hoven (Fig. 317), SS physician at the Buchenwald concentration camp, based his thesis about treatment of pulmonary tuberculosis by inhalation of coal dust on his research at the camp. In the introduction, he averred that "a true decision about the unresolved problems can only be based on experiments on humans." Thirty-three "patients" recruited for his study had to inhale coal dust; 10 other prisoners with tuberculosis served as controls. Three members in the treatment group and two in the control group died, that is, were killed, after exactly 10 or 25 days, those specific times being chosen to enable Hoven to "tidy up" his study with the results of autopsies. Additional experiments on 18 patients followed, but a valid statistical analysis of the study was impossible. Incredibly, Hoven concluded that inhalation of coal dust was an effective treatment for pulmonary tuberculosis and his thesis was judged to be "very good" by the medical faculty of the University of Freiburg.[10]

The Elimination of the Fatal Genetic Find

The substandard quality of studies conducted by the SS was due, in large part, to the ideological background of those who performed them. The SS was interested chiefly in studies that corresponded to and validated its own warped views of the world. The impact of racial factors on the soundness of the population was vastly overemphasized, and genetics were thought to be of prime importance in disease, even in infectious processes such as tuberculosis. When SS physician, Kurt Heissmeyer, sought to prove the dominance of genetic factors in the pathogenesis of tuberculosis by inoculating tubercle bacilli into the skin and bronchi of test subjects, he was granted immediate approval by his superiors. Heissmeyer explained the necessity of those experiments in appropriate Nazi terminology thus:

Following the establishment of the ideological concept of 'people and race' it no longer is tenable to explain the pathogenesis of tuberculosis through experiments on animals because, in that instance, the role of the constitution for the development of tuberculosis is either denied, or the constitution of the animal is equated with that of a human being.[11]

The Nazi ideology of "people and race" was intertwined with popular concepts about natural healing such as "biological diets" and bathing in water of increasing temperatures, all of which were thought to "enable the organism to restore its inner order."[12] Coupled with these beliefs was contempt for official medicine and its seemingly impersonal modes of treatment. Many leading Nazis were proponents of natural healing, among them the Führer's Deputy, Rudolf Hess, and the head of the SS and the Gestapo, Heinrich Himmler (Fig. 318). Himmler reserved for himself all decisions about experiments on humans by the SS and was a major influence in the recruitment of subjects for research. Any absurd study was allowed if it suited Himmler's notions about health and disease.

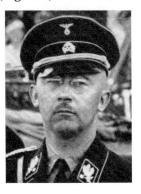

FIG. 318
*Heinrich
Himmler
(1900-1945)*

Himmler was a believer in the validity and effectiveness of "biochemical therapy," a mode of treatment based on the assumption that diseases result from disturbances in the equilibrium of salts within tissue and that these disturbances can be corrected by application of the deficient salts in homeopathic dilutions. To prove that concept, 40 inmates of the Dachau concentration camp who suffered from phlegmon or sepsis, were treated with biochemical agents. All of those with sepsis died. The top physician of the SS, Ernst Grawitz, informed Himmler of these preliminary results, pointing out that "a therapeutic effect on the course of the disease could not be observed" and suggesting that the experiments be terminated. Himmler's response was harsh. "I am convinced," he wrote in a letter to Grawitz in September 1942, "that you, having been granted the title of professor and, if I am not mistaken, making use of it with great pleasure, will find in these experiments an opportunity to make a scientific contribution and lay belatedly the foundation of that title."[13] Grawitz, who later was credited with having proposed gas chambers as an efficient method for achieving the "Final Solution," got the message. At Himmler's insistence, biochemical therapy continued to be studied at Dachau. Forty more test subjects, most of them Polish clergymen, had pus injected into their skin and veins, and then were treated either with sulfonamides or with biochemical agents. Most of the subjects in the latter group soon were dead.[14]

In order to improve the quality of the "people's community" by preventing propagation of inferior human beings, the SS conducted extensive research on methods of sterilization that could be used on a mass scale. In a letter to Himmler, dermatologist Adolf Pokorny proposed to study the effects of caladium sequinum, a drug obtained from a North American plant. His appeal to Himmler could not have been more compelling: "If, on the basis of this research, it were possible to produce a drug which, after a relatively short time, effects an imperceptible sterilization of human beings, then we would have a powerful new weapon at our disposal. The thought alone that the 3 million Bolsheviks, who are at present German prisoners, could be sterilized so that they could be used as laborers but be prevented from reproduction, opens the most far-reaching perspectives."[15] As a result of Pokorny's suggestion, a number of experiments were conducted on internees at concentration and extermination camps for the purpose of testing the effec-

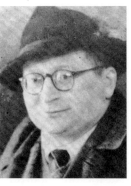

FIG. 319
*Carl Clauberg
(1898-1957)*

tiveness of caladium sequinum. Other methods of sterilization tried on prisoners included irradiation of the genitalia with X-rays and injection of them with irritating solutions. The most wide-ranging experiments were performed by gynecologist Carl Clauberg (Fig. 319) who, in the late 1920s, had made important contributions to the production synthetically of female sex hormones (progesterone). Clauberg was director of a department of gynecology in Königshütte, a small city in Upper Silesia not far from Auschwitz.[16] In the summer of 1942, at his own request, he began to experiment with forms of sterilization using inmates of that camp, eventually sterilizing several thousand Jews and Gypsies. In 1943, Clauberg informed Himmler that, using injections of supercooled carbon dioxide, he could sterilize 1,000 women per day with a staff of only 10 men.[17]

The Heritage of Ancestors – Research in Support of Nazi Ideas

The SS had its own organization for research, by the name of Heritage of Ancestors (Ahnenerbe). Fields of research under its auspices ranged from history to classic philology and from geology to entomology. In each of those arenas, research was designed to substantiate and enhance existing concepts of National Socialism. Because Heritage of Ancestors lacked distin-

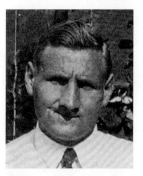

FIG. 320
*August Hirt
(1898-1945)*

guished physicians, its medical branch was small. Nonetheless, it received special attention and support from the president of the organization – none other than Heinrich Himmler himself. In 1941, Himmler induced August Hirt (Fig. 320), chairman of anatomy at the University of Strassburg, to join the organization. The bait was the opportunity to conduct experiments on "prisoners and professional criminals" at the concentration camp at Natzweiler. Hirt, the most renowned physician of Heritage of Ancestors, used that opportunity to study the effects of mustard gas on the human body and the possibilities of preventing the effects of it by administration of high doses of vitamin A. Many prisoners died in the course of these studies. When Hirt accidentally exposed himself to the gas and had to be hospitalized, Himmler sent his best wishes, together with five kilograms of apples and 10 kilograms of oranges.[18]

Himmler fulfilled another wish of Hirt's, namely, to organize a collection of Jewish skulls at the University of Strassburg. In this regard, Hirt suggested to Himmler that all "Jewish-Bolshevist commissaries" arrested by the army should be turned over to the field police and guarded "until the arrival of a special commissioner . . . charged with safeguarding the material. He should be a junior medical officer or student in the Armed Forces or even the Military Police, and should be provided with an armored car and driver. It will be his job to prepare a previously determined series of photographs and anthropological measurements, and to establish, insofar as is possible, descent, birth dates, and other vital statistics. Subsequently, when the death of these Jews has been effected – the head must not be injured – he severs the heads from the bodies and sends them on to their destination, immersed in specially constructed air-

tight tin containers filled with preserv-
ative."[19] Himmler found this to be a
worthy project and instructed the executive secretary of Heritage of Ancestors, Wolfram Sievers (Fig. 321), "to
support Prof. Hirt in every possible
way."[20] Because of logistic difficulties,
Sievers (who later was nicknamed "The
Nazi Bluebeard") never did supply Hirt
with the heads of Jews. Instead, he sent

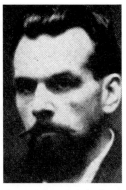

FIG. 321
*Wolfram
Sievers
(1905-1948)*

him 115 living prisoners from Auschwitz. After arrival at
Natzweiler, the prisoners were photographed, measured, X-
rayed, and given blood tests; then they were gassed to preserve
their corpses for posterity[21] (Fig. 322, 323).

Studies in anthropology and racial hygiene were supported
by the SS until the end of the war. The most notorious were

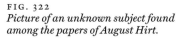

FIG. 322
*Picture of an unknown subject found
among the papers of August Hirt.*

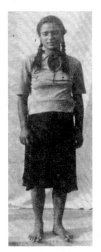

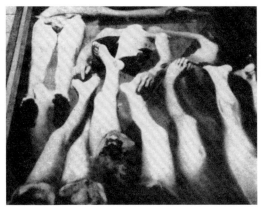

FIG. 323
*Collection of
corpses of Jews at
the Institute of
Anatomy of the
University of
Strassburg.*

FIG. 324
Josef Mengele
(1911-1979)

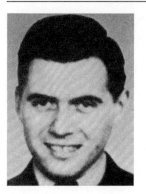

FIG. 325
Otmar von
Verschuer
(1896-1969)

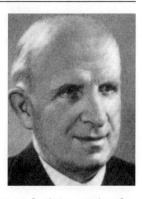

those of the "Angel of Death," Josef Mengele (Fig. 324), who served as a physician at Auschwitz from May 1943 until the liberation of the camp in 1945. Mengele had been an assistant of Otmar von Verschuer (Fig. 325), one of the leading geneticists in the world and director of the prestigious Kaiser Wilhelm Institute for Anthropology, Human Genetics, and Eugenics in Berlin. In collaboration with Verschuer, Mengele performed a variety of comparative studies on twins (Fig. 326, 327). In one experiment, a set of twins was inoculated with typhus bacilli in order to determine whether the siblings reacted in the same way to the infection or differently. In other studies, spinal fluid and blood from one twin were transferred to the other; and, in one, arteries of twins were interconnected to create a common circulatory system.[22] Mengele himself selected his subjects, even when he was not officially on duty, from among incoming prisoners on their arrival at the railway station in Auschwitz. Standing on the ramp in an impeccable uniform, he decided, with an elegant wave of his hand, who was to live and who was to die. Twins for his studies were set apart from other prisoners. Mengele also searched for persons with "interesting" malformations in order to enrich the Central Collection of Genetic Biology at Verschuer's institute in Berlin. Like a collector of butterflies or stamps, he looked for rare specimens, such as heterochromatic eyes and skeletons of dwarfs[23] (Fig. 328).

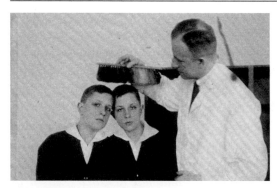

FIG. 326
Twins used for research by Otmar von Verschuer at the Kaiser-Wilhelm Institute in Berlin (1930)

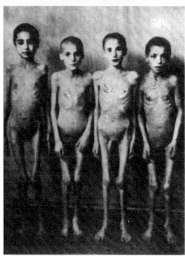

FIG. 327
Twins used for research by Josef Mengele at the extermination camp at Auschwitz.

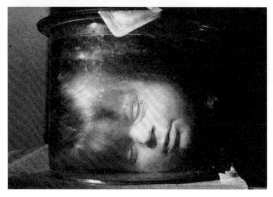

FIG. 328
Skeletons, eyeballs, embyros, and heads of children were collected by Mengele and sent to Verschuer's institute in Berlin.

The Abuse of Man

Collecting Rare Specimens

Many scientific endeavors of that era were undertaken in the same spirit as collecting in general. When a rare material was encountered, it was plucked if only to prevent it from being wasted. If people were to be killed anyway, why not take their eyeballs? And if corpses became available in unanticipated numbers, why not make use of them? Hermann Stieve (Fig. 329), chair of anatomy at the University of Halle and founder of the *Journal for Microscopical Anatomic Research* (*Zeitschrift für Mikroskopisch-Anatomische Forschung*), was hailed for his studies on anatomic attributes of the ovary. In a letter to the curator of the University of Halle in 1931, he had complained petulantly that "it is extremely difficult to get hold of ovaries of healthy girls." In 1935, Stieve became Director of the Institute of Anatomy and Anatomic Biology of the University of Berlin, and there his problems in regard to acquisition of material for study soon were resolved. He was supplied with all the bodies he needed from among the prisoners executed at the penitentiaries of Brandenburg and Berlin-Plötzensee. All victims of Nazi "justice" went through Stieve's hands, and the extraordinary quantity of them enabled him to advance his career. While other anatomists were laboring over the ovaries of mice or rabbits, Stieve conducted his studies on ovaries of freshly killed

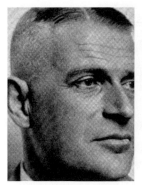

FIG. 329
*Hermann
Stieve
(1886-1952)*

girls and young women. His conclusion was that "the architecture of the human ovary is described incorrectly in virtually all textbooks of gynecology, anatomy and histology" because "the description is based on observations of ovaries of elderly women." Stieve also examined the effects of emotional stress on the function of the uterus, and the authenticity of his observations could not be called into question – women waiting to be executed had more than enough stress to assess those effects.[24]

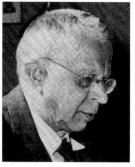

FIG. 330
Julius Hallervorden (1882-1965)

Like Stieve, neuropathologist Julius Hallervorden, of the Kaiser Wilhelm Institute for Brain Research in Berlin (Fig. 330), became a "passive" beneficiary of Nazi politics. Without having to do harm to patients himself, he was able to conduct extensive research on human brains by ordering them by the hundreds from victims of the euthanasia program. When interrogated about his research after the war, Hallervorden's total lack of remorse showed through chillingly by virtue of how indifferent he was to the method by which material was procured. This is what he said:

I heard that they were going to do that, and so I went up to them and told them: 'Look here now, boys, if you are going to kill all these people, at least take the brains so that the material could be utilized.' They asked me: 'How many can you examine?' and so I told them an unlimited number – 'the more the better.' I gave them fixatives, jars, and boxes and instructions for removing and fixing the brains and then they came bringing them like the delivery van from the furniture company. There was wonderful material among these brains, beautiful mental defects, malformations, and early infantile disease. I accepted these brains of course. Where they came from and how they came to me, was really none of my business.[25]

The Reich's Office of Research – a Tool of War

With the exception of studies related to Nazi ideology, such as racial hygiene, and realms of research that profited by chance from the copious material then becoming available, medical research under the Nazis was restricted almost exclusively to subjects relevant to the war. As early as September 1937, all chairs of departments of medicine in Germany were obligated to report to the authorities any work in progress concerning "war medicine," which, henceforth, would be supported chiefly by the Reich's Office of Research.[26] When the war began two years later, studies of aspects of medicine significant in war were intensified and adjusted to meet the immediate demands of the military. The problems confronted by the military, however, were not easy to solve. When methods and ideas were lacking, the Nazis tried to overcome the deficiency by making use of an opportunity not open to their enemies, namely, unscrupulous experiments on humans.

Prisoners-of-war, for example, were used as test cases for studying the effects of various types of poison and ammunition on the human body. In August 1941, the consultant in forensic medicine to the Academy of Military Medicine, Gerhart Panning, ordered Russian prisoners to be shot in different parts of their bodies, using bullets with great explosive force that had been manufactured in Russia. The victims suffered from agonizing pain before they were killed and were dissected on the spot.[27] When Panning published the results of his studies in the journal, *Der Deutsche Militärarzt* (*The German Military Physician*), he concealed the fact that he had tested the ammunition on live prisoners, claiming instead to have studied the effects on "Soviet corpses found with shots from the rear," as if to suggest that the Russians had been killed intentionally by their own comrades. The shocking injuries caused by the Russian bullets prompted Panning to assert piously, and ironically, that "it is an indubitable violation of the law of nations to use such bullets on human beings"[28] (Fig. 331, 332). At Buchenwald, in 1943 and 1944, various poisons were administered secretly in food given to Russian prisoners while German doctors stood behind a curtain to observe their reactions. Some of the prisoners died immediately and those who survived were killed in order that autopsies could be performed on their bodies.[29]

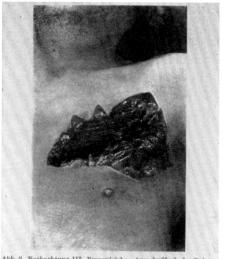

FIG. 331
Photograph in Panning's article about the physical effects of Russian ammunition. The original caption reads: "Observation III. Russian corpse. Exit hole in the left chest measuring 16x13 cm, with an entrance hole on the left back measuring 0.5 cm."

Abb. 2. Beobachtung III, Russenleiche. Ausschußloch der linken Brustseite mit 16 : 13 cm, bei 0,5 cm großem Einschußloch der linken Rückenseite. Sprenghöhle mit Schmauchablagerung von der Lunge bis in die Ausschußweichteile erstreckt.

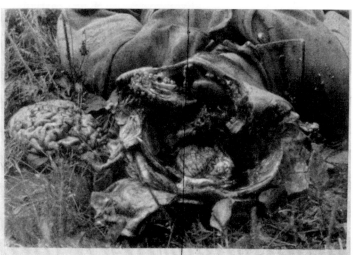

Abb. 3. Beobachtung VI, Russenleiche. Vollständige Sprengung und Enthirnung bei Schädelschuß mit 0,5 cm großem Hauteinschuß am Hinterhaupt.

FIG. 332 *Photograph in Panning's article about the physical effects of Russian ammunition. The original caption reads: "Observation VI. Russian corpse. Complete explosion and destruction of the brain following a shot in the head with an 0.5 cm entrance hole in the skin of the occiput."*

The Abuse of Man

A "Higher Form of Killing"

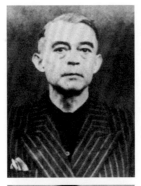

FIG. 333
Kurt Blome
(1894-1969)

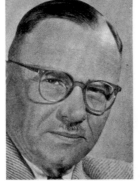

FIG. 334
Carl Moncorps
(1896-1952)

Agents of biological warfare were studied in a secret laboratory in Posen that was directed by the deputy of the Reich's Leader of Health, Kurt Blome (Fig. 333). Although biological warfare was rejected publicly by Hitler, the army command had consented to having the laboratory constructed and various experiments conducted there. Disguised as "cancer research," Blome's studies, in an effort to develop biological weapons, exposed prisoners to contagions such as plague bacilli.[30]

Extensive research was carried out on agents of chemical warfare that had been proven to be effective in action during World War I. In his acceptance speech for the Nobel Prize (won for his synthesis of ammonia) in 1918, German chemist Fritz Haber had referred to poison gas as "a higher form of killing."[31] To improve techniques of chemical warfare, studies were conducted by the SS, various branches of the army, and several departments in German universities. One such study, performed at the University of Münster by the chairman of dermatology, Carl Moncorps (Fig. 334), sought methods whereby neurotoxic substances could penetrate the skin without any trace of their having done that. The methods and the results of that study are not known.[32] In the gas chamber of the German army in Berlin-Spandau, prisoners were exposed to different types of poison gas, including phosgene, mustard gas, and two highly neurotoxic substances (nerve gases), Tabun and Sarin. Photographs of the effects of those substances on humans were published in 1944 by the leading toxicologist of the army, Wolfgang Wirth, in a booklet called *Injuries by Chemical Warfare Agents*[33] (Fig. 335, 336). Agents of chemical warfare were tested also in prisoners of the concentration camp at Natzweiler, where a gas chamber had been installed specifically for that purpose. In the summer of 1943, Otto Bickenbach of the University of Strassburg (Fig. 337) exposed some 150 prisoners to phosgene, a suffocating highly poisonous gas. Approximately 40 test subjects died and those who survived were transferred to the concentration camps at Auschwitz, Belsen, and Lublin.[34] After the war, Bickenbach acknowledged that "experiments on human material go directly against medical ethics. Nevertheless, I carried them out, and particularly because I was aware of the horrors of the gas war."[35]

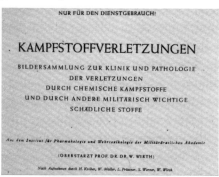

NUR FÜR DEN DIENSTGEBRAUCH!

KAMPFSTOFFVERLETZUNGEN

BILDERSAMMLUNG ZUR KLINIK UND PATHOLOGIE
DER VERLETZUNGEN
DURCH CHEMISCHE KAMPFSTOFFE
UND DURCH ANDERE MILITÄRISCH WICHTIGE
SCHÄDLICHE STOFFE

Aus dem Institut für Pharmakologie und Wehrtoxikologie der Militärärztlichen Akademie

(OBERSTARZT PROF. DR. DR. W. WIRTH)

Nach Aufnahmen durch H. Kreiber, W. Müller, L. Präuner, S. Werner, W. Wirth

FIG. 335
Title page of the booklet "Injuries by Chemical Warfare Agents" (Kampfstoffverletzungen) by Wolfgang Wirth.

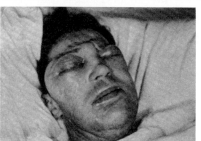

FIG. 336 *Photograph from Wirth's booklet on chemical warfare agents: massive edema following exposure to a solution of derivatives of arsenic.*

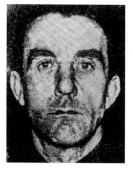

FIG. 337
*Otto Bickenbach
(1901-1971)*

The Abuse of Man

Testing the Limits at High Altitudes

When British fighter planes, in the spring of 1941, began to succeed in attacking German planes from ever greater heights, the Luftwaffe intensified its efforts to reach higher altitudes of flying. This endeavor was associated with increased risk for pilots especially if air pressure in a plane was lost during combat. In order to develop a system for saving pilots in such emergencies, the Luftwaffe had to learn more about responses and limits of humans in low ambient air pressure.[36] Studies on volunteers from the air force had revealed that an altitude of 11,000 meters could be tolerated for less than one minute before death became imminent. The effects of exposure to higher altitudes and for longer periods of time had been studied only in animals. In a letter to Himmler in May 1941, Sigmund Rascher (Fig. 338), a Luftwaffe physician and member of the SS, deplored the fact "that, unfortunately, no experiments with human material have been performed because such experiments are very dangerous and nobody volunteers for them."[37] Rascher was referring to experiments associated with severe side effects and even death. To make such risky experiments possible, Rascher asked Himmler to provide "two or three professional criminals," explaining the reason in these words: "The experiments that, as a matter of course, may lead to death of test subjects would be carried out

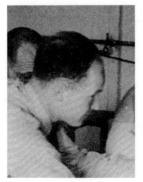

FIG. 338
Sigmund Rascher (1909-1945)

under my supervision. I have discussed this issue absolutely confidentially with the deputy physician of the air force who performs those experiments, and he also believes that the problems under consideration can only be clarified by experiments on humans . . ." Rascher added, parenthetically, that "imbeciles could also be used as research material."[38]

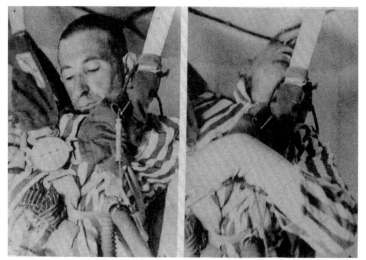

FIG. 339
*Experiment on
the effects of
exceedingly
low atmos-
pheric
pressure at the
concentration
camp at
Dachau.*

Himmler, who was acquainted with Rascher's wife, granted the physician his full support and, in that spirit, an air force laboratory was established for him at Dachau. Healthy Poles, Russians, and Jews were selected as test subjects. Hanging in a parachute in a low-pressure chamber from which air was exhausted by vacuum pumps, the subjects were exposed to pressures corresponding to altitudes of up to 21 kilometers, left dangling for varying lengths of time, and then raised and dropped at different speeds. Among the consequences were pareses, blindness, insanity, and death. Some experiments were carried out for the expressed purpose of studying the mechanisms of death. Autopsies were performed immediately on conclusion of these experiments so that Rascher could examine the internal organs of test subjects while they were still functioning[39] (Fig. 339). The experiments revealed that although unconsciousness set in within a few seconds after a rapid decrease in air pressure, test subjects actually were able to survive at high altitudes for longer periods of time than had been supposed. On the basis of these findings, Siegfried Ruff, who oversaw Rascher's experiments, developed, in 1943, an ejector seat that could be activated by a pilot before unconsciousness occurred. Ejection was followed by the automatic, but delayed, opening of a parachute, thereby enabling the falling pilot to reach a higher pressure more quickly. Beginning in 1944, the ejector seat was placed in all new German fighter planes, and, after the war, the Allied nations adopted Ruff's concept for the rescue of pilots of disabled planes.[40]

Another problem confronting the air force was loss of pilots who had been shot down over the English Channel and who were not picked up by German vessels in time to prevent death from hypothermia. The questions posed involved the length of time humans could survive in icy water and how long they could go drinking either seawater or nothing at all. Both issues were examined at Dachau. In one series of experiments conducted by Rascher in collaboration with Ernst Holzlöhner, professor of physiology at the University of Kiel, test subjects were submerged partially in basins of icy water while their body temperature, respiration, and heart action were monitored carefully. Samples of blood, urine, and spinal fluid were taken at regular intervals. Test subjects usually died after six to eight hours, that is, when their body temperature had hit 28° to 25°C [41] (Fig.

FIG. 340
Experiment on freezing at the concentration camp at Dachau. The physicians conducting the experiment are Ernst Holzlöhner (left) and Sigmund Rascher (right).

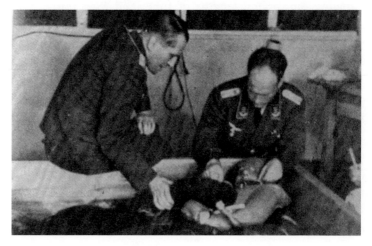

340). Another group of prisoners had to drink seawater alone for more than two weeks. As usual, body functions were monitored closely: the temperature was controlled, the liver biopsied, and the blood and spinal fluid sampled regularly. Many test subjects went mad from thirst. The wife of chief investigator, Wilhelm Beiglböck of the University of Vienna (Fig. 341),

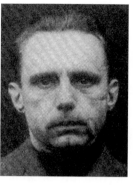

FIG. 341
*Wilhelm
Beiglböck
(1905-1963)*

feared for her husband's safety because the prisoners had fits of raving madness. Nevertheless, no prisoner was allowed, for any reason, to withdraw from the study.[42]

As the war went on, an increasingly serious difficulty for the German forces was injuries that soldiers inflicted on themselves, *sub rosa*, in order to keep from being sent to the front. To recognize such lesions induced factitiously, studies were conducted on prisoners at Auschwitz concerning different ways of producing injuries artificially. Subsequently, about half of the test subjects died. Most of the tests involved cutaneous wounds produced by serious burns, injection of gasoline, and ingestion

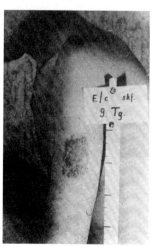

FIG. 342
Jewish victim of tests about wounds inflicted deliberately at the extermination camp at Auschwitz.

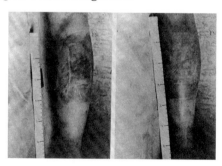

FIG. 343
Test subjects with severe burns of the skin that were biopsied and the tissue examined histopathologically at the University of Breslau.

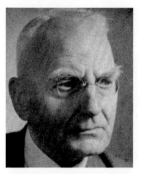

FIG. 344
Heinrich Löhe
(1877-1961)

of picric acid (which produced yellowish discoloration of the skin reminiscent of hepatitis). Biopsy specimens taken from the involved skin were sent to the University of Breslau to be assessed there histopathologically (Fig. 342, 343). The results of this research were to be presented at a congress of the consulting physicians of the Academy for Military Medicine in April 1945. The program was to include lectures on "Pharmacological Comments About Self-Afflicted Injuries" by toxicologist, Wolfgang Wirth, and "Induction and Simulation of Internal Diseases" by dermatologist, Heinrich Löhe (Fig. 344). Because the German armed forces were in rout and disarray as the war was coming to its end, the congress never convened.[43]

Infectious Diseases and Vaccine Studies

The most serious medical problems for German troops throughout the war were infections, ranging from phlegmon and gas gangrene to spotted fever, malaria, and hepatitis. For example, hepatitis was highly prevalent among German troops in southern Russia, where it caused "a reduction of companies of up to 60 percent for up to six weeks," as reported in a letter to Himmler in June 1943 by the leading physician of the SS, Ernst Grawitz.[44] The cause of hepatitis was not known, although the contagiousness of it was obvious. Preliminary studies at the University of Breslau on inoculation of psychiatric patients with tissue of hepatitis had been published in 1942 by Hans Voegt in the *Münchener Medizinische Wochenschrift*. Voegt commented that among the findings were "more or less severe damage of the liver two to four weeks after the inoculation in all test subjects."[45] Voegt's superior, Kurt Gutzeit, professor of internal medicine at the university, encouraged another of his assistants, Arnold Dohmen, to study hepatitis by inoculation experiments. Dohmen originally tried to avoid using human subjects by doing experiments on animals, but Gutzeit was determined "to wake him up from his lethargy on animal experiments." In a letter to another assistant in 1944, Gutzeit expressed his amazement at "how curious it is that the step from animal to human being is so difficult; but after all, experiments on humans are the essential point." At last Dohmen agreed and asked the SS to provide "eight young prisoners sentenced to death." He was given eleven Jewish children and adolescents between ages nine and 19 years. Dohmen inoculated cultures of viruses into the duodenum of the youngsters and then performed repeated liver biopsies to study the effects. Nothing of consequence was learned.[46]

In order to develop a vaccine against malaria, large-scale experiments on humans were conducted by Claus Schilling, former director of the department of tropical medicine of the Robert Koch Institute in Berlin. Schilling had retired in 1936, but continued his research. He had succeeded, according to his own testimony, in producing "complete immunity against malaria in two persons by combining inoculations of living parasites with chinine." On the basis of this weak claim, the entire concentration camp at Dachau was placed at Schilling's disposal and scores of prisoners were infected with malaria. Many test subjects died in vain because no effective method to induce immunity against malaria could be developed. Following the war, Schilling defended his research by this rationalization: "I admit that human beings had to suffer from those experiments, but the interest of science to prevent that disease and to rescue millions rated much higher"[47] (Fig. 345).

Typhus, a disease transmitted by lice, was extraordinarily prevalent in concentration and extermination camps and in overcrowded Jewish ghettos; it became a problem, too, for Ger-

FIG. 345
Malaria being studied
via intravenous injec-
tions of contaminated
blood at the concentra-
tion camp at Dachau.

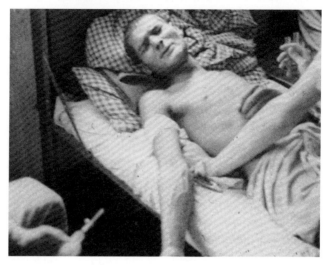

FIG. 345
Malaria being studied via intravenous injections of contaminated blood at the concentration camp at Dachau.

man troops. In the camps, epidemics of typhus were countered by killing all inmates on those blocks in which the disease was rampant. Effective treatment for typhus did not exist, and vaccines were expensive and associated with significant side effects. Several German pharmaceutical firms raced to develop new vaccines and drugs in anticipation of highly lucrative sales, and all of them insisted that their products be included in experiments conducted in humans by the SS. Eugen Haagen (Fig. 346), director of the Institute of Hygiene at the University of Strassburg, whose work previously on vaccination against ty-

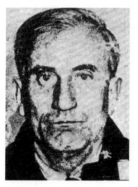

FIG. 346
*Eugen Haagen
(1898-1972)*

phus had resulted in his being named a candidate for a Nobel Prize, tested the new vaccines on inmates of the extermination camp at Natzweiler. Following experimental vaccination, prisoners were inoculated with virulent typhus bacilli in order to determine the efficacy of the vaccines.[48] When those experiments were criticized by members of Haagen's own institute, his assistant, Helmut Gräfe, explained everything by saying, "We only use Poles, not Alsatians. Poles are not humans."[49] In the extermination camp at Buchenwald, a large laboratory was established specifically for the study of typhus. At least 1,000 prisoners were infected artificially; some received vaccines or drugs prior to or following infection, whereas others served as controls and went untreated. Still others were used exclusively as culture media, that is, they were infected for the sole purpose of having sufficient quantities of contagious blood available. More than 250 prisoners at Buchenwald died as a direct result of these experiments.[50]

The Sulfonamide Trials

The pharmaceutical industry used the unique opportunities that existed in concentration and extermination camps for numerous other studies as well. For a brief period, pharmacokinesis, side effects, and effectiveness of new drugs could be assessed cheaper and faster than ever before or since. The group of drugs studied most intensely was sulfonamides. Following their introduction in 1935 by Gerhard Domagk, who won a Nobel Prize for his work in 1939, many derivatives of sulfonamides had been developed and were waiting to be tested in a clinical setting. In Germany, studies concerning the efficacy of sulfonamides were done chiefly by dermatologists. One of the most prolific investigators in this area was the chairman of dermatology at the University of Düsseldorf, Hans Theo Schreus (Fig. 347), who, in 1941, demonstrated through animal experiments the therapeutic value of several new derivatives of sulfonamides. By contrast, surgeons, resenting the intrusion of dermatologists into their

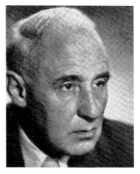

FIG. 347
Hans Theo Schreus (1892-1970)

sphere, tended to minimize the value of sulfonamides and emphasize the primacy of surgery in treating infections of wounds sustained during combat. At a time when British soldiers were carrying sulfonamide tablets for immediate ingestion in the event of being wounded, German military physicians were still debating whether use of these drugs should be adopted. For example, Ferdinand Sauerbruch, the inventor of the "iron lung" for use in open thoracic surgery, stated, at a meeting in 1942 of the Academy for Military Medicine in Berlin, that sulfonamides veil "surgical activities and pander to superficiality."[51]

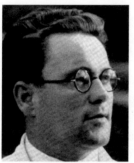

FIG. 348
Karl Gebhardt
(1897-1948)

In May 1942, Reinhard Heydrich, head of the SS Security Police and The Reich's Protector of Bohemia and Moravia, was wounded severely in an attempted assassination in Prague and died of sepsis eight days later. His physician, Karl Gebhardt (Fig. 348), a major general in the Waffen-SS, President of the German Red Cross, and personal physician to Heinrich Himmler, was criticized for having failed to prevent the fatal infection by administering sulfonamides.[52] Gebhardt reacted to the criticism with a study on sulfonamides of his own. For that endeavor, he did not utilize the numerous soldiers who suffered from gas gangrene and other infections, but instead copied the animal experiments conducted by Schreus in 1941. There were two major differences, however, between these sets of experiments. First, in order to exonerate himself, Gebhardt deliberately sought to demonstrate that sulfonamides were not helpful in treating infected wounds. In order to achieve that "proof," he administered the drug for too short a period of time and in a dose too low to be effective. Second, Gebhardt did not use animals for his experiments; his tests subjects were female inmates of the concentration camp at Ravensbrück.[53]

Gebhardt induced gas gangrene artificially on these incarcerated women by cutting deep wounds through the skin and down to the bone, and by inoculating the wounds with cultures of bacteria and splinters of glass and wood. Some test subjects were treated with sulfonamides, others comprised the control group and went untreated. One of Gebhardt's assistants, derma-

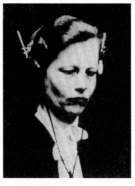

FIG. 349
Herta Oberheuser (born 1911)

tologist Herta Oberheuser (Fig. 349), described the study almost gleefully. "In August 1942," she said, "the so-called guinea-pig operation started in our section; I call it the experiment with living objects. I was in charge of the treatment and management of so-called guinea-pigs in section I." The guinea pigs she referred to were female "Polish political prisoners who were to be executed." Oberheuser described how the women were examined and reported that "we used exclusively healthy women for experimental purposes. The first experiment conducted by us was an attempt to produce gas gangrene in healthy women through inoculation of bacteria. This included the deposit of foreign bodies such as wood. I believe that only three women died as a consequence of the experiments. We identified weakness of the circulation as the cause of death"[54] (Fig. 350).

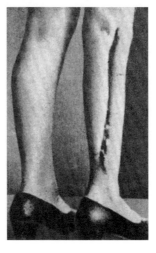

FIG. 350
Victim of medical research at the concentration camp at Ravensbrück.

Herta Oberheuser had started to work with sulfonamides during her residency under Chairman Hans Theo Schreus in the department of dermatology of the University of Düsseldorf. During the time she was assigned to Ravensbrück, she visited Schreus repeatedly, presumably to discuss with him the results of her studies. She also tried to persuade assistants in the skin clinic in Düsseldorf to join her at Ravensbrück, beckoning them with the promise that "anything" could be done in that concentration camp. "Anything" included the implantation of plastic membranes into the meninges, excision of muscles, smashing of bones for the purpose of studying regeneration of them, and experimental transplantations of bone, ranging from small fragments to an entire shoulder.[55] Oberheuser attended to persons who were operated on, insisting on "systematic non-care" for them, and she, herself, killed several subjects deliberately by injections of gasoline.[56]

Another dermatologist who worked on sulfonamides was Josef Vonkennel (Fig. 351), chairman of the department of dermatology at the University of Leipzig and consultant dermatologist to the armed SS squadrons (Waffen-SS). Vonkennel was the only dermatologist whose research was thought to be important enough to be funded by the government in the last year of the war. In the SS Research Institute V, established as a separate branch of his clinic, Vonkennel and his assistant, Joseph Kimmig (Fig. 352), developed diaminodiphenylsulfone, a sulfonamide with antibiotic and anti-inflammatory properties, that still is used widely for treatment of such disparate diseases as leprosy and dermatitis herpetiformis. To test the efficacy of

FIG. 351
*Josef
Vonkennel
(1897-1963)*

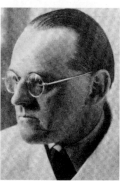

FIG. 352
*Joseph
Kimmig
(1909-1976)*

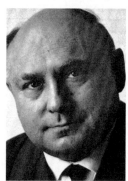

the drug, Vonkennel initiated tests on inmates at Buchenwald.[57] The camp was located near Leipzig, and Vonkennel went there regularly by car to supervise the experiments, while his chauffeur, a brother of Joseph Kimmig, waited outside the camp for Vonkennel's return.[58] The experiments included application of poison gas to the skin of prisoners in order to produce severe burns that then were treated with diaminodiphenylsulfone. Several test subjects died in this process.[59]

The Impersonality of Abuse Experimentally

Experiments in humans under the Nazis far exceeded anything that had gone on before. These experiments were not the work of a "minority of German doctors – a macabre 'order,'" as German medical officials claimed self-righteously after the war, but were part and parcel of the entire field of medical research during the Third Reich.[60] Most of those who performed or supervised experiments on humans were members of highly respected institutes, including no small number of leading universities. Many were specialists of worldwide repute. They performed their research without remorse and without emotional investment in the fate of their test subjects. It was official Nazi policy to conduct the necessary, albeit cumbersome, task of killing millions of "inferior human beings" in the most unemotional and impersonal manner possible. SS guards at Auschwitz even had to sign an oath not to brutalize prisoners for their own amusement. This oath stated that "Only the Führer decides about life and death of enemies of the state. Therefore, no National Socialist is entitled to lay hands on an enemy of the state. Each prisoner must be punished only by the commander."[61] To be sure, the oath was not always honored, but many SS men avoided unnecessary contact with prisoners. Even the notorious Josef Mengele was reported never to have hit or whipped a prisoner himself. Instead, he killed his victims in the manner of a man of science, on a dissecting table with a syringe in his hand.[62, 63]

This same attitude of distance, imperviousness, and cold professionalism characterized all research on human beings at the time. Experiments were performed as matter-of-factly as ordinary surgical procedures or routine autopsies. Only the technical quality of the procedure mattered; a test subject was just another case, another number. The impersonal relationship between researcher and test subject was but a slight exaggeration of the situation physicians had become accustomed to in the normal course of their professional life in hospitals. They had been trained to perform medical procedures without emotion. That their efforts in hospitals were designed to help individual human beings under their care, whereas experiments in concentration and extermination camps brought about deliberate destruction of individual lives, was for them a minor difference that could be rationalized easily.

Because physicians felt no empathy for their test subjects or suppressed any such feelings as soon as they surfaced, there was little, if any, thought given to the inordinate harm being inflicted on them. In contrast with patients in hospitals, inmates of concentration and extermination camps were not thought of as human beings with dignity, needs, and hopes of their own. In fact, having been transported to such a camp like animals in dirty cattle cars devoid of sanitary facilities, having lived without any privacy whatever for months in overcrowded barracks infested with lice, and having been brought low by hunger, fear, sickness, to say nothing of incessant humiliation, any personal dignity that a test subject might still have left no longer was apparent. For most of these pitiful creatures, neither hopes nor prospects remained. Barely able to maintain their miserable lives, not regarded as human, they were perceived – as the poignant name given to them by physicians in the camps implied – as "human guinea pigs."

CHAPTER 15

RESEARCH BY THE JAPANESE IN OCCUPIED CHINA

The events in Germany between 1933 and 1945 are unique in history. The systematic extermination of six million Jews, along with many thousands of Roma and Sinti Gypsies, mentally disabled and chronically ill persons, homosexuals, and political opponents of all kinds, in a cold-blooded, punctiliously planned, and efficient manner, required more than the will of one brutal dictator. It became possible only through the deadly constellation of various factors, among them an extraordinarily organized bureaucracy, a well trained personnel, an exquisitely injured national pride, a widespread mentality of militarism, a long tradition of imposed order and reflexive obedience to authority, the total surveillance in a totalitarian state, and, above all, the conviction of the superiority of a nation predicated on an immutable ideological foundation.

Although this array of factors came together in singular fashion in Nazi Germany, each of them was at play at various times elsewhere in the world. In Japan, especially, the conditions in many ways resembled those in Nazi Germany. Militarism was an essential element of Japanese culture, just as it was in Germany, but to an even greater extent. In fact, Japan had been under a military dictatorship since the Middle Ages, and the bushido, or code of samurai warriors, was held to be the highest form of virtuous conduct. The bushido demanded strict obedience to orders by superiors, even to the extent of committing suicide in cases of misconduct. The tradition of unfailing obedience was furthered by remnants of feudal structures that throughout the early part of the twentieth century still dominated life in the Japanese countryside. Like people of most developed nations, including Germany, the Japanese were convinced that they were special, and, therefore, destined to accomplish an important mission in the world. This belief had been nourished by centuries of isolation and isolationism and had a strong ideological foundation in Shinto religion, which stressed the racial superiority of the Japanese and ordained worship of the Japanese emperor as a divinity. Although Japan had emerged from the First World War as a leading military and political power, many Japanese citizens, like their German counterparts, believed that their country was denied its proper and deserved role in the world. As in Germany, a democracy was established in post-World War I Japan, but it was rejected by large parts of the population who longed for return to the safety and order of the former autocratic system. That democracy was staggered by the constant threat of a military coup d'état and assassinations of liberal politicians by right-wing terrorists. As in Germany, an economic crisis in the 1920s was attributed to flaws inherent in democracy, and this became the springboard for radicalism by various ultranationalist groups. Political turbulence and fear of communists – again, just as happened in Germany – resulted in laws that restricted personal and political freedoms, and were used to imprison political opponents. Eventually those laws paved the way for a totalitarian state.[1]

In the first decades of the twentieth century, Japan was replete with contradictions and opposing currents, a consequence of the rapid modernization of the country and the adop-

tion of Western culture and technology. Although strict observance of traditional mythology, chief among them the divinity
of the emperor, was enforced at schools, an avalanche of trans-
lations of Western writers, ranging from Adam Smith to Marx
and Goethe to Tolstoy, swamped the country. As new concepts,
such as "equal rights," "liberalism," "socialism," and "pacifism,"
were gaining momentum, the oligarchic rule by so-called elder
statesmen, nobility, and military leaders came to be replaced by
cabinets formed by members of particular parties. Universal
suffrage was granted in 1925.[2]

There also was a change in Japanese foreign policy. Since the
end of the nineteenth century, Japan had expanded its influence on the Asian mainland, mostly at the expense of China.
Because of modern military technology, the First Sino-Japanese War, in 1894 -1895, was won by the Japanese in six weeks,
and the Chinese Ching regime had to grant Taiwan and the
Pescadores Islands to Japan, along with a large monetary in-
demnity. Ten years later, Japan won its second modern war,
against Russia, this time in less than eighteen months, and by
virtue of the victory was awarded a lease on the Liaotung Penin-
sula of Manchuria and the southern half of Sakhalin Island.
The Japanese triumph also ended a long-term quarrel with
Russia about which country should control Korea; in 1910,
Korea was annexed officially by Japan. During World War I,
Japan seized the German-held Marshall, Caroline, and Mari-
ana Islands in the Pacific Ocean and forced China to grant it far-
reaching economic rights in Manchuria and Kwangtung
provinces. To protect its investments in that area, the War Ministry in Tokyo in 1919 established a Kwangtung Army. With the
end of World War I, however, the aggressive policy of Japan
began to soften. Japan became a charter member of the League
of Nations, signed a treaty on naval disarmament, and pledged
to respect the territorial integrity and sovereignty of China. For
the first time in many years, spending for the military was cut

by the Japanese government, and the army was reduced in size by four divisions.[3]

The emergence of democracy and liberalism in Japan was accompanied by a rise in corruption and a series of financial scandals and bank failures. Party politics were influenced greatly by a few wealthy families, called the zaibatsu, whose companies controlled most of the coal, steam engine, pulp, and aluminum industries. At the same time, small economic enterprises were collapsing. The downturn in the economy – caused by the closure of munitions factories after the war, widespread boycotts of Japanese goods by China, discriminatory tariffs enacted by other countries, a devastating earthquake in 1923, and the tidal-wave effect of the Wall Street crash in 1929 – resulted in soaring inflation. Peasant families were starving and destitute farmers and fishermen were forced to sell their daughters into prostitution. These events, combined, agitated the military, especially junior and mid-level officers who came largely from the rural agrarian class. Dismayed by the apparent inability of liberal bourgeois democracy to deal with the social and political problems of the day, they turned increasingly to solutions proposed by the dictatorships in Italy and Germany, where liberation from the defeatism of democracy seemed to inaugurate a new era of economic prosperity and social stability. Because these young military men were nurtured in a xenophobic society, they were not disturbed by Hitler's avowed racism and they attempted to establish a Japanese version of National Socialism.[4]

Expansion by Conquest

One idea that the Japanese military shared with the National Socialists was belief in the necessity, for the survival of the nation, of expansion by conquest. Japan was poor in arable land and, despite an increase in the yield per acre, it relied increasingly on imported foodstuff to feed its growing population. In his book, *Addresses to Young Men*, Lieutenant Colonel Hashimoto Kingoro wrote as follows: "There are only three ways left to Japan to escape from the pressures of surplus population ... emigration, advance into world markets, and expansion of territory. The first door, emigration, has been barred to us by the anti-Japanese immigration policies of other countries. The second door ... is being pushed shut by tariff barriers and the abrogation of commercial treaties. What should Japan do when two of the three doors have been closed against her?"[5]

Such ideas fell on fertile soil, especially among officers of the Kwangtung Army stationed in Manchuria, far from interference by meddling Japanese politicians. On September 18, 1931, young officers blew up the tracks of the Japanese-owned railway, blamed that "incident" on Chinese saboteurs, and used it as a pretext to seize all of Manchuria. The central government in Tokyo accepted "reluctantly" the independent actions of its insubordinate military officers and created a thinly disguised facade of legitimacy by installing Pu Yi, the last emperor of China, as a puppet ruler of what was then called the independent state of Manchoukuo. Three months later, on May 15, 1932, the assassination of Japan's Prime Minister, Inukai Ki, by officers and cadets of the army marked the end of government by a cabinet formed of members of political parties and the return to military dictatorship in Japan.[6]

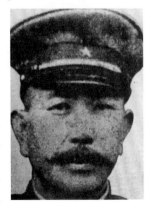

FIG. 353
Ishii Shiro
(1892-1959)

It also marked a turning point in the meteoric career of Ishii Shiro (Fig. 353), a major in the medical corps of the Imperial Army, and an arrogant, eccentric, ambitious, and highly capable physician with excellent connections to both leading representatives of Japanese medical schools and those in the top echelon of the army. In the spirit of the Chinese proverb that "Great doctors tend their country, good doctors tend people, and lesser doctors heal illnesses," Ishii studied prospects for biological warfare and succeeded in arousing the interest of his superiors. Put in charge of research on biological warfare at the Army Medical School in Tokyo, Ishii achieved some success with his experiments. He believed, however, that the ultimate test for feasibility of biological warfare lay in human experimentation, which could not be carried out in the densely populated capital of the Empire. "There are two types of biological warfare, A and B," he said. "A is assault research, and B is defense research. Vaccine research is of the B type, and this can be done in Japan. However, A type research can only be done abroad."[7]

With the seizure of Manchuria, A-type research became possible. In August 1932, Ishii was assigned to the newly acquired colony and given *carte blanche* to begin his work. Provided with abundant and readily available funding, the best technical equipment that money could buy, and command over a unit of 300 men, Ishii established a research base in Beiyinhe, an isolated village located near one of the major railroad lines. A large zone in the village was cordoned off by the Japanese, inhabitants were ordered to leave their homes within three days, and most of the buildings were burned. Local Chinese peasants were then drafted to construct a prison with laboratories, buildings for experimental animals, a crematorium to dispose of carcasses of animals and humans, warehouses, a canteen, and homes for the members of Ishii's unit.

The prisoners included Chinese guerrillas, underground anti-Japanese workers, and "suspicious persons" rounded up by the police. They were confined to tiny cells and handcuffed and shackled most of the time, but they were fed a diet far superior to that of ordinary Chinese peasants so they would be able to withstand the experiments to which they were subject-

ed. At that time, Ishii concentrated his efforts on three contagions – anthrax, glanders, and plague. Plague bacilli were recovered from fleas harvested at the Manchurian-Soviet border,
where plague was endemic, and the bacilli were injected into
prisoners, who soon grew delirious with fever and died within a
few days. Prisoners also were used for other types of experiments that addressed such issues as reactions to poison gas,
blood loss, hunger, thirst, and cold. Lieutenant General Oka-
mura Yasutsugu, Deputy Commander in Chief of the Kwangtung Army, was impressed especially by Ishii's studies on frostbite. Following a visit to the camp, he informed his superior that
"the best treatment for frozen limbs is soaking in water at 37°C,"
a finding "based on invaluable data from *in vivo* experiments
with humans who were frozen repeatedly and then defrosted."[8]

Ishii attached great importance to the secrecy of his operation. An area of 250 meters around the camp was declared off
limits to local residents, and anyone caught within this perimeter was punished severely by camp authorities. In the fall of
1934, however, a rebellion of prisoners and a mass escape ended
the efforts at secrecy. A year later, the ammunition dump of the
camp exploded, causing great damage. As a consequence, Ishii
abandoned the Beiyinhe facility in 1937.[9]

By that time, tensions between Japan and China had heightened even further. The ease of acquisition of Manchuria, the
lack of a strong reaction by other military powers, and the hostile response of Chinese nationalists strengthened the position
of radical Japanese expansionists. Moreover, worries about the
gradual consolidation of China under Chiang Kai-shek induced
the Japanese to accelerate the aggression. They considered a
military strike to be crucial before China grew too strong to be
conquered, and they used incidents of no real importance as excuses for staging major military operations. Shortly after the establishment of Manchoukuo in 1932, a Shanghai mob attacked
five Japanese Buddhist priests, leaving one of them dead. Japan

immediately retaliated by bombing Shanghai and killing tens of thousands of civilians. When the slaughter in Shanghai aroused worldwide criticism, Japan responded by withdrawing from the League of Nations. In the summer of 1937, shots were fired at Japanese soldiers garrisoned by treaty in the Chinese city of Tientsin, near Beijing (Peking). Using the incident as a pretext to initiate hostilities, the Japanese army in Manchuria moved troops into the area, precipitating another Sino-Japanese War, which never was declared formally. Japanese forces quickly overran northern China and advanced to the south, reaching Nanking, the newly established capital of the Republic of China, in December 1937.[10]

An Orgy of Cruelty

When Nanking fell, Japanese troops began an orgy of cruelty that even exceeded anything that happened under Nazi rule in Europe. Within a few weeks, some 300,000 Chinese noncombatants were murdered, a death toll far greater than from the atomic blasts of Hiroshima and Nagasaki combined (Fig. 354, 355). Tens of thousands of young men were rounded up and herded to the perimeter of the city, where they were mowed down by machine guns, used for bayonet practice, or soaked with gasoline and burned alive. Chinese captives were lined up and used for beheading contests with samurai swords, contests that were covered avidly in the Japanese media (Fig. 356). For days, the Yangtze River ran red with blood, and for months the city streets were heaped with corpses (Fig. 357). An estimated 20,000 to 80,000 Chinese women were raped, often by gangs of Japanese soldiers, and after the act was consummated, they were disemboweled, nailed alive to walls, or forced into prostitution for the benefit of soldiers. Fathers were forced to rape their daughters, and sons their mothers, while other family members watched (Fig. 358). Live burials, castration, carving

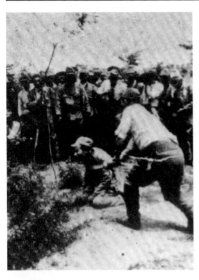

FIG. 354
Massacres at Nanking: thousands of Chinese men and women were beheaded by sword.

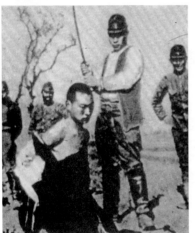

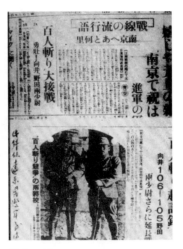

FIG. 355
Massacres at Nanking: beheading of captives was turned into a sport.

FIG. 356
Headline of the newspaper, Japan Advertiser: "Contest to Kill First 100 Chinese with Sword Extended When Both Fighters Exceed Mark – Mukai Scores 106 and Noda 105."

FIG. 357
Corpses of citizens of Nanking thrown by Japanese troops into the Yangtse river.

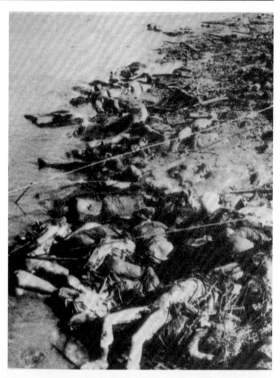

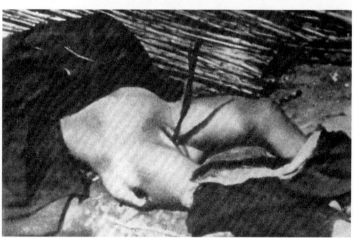

FIG. 358 *Nanking woman after having been raped and mutilated.*

up of organs, and roasting of human flesh became routine; even more diabolical tortures, such as hanging people by their tongues on iron hooks, were invented and practiced.[11]

The purported bases for this outburst of violence and sadism were many, among them the violence and suppression Japanese soldiers themselves had to endure throughout their training, and the explicit order, issued from the headquarters of Commander in Chief, Prince Asaka Yasuhiko, an uncle of Emperor Hirohito, to "kill all captives."[12] The most important motivation, however, was the unmitigated contempt for the Chinese that had been cultivated by decades of Japanese propaganda and was furthered by the lack of resistance by the Chinese, despite their great numerical superiority. To members of the Imperial Army, the Chinese were an inferior race, and murder of these "subhumans" carried no more moral weight than did squashing a bug. A Japanese general told a western correspondent that "to be frank, your view of the Chinese is totally different from mine. You regard the Chinese as human beings while I regard the Chinese as pigs." Some Japanese soldiers even considered pigs to be more valuable than Chinese humans "because a pig is edible."[13]

The Legacy of Ishii Shiro

With this attitude prevalent in the Imperial Army, it is not surprising that medical experiments on the Chinese were performed without restriction or remorse. On his trips to Japan, Ishii boasted of his experiments, and, although he insisted on strict secrecy in Manchuria, he did not shrink from showing pictures of his work on human subjects during his lectures at Japanese medical colleges and universities. Ishii was a fascinating lecturer, impressive by virtue of his intelligence, exuberant personality, devil-may-care attitude, and obvious capability to achieve the unusual. On his lecture trips, he recruited promising young scientists who followed him to Manchuria because they were paid well and hoped to advance their careers with newly acquired experiences.[14] That those experiences would include the murder of scores of humans did not deter them because most test subjects were "lowly" Han Chinese. Furthermore, they believed implicitly that advanced research was not to be inhibited by ethical restraints and that the end justified the means. For those who might harbor any doubts, Ishii supplied this rationalization in a speech to his unit in 1938:

Our god-given mission as doctors is to challenge all varieties of disease-causing microorganisms, to block all roads of intrusion into the human body, to annihilate all foreign matter resident in our bodies, and to devise the most expeditious treatment possible. However, the research work upon which we are now about to embark is the complete opposite of these principles, and may cause us some anguish as doctors. Nevertheless, I beseech you to pursue this research, based on the dual thrill of 1), a scientist to exert efforts to probe for the truth in natural science and research into, and discovery of, the unknown world and 2), a military person, to successfully build a powerful military weapon against the enemy.[15]

Ishii fascinated not only students and coworkers, but also his superiors in the military. His bad habits, such as heavy drinking and womanizing, were excused as the eccentricities of an unusual man. He was promoted every three years, ultimately reaching the rank of Lieutenant General; his financial resources increased steadily and exceeded that of generals commanding many divisions; some 5,000 men were placed under his direct command, among them 300 to 500 doctors and scientists.[16] In 1936, Ishii was appointed chief of the "Anti-Epidemic Water Supply and Purification Bureau" whose official purpose was to supply the Japanese army with clean drinking water. The bureau was an ideal cover for Ishii who, in time, built up units for conducting his research all over China.

15 · Research by the Japanese

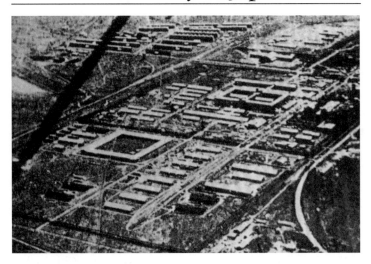

The Infamous Unit 731 and Biological Warfare

Ishii's main facility for research was created in Manchuria and
its dimensions were breathtaking. In a region called Pingfan,
thousands of acres were expropriated by the Japanese; at least
eight villages were evacuated and partially torn down, and a
new city was built with a perimeter of more than six square kilometers, rivaling Auschwitz-Birkenau in size (Fig. 359). The
new "city" consisted of at least 76 buildings, an airfield, a power
plant, recreational facilities, dormitories for civilian workers,
two prisons, a munitions dump, barns for test animals, a huge
farm that produced fruit and vegetables for the staff and plants
for experiments in biological warfare, and laboratories for different modes of research.[17] The Pingfan Research facility became known as Unit 731, a name that should be remembered
forever in the history of cruelty to man.

One section of the facility was devoted to the development of
various types of bombs for biological warfare. In another section, all kinds of pathogens were produced, including, but not
limited to, the causative organisms of plague, cholera, typhoid,

and paratyphoid fevers, dysentery, anthrax, glanders, tetanus, and gas gangrene. To produce sufficient numbers of organisms, four boilers had been installed, "each of one-ton capacity, for the preparation of the culture medium for the bacteria, and 14 autoclaves for sterilizing the medium." When operating at full capacity, the production division could "manufacture as much as 300 kilograms of plague bacteria monthly, . . . 500-600 kilograms of anthrax germs, or 800-900 kilograms of typhoid, paratyphoid, or dysentery germs, and as much as 1000 kilograms of cholera germs." Another section of the Pingfan factory was responsible for storage and maintenance of the enormous quantity of germs; yet another was for training of newly assigned personnel.[18]

The subordinate work at Pingfan was assigned to Chinese laborers. Ten to fifteen thousand local peasants were recruited between 1936 and 1945, and more than one-third of them died of exhaustion and maltreatment (Fig. 360). During construction of the facilities, Chinese laborers were informed, in order to conceal the true purpose of Pingfan, that the Japanese were building a lumber mill. Thus, human test subjects soon were referred to sarcastically as "logs" by Ishii and his staff. Every other

FIG. 360
Instruments of torture employed at Pingfan to discipline Chinese workers.

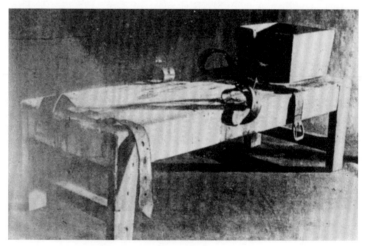

day, soldiers from nearby Harbin delivered eight or more "logs" who had either been arrested for some sort of crime, such as smoking opium or vagrancy, or, when the demand for human specimens increased, had been picked up while walking on the streets of Harbin. "Logs" usually were delivered at night and stored in two prisons that had been erected in the center of a huge, rectangular administration building, shielded from curious eyes. If "logs" survived an experiment, they sometimes were used again, but rarely for longer than a month. Ultimately, all test subjects were "sacrificed."[19]

Among the types of research performed on human beings at Pingfan was the development of new vaccines. For example, a cholera vaccine produced with ultrasonic equipment was compared with a conventional vaccine by forcing test subjects to drink copious quantities of cholera-infected milk, after they had been inoculated by one or the other of the vaccines. A third group of test subjects was infected without having been vaccinated at all. All subjects in the latter group and some of those who had received the conventional vaccine died, whereas persons who had received the new vaccine did not develop signs of cholera. Henceforth, the ultrasonically-produced vaccine was used for prevention of cholera in Japanese troops.[20]

Numerous studies were given to the destructive aspects of biological warfare. Test subjects were injected with all kinds of pathogens, and their reactions were monitored closely. Nearly invariably, experiments were supplemented by findings at autopsy; if subjects did not succumb to the infection, they were killed by beheading, electric current, injections of potassium cyanide, or other means. Not infrequently, dissection of subjects proceeded while they were still alive. One pathologist recalled that experience in these words: "I cut him open from the chest to the stomach and he screamed terribly and his face was twisted in agony. He made this unimaginable sound, he was screaming so horribly. But then finally he stopped. This was all

FIG. 361
Scientists of Unit 731 with two of their Chinese victims.

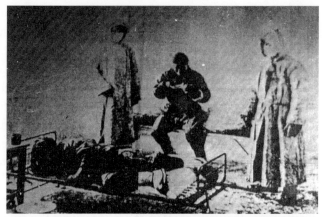

FIG. 362
Japanese pathologists after a vivisection on a Chinese test subject.

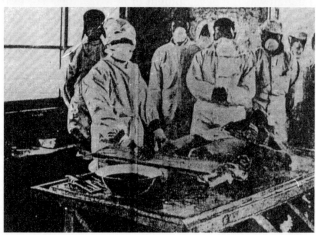

in a day's work for the surgeons, but it really left an impression on me because it was my first time"[21] (Fig. 361, 362, 363, 364).

Most of the data acquired through these studies already were well known and established firmly. There was no need, for example, to reexamine the natural course of common diseases like typhus and smallpox. In the case of a rare disease, such as epidemic hemorrhagic fever, some new knowledge was acquired concerning modes, signs, and symptoms of the infection, but the same information could have been gained through

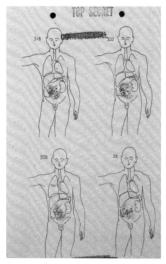

FIG. 363
Diagram of
autopsy
findings in
four Chi-
nese sub-
jects infect-
ed with
glanders.

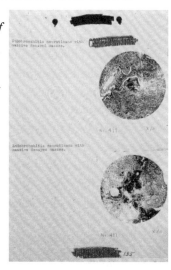

FIG. 364
Photographs
of histo-
pathologic
findings in
Chinese test
subjects in-
fected with
anthrax.

experiments in animals and by observation of patients who had acquired the diseases naturally. In fact, at the time the experiments were carried out, several outbreaks of epidemic hemorrhagic fever in China could have provided ample material come by naturally for study. Kitano Masaji (Fig. 365), who succeeded Ishii in 1942 as commander at Pingfan and who infected experimentally more than 100 persons with the disease, noted that the mortality of epidemic hemorrhagic fever in the general population was between 15 percent and 30 percent. He called attention to the fact that "mortality in experimental cases was 100 percent due to the procedure of sacrificing experimental subjects."[22]

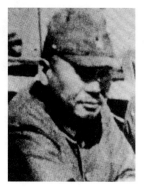

FIG. 365
Kitano Masaji

In addition to the qualitative assessment of reactions to infectious agents, laboratory studies on human subjects also concerned the quantity of organisms needed to produce reactions and the techniques by which germs could be administered unnoticed by the victims. For example, test subjects were fed cookies containing plague bacteria and chocolates filled with anthrax bacteria.[23] Another type of human experiment, conducted outside the laboratory, was the open-air study, carried out at a secret airfield built for this purpose at Anda, north of Harbin. These experiments generally involved tying subjects to stakes in the ground while an airplane dropped bombs filled with infectious germs that exploded at different altitudes above them.[24] Other airplanes, outfitted with canisters containing bacteria and nozzles, sprayed bacteria in a fine mist around the struggling captives.[25]

Yet another type of experiment, conducted on a much larger scale, was the field test in which both civilian and military contingents were exposed unwittingly to pathogens (Fig. 366). The largest field test was conducted in 1942 in the Chekiang province in Eastern China, where resistance against the Japanese occupation remained unbroken. Two biological warfare units, one in Pingfan (Unit 731) and the other in Nanking (Unit Ei 1644) (Fig. 367), pooled their resources and know-how for a massive bacteriological attack. Bottles labeled "water supply"

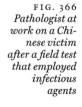

FIG. 366
Pathologist at work on a Chinese victim after a field test that employed infectious agents

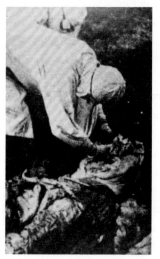

were filled with the germs of typhus and paratyphus and delivered to people's homes and dropped into wells and marshes. Epidemics soon ravaged the region, taking a toll of many thousands. The field test, however, was only partially successful because Japanese troops also were affected by the epidemics. Ten thousand troops became ill and at least 1,700 died.[26] In the vicinity of Changchun, the capital of the puppet state of Manchoukuo, devastating

15 · Research by the Japanese

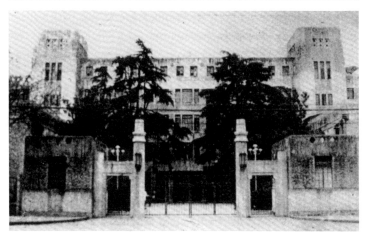

FIG. 367
*Headquarters
in Nanking of
the biological
warfare unit Ei
1644.*

outbreaks of plague resulted from field tests by the local biological warfare branch (Unit 100) that operated independently of Ishii's group.[27] In many regions of China, epidemics of diseases, unknown previously, continued to erupt for many years after the war.[28]

Like Germany, Like Japan

In addition to matters that pertained to biological warfare, many other medical problems were explored by Japanese physicians, who made ample use of new possibilities provided for them by virtue of the unlimited supply of human material for their experiments. Subjects and methods of research resembled closely those in Nazi Germany. For example, Hisato Yoshimura, who, after the war, became president of the medical faculty of the University of Kyoto, studied frostbite using basically the same techniques employed at the concentration camp at Dachau by Sigmund Rascher. According to later testimony by some of Yoshimura's subordinates, "... at times of great frost, with temperatures below -20°, people were brought out from the detachment's prison into the open. Their arms were bared and made to freeze with the help of an artificial current of air.

This was done until their frozen arms, when struck with a short stick, emitted a sound resembling that which a board gives out when it is struck." Prisoners were then subjected to various methods of treatment for their frostbite, such as exposure of frozen limbs to water of varying temperatures and amputation of limbs, before they were ultimately "sacrificed." In 1952, Yoshimura published some of his findings in a Japanese textbook of physiology, including the results of an experiment in which newborns were plunged into water of 0°C for 30 minutes. At least three neonates immersed in this fashion were killed.[29]

Physiological responses to thirst and problems related to flying at high altitudes were studied at Pingfan in the same manner as at they were at Dachau.[30] Studies on the effects of mustard gas at Beiyinhe and Pingfan were similar to those performed at the Natzweiler concentration camp.[31] Not infrequently, the experiments had no real military purpose and were undertaken merely to satisfy curiosity. In some of these "studies," for example, horse urine was injected into human kidneys, air was injected into veins, and test subjects were hung upside down to determine the time it would take for a person in that position to choke to death.[32] Like Nazi physicians, members of Ishii's unit killed healthy persons – chiefly pregnant women and prepubescent boys – to enrich their collections of anatomic specimens.[33] Reminiscent of Nazi experimentation, results often were published under the heading of "animal experiments," with human test subjects transformed magically into "Manchurian monkeys" or "Taiwan monkeys."[34] Human experimentation also was carried out on prisoners of war, such as on "the immunity of Anglo-Saxons to infectious diseases" at the prison camp at Mukden in Manchuria.[35] As in Nazi Germany, much of the research was of poor scientific quality, for example, the same test subject often was used for several consecutive experiments – such as exposure to poison gas, followed by injection of a sublethal dose of potassium cyanide and then by exposure to high voltage – all of which rendered data derived from the subsequent experiments meaningless.[36] American experts who later scrutinized the data accumulated by Japanese scientists considered them to be "not of significant value." Although the United States in 1943 was the last major power to embark on biological warfare research, the experts concluded that "within one year of the establishment of its program, the level of US expertise already exceeded that of the team at Unit 731."[37]

Parallels between Japan and Nazi Germany did not end with the loss of the war. In the postwar period, the pattern of behavior of physicians in both countries was similar indeed. In Germany, most physicians denied any knowledge of concentration camps, extermination of Jews, and use of human beings for purposes of medical research. In Japan, members of Ishii's staff and other biological warfare units insisted that their work never had involved human test subjects.[38] German physicians lent support to one another by providing affidavits that their colleagues always had been opposed to the Nazis and had never been engaged actively in the Nazi movement.[39] In Japan, scientists who admitted participation in studies on biological warfare denied knowledge of activities on the part of colleagues and averred that neither the military leaders nor the Emperor had been informed about the research.[40] In Germany, physicians who had participated in abominable human research suddenly flaunted high ethical convictions. A prime example was that of Otmar von Verschuer who, in 1944, had written about the "racial war" against "World Jewry" and had demanded as a "political priority of the present, a new, total solution of the Jewish problem." After the war he suddenly bemoaned the "misuse of science" by the Nazis and the "dreadful annihilation of Jews."[41] Likewise, Verschuer's Japanese colleague, Kitano Masaji, who had succeeded Ishii Shiro as commander at Pingfan in 1942 and had expanded human experimentation there, proclaimed a few years later that "a bacteriological weapon is a misuse of science."[42] In Germany, many former Nazis had highly successful postwar careers. Verschuer, for example, became chairman of human genetics at the University of Münster and Josef Vonkennel assumed the chair of dermatology at the University of Cologne.[43] The same was true for former coworkers of Ishii. Kitano Masaji became director of the Tokyo branch of the Japanese Blood Bank; Tachiomaru Ishikawa, the chief pathologist at Pingfan who dissected countless prisoners while they were still alive, rose to the position of dean of the medical faculty at the University of Kanazawa; Okamoto Kozo, who performed numerous vivisections at Pingfan, was made director of the medical faculty of the University of Tokyo.[44]

Human experimentation in Japan, as in Germany, did not emerge merely as a consequence of deviation from accepted ethical standards by a small "macabre order" of physicians. Despite all claims to the contrary after the war, the studies performed by Ishii, Kitano, Ishikawa, and countless of their coworkers, were given full approval by leading representatives of Japanese medicine and by the Japanese medical profession at large.

CHAPTER 16

EXPERIMENTS ON HUMANS BY THE ALLIES

Throughout history, the most devastating element in times of war has been infectious diseases. Poor diet and poor hygienic conditions often led to epidemics that were responsible for more fatalities than did injuries on the battlefield. In the late nineteenth and early twentieth centuries, medical research was recognized increasingly as an important aspect of a war effort and it was undertaken without the restraints usually imposed on scientists in civil life.

The importance of medical research in time of war was not lost on the Allied nations, which engaged in human experimentation that concerned many and diverse medical problems. The types and full extent of experiments on humans in the Soviet Union are not known. That such experiments were performed, however, is beyond doubt, and the insignificance attached to an individual in the states of the Soviet Republic seems to indicate that requirements for consent were not observed rigorously. Evidence for that assumption is provided by a few stories of studies by Soviet medical men and basic scientists that trickled out in later years. In 1940, the Russian virologist, A.A. Smorodintsev, injected blood or urine of people with epidemic hemorrhagic fever into mentally defective patients and succeeded in transmitting that often fatal disease.[1] Investigation of other matters, such as agents of chemical and biological warfare, must have been even more common. During the Stalin period, the Soviet police often plucked people off the streets and took them to dreaded Lubyanka Prison in Moscow, where KGB headquarters was housed. Many thousands were killed there, and many of them were obliged to undergo painful experiments before being put to death. Although such experiments continued to be conducted well into the 1970s, the worst offenses of the KGB in this regard appear to have occurred in the 1930s and 1940s.[2]

In Great Britain and the United States, experiments were carried out chiefly on "volunteers." The meaning of "volunteer," however, varied considerably, ranging from inmates in penitentiaries and soldiers threatened by court martial to individuals who offered themselves, at their own initiative, with no coercion whatsoever. British biochemist, Hans Adolf Krebs (Fig. 368), a Jewish refugee from Germany who shared the 1953 Nobel prize in medicine with Fritz Lipmann for discovery of the citrate acid cycle, used conscientious objectors at the Sorby Research Institute in Sheffield, England, for studies on diet. In 1946 he informed the British Medical Research Council that

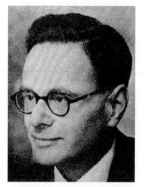

FIG. 368
*Hans Adolf
Krebs
(1900-1981)*

"some of the volunteers come to the Institute with the express wish to take part in experiments which involve risks to life and limb. They do not wish to evade military service to get a 'soft' job. It is their intention to do something which is, in a way, comparable with military service, in that it is work for the good of the community, associated with some dangers."[3]

16 · Experiments by the Allies

Conscientious Objectors Go to War

In contrast to the situation in the United States, where conscientious objectors were put in jail unless they could provide convincing religious motives for their stance, the British accepted many reasons of conscience as grounds for refusal to join the military. Once those reasons had been approved by a special body, objectors could choose various forms of work for the public good, including service as a guinea pig. In Sheffield, the medical entomologist and ecologist, Kenneth Mellanby, who in the 1960s would become one of the first scientists to call attention to the environmental effects of pollution, took advantage of this fortuitous situation. At the Sorby Research Institute, he embarked on a study of scabies, an intensely pruritic skin disease caused by the female mite, *Sarcoptes scabiei*, a malady that had spread rapidly in the first years of the war. By the end of 1941, between one and two million people throughout Britain were thought to be infected with scabies; military authorities were worried because of "a shockingly large amount of absence from duty" engendered by the infestation.[4] Mellanby studied the transmission of the mite by having objectors don the underwear of patients with scabies and sleep in the same bed with them. He examined the course of the disease by letting objectors go untreated for up to nine months, and he then studied the efficacy of various experimental therapeutic modalities. Mellanby emphasized that objectors submitted themselves to these experiments voluntarily, but he admitted that "the war has given us opportunities for carrying out investigations which would have been impossible under other circumstances."[5]

Once the studies on scabies were under way, Mellanby and his colleagues turned to other subjects, among them studies on vitamins A and C. To produce deficiencies of these vitamins, test subjects were given "a very dull and restricted diet, with no breaks or periods of alleviation, for a stretch of practically two years, which must quite easily be the world's record for such an experiment."[6] Depletion of vitamin A caused only minor problems, but lack of vitamin C resulted in the well known signs of scurvy. At that stage, several experiments were carried out on those subjects. Mellanby explained that "one of the more unpleasant experiments was on wound healing. A 3 cm cut was made deep into the flesh of a thigh. This was allowed to heal and then the weight needed to open the wound again was measured. Deprived individuals healed less well, but no protective effect of high intakes of the vitamin were detected."[7]

Other research projects of a nature questionable ethically included attempts by H.N. Greene of the University of Sheffield to induce shock through injection of a toxin, resulting in "many somewhat alarming experiences."[8] Studies on the efficacy and side effects of antimalarial drugs involved conscientious objectors being infected with "a virulent strain of malignant tertian malaria, which is often fatal."[9] As a consequence of the artificially induced infection, "a substantial proportion [of test subjects] developed clinical malaria and were unpleasantly ill."[10]

British Experimentation in the Empire

More extensive experiments in humans were conducted by British scientists in other parts of the Empire. Together with a native physician, two medical officers of the British Armed Forces in India reported in 1942 on "transmission of Indian kala-azar to man by the bites of *Phlebotomus argentipes.*" Kala-azar, which literally means "black death," is a severe systemic disease caused by the parasite, Leishmania donovani, and is characterized by fever, weakness, fatigue, emaciation, anemia, enlargement of the liver and spleen, generalized lymphadenopathy, and hyperpigmentation of the skin. At the time the experiment was performed, no successful treatment was available for Kala-azar. According to the authors, all test subjects were volunteers, namely, "healthy Khasi males," none of whom "had ever left the non-endemic area of the Khasi hills." Whether these "volunteers" had been informed of the nature and consequences of the experiment was not mentioned.[11]

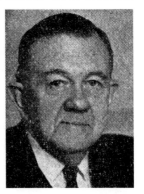

FIG. 369
*Neil Hamilton
Fairley
(1891-1966)*

In Australia, methods for prophylaxis and treatment of malaria were studied by Neil Hamilton Fairley (Fig. 369), who eventually would become a respected professor of tropical medicine at London University and president of the Royal Society of Tropical Medicine and Hygiene.[12] At the Land Headquarters Medical Research Unit at Cairns, Queensland, human subjects "were given various prophylactic courses of drugs, and were subjected to different degrees of infection by malarial parasites. In order to find out whether protection which seemed effective in unstressful conditions would be equally effective during hostilities, the volunteers were subjected to cold, to exhaustion and even to the effects of alcoholic excess."[13] Up to two pints of blood were removed in order to simulate loss of blood from injuries, insulin was injected to mimic starvation, and adrenalin was given to heighten the level of emotion needed to emulate that experience in battle.[14]

For his research, Fairley made use of "an unending supply of volunteers from the army."[15] Among his subjects were Jewish refugees from Germany and Austria who had been ejected from Britain and sent forthwith to Australia. On their arrival in Australia, they were interned in a camp where, in order to be freed, they were given the opportunity of volunteering for the Army. As interned aliens, however, they were denied the right to active duty and, therefore, signed up for the military's medical experiments. They were given little, if any, information about risks associated with the experiments; some of the refugees could not even communicate in English, so they had no idea of what to expect.[16] Likewise, soldiers who returned from combat infected with malaria participated in trials of experimental drugs without being informed that a new, effective drug, Atabrine, already was in use. The trials conducted by Fairley demonstrated the efficacy of chloroquine, which still is used for prevention and treatment of malaria and for a variety of other diseases. The drug created a windfall for the pharmaceutical company that produced it, but when, after the war, a soldier inquired about remuneration for the "guinea pigs," he was told that it was not appropriate to seek an award when so many others had suffered hardship or lost their lives.[17]

Chemical Warfare

Another British physician, Fred S. Gorrill (Fig. 370), headed a research unit in Australia that examined properties of agents of chemical warfare in tropical climates. Although Great Britain had signed and ratified the 1925 Geneva Convention that banned chemical weapons, it had continued research on them under the pretext of preparation defensively against the event of chemical attack. By the beginning of the Second World War, chemical weapons, such as mustard gas, had been studied extensively. Long-term effects of exposure to mustard gas – such

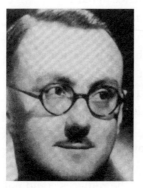

FIG. 370
Fred S. Gorrill

as chronic bronchitis, emphysema, susceptibility to tuberculosis and other infectious diseases, and development of various types of cancer – had not yet been certified fully. Victims of gas attacks in World War I, however, had already demonstrated that mustard gas had capability to affect every system of the body.[18] In 1933, English novelist H.G. Wells wrote of mustard gas in his book, *The Shape of Things to Come*, and this is some of what he said:

Steadily but surely it killed every living substance with which it came into contact; it burned it, blistered it, rotted it away. It is doubtful if any of those affected by it were ever completely cured. Its maximum effect was rapid torture and death; its minimum, prolonged misery and an abbreviated life.[19]

Although mustard gas was known to be absorbable and to exert toxic effects on all internal organs, scientists who engaged in research about chemical warfare tended to minimize the risks of it. They adhered to the concept that chemical weapons were more "humane" than traditional modes of warfare because the number of casualties caused by them was fewer. Long-term consequences of poisoning with mustard gas were ignored and short-term effects were trivialized. Because of superficial similarities they had in common, such as erythema and blistering of the skin, poisoning with mustard gas was compared to a severe sunburn. Measures to prevent the "sunburn" – such as wearing protective clothing and applying protective ointments – had been tested on human subjects throughout the 1920s and 1930s at the British biological warfare research center in Porton Down, at Salisbury, and scientists there were confident that they could handle chemical attacks.[20] All data, however, had been acquired under the moderate climatic conditions of Europe. How chemical weapons acted in a hot, humid environment was not known. When, in 1942, Fred Gorrill carried out preliminary studies on volunteers of the Australian army, he noted that the toxicity of phosgene, lewisite, mustard gas, and other agents was much greater than he had anticipated. Following exposure to chemical agents in a gas chamber, test subjects developed severe burns, leading to detachment of their entire skin, loss of nails, and agonizing pain[21] (Fig. 371, 372). Alarmed by these findings, the War Cabinet commissioned Gorrill to establish a research center for

FIG. 371
*Test subject
with burns
secondary to
contact with
nitrogen
mustard.*

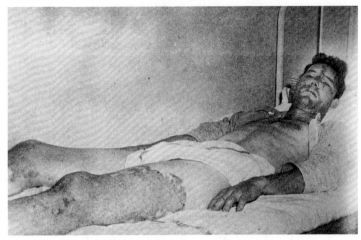

chemical warfare in Queensland, where he was charged with carrying out large-scale experiments on humans.

The "volunteers" for these experiments were Australian soldiers, young in age and low in rank, recruited from nearby military holding camps. These men had joined the armed forces with the desire to help defend their homeland. Increasingly bored with routine marches in Queensland, they were eager to get into action; when word spread about a secret mission, they

FIG. 372
*Test subject
with burns sec-
ondary to con-
tact with nitro-
gen mustard.*

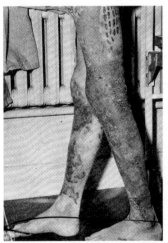

volunteered for what they believed would be a combat assignment. On arriving at the research camp, many volunteers were completely unaware of what was in store for them.[22] Others had been informed about the experiments, but in a vague and deceptive way. For example, a call for volunteers that circulated among Australian troops in 1943 read as follows:

(a) Volunteers are required to take part in experiments with gas.

(b) These experiments are directed to proving the effectiveness of our defensive equipment.

(c) There is a small element of risk of burns and blisters but no risk of permanent injury.

(d) The period volunteers will be away from units will usually be 3-4 weeks.

(e) Volunteers must undertake to preserve secrecy about the whole matter.[23]

Considering the knowledge that already existed about chemical warfare agents and the severe effects encountered in the most recent experiments, the information provided to the recruits was fraudulent. Once soldiers had volunteered, however, there was no way out; orders had to be followed, and letting one's mates down was considered to be a breach of honor. Moreover, volunteers were offered incentives, such as a free bottle of beer each day, extra leave, and a few shillings added to their pay.[24] Many volunteers, through their inexperience and failure to resist, paid a terrible price for these meager emoluments because much of the defensive equipment being tested proved worthless. In the heat of Queensland, the dyes in British protective clothing released aniline, which was toxic to the subjects being tested. When other types of protective clothing were tried out in a gas chamber, they were found to be penetrable by mustard gas, leading to severe burns of the scrotum, arms, and legs. Likewise, high concentrations of mustard gas gained entry to the rubber components of standard respirators, causing injuries to eyes and skin.[25]

Because of the immense number of American casualties in the Pacific islands, where the Japanese were entrenched in foxholes and complex concrete tunnels resistant to conventional bombardment, the Allies began to consider the possibility of initiating chemical attacks in that theater of war. To procure data about various aspects of chemical warfare, Gorrill and his team staged unprecedented experimental attacks on the Brook Islands, a group of small coral islands off the Queensland coast. The aim was to determine how many tons of mustard gas per square mile were required to injure troops and how much time must elapse before troops in either protective clothing or ordinary battle dress were able to occupy the area. While tons of mustard gas bombs were being dropped on the island, volunteers were left in Japanese-style dug-outs[26] or brought ashore after predetermined intervals for varying periods of time. They were equipped with different kinds of protective clothing, ranging from a full double layer, worn by the research team, to none at all.[27] On the island, volunteers were instructed to measure concentrations of mustard gas and to engage in various physical exercises. In order to duplicate a battle situation, they had to traverse the contaminated jungle again and again, were not allowed to wash or change their contaminated uniforms for up to a week, and were barred from receiving any medical treatment.[28] The consequences were devastating. Many volunteers displayed signs of extensive systemic toxicity, such as violent nausea and vomiting, severe headaches, burns with widespread blisters, and loss of nails and teeth.[29] Several subjects died as a result of these tests[30] (Fig. 373, 374).

FIG. 373
Test subject in full protective gear during chemical warfare trials on the Brook Islands.

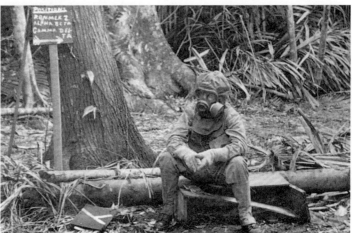

16 · Experiments by the Allies

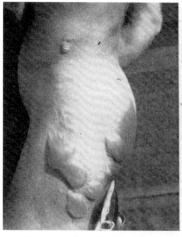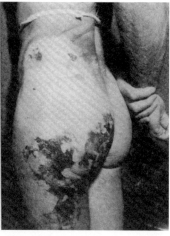

FIG. 374
*Burns on the
buttocks follow-
ing contact
with nitrogen
mustard on the
Brook Islands.*

The Brook Islands trials were successful from a military standpoint and allowed Gorrill to conclude that Japanese fortifications on Pacific islands were vulnerable to chemical attack.[31] The Allies, however, never made use of that information, so that the suffering of some 2,000 Australian volunteers ultimately was for naught. When test subjects later developed chronic bronchitis, cancer, and other sequelae, their claims of being victims of chemical warfare were not believed to be legitimate. Because the trials had been conducted in secret and the data remained classified, only a few succeeded in obtaining compensation in the form of a modest pension.[32] The scientists responsible for the experiments fared much better. Their wartime scientific work gained them respect and helped foster their careers. For example, David Sinclair (Fig. 375), Gorill's second-in-command, published numerous articles on the effects of mustard gas in scientific periodicals, such as the *British Medical Journal*[33] and the *British Journal of Dermatology*.[34]

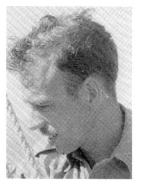

FIG. 375
David Sinclair

Gorrill, himself, eventually became director of the British pharmaceutical company, Glaxo.[35]

Mobilizing Medical and Chemical Research in Wartime America

Gorrill's trials regarding chemical warfare in Queensland were carried out not only with the backing of British and Australian authorities, but also with massive support from the U.S. Army, which provided protective clothing, chemical weapons, barges, and airplanes. This type of cooperation among the Allies was common, although most war-related research was conducted strictly on a national basis. The United States had its own research program on chemical warfare, and a report produced in 1993 by the American Institute of Medicine suggests that more than 60,000 volunteers may have participated in experiments on humans during the Second World War. As in Australia, "volunteers" were soldiers who were not informed openly, directly, and truthfully about the nature of the experiments. Some had agreed to test "summer clothing" and were horrified to find themselves wearing it in gas chambers. Those who became sick were threatened with court martial "if they did not continue the test and re-enter the gas chambers." Moreover, they were told "that they would be sent to prison if they ever revealed their participation in these tests."[36]

The research program instituted in the United States during the war was more extensive and ambitious than that of any other country. Shortly before entering the war, President Franklin D. Roosevelt established the Office of Scientific Research and Development, which oversaw the work of two committees, one directed to research on weapons and the other aimed at problems of a medical nature. The Committee on Medical Research had the job of "mobilizing the medical and scientific personnel of the nation; recommending contracts to

16 · Experiments by the Allies

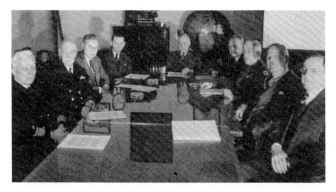

FIG. 376
The Committee on Medical
Research in 1945. From
left to right: R. E. Dyer,
Assistant Surgeon General
and Director of the Na-
tional Institute of Health;
Harold W. Smith; A.B.
Hastings; C.S. Keefer; A.N.
Richards, Chairman; L.H.
Weed, Vice-Chairman;
Brig.- Gen. J.S. Simmons;
A.R. Dochez; I. Stewart,
Secretary.

be entered into with universities, hospitals and other agencies
conducting medical research activities; and submitting recommendations with respect to medical problems related to the national defense."[37] Chief among these problems was finding antidotes for diseases – such as influenza, malaria, and dysentery –
that were particularly ruinous to troops (Fig. 376).

Thus began what Chester Keefer, one of the mainstays of the
Committee on Medical Research, later described as "a novel experiment in American medicine, for planned and coordinated
medical research had never been assayed on such a scale."[38]
Over the next four years, the Committee recommended for
funding some 600 research proposals, many of them involving
human subjects, to the Office of Scientific Research and Development. That Office, in turn, contracted with investigators at
135 universities, hospitals, research institutes, and industrial
firms to conduct the investigations. The committee utilized the
services of approximately 17,000 medical doctors and 38,000
scientists and technologists. Between 1941 and 1947, the U.S.
government appropriated $25 million for medical research. At
that time, it was an extraordinary sum which allowed hospitals,
colleges, and corporate institutions to employ scientists and
technicians in ample numbers and to endow them with the
most advanced instruments of technology.[39]

The need to establish adequate research facilities rapidly for broad-scale clinical investigations became a major hurdle. The most obvious solution was the use of existing military facilities and military personnel, especially because the risks of medical experiments paled before the dangers of battle. Soldiers, however, were considered to be too valuable to be "wasted" on medical research; studies involving military personnel were the exception.[40] As in Great Britain, some of the most critical experiments – such as studies concerning the reactions of the human body to high altitudes, freezing, and starvation – were performed on conscientious objectors.[41] But the bulk of medical research was conducted in penal institutions, where confinement and control of prisoners offered ideal conditions for trials on human beings.[42]

Captive Volunteers

A precedent for medical experiments on prisoners already had been established in the United States early in the twentieth century. Stereotypical of these were the cholera inoculations of prison inmates in the Philippines in 1906 by Richard Strong, and the study of pellagra in 1915 by U.S. Public Health official, Joseph Goldberger, at a prison farm in Mississippi. During World War II, however, research using penitentiary inmates in the U.S. escalated from episodic investigations by individual physicians to a national endeavor involving vast numbers of medical doctors. Throughout the country, prisoners were solicited for trials by virtue of appeal to their patriotism. Newspapers proclaimed proudly that "these one-time enemies to society appreciate to the fullest extent just how completely this is everybody's war."[43] Although patriotism surely played some role in the decision of prisoners to participate in trials, an equally (or more) compelling motive was the expectation of a reward for their services. Even when the wardens emphasized that a convict's participation in a research project would in no way "secure or enhance his chance" for early release, prisoners were "all sure that some means would be found to give consideration." And they were right; most prison volunteers eventually received parole.[44]

The inducements of patriotism combined with self-interest resulted in a nearly limitless supply of volunteers from prisons. In New York, for example, scores of inmates at Sing Sing Prison volunteered for daily doses of unfamiliar drugs in order to help the army determine whether a soldier could carry a full workload while under the influence of a particular medication. New Jersey prisons supplied the army with volunteers for a series of inoculation experiments on sleeping sickness, sandfly fever, and dengue fever. In El Reno, Oklahoma, 300 prisoners participated in an effort by the National Institute of Health "to determine the amount of toxoid necessary to immunize men against the organism that causes gas gangrene."[45] In Terre Haute, Indiana, 185 inmates of the U. S. Penitentary were enlisted in experiments on gonorrhea that consisted of deliberate infection of three groups of men; one treated with sulfonamides; another with topical agents; and a third not at all, the latter serving as controls.[46] In the summer of 1942, the U.S. Navy, with the support of Edward Joseph Cohn, a distinguished biochemist at Harvard, recruited volunteers from a state prison in Norfolk, Massachusetts by telling the prisoners that because the war had created a shortage of plasma, they were needed to test a substitute derived from beef blood. Sixty-four volunteers, most of whom had less than two years to serve until parole, were injected with an ounce of purified beef blood. Twenty prisoners became extremely ill from serum sickness "with high fever, rashes, and joint pains. One was dead."[47]

The most pressing medical problem at the time for the U.S. military was malaria, "an enemy even more to be feared than the Japanese."[48] The disease was debilitating and deadly, and the incidence ran high in the Pacific theater. Moreover, the

Japanese controlled the major supply of quinine, one of the few known effective antidotes for malaria. To establish alternative modalities of treatment, large-scale experiments on prisoners were carried out at several U.S. penitentiaries. In Atlanta, Georgia, for instance, 2,000 prisoners volunteered to become "human guinea pigs and undergo malarial infection and treatment with new drugs that were untried on the human system." Eventually, 130 men were enrolled in the study: "One hundred and five were infected with mosquito-induced, temperate-zone vivax malaria, 15 were inoculated by bites of mosquitoes that had been infected with a New Guinea strain of vivax malaria, and the remaining 10 men given one or more intravenous injections of blood taken from other malaria volunteers during attacks of malaria or during a latent phase of their infection."[49]

In September 1944, Alf S. Alving (Fig. 377) of the University of Chicago asked inmates at the Stateville Penitentiary in Illinois "to volunteer as experimental subjects in an effort to find a cure for malaria." All participants had to sign a waiver that read as follows: "I hereby accept all risks connected with the experiment and on behalf of my heirs and my personal and legal representatives. I hereby absolve from such liability the University of Chicago and all the technicians and assistants taking part in the above-mentioned investigations. I hereby certify that this offer is made voluntarily and without compulsion." In the

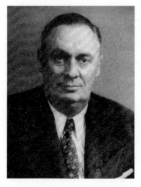

FIG. 377
*Alf S. Alving
(born 1902)*

course of two years, more than 400 prisoners were subjected to bites by infected mosquitos. The results were a series of cycles of recovery and relapse, the latter being attended by high fevers, nausea, vomiting, and aches and pains, plus innumerable blood tests.[50] One prisoner died of a heart attack after several bouts of high fever[51] (Fig. 378, 379).

16 · Experiments by the Allies

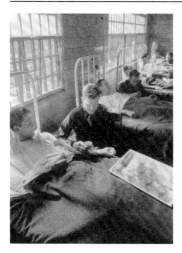

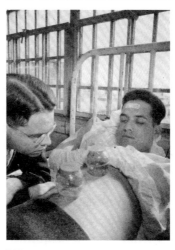

FIG. 378
Malaria experiment during World War II at Stateville Penitentiary in Illinois: Systematic infection of prisoners with malaria.

FIG. 379
Malaria experiment during World War II at Stateville Penitentiary in Illinois: Infected mosquitos being placed on the abdomen of a prisoner.

Although prisoners were required to sign waivers absolving researchers from culpability and liability, they usually were not informed fully about the risks associated with the experiments. Exceptions were made only when researchers and administrators of the Committee on Medical Research sensed the possibility of serious adverse reactions from the public. Such was the case in regard to the Terre Haute gonorrhea experiments. Before the study was begun at the U.S. Penitentiary, the ethical, legal, and political implications of it were discussed comprehensively. Its significance for the war effort was assessed by calculating the loss from gonorrhea of "man days per year," which was found to be equivalent to "putting out of action for a full year the entire strength of two full armored divisions or of ten aircraft carriers." Although the arguments in favor of the study were compelling, Alfred Newton Richards (Fig. 380), chairman of the Committee on Medical Research, resolutely insisted that "when any risks are involved, volunteers only should be utilized

FIG. 380
*Alfred Newton
Richards
(1876-1966)*

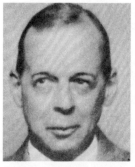

as subjects, and these only after the risks have been fully explained and after signed statements have been obtained which shall prove that the volunteer offered his services with full knowledge and that claims for damages will be waived. An accurate record should be kept of the terms in which the risks involved were described."[52] Considering the urgency of wartime, these provisions were remarkably strict and they indicate that at least some physicians were aware of ethical boundaries of research. Whenever public scrutiny was considered to be unlikely, however, ethical scruples were overridden by a mentality rooted in the conditions of war. Because medical investigations were integral to the military effort, the rules of the battlefield were applied to the laboratory, and the requirement for obtaining informed consent of test subjects was lost in the fray.[53]

Taking Advantage of Vulnerable Populations

Consequently, not only prisoners, but also inmates of orphanages and institutions for the mentally retarded, became subjects of the war effort. Merlin Cooper and B. K. Rachford of the Cincinnati Children's Hospital injected "killed suspensions of various types of [the] shigella group of bacteria" into veins, muscles, and subcutaneous fat of inmates at the Ohio Soldiers and Sailors Orphanage in an attempt to immunize them against dysentery. The test subjects – boys and girls between the ages of 13 and 17 – experienced serious side effects. Following intravenous injection of ten million bacteria of dysentery, the researchers made the following observation: "The systemic reaction was profound and began within less than 30 minutes. It was essentially the same in all of the boys. The skin was pale and ashy grey in color. The blood pressure was not altered but the temperature sky-rocketed to 105°F and up in spite of measures to counteract the rise. Severe pounding headache and a constricting type of backache were almost universal complaints. The bulbar conjunctivae were hyperemic. Rapidly, nausea, vomiting and watery diarrhea ensued. Fever persisted for 24 hours and when it subsided the subjects were exhausted." In other boys, bacteria of dysentery were injected subcutaneously in gradually increasing dosages "until it appeared that systematic reaction, local reaction, or both were limiting factors."[54]

Werner Henle of the University of Pennsylvania School of Medicine tested vaccines for experimentally induced flu on several hundred residents at a nearby state facility for the retarded at Pennhurst. At periods of three or six months following administration of the vaccine, test subjects were infected with influenza by fitting an aviation oxygen mask over their faces and having them inhale a gaseous preparation of the virus for four minutes. Other residents of the institution served as controls and were infected without being vaccinated. As expected, those who contracted the disease experienced high fevers, aches, and pains. A group of residents who had received the vaccine in a mineral oil base had nodules at the site of injection for between six to twelve months, and two had fulminant abscesses, one requiring reconstructive surgery.[55] A similar study with experimental vaccines for flu was performed on residents of Michigan's Ypsilanti State Hospital by microbiologist Jonas Salk, who observed that "in the unvaccinated group, 11, or 41 percent, . . . had temperatures of 100 or more and 6, or 22 percent, had temperatures of 101 or above. In the 69 vaccinated individuals, 7, or 10 percent, had temperatures between 100 and 100.9."[56] At the Manteno State Hospital in Illinois, patients who were psychotic or retarded mentally were included in the malaria program conducted by Alf Alving. After they were infected with malaria, they were treated with a variety of unproven experimental drugs.[57]

The Abuse of Man

The Manhattan Project

Medical experiments were carried out, too, on unsuspecting patients in American hospitals. The most glaring example of this abuse was a series of secret experiments involving intravenous injections of solutions of plutonium and other radioactive substances. In the effort with dispatch to build atomic bombs that would be dropped in August 1945 on Hiroshima and Nagasaki, the U.S. Army had instituted an extensive research program designated the Manhattan Project. The key substance requisite for achieving that desideratum, plutonium, had been isolated in 1941 at the University of California at Berkeley, and the biological hazards of it were still unknown. Because the scientists involved in the Manhattan Project were at great risk of becoming contaminated, leading radiologists were charged with studying the pharmacokinetics of plutonium and determining the highest dose of it tolerable – that is, one that would not result in impairment of health.

Louis Hempelmann (Fig. 381) was responsible for all health and safety aspects of the construction site for the bomb at Los Alamos, New Mexico. In a memo on August 25, 1944, to the head scientist of the Manhattan Project, J. Robert Oppenheimer, Hempelmann noted that following the establishment of chemical methods for the detection of minute amounts of

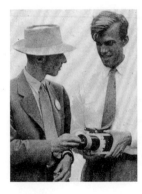

FIG. 381
Louis
Hempelmann
(1914-1993,
right) and
J. Robert
Oppenheimer
(left) examin-
ing a Geiger
Counter at a
nuclear test
site in
September
1945.

plutonium and a series of experiments on animals, "tracer experiments on humans to determine the percentage of plutonium excreted daily" would have to be performed.[58] By January 1945, the chemist Wright Langham (Fig. 382) had developed a method for detection of plutonium; experiments on dogs, rats, mice, and rabbits had indicated that plutonium was deposited in the liver and bone marrow, organs highly vulnerable to the effects of radiation.[59] The scientists of the Manhattan Project refrained, therefore, from performing experiments on themselves. "We considered doing such experiments at one time,"

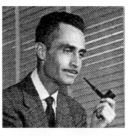

FIG. 382
Wright
Langham
(1911-1972)

Langham wrote in 1952, "but plutonium is considered to be sufficiently potentially dangerous to discourage our doing absorption experiments on ourselves."[60]

Instead, the scientists found other human test subjects, who were described in official documents as being "hopelessly sick" or "terminal."[61] This, however, was not exactly the case. Of 18 test subjects injected with plutonium between April 1945 and July 1947, seven survived for more than 10 years. These long-term survivors were exposed to cumulative doses of up to 1,000 rem of radiation. Some of them eventually developed diseases that may well have been related to the effects of radiation, such as cancer, fatal infections, and degeneration of bones. The diseases for which the test subjects had been hospitalized originally ranged from bone fractures to gastric ulcers, hemophilia to Addison's disease, and scleroderma to dermatomyositis (Fig. 383, 384). At the principal research facility of the program located at the University of Rochester in New York, patients with malig-

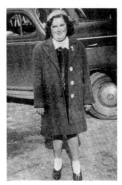

FIG. 383
18-year-old girl
with Cushing's
disease who was
injected with plu-
tonium at the
University of
Rochester in No-
vember 1945.

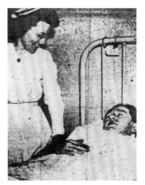

FIG. 384
48-year-old
patient with
hemophilia
during his 38th
trip to the hos-
pital at the
University of
Rochester fol-
lowing injec-
tion of him
with plutoni-
um in October
1945.

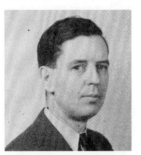

FIG. 385
Samuel Bassett

nant neoplastic diseases were excluded specifically from the plutonium trials because, as the responsible physician, Samuel Bassett (Fig. 385), explained, "their metabolism might be affected in an unknown manner."[62]

Bassett received the protocol for the study, and the vials containing plutonium from Wright Langham of Los Alamos. Patients – referred to as "HP" or "human products" – were given injections which contained five times the amount of plutonium that had been declared safe in humans. Prior to the injections, and for weeks or years following, the subjects had to provide ongoing samples of urine and feces, were X-rayed often, and had countless blood tests performed on them. Biopsy specimens also were obtained and autopsies performed whenever a subject died. The extensiveness of the examinations caused some test subjects to suspect that they had been used as guinea pigs, but they never were told that. According to Hempelmann, a "deliberate decision was made not to inform the patient of the nature of the product that was injected;"[63] the scientists saw to it that no mention ever was made in hospital records.[64]

The doses of plutonium given in experiments performed by different branches of the Manhattan Project were not consistent. At the University of Chicago's Billings Hospital, a 56-year-old woman with metastatic breast carcinoma was injected with 94.91 micrograms of plutonium, nearly one hundred times more than the amount scientists thought a healthy human body could tolerate. Almost immediately after the injection, she began to vomit and was unable to eat, drink, or retain anything; 17 days later she died.[65] Envious of the superior data being generated by the branch in Chicago, Langham asked his colleague, Samuel Bassett, to administer higher doses to his test subjects, arguing that "this would permit the analysis of much smaller samples and would make my work considerably easier."[66]

16 · Experiments by the Allies

At the University of California at Berkeley, Joseph Hamilton (Fig. 386), one of the first physicians to join the Manhattan Project, made this suggestion in September 1945: "The next human subject that is available is to be given, along with plutonium 238, small quantities of radioyttrium, radiostron-

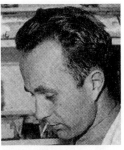

FIG. 386
*Joseph
Hamilton
(1907-1957)*

tium, and radiocerium. This procedure has in mind two purposes. First, the opportunity will be presented to compare in man the behavior of these three representative long-lived fission products with their metabolic properties in the rat, and second, a comparison can be made of the differences in their behavior from that of plutonium."[67]

The "next human subject" was a four-year-old Australian boy suffering from metastatic osteogenic sarcoma. He had been brought to California for treatment by his mother, who was desperate. Transportation had been organized by the U.S. Army and by the American Red Cross. On arrival in San Francisco, the mother and her son were met by a crowd of reporters and photographers. While American newspapers were displaying triumphantly one-page banner headlines like "Mercy Flight Brings Aussie Boy Here," the child was taken to a hospital, separated from his mother, and injected with a cocktail of radionuclides. The rate at which these substances were metabolized was determined by blood tests, examinations of urine and feces, and biopsies of bone, muscle, and connective tissue. Afterwards, the boy was released from the hospital, his tumor still increasing in size. Without any further medical help, he and his mother returned to Australia, where the boy died, in pain so excruciating that he screamed incessantly, in January 1947.[68]

In a series of lectures given to select audiences in the fall of 1946, Stafford Warren (Fig. 387), medical director of the Manhattan Project, spoke of plutonium as "probably the most toxic

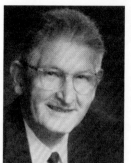

FIG. 387
*Stafford L.
Warren*
(1896-1981)

metal known. You need only to absorb a few micrograms of plutonium and other long-life fission materials, and then know that you are going to develop a progressive anemia or a tumor in ... five to fifteen years. This is an insidious hazard and an insidious lethal effect hard to guard against."[69]

Alarmed by these notions and by new guidelines for human experimentation being advanced by the American Medical Association (AMA) in connection with the trial of Nazi doctors at Nuremberg in 1947, the general manager of the newly formed Atomic Energy Commission, Carroll Wilson, set forth rules for experiments with radioactive materials on humans. In a letter to Warren on April 30, 1947, Wilson approved a "program for obtaining medical data of interest to the Commission in the course of treatment of patients" under the condition that treatment "will be administered to a patient only when there is expectation of a therapeutic effect ... It should be susceptible of proof from official records that, prior to treatment, each individual patient, being in an understanding state of mind, was clearly informed of the nature of the treatment and its possible effects, and expressed his willingness to receive the treatment." Moreover, Wilson required that "in every case at least two doctors should certify in writing (made part of an official record) to the patient's understanding state of mind, to the explanation furnished him, and to his willingness to accept the treatment."[70]

In brief, Wilson required informed consent for any form of experimental therapy and he forbade nontherapeutic experiments on humans. Despite these rules, Joseph Hamilton continued to inject patients with radionuclides, at the same time, ironically, that Nazi physicians were being tried in Nuremberg for unethical human experimentation.[71]

CHAPTER 17

THE NUREMBERG CODE

"**W**ar is hell." That dictum by General William Tecum-
seh Sherman not only guaranteed the hero of the
Union in the American Civil War fame that would
be lasting, but served also to justify anything done in wartime in
order to secure victory ultimately. As warfare became more and
more technological and devastating, however, most nations
agreed that some rules should be observed, no matter how hellish the conflagration. On the initiative of Swiss philanthropist
Jean-Henri Dunant (Fig. 388), an international conference
convened in Geneva in 1863 for the purpose of creating a neu-
tral organization that would aid wounded soldiers of all countries in times of war. One year later, the International Red Cross
was established, and the Geneva Convention laid down rules
for the treatment of military wounded and for the protection of

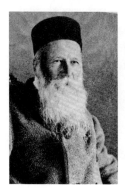

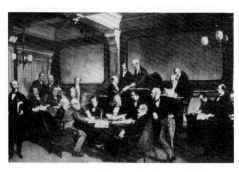

FIG. 389
Founding of the
International
Red Cross at the
Geneva Con-
vention on Au-
gust 22, 1864
(Painting by
C.E. Armand-
Dumaresq).

FIG. 388 *Jean-Henri Dunant (1828-1910)*

medical personnel and hospitals during war. (Fig. 389) At the 1899 Hague Conference in the Netherlands, customs and laws of warfare were revised to eliminate unnecessary suffering on the part of all concerned, be they combatants, noncombatants, or neutrals. Certain measures of warfare were banned, and a mechanism for the option of arbitration of controversial issues between nations was established in the form of the Permanent Court of Arbitration, known popularly as the Hague Tribunal. Subsequently, the provisions of the Geneva and Hague Conventions were revised and amended several times, specifying the rights and duties of neutrals, establishing rules to protect populations of civilians, and imposing restrictions on the use of various types of warfare.

In time, most signatories to the both conventions ignored some of the provisions of them. One glaring example was ongoing research in biological warfare that had been outlawed specifically by the Geneva Convention.[1] Violations of rules of warfare by the Axis powers of World War II, however, were excessive in the extreme. The United Kingdom, the United States, and the Soviet Union responded to the "atrocities, massacres, and cold-blooded mass executions which are being perpetrated by the Hitlerite forces in the many countries they have overrun" by warning their enemies of future consequences. In a "Declaration on German Atrocities" released in Moscow on November 1, 1943, Franklin D. Roosevelt, Winston Churchill, and Joseph Stalin

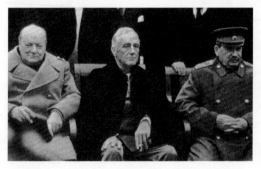

FIG. 390
*Churchill,
Roosevelt, and
Stalin (from
left to right) at
the Yalta
Conference in
1945.*

(Fig. 390) issued this warning:

Those German officers and men and members of the Nazi party who have been responsible for, or have taken a consenting part in the above atrocities, massacres, and executions, will be sent back to the countries in which their abominable deeds were done in order that they may be judged and punished according to the laws of these liberated countries and of the free governments which will be created therein.[2]

When, following the armistice, this proclamation was translated into practice, many physicians who had been involved in unethical experiments on humans were tried by a court in the region in which they had conducted their research. Claus Schilling was sentenced to death by a U.S. military court in Dachau in 1945 for his malaria experiments and was executed in 1946. Johann Paul Kremer, the "muscle collector" of Auschwitz was sentenced to death by a court in Krakow, Poland in 1947 (he was pardoned in 1958). Carl Clauberg, who sterilized thousands of Auschwitz prisoners, was sentenced to 25 years in prison by a Soviet court in 1948 and was released in 1955. Otto Bickenbach, of phosgene infamy, and Eugen Haagen, who mercilessly carried out countless vaccination experiments at Natzweiler, were sentenced to life by a French court in Metz in 1952 and were given amnesty after only three years.[3]

War Criminals on Trial

The Moscow Declaration by the Allies in November 1943 stated, too, that "The above declaration is without prejudice to the case of the major criminals, whose offenses have no particular geographical localization and who will be punished by the joint decision of the Governments of the Allies."[4] The decision came in the form of the London Agreement of August 8, 1945, in which the United States, Great Britain, France, and the Soviet Union established an International Military Tribunal composed of one judge and one alternate judge from each nation, the charge of that tribunal being to try war criminals. The crimes of defendants fell into three general categories: against peace by planning, initiating, and waging of aggressive war; against the laws and customs of war as embodied by the Hague Conventions; against humanity, such as the extermination of ethnic or religious groups and other atrocities committed on a large scale against civilians.

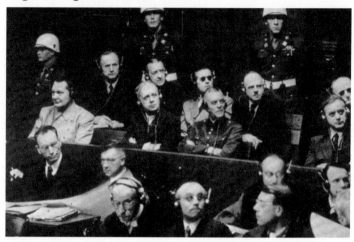

FIG. 391 *The chief defendants at the Nuremberg Trials of German war criminals. Behind the barrier, from left to right: Hermann Göring, Joachim von Ribbentrop, Wilhelm Keitel, Alfred Rosenberg. Back row: Karl Doenitz, Erich Raeder, Baldur von Schirach, Fritz Sauckel, Alfred Jodl.*

Twenty-one leading representatives of the Nazi regime were indicted, among them the former Prime Minister of Prussia and head of the Luftwaffe, Hermann Göring, Field Marshal Wilhelm Keitel, and the Führer's "deputy," Rudolf Hess. The War Crimes Trial began in Nuremberg on November 20, 1945, and ended on October 1, 1946. Three defendants were acquitted, seven received prison terms ranging from 10 years to life, and twelve were sentenced to death by hanging (Fig. 391). More important than those individual sentences, however, were the principles on which the judgments were based. In accordance with the London Agreement, planning or initiating an aggressive war became a crime under international law, for which individuals, and not merely states, could be held accountable. The tribunal rejected the contention of some defendants that they were not legally responsible for their acts because they had simply carried out the orders of superiors. The principle was clear, namely, "the true test is not the existence of the order, but whether moral choice was in fact possible." In 1946, the General Assembly of the United Nations adopted unanimously the Principles of International Law recognized by the Charter of the Nuremberg Tribunal. This document stated that international war crimes and crimes against humanity are acknowledged as violations, and that those who commit these acts can be tried and punished by an international tribunal, even if their acts were not in violation of their own domestic law, and even if they were acting under orders of a superior.[5]

Doctors on Trial

Following the conclusion of the first Nuremberg Trial, 12 more trials were held by the United States alone under the authority of Control Council Law No. 10, which resembled closely the London Agreement but provided for War Crimes Trials in each of the four zones of occupied Germany. The most important of these was the Doctors' Trial, which took place between December 9, 1946, and August 20, 1947. Twenty physicians and three non-medical officials who had participated in medical experiments in humans were "charged with murders, tortures, and other atrocities committed in the name of medical science."[6]

The decision of the Americans to conduct a public trial of Nazi physicians was controversial. The French, especially, favored an international scientific commission for assessing experiments conducted on humans by the Nazis and suggested that it be established at the Institute Pasteur in Paris. In preparation for the proposed international commission, a French committee was established in June 1946. It consisted of four physicians, one biologist, and the director of the Service de

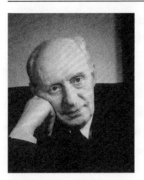

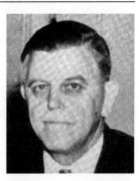

Recherches des Criminels de Guerre. In like manner, a British Advisory Committee for Medical War Crimes was founded under the direction of Lord Charles Moran, personal physician to Churchill and President of the Royal College of Physicians (Fig. 392). In the summer of 1946, international experts met in Paris "to discuss war crimes of medical nature." The head of the American delegation was Andrew Conway Ivy (Fig. 393), a noted physiologist and research scientist, chairman of the department of clinical science at the University of Illinois, scientific director of the Naval Medical Research Institute, and executive director of the National Advisory Cancer Council. Ivy was ambivalent about trying Nazi physicians in court. Although the monstrosity of some of their experiments was beyond doubt, he feared that "unless appropriate care is taken, the publicity associated with the trial may so stir public opinion against the use of humans in any experiment whatsoever that a hindrance will thereby result to the progress of science."[7]

The reservations of Ivy were shared by other physicians. Lord Moran, who was elected president of the International Scientific Commission, proposed that all documents concerning Nazi medical experiments be collected at the Institute Pasteur, where they would be analyzed scientifically prior to publication of them. The reservations of physicians, however, were overruled by politics. The American government wanted the War Crimes Trials to attract great attention, with resultant publicity, and believed that a trial of physicians surely would bring swift punishment. The British government, hard-pressed fiscally, was pleased to leave the costly War Crimes Trials to the Americans. Once the Doctors' Trial in Nuremberg began, American support for the International Scientific Commission ceased. The Commission, lacking financial means to accomplish its task, lingered for a few more months and was dissolved in 1947.[8]

The Americans soon discovered that the Doctors' Trial was not going to be so easy after all. The prosecution team of the United States did not have the knowledge or expertise that some European countries had vis-à-vis the specifics of the Nazi experiments. Following the armistice, most of the documents about unethical experiments on humans by the Nazis had been collected by French and British physicians, one example of that being a precise account of the experiments with sulfonamides at the Ravensbrück concentration camp. This deficiency of the Americans revealed itself in a selection of defendants that was arbitrary.[9] Among the physicians tried in Nuremberg were the highest echelon of the medical services of the Nazi party, the SS, and the German army. These included Karl Brandt, personal physician to Adolf Hitler and the Reich's Commissioner for Health and Sanitation; Karl Genzken (Fig. 394), chief of the medical department of the Waffen SS; Karl Gebhardt, Heinrich Himmler's physician and chief surgeon of the Staff of the

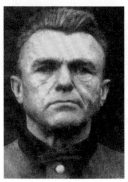

FIG. 394
Karl Genzken
(1885-1957)

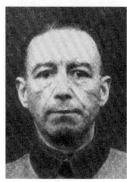

FIG. 395
Siegfried Hand-
loser (1885-
1954)

Reich's Physician SS, and Siegfried Handloser (Fig. 395), chief of the Medical Services of the Armed Forces. Some of the other defendants, however, had played only minor roles in medical experiments. Dermatologist Adolf Pokorny, for example, was indicted for the sole reason of having suggested, in a letter to Himmler, the mass sterilization of Russian prisoners of war (Fig. 396). Even more regrettable was the fact that many other physicians who had participated actively in the planning and execution of cruel medical experiments went scot-free.

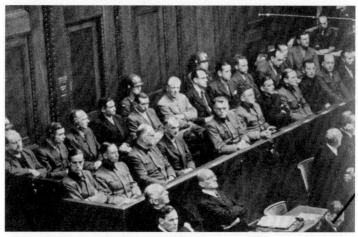

FIG. 396 *Defendants at the Nuremberg Doctors' Trial. Left to right, front row: Karl Brandt, Siegfried Handloser, Paul Rostock, Oskar Schröder, Karl Genzken, Karl Gebhardt, Kurt Blome, Joachim Mrugowsky, Rudolf Brandt, Helmut Poppendick, and Wolfram Sievers. Left to right, back row: Gerhard Rose, Siegfried Ruff, Viktor Brack, Hans Wolfgang Romberg, Hermann Becker-Freysing, Georg August Weltz, Konrad Schäfer, Waldemar Hoven, Wilhelm Beiglböck, Adolf Pokorny, Herta Oberheuser, and Fritz Fischer.*

One example of criminality going unpunished is Hans Reiter (Fig. 397), who had been president of the Reich Health Office and instrumental in initiating cruel typhus experiments at the Buchenwald extermination camp. But Reiter was not held responsible for any crimes; instead, he continued to work as a respected physician, published research papers, and was honored at international meetings of rheumatologists, where he spoke often about the syndrome that came to bear his name.[10] Another example is dermatologist Josef Vonkennel who also had conducted questionable experiments at Buchenwald, but after the war was able to continue a successful academic career as chairman of the department of dermatology at the University of Cologne.[11] Even Otmar von Verschuer, mentor of Josef Mengele, went

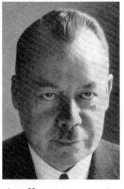

FIG. 397
Hans Reiter
(1881-1969)

untouched. He continued his career as chair of human genetics at the University of Münster, was lionized in international academic circles, and, in 1961, was an honored guest at the Second International Conference of Human Genetics in Rome.[12] Mengele himself evaded prosecution by changing his identity and fleeing Europe. Like many other former Nazis, he spent the rest of his life *incognito* in South America.

Some Nazis who were responsible for medical experiments in concentration and extermination camps devised another escape route from what would have been certain condemnation by their peers. Among them was Hans Eppinger (Fig. 398), professor of internal medicine at the University of Vienna and a highly esteemed specialist in diseases of the liver. In 1944, Eppinger had been involved in the seawater experiments at Dachau. When interrogated in 1946 about those studies, Eppinger resorted to an old trick used by scientists as a means of defending themselves against charges of unethical experiments in humans – he tried to attach a compelling therapeutic dimension to his studies, stating that "seawater has been regarded as a highly effective therapeutic agent since antiquity." When he realized that this cynical maneuver

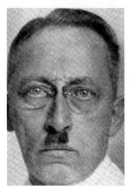

FIG. 398
Hans Eppinger
(1879 -1946)

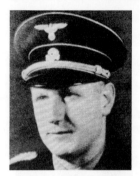

FIG. 399
*Leonardo
Conti
(1901-1945)*

would not prevent him from being prosecuted, he killed himself in September 1946.[13] Leonardo Conti (Fig. 399), the Reich's Leader of Health, committed suicide in October 1945, leaving behind a note that read thus: "I depart from life because I have made an incorrect statement under oath. I was out of my mind. For months, I have suffered from the most terrible depressions, thoughts about death, fears, and visions, although I have never been a coward."[14]

A Forum To Educate the German People

Signs of remorse that surfaced in Conti's letter, however, were an exception. The defendants at the Doctors' Trial at Nuremberg all insisted that they had done nothing wrong, and that their prosecution in a public forum was nothing but propaganda on the part of the victors. In some respects, the latter con-

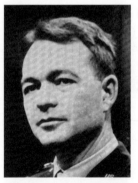

FIG. 400
*Telford Taylor
(1908-1998)*

tention was correct. The Americans used the Nuremberg Trials for calling attention to the misdeeds of the Nazis in a deliberate effort to educate the German people about the crimes perpetrated by their countrymen. In his opening statement to the Doctors' Trial on December 9, 1946, Chief Counsel for War Crimes, Telford Taylor (Fig. 400), said this:

This case, and others which will be tried in this building, offers a signal opportunity to lay before the German people the true cause of their present misery. These defendants and others turned Germany into an infernal combination of a lunatic asylum and a charnel house. Neither science, nor industry, nor the arts could flourish in such a foul medium. The country could not live at peace and was fatally handicapped for war. I do not think the German people have as yet any conception of how deeply the criminal folly that was Nazism bit into every phase of German life, or of how utterly ravaging the consequences were. It will be our task to make these things clear. That murder should be punished goes without saying, but the full performance of our task requires more than the just sentencing of these defendants. Their crimes were the inevitable result of the sinister doctrines which they espoused, and the same doctrines sealed the fate of Germany, shattered Europe, and left the world in ferment. Wherever those doctrines may emerge and prevail, the same terrible consequences will follow. That is why a bold and lucid consummation of these proceedings is of vital importance to all nations. That is why the United States has constituted this Tribunal.[15]

Despite, or rather in keeping with, the explicit intention of the prosecution to use Nuremberg as a forum to educate the German people, the Doctors' Trial was not a mock trial. After 12 years of violation of basic principles of ethics and of law in Nazi Germany, the accused were given every opportunity by the American judges to defend themselves. During the 133 days of trial spent on the presentation of evidence, 32 witnesses gave oral evidence for the prosecution, whereas 53 witnesses, including the 23 defendants, testified for the defense. The prosecution put in evidence a total of 507 exhibits, including affidavits, reports, and documents; the defense put in 901 of them. Requests by the defense for attendance at the trial of persons who had given affidavits on behalf of the prosecution were granted whenever possible, with those witnesses being brought to Nuremberg for interrogation or cross-examination by counsel for the defense (Fig. 401). Throughout the trial, great latitude in presenting evidence was allowed to the defense counsel, even to the point of placing in evidence matters with only scant probative value[16] (Fig. 402).

The prosecution averred that the experiments conducted in

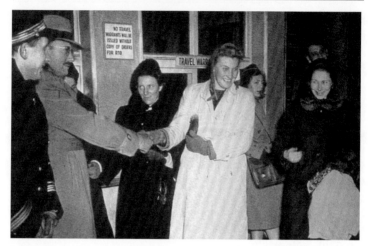

FIG. 401
Leo Alexander greeting survivors of the experiments at the concentration camp at Ravensbrück in Nuremberg at the train station.

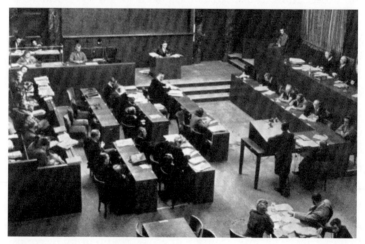

FIG. 402
The courtroom of the Nuremberg Doctors' Trial.

prisons and concentration and extermination camps had "revealed nothing which civilized medicine can use . . . the moral shortcomings of the defendants and the precipitous ease with which they decided to commit murder in quest of 'scientific results' dulled also that scientific hesitancy, that thorough thinking-through, that responsible weighing of every single step which alone can ensure scientifically valid results."[17] The defense countered by praising the value of the results of the wartime studies. In regard to the typhus program at Buchenwald, Gerhard Rose (Fig. 403), Brigadier General in the Medical Service of the Air Force and head of the department of tropical medicine at the Robert Koch Institute, emphasized that the experiments "showed that the useful vaccines did not protect against infection, but almost certainly prevented death." Rose went on to make the following claim dramatically: "One thing is certain, that the victims of this Buchenwald typhus test did not suffer in vain and did not die in vain. There was only one choice, the sacrifice of human lives, of persons determined for that purpose, or to let things run their course, to endanger the lives of innumerable human beings who would be selected not by the Reich's Criminal Police Office but by blind fate."[18] The counsel for defendant Joachim Mrugowsky (Fig. 404), who had been chief of the Hygienic Institute of the Waffen SS, pointed out that ". . . 154 deaths from the typhus experiments have to be compared with

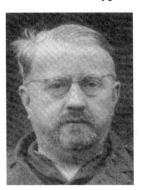

FIG. 403
Gerhard Rose
(1896-1992)

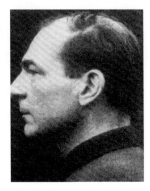

FIG. 404
Joachim
Mrugowsky
(1905-1948)

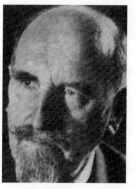

FIG. 405
Franz Volhard
(1872-1950)

the 15,000 who died of typhus every day in the camps for Soviet prisoners of war, and the innumerable deaths from typhus among the civilian population of the occupied eastern territories and the German troops."[19]

The seawater experiments at Dachau were classified by the prosecution as a "ghastly failure." According to Telford Taylor, the problems studied in these experiments "could have been solved simply and definitely within the space of one afternoon" by consulting a "thinking chemist."[20] A witness for the defense, Franz Volhard (Fig. 405), head of internal medicine at the University of Frankfurt and well known for his discovery of the enzyme, lipase, rejected Taylor's contentions, contending "that, scientifically speaking, the planning was excellent." In Volhard's view, the results of the study could not have been obtained in any other way and were of great importance. Eppinger's finding "that the drinking of small quantities of seawater up to 500 cc given over a lengthy period turned out to be better than unalleviated thirst" was cited by Volhard as "a wonderful thing for all seafaring nations."[21]

The Legal Status of Human Experiments

More important than the controversial scientific value of the

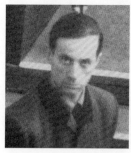

FIG. 406
Karl Brandt
(1904-1948)

experiments was the question of whether medical tests conducted on nonvolunteers had any legal standing. When asked by the head of the prosecution staff, James McHaney of Little Rock, Arkansas, whether such experiments were criminal acts, defendant Karl Brandt (Fig. 406) replied, "There are three aggravating factors with respect to the question of the criminal element in experiments: their involuntary character, the lack of necessity for them, and the danger involved." According to Brandt, experiments that were deemed important to the future of mankind and were not dangerous to the subjects should be permissible in the absence of consent. Brandt believed, however, that the danger to which test subjects were exposed was a secondary consideration. "The critical factor in the posing of an experiment," he declared, "is the question of whether the experiment is important or whether it is unimportant."[22] In the case of a dangerous experiment on nonvolunteers, the importance of the experiment had to be determined by "some superior authority . . . In such a case I am of the opinion that the individual or government institution determining their importance must also undertake to relieve the physician of responsibility in the event of a fatal outcome of the experiment . . . From this moment on the physician is only an instrument, in about the same way as is an officer in the field who is ordered to take a group of three or five soldiers without fail to a position where they will perish, fall."[23]

In the opening statement for the prosecution, Taylor had announced his intention "to pass very briefly over matters of medical ethics, such as the conditions under which a physician may lawfully perform a medical experiment."[24] In the course of the trial, however, it soon became evident that matters of medical ethics and legalities could not be covered briefly. Throughout their testimony, the defendant physicians stressed the lack of universally accepted principles for carrying out experiments on humans. The defense counsel cited 60 published studies involving human test subjects conducted throughout the world, with particular emphasis on research among populations in penitentiaries in the United States.[25] The conclusion of the defense was stated in these words: "Experiments which time and again have been described in international literature without meeting any opposition do not constitute a crime from the medical point of view ... The authors of those reports on their human experiments gained general recognition and fame; they were awarded the highest honors; they gained historical importance. And in spite of all this, are they supposed to have been criminals? No! In view of the complete lack of written legal norms, the physician, who generally knows only little about the law, has to rely on and refer to the admissibility of what is generally recognized to be admissible all over the world."[26]

In opposition to the contentions of the defense, the prosecution focused its arguments concerning ethical standards for the conduct of human experimentation on the testimony of three medical expert witnesses. One was Leo Alexander (Fig. 407, 408), a Boston neurologist and psychiatrist who, in the summer of 1945, as an officer in the United States Army, had investigated medical and research activities carried out during the war in Germany. In 1946, Alexander had been appointed consultant to the Secretary of War, serving in the Office of the Chief Counsel for War Crimes. Another witness was Andrew Ivy, who had been nominated as a consultant to the Doctors' Trials by the Board of Trustees of the American Medical Association (AMA). The third witness was Werner Leibbrand (Fig. 409), a German historian of medicine who had been persecuted by the Nazis for being married to a Jew and for being a member of the

FIG. 407
Leo Alexander
(1905-1985)

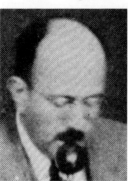

FIG. 408
Leo Alexander
demonstrating
a scar on the leg
of a Polish
woman as a re-
sult of studies
on her with sul-
fonamides in
experimental-
ly-induced gas
gangrene.

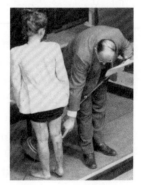

Association of Socialist Physicians.[27]

In his testimony, Leibbrand emphasized the existence of inviolable ethical principles in medicine that extended from the time of Hippocrates to the twentieth century. Those principles, he insisted, had been disregarded flagrantly by the defendants. When pressed by Robert Servatius, counsel for Karl Brandt, Leibbrand admitted that experiments by Americans on prisoner volunteers, such as in the malaria study at the Stateville Prison in Illinois, also represented breaches of those principles. In Leibbrand's view, declarations by prisoners of their willingness to undergo experiments were not adequate because "as prisoners they were already in a forced situation."[28] Obviously, this statement by a witness of their own was highly embarrassing to prosecutors, but Andrew Ivy compensated for the potential disaster. Ivy was determined to ensure that Nazi medical experiments would be viewed as isolated aberrations and not as a reflection of medical science in general. He was prepared to say whatever was necessary to prevent the Doctors' Trial at Nuremberg from affecting deleteriously research practices in the United States, even to the point of stretching the truth.[29]

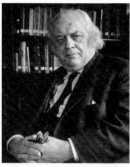

FIG. 409
Werner
Leibbrand
(1896-1974)

Principles and Shortcomings of Ivy

After his first meeting with the Nuremberg prosecutors in the summer of 1946, Ivy had written reports for the AMA and Nuremberg prosecution team in which he set forth rules for what he deemed to be acceptable medical reseach. Many of these rules were later included, almost *verbatim*, in the Nuremberg Code, which was to become the international standard for the conduct of medical research. Ivy stressed such concepts as the necessity for uncoerced consent, justification of new studies by previous experimental work, and avoidance of needless risk.[30] Hoping to rebut Leibbrand's testimony concerning American experiments on prisoner volunteers, Ivy contacted the Governor of Illinois, Dwight H. Green, and persuaded Green to appoint him chairman of a committee to examine the ethics of the malaria research at Stateville Prison.[31] Ivy also succeeded in inducing the AMA to issue guidelines for experiments on human beings,[32] something that Walter B. Cannon had not been able to achieve 30 years earlier. This is what the AMA guidelines stated: "In order to conform to the ethics of the American Medical Association, three requirements must be satisfied: (1) the voluntary consent of the person on whom the experiment is to be performed; (2) the danger of each experiment must be previously investigated by animal experimentation; and (3) the experiment must be performed under proper medical protection and management."[33] Compared with earlier regulations, such as the guidelines promulgated in Germany in 1931, the AMA principles were somewhat primitive, lacking provisions for informed consent and the protection of particularly vulnerable populations. Nevertheless, they surely could enable medical research conducted in the United States to be distinguished sharply from medical experiments performed in Nazi Germany.

In his testimony before the Nuremberg court, Ivy invoked the Hipporatic Oath, referring to it as "The Golden Rule of the medical profession." Although that Oath does not mention the relationship between a researcher and a test subject, it does set forth the responsibilities of a physician to other physicians and to patients; its applicability, therefore, to the experiments under consideration at Nuremberg was obvious. Never before, with the exception of experiments conducted by the Japanese, had the principle of *primum non nocere* been violated more willfully or conspicuously than in Nazi experiments, in which so many physicians displayed utter indifference to the suffering of persons under their care. According to Ivy, the Hipprocratic Oath "states how one doctor would like to be treated by another doctor in case he were ill. And in that way how a doctor should treat his patients or experimental subjects. He should treat them as though he were serving as a subject."[34] That directive certainly had not been followed by the defendant physicians.

Because every physician should be bound personally by the Oath of Hippocrates, Ivy asserted, the state could not assume moral responsibility for a doctor to his patient or to an experimental subject, as had been argued by Karl Brandt. In order to set research practices in the United States apart from Nazi experiments, Ivy gave as example the new AMA guidelines. When the defense noted that those guidelines had been published 19 days after the opening arguments by the prosecution, Ivy countered that it did not matter, and that such guidelines had always been accepted "as a matter of common practice in America."[35] Ivy also made reference to the "committee appointed by Governor Green in the State of Illinois to consider the ethical conditions under which prisoners and penitentiaries may be used ethically as subjects in the medical experiments," conveying the impression that the committee had thought carefully and for long before approving the malaria experiments at Stateville prison. He went so far as to read the conclusions of the commit-

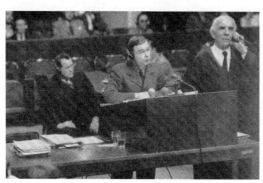

FIG. 410
The defendant, Siegfried Ruff, cross-examining Andrew C. Ivy. The tribunal at Nuremberg permitted defendants to question witnesses directly.

tee into the record of the trial. Ivy, however, did not volunteer the fact that the prestigious Green Committee never actually had met. When the defense discovered that the Green Committee had only been formed in December 1946, Ivy backtracked, insisting that the establishment of it had nothing to do with the Nuremberg Trial[36] (Fig. 410).

The defense learned, too, that Ivy himself had conducted medical experiments on conscientious objectors, who had been given the choice of either participating in the experiments or being subjected to prison or enforced labor. On cross-examination, Ivy advised that he had used those conscientious objectors as test subjects because he considered it to be "their duty."[37] Ivy also stated that the reason for using conscientious objectors and prisoners for medical research, "instead of teachers and businessmen," was that "these individuals had no other duties to perform. Their time was fully available for purposes of experimentation."[38] When counsel for the defense, Robert Servatius, challenged the claim that all prisoner volunteers in America had exposed themselves to deadly diseases solely for reasons of patriotism, Ivy replied that this assertion was "entirely reasonable" because there was no reason why "a prisoner in a penitentiary should not be patriotic or love his country."[39] When Servatius suggested that another reason for prisoners to volunteer might have been offers of money, Ivy responded that the real motivation for participating in experiments had been ". . . to serve for the good of humanity."[40]

In spite of Ivy's stonewalling, Servatius was able to point out that "there is a mixture of voluntariness and compulsory expiation, 'purchased voluntariness.' The subject gives his consent because he is to receive money, cigarettes, a mitigation of punishment etc. If one compares the actual risk with the advantage granted, one cannot admit the consent of these 'voluntary prisoners' as legal, in spite of all the protective forms they have to sign, for these can only have been obtained by taking advantage of inexperience, imprudence, or distress. Looking through medical literature, one cannot escape the growing conviction that the word 'volunteer,' where it appears at all, is used only as a word of protection and camouflage."[41] Gerhard Rose added this thought: "Aside from self-experiments of doctors, which represent a very small minority of such experiments, the extent to which subjects are volunteers is often deceptive. At the very best they amount to self-deceit on the part of the physician who conducts the experiments, but very frequently to a deliberate misleading of the public."[42]

Overall, the Doctors' Trial at Nuremberg did bring attention to problems unresolved concerning experimentation on humans, including the dubious nature of "voluntary consent" to risky medical experiments and the exploitation of populations who are unable to make enlightened rational decisions. The defendants also reminded the world of the timeworn arguments used to justify experiments on humans, such as the importance of those experiments to the progress of science, the role of the physician as a "warrior against disease" who should not be judged by the standards of civil life, and the insignificance of the suffering of a few test subjects in comparison with the benefit potentially to millions.

Alexander's Memorandum on Ethics

Because of the many unresolved questions related to human experimentation, the tribunal considered it important to establish criteria for acceptable research. One source for these criteria were the principles compiled by Andrew Ivy at the beginning of the trial. Another was a memorandum by Leo Alexander, titled "Ethical and Non-Ethical Experimentation on Human Beings," that was submitted to the Chief Counsel for War Crimes and the court on April 15, 1947. Alexander's first and foremost requirement concerned the importance and nature of consent that was informed and voluntary. In the memorandum of Alexander were these lines:

Legally valid voluntary consent of the experimental subject is essential. This requires specifically:

a. The absence of duress;

b. Sufficient disclosure on the part of the experimenter and sufficient understanding on the part of the experimental subjects of the exact nature and consequences of the experiment for which he volunteers to permit an enlightened consent.

In the case of mentally ill patients, for the purpose of experiments concerning the nature and treatment of nervous and mental illness, or related subjects, such consent of the next of kin or legal guardian is required; whenever the mental state of the patient permits (that is, in those mentally ill patients who are not delirious or confused), his own consent should be obtained in addition.[43]

Other requirements specified by Alexander involved "the nature and purpose of the experiment [which] must be humanitarian, with the ultimate aim to cure, treat, or prevent illness;" and that there be no "a priori reason to believe that death or disabling injury of the experimental subject will occur." Additionally, adequate preparations had to be made "to aid the experimental subject against any remote chance of injury, disability, or death," obligating the experimenters to possess a high degree of skill. The experiments should never be "random and unnecessary in nature," and, if involving significant risk, they should be performed "only if the solution is not accessible by any other means." Also,"the degree of risk taken should never exceed that determined by the humanitarian importance of the problem," and risky experiments were acceptable only if the experimenter himself participated as a test subject.[44]

The Nuremberg Code

These principles were considered important enough by the court to be included in the process whereby judgment was ren-

17 · The Nuremberg Code

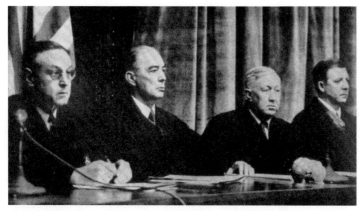

dered (Fig. 411). Several changes were made, however, including the addition of two provisions for prompt termination of an experiment at the discretion of the investigator or at the request of a test subject. One section of Alexander's memorandum that dealt with measures for safeguarding experimental subjects against injury or death was split into three separate points, bringing to 10 the total number of requirements laid out by the Nuremberg Code. The most important change concerned the requirements for consent. The judges deleted from Alexander's memorandum provisions for proxy consent on behalf of incompetent subjects, most likely because this problem was unrelated to the experiments under consideration at the trial. The provisions for the validity of consent became even more strict and were set forth as follows:

The voluntary consent of the human subject is absolutely essential. This means that the person involved should have legal capacity to give consent; should be so situated as to be able to exercise free power of choice, without the intervention of any element of force, fraud, deceit, duress, over-reaching, or other ulterior form of constraint or coercion; and should have sufficient knowledge and comprehension of the elements of the subject matter involved as to enable him to make an understanding and enlightened decision. The duty and responsibility for ascertaining the quality of the consent rests upon each individual who initiates, directs or engages in the experiment. It is a personal duty which may not be delegated to another with impunity.[45]

The 10 points that came to be known as the Nuremberg Code were claimed, incorrectly, to represent the accepted international standards for human experimentation. Before listing the points, the judges stated that "all agree that certain basic principles must be observed in order to satisfy moral, ethical, and legal concepts."[46] On the basis of the provisions of the Nuremberg Code, however, many other physicians and scientists throughout the world should have been condemned for violations of ethical experimentation in humans. The judges surely must have recognized this, but they also saw the great need to clarify the limits of acceptable experimentation in a legal context to aid in future judgments of violations and to ensure that no researcher in the future could argue that he was not aware of them. In regard to the Doctors' Trial itself, strict application of the Nuremberg Code was hardly neccessary because what had been done in Nazi Germany exceeded by far the narrow limits of the Code. As pointed out in the final judgment, "these ten principles were much more frequently honored in their breach than in their observance."[47]

What set Nazi medical experiments apart from those of Americans was not the research itself or the quality of it, but the woeful lack of respect given to an individual test subject by the Germans. In the United States, no ethnic or political groups had been subjected to wholesale savagery, the experiments had not been deliberately cruel, and death had never been regarded as an acceptable end point of a study.[48] Moreover, the zeal exhibited by the Nazi defendants in performing cruel experiments belied the notion that they were forced by powerful government officials to do the state's bidding. In point of fact, any German physician had the right to refuse to participate in experiments on humans without having to face unpleasant consequences.[49] Accordingly, the chief prosecutor in the Doctors' Trial, James M. McHaney, emphasized in his closing argument these points:

These defendants are, for the most part, on trial for the crime of murder . . . It is only the fact that these crimes were committed in part as a result of medical experiments on human beings that makes this case somewhat unique. And while considerable evidence of a technical nature has been submitted, one should not lose sight of the true simplicity of this case.[50]

The experiments under consideration in Nuremberg fulfilled the criteria for both war crimes (such as "murder or ill-treatment of prisoners of war") and for crimes against humanity (such as "torture or other inhumane acts committed against any civilian population"[51]). For seven of the 23 defendants – including Kurt Blome, Siegfried Ruff, and Adolf Pokorny – participation in those crimes could not be proven "to the exclusion of every reasonable doubt," and they were acquitted. Nine defendants – among them Herta Oberheuser, Fritz Fischer, Wilhelm Beiglböck, and Gerhard Rose – were sentenced to prison terms ranging from 10 years to life. Seven – Karl Brandt, Karl Gebhardt, Rudolf Brandt, Joachim Mrugowsky, Wolfram Sievers, Viktor Brack, and Waldemar Hoven[52] were sentenced to death (Fig. 412).

The 10 principles of the Nuremberg Code were used as a template against which the acts of some of the defendants could be judged; they were not essential for the final reckoning in

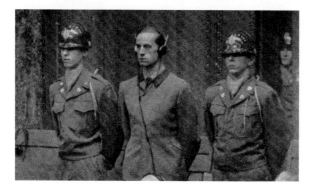

FIG. 412
The leading defendant, Karl Brandt, being sentenced to death by hanging.

these trials.[53] Their inclusion, however, meant that for the first time rules for the conduct of experiments on human beings were established firmly by law. The Nuremberg Code was not just another fatuous framework to guide experimentation on human test subjects. It was a legal document that could serve to enforce ethical standards by holding researchers accountable, personally, for any and all breaches of its strictures.

CHAPTER 18

THE AFTERMATH OF NUREMBERG

With the promulgation of the Nuremberg Code, regulations concerning medical experiments on human beings at long last acquired legal force. The Code's standing in international law was not on the same level as the Nuremberg Principles, adopted in 1950, which concerned crimes against peace, crimes against the laws and customs of war, and crimes against humanity. The principles that emerged from the War Crimes Trials conducted by the four victorious powers were endorsed by the General Assembly of the United Nations. In contrast, the Nuremberg Code was stipulated by American judges only; it could be used, however, by courts to set criminal and civil standards of conduct in the United States.

Nevertheless, no court in the United States, to date, has ever awarded damages to someone injured in a medical experiment or punished someone who conducted such an experiment on the basis of a violation of the Nuremberg Code.[1] Ironically, it was the very difference between Nazi medical experiments and those conducted in free, civilized societies that allowed physician-scientists, the bodies responsible for forging policies about medicine, and the courts to neglect the implications of the Code in regard to practices of research in their own countries. The Nuremberg Code was considered to be a worthwhile system of principles for barbarians, but not to be necessary for ordinary physicians (who, it was assumed, generally knew right from wrong).[2] But the fact that the experiments on trial in Nuremberg had been possible in what had been a highly cultivated nation should have been a warning that barbarism knows no borders; the methods utilized by Nazi physicians to defend themselves should have made it clear that even the most brutal acts can be rationalized on the altar of utilitarianism.

Utilitarianism – the concept that the means must be judged by the ends – soon overwhelmed the profound respect for ethical values that had surfaced briefly during the Nuremberg Trials. As soon as general insistence on ethical standards began to feel burdensome, the rules of conduct were changed. For example, in the War Crimes Trials conducted by the International Military Tribunal, Far East, in Tokyo from 1946 to 1948, 25 major Japanese war criminals were indicted, among them four former prime ministers and a number of career diplomats, foreign office officials, and high-ranking Army and Navy officers. All were found guilty, and seven were sentenced to be hanged (Fig. 413). Japanese physicians, however, who had committed atrocities in the name of science, were not brought to trial, even though the cruelty and magnitude of their experiments had, in many ways, surpassed those of the Nazis. With relations between the United States and the Soviet Union becoming in-

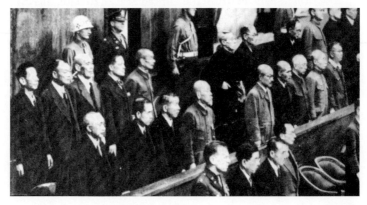

FIG. 413
Defendants of the War Crimes Trial conducted by the International Military Tribunal Far East in Tokyo. In the front row, fifth from right, is former premier Hideki Tojo, who was sentenced to death and executed in December 1948.

creasingly hostile, the U.S. military government in Japan under General Douglas MacArthur sought determinedly to obtain data that derived from research on biological warfare conducted by the Japanese. Those data were offered by Ishii Shiro under the condition that he and his colleagues be granted immunity from prosecution.[3] The offer was accepted.

In retrospect, Ishii actually had little of value to present to the U.S. military. According to a memorandum of 1982 in the archives of the U.S. Research Center for Biological Warfare at Fort Detrick, "Scientists in the U.S. program said the information was not of significant value, but it was the first data in which human subjects were described. Even without Ishii's help, the U. S. Biological warfare research program would have surpassed that of Unit 731 within a year."[4] By disclosing information gradually and in tantalizing bits, Ishii made American scientists believe that much more was coming. After receiving one of these bonbons of information in December 1947, the Chief of Basic Sciences at Fort Detrick, Edwin V. Hill, made this declaration jubilantly: "It represents data which have been obtained by Japanese scientists at the expenditure of many millions of dollars and years of work. Information has accrued with respect to human susceptibility to those diseases as indicated by specific infectious doses of bacteria. Such information could not be obtained in our own laboratories because of scruples attached to human experimentation. These data were secured with a total outlay of 250,000 Yen to date, a mere pittance by comparison with the actual cost of the studies."

My Enemy, My Ally

This utilitarian attitude superseded all ethical considerations. Although American Intelligence was fully aware of the nature of the experiments performed by Ishii and his staff, and that American prisoners of war had been used in those studies, it was willing to overlook these infractions in order to procure data from the Japanese. For example, an officer of the Army Intelligence (so-called G-2) noted in a report in January 1947 that "Ishii had his assistants inject bubonic plague bacilli into the bodies of some Americans in Mukden, Manchuria, as an experiment." Evidently unruffled by this atrocious behavior, the officer commented matter-of-factly that "naturally, the results of these experiments are of the highest intelligence value."[6]

The attempt to procure information thought to be valuable was one reason the U.S. government refrained from trying Japanese physicians for war crimes and for crimes against humanity. Another reason was the lessons learned from the Nuremberg Trials. Just as Nazi physicians had defended themselves by pointing out publicly questionable experiments on humans conducted in American penitentiaries, so would a trial of Japanese physicians inevitably result in a very visible and highly undesirable discussion of biological warfare about which American researchers had been engaged. Information about biological warfare was said by the U.S. Military to be "of a highly sensitive nature" and that "every precaution must be taken to maintain its secrecy."[7] Moreover, the military promoted the disturbing thought "that the USSR possesses only a small portion of this technical information, and since any 'war crimes' trial would completely reveal such data to all nations, it is felt that such publicity must be avoided in interests of defense and security of the U.S."[8]

As a result, American investigators of war crimes, who already had collected comprehensive material concerning Ishii and his horrendous work, were placed under the control of Intelligence and ordered to make no effort toward prosecution or "any form of publicity of this case without G-2 concurrence."[9] Consequently, at the Tokyo War Crimes Trials, biological warfare played no role. Ishii retired with a handsome pension, and many of his former coworkers advanced to key positions in postwar Japan. Associates of Unit 731 headed up Japan's Medical Association and National Cancer Center, became Surgeon General of the reformed armed forces, acquired leading positions in pharmaceutical companies, and staffed the medical faculties of universities of Tokyo, Kyoto, and Osaka, and many other medical schools.[10]

The beginning of the Cold War turned many former enemies into allies, no matter how heinous their crimes had been. The U.S. military sought the expertise of scientists, not only from Japan, but from the former Nazi regime as well. Between 1945 and 1955, a program called Project Paperclip, established by the U. S. Joint Intelligence Objectives Agency, employed 765 German and Austrian scientists, engineers, and technicians, including four defendants at the Nuremberg Doctors' Trial. Konrad Schäfer, who had been involved in the seawater experiments at Dachau, was invited to Randolph Field, Texas to work for the U.S. Air Force. Kurt Blome, former head of a German research program devoted to biological warfare, was given a position as camp doctor at the U.S. European Command Intelligence Center in Oberursel near Frankfurt.[11] Other former Nazis became recruits for Project Paperclip, among them being Hubert Strughold, who was involved in the high altitude experiments at Dachau, and who eventually became "the father of American space medicine," and rocket scientist Wernher von Braun, a former member of the SS, who was brought to the U.S. for the purpose of directing technical development of the Army's ballistic missile program and continued his work there, galvanizing the American space program. Because President Harry S. Truman had signed an executive order banning former Nazis from American shores, the records of Project Paperclip recruits were rewritten, omitting embarrassing associations politically and emphasizing only the most banal of wartime activities. On the basis of these adjusted records, there was no reason to deny German scientists a visa for immigration to the

United States. Utilitarianism triumphed, and ethical considerations that so recently had dominated the Nuremberg Trials no
longer were in vogue.[12]

Utilitarianism Rules

This mode was true not only for the military, but also for academic medicine. Many witnesses of the Nuremberg Trials soon returned to the forefront of human experimentation. In Great
Britain, Kenneth Mellanby, who had observed the Doctors'
Trial as a correspondent for the *British Medical Journal*, called
for clinical studies on humans in an "institute for human biology."[13] He also defended certain Nazi research, designating the
subjects of the malaria experiments "quite genuine volunteers"
at "reasonably humane" Dachau. Mellanby referred to the typhus experiments at Buchenwald as an "important and unique
piece of medical research," and justified the use of results of
those studies by declaring, "The victims were dead; if their suf-
ferings could in any way add to medical knowledge and help
others, surely this would be something that they themselves
would have preferred."[14] The results of experiments on humans
performed in the Third Reich eventually found their way into
the international medical literature, usually without any note of
the circumstances under which the findings were generated.
For example, the freezing experiments conducted by Sigmund
Rascher at Dachau were referred to 44 times between 1955 and
1984 in such prestigious medical publications as the *Lancet*, the
British Medical Journal, and the *Journal of the American Medical Association*.[15]

In the United States, Andrew Ivy reaffirmed his stance that
experiments on prisoners were wholly acceptable. In an article
titled, "The History and Ethics of the Use of Human Subjects in
Medical Experiments" that appeared in the journal *Science* in
1948, Ivy refrained from mentioning the first requirement of

the Nuremberg Code, which stipulated that volunteerism in medical experiments must not be coerced. He also failed to marshal the argument of the counsel for the defense at Nuremberg, namely, that imprisoned individuals, by definition, are unable to exercise free will. According to Ivy, true volunteerism existed when a prisoner was "able to say 'yes' or 'no' without fear of being punished or of being deprived of privileges due him in the ordinary course of events." Ivy acknowledged that "a reduction of sentence in prison, if excessive or drastic, can amount to undue influence" but emphasized that the purpose of the parole system was to reward prisoners for meritorious service. "Serving as a test subject in a medical experiment," he argued, "is obviously an act of good conduct, is frequently unpleasant and occasionally hazardous, and demonstrates a type of social consciousness of high order when performed primarily as a service to society." Therefore, "service as a subject in a medical experiment" should be "encouraged and rewarded."[16] By emphasizing voluntary consent and social consciousness, Ivy gave medical research on prisoners the seal of legitimacy ethically. His position was adopted by the "committee appointed by Governor Dwight H. Green of Illinois," in which Ivy was chairman, and was published as official policy in an editorial in *JAMA* in 1948.[17]

Controversial Views

Beginning in the 1950s, the limits ethically of medical research were discussed at a variety of conferences and in numerous articles in the scientific literature. Sensitivity existed in some quarters regarding the use of vulnerable populations for medical research. In 1943, in the midst of the war, the President of the National Academy of Science, Frank Jewett, had questioned whether prisoners were capable of giving true voluntary consent to an experiment.[18] In 1953, Duncan Leys of Bickley, Kent, compared the then current attitude of British physicians with those of Nazi doctors in concentration and extermination camps and made this observation: "The magnitude and crudity of their 'experiments' must not be allowed to blunt sensitivity to breaches of the medical ethic made on a smaller scale and with greater plausibility. Of this nature are experiments performed upon condemned criminals, with or without the victim's consent, upon conscientious objectors to military service, upon persons with chronic mental illness or deficiency or incurable disease of any kind."[19] Likewise, a memorandum in 1955 of the Public Health Council of the Netherlands stated this unambiguously: "Experiments on children; in institutions for children, old people, etc.; on the insane; or on prisoners, which involve dangerous risks, inconvenience or pain are not approved. All experiments on the dying under any circumstance are disapproved."[20]

The use for medical research of patients who were dying was highly controversial. Some pragmatic authors considered that, in "patients with incurable, inexorably fatal afflictions . . . an unprecedented opportunity exists for the wider study of these individuals in pharmacologic, physiologic, and other medical investigations."[21] Others countered that "the description 'hopelessly incurable' . . . does not specify the time element – hopeless within hours, days, months, years? And, if months or years are concerned, do all experts agree on the status of their respective sciences and deny the possibility of discovering effective agents

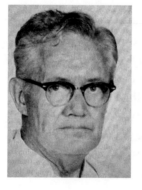

within such a period?" Moreover, the use of the "hopelessly incurable" for medical research created "the paradox that the healthier the patient, the more he should be the concern of his physician; the sicker, the less."[22] Henry Knowles Beecher, a renowned and controversial anesthesiologist and researcher at Harvard University (Fig. 414), warned against choosing "individuals who may die suddenly or who seem to be in imminent danger of death . . . as subjects for experimentation, however harmless the planned procedure may be. If death occurs during such an experiment, it would cast a shadow over a potentially valuable agent or useful technique, not to mention placing the investigator in a most unhappy predicament, where, although innocent, he may appear guilty."[23] The primary concern of the man who, in 1966, would write the classic *Ethics and Clinical Research,* appeared to be mostly research and science, rather than the patient.

Nurses, medical students, and other persons who were likely to be "conditioned by idealistic impulses" also were controversial as test subjects.[24] The medical literature is replete with examples of professors who used coercive influence on students to get them to undergo risky experiments. Among the earliest of those professors was François-Joseph-Victor Broussais who, in the early nineteenth century, induced three medical students to inoculate themselves with pus of lesions of syphilis.[25] Between 1850 and 1851, Joseph Alexandre Auzias-Turenne of Paris was responsible for the death of a young German physician by accepting the offer of the acolyte to subject himself to experimental syphilization.[26] Franz Rinecker of Würzburg produced syphilis experimentally in 1852 in two young physicians of his department, both of whom were eager to help their mentor.[27] Elias Metchnikoff of Paris, in 1906, persuaded one of his medical students to inoculate himself with syphilis, using as a safeguard a calomel ointment that, unfortunately, proved ineffective.[28] Beecher got it right in 1959 when he wrote that "laboratory personnel and medical students are captive groups, not so seriously . . . as prisoners of war perhaps, but nonetheless available for certain kinds of subtle coercion. A volunteer should be just that, not one who may be subject to fear of the consequences if he does not cooperate."[29] Michael Boris Shimkin, a leading cancer researcher at the National Cancer Institute and the University of California at San Francisco, concluded that "the human experimental subject must not be selected upon any basis such as race, religion, level of education, or economic status."[30]

For individuals of depressed economic status, the offer of financial compensation for participation in medical experiments clearly was a coercive factor that could compromise the quality ethically of a study. As early as 1762, Lord Henley had observed that "necessitous men are not, truly speaking, free men, but, to answer a present exigency, will submit to any terms that the crafty may impose upon them."[31] Although the problem posed by financial incentives to persons being recruited for medical experiments was acknowledged and even debated, the question remained how test subjects were to be procured "if the various special social groups cited above are to be excluded on ethical grounds as sources of volunteers." Moreover, "if it is unethical that volunteers for non-therapeutic experimentation should be influenced by hopes of some kind of personal gain, what are the motives that would otherwise incite them to volunteer?"[32]

Even the use of volunteers who were just and only that was problematic. Numerous studies showed conclusively that an unusually high incidence of severe psychological maladjustment existed among volunteers for medical experiments.[33] This was especially true for volunteers who gave reasons other than financial for participation. These subjects volunteered for reasons "frequently related to their maladaptive patterns,"[34] such as "thrills," "kicks," relief from boredom, and satisfaction of their self-destructive urges. In brief, "normal" volunteers were far from normal in a high percentage of cases.[35] For some investigators, however, the latent psychopathology that drove people to volunteer for what might be dangerous studies was a welcome lifesaver in the turbulent seas of human experimentation. Researchers counted on "the help of individuals now willing to risk life or limb on the speedway or in the ascent of the [sic] Mount Everest" and sought to "institutionalize a not uncommon appetite for adventure consistent with acceptable moral

standards" for the sake of recruiting volunteers for medical research.[36] Others suggested that there should be "compulsory
experimentation," noting that because more deaths were
caused by disease than by wars, "there is no significant difference between general recruitment when a war breaks out and
the mobilization of society for the sake of fighting sickness."[37]
Although such arguments did not find wide acceptance, the
need for test subjects in medical research overrode scruples,
and the possibility of some "subtle coercion" in recruiting them
was accepted with nary a blink.

The Declaration of Geneva

The detachment of human experimentation from the strict requirements of the Nuremberg Code was furthered by the World
Medical Association (WMA). Founded in September 1947 at
the headquarters of the British Medical Association in London,
it was hoped that the WMA would, in case of another war, "act
as a brake upon medical war crimes."[38] Among the first initiatives of the World Medical Association was the creation of a
"physician's oath" to affirm his or her dedication to the profession. That restatement of the Hippocratic Oath presented at
the Second General Assembly of the World Medical Association
in 1948, became known as the Declaration of Geneva. The
recital of the Declaration by every newly qualified physician
was expected to have a beneficial effect on attitude toward medical practice, especially in "view of the recent war crimes and the
continued troubled state of the world." The recent atrocities in
Nazi Germany were recalled in a passage in the Declaration
that read as follows:

I will not permit considerations of religion, nationality, race, party
politics or social standing to intervene between my duty and my
patient; I will maintain the utmost respect for human life, from the
time of its conception. Even under threat, I will not use my knowledge contrary to the laws of humanity.[39]

The issues of medical research and the relationship between researcher and test subject were not addressed at all in the Declaration of Geneva. Five years later, however, the WMA began to consider guidelines concerning experiments on humans; at the Eighth General Assembly in Rome in 1954, a Resolution on Human Experimentation was adopted. It differed substantially from the Nuremberg Code in that it was broader in scope, establishing as it did practical principles for biomedical research that included proxy consent in the case of persons not able to answer for themselves and making a distinction between sick and healthy subjects. These considerations had not been important at the Nuremberg Doctors' Trial and, therefore, had not been stressed sufficiently at that time. At the same time, the emphasis of the Nuremberg Code on voluntary consent of test subjects was much weakened in the Resolution on Human Experimentation and the importance of the conscience of the experimenter was considerably strengthened in it (Fig. 415).

For example, regulations concerning consent were not addressed in the first, but in the last, of the five principles adopted and were worded much less stringently than in the Nuremberg Code. Consent by proxy was specified in these words:

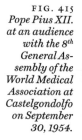

FIG. 415
*Pope Pius XII.
at an audience
with the 8ᵗʰ
General Assembly of the
World Medical
Association at
Castelgondolfo
on September
30, 1954.*

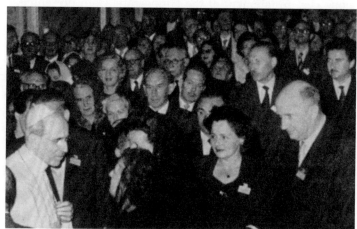

It should be required that each person who submits to experimentation be informed of the nature of, the reason for, and the risk of the proposed experiment. If the patient is irresponsible, consent should be obtained from the individual who is legally responsible for the individual. In both instances, consent should be obtained in writing.

The first principle of the Resolution required that experiments be conducted by qualified scientists who adhere to the general rules of respect for an individual. The second principle called for publication with "prudence and discretion" of results of medical experiments. The third principle addressed experiments in healthy subjects. It necessitated that they be "fully informed," but also mandated that "the paramount factor in experimentation on human beings is the responsibility of the research worker and not the willingness of the person submitting to the experiment." In regard to experiments on sick subjects, the fourth principle stated that ". . . one may attempt an operation or treatment of a rather daring nature. Such exceptions will be rare and require the approval either of the person or his next of kin. In such a situation it is the doctor's conscience which will make the decision." In brief, the guidelines of the World Medical Association focused on the responsibilities of researchers, rather than on the rights of test subjects.[40]

Critics of the Nuremberg Code

In those years, the Nuremberg Code was criticized by physicians on a number of grounds. For example, the fifth rule forbade experiments if there was "an a priori reason to believe that death or disabling injury will occur," with the exception of "experiments where the experimental physicians also serve as subjects." Although some physicians felt that participation of the investigator "as a subject in any project having even remote possibilities of hazard" might be desirable "as evidence of his good faith,"[41] the majority of them rejected self-experimentation. One reason was that self-experiments were thought to be flawed scientifically "whenever judgment can enter into the conclusions drawn."[42] Moreover, as the U.S. National Conference on the Legal Environment of Medical Sciences of 1964 concluded, "if an experiment is morally contraindicated, under basic human considerations . . . the participation of the investigator would not morally rectify it."[43]

The sixth rule of the Nuremberg Code, which stated that "the degree of risk . . . should never exceed that determined by the humanitarian importance of the problem to be solved by the experiment," was criticized as "presumptuously evaluating the ultimate significance of one's own research."[44] Rule number two, which declared that ". . . the experiment should be such as to yield fruitful results for the good of society, inprocurable by other methods or means of study, and not random and unnecessary in nature," was judged to be vague. In a report to the Council on Drugs of the American Medical Association in 1959, Henry Beecher queried the meaning of the phrase "unnecessary in nature." He also rejected the phrase "for the good of society" as being "unsavory," pointing out that "the scientist or physician has no right 'to choose martyrs for society.'" He went on to say this: "Any classification of human experimentation as 'for the good of society' is to be viewed with distaste, even alarm. Undoubtedly all sound work has this as its ultimate aim, but such high-flown expressions are not necessary and have been used within recent memory as cover for outrageous ends." Beecher also criticized the rejection by the Nuremberg Code of random experiments. In his view, "anesthesia, X-rays, radium, and penicillin, to mention a few products of 'random' experimentation, seem to justify the disallowed approach. Most of the epoch-making discoveries in science have been unexpected."[45]

Beecher also took on the third rule of the Code, which said that "The experiment should be so designed and based on the results of animal experimentation and a knowledge of the natural history of the disease or other problem under study that the anticipated results will justify the performance of the experiment." Beecher asked, ". . . if the anticipated results fail to justify the performance of the experiment, has the investigator necessarily been guilty of wrong behavior? Who can guarantee the success of any new experiment?"[46]

Other criticism of the Nuremberg Code was aimed at the rule that was first and foremost, namely, that which concerned consent. As a prerequisite for obtaining valid consent, the Code required that test subjects be informed of "the nature, duration, and purpose of the experiment; the method and means by which it is to be conducted; all inconveniences and hazards reasonably to be expected; and the effects upon his health or person which may possibly come from his participation in the experiment." In principle, these demands were neither new nor controversial, but they were not easy to fulfill. As early as 1910, Paul Ehrlich emphasized the duty of the chemotherapeutist to "tell his patient what possibilities of risk exist and how frequent they are." Later he admitted that it was impossible to give such information accurately until sufficiently large case evidence was available.[47] Even if such information were available, it was not always possible to communicate it to the test subject. As Otto E. Guttentag of the University of California at San Francisco pointed out in 1953, ". . . one only has to think of present-day specialization in medicine in order to realize that the patient is frequently not able to grasp all the implications of a certain procedure so far as his health is concerned."[48] In the same year, the British Medical Research Council made this statement:

To obtain the consent of the patient to a proposed investigation is not in itself enough. Owing to the special relationship of trust which exists between a patient and his doctor, most patients will consent to any proposal that is made. Further, the considerations involved are nearly always so technical as to prevent their being adequately understood by one who is not himself an expert.[49]

These considerations led some authors to conclude that no one should be accepted as a volunteer for a medical experiment who was not "at least at the level of a graduate student and who has investigated for himself the nature and possible dangers of the drug or procedure involved."[50] That provision not only would have made studies in diseased subjects impossible, but would have brought those in healthy individuals to a virtual standstill. In addition, in many instances, it could have led to invalid data. Beecher recognized correctly that "for some types of investigation, especially when subjective factors are involved, it is essential to have subjects who know nothing about the expected results and have no vested interest in the outcome."[51]

The problem of subjectivity entering into the assessments in clinical studies made adherence to the first rule of the Nuremberg Code exceedingly difficult. "Explicit observance of point one," Beecher advised, "would require detailed explanation to the participating subject with the inevitable result that he would become self-conscious and introspective. An abundance of evidence in the field of study of subjective responses has shown that such introspection has produced misleading results. The use of placebos in therapy, occasionally necessary for the guidance of the able, responsible physician as well as the treatment of the patient, could hardly be tolerated under a strict observance of the point in question." Beecher also advised that rigid interpretation of the clause of the Nuremberg Code dedicated to consent "would effectively cripple, if not eliminate, most research in the field of mental disease, which is one of the two or three greatest medical problems."[52]

Even in the ideal circumstance of a competent test subject being aware fully of all possible implications of an experiment, the importance of consent in the Code was qualified. In a statement read before the First International Congress of the Histopathology of the Nervous System on September 14, 1952,

Pope Pius XII (Fig. 416) asserted that "the patient cannot confer rights he does not possess." In the Pope's view, the patient was "not absolute master of himself, of his body or of his soul ... He has the right of use, limited by natural finality, of the faculties and powers of his human nature. Because he is a user and not a proprietor, he does not have unlimited power to destroy

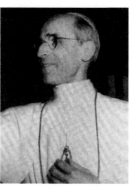

FIG. 416
*Pope Pius XII.
(1876-1958)*

or mutilate his body and its functions." The Pope concluded that the patient had "no right to involve his physical or psychic integrity in medical experiments or research when they entail serious destruction, mutilation, wounds or perils."[53]

Because of problems inherent in the Nuremberg Code and in other similar guidelines, some authors rejected any codified regulation of experiments on humans. James Macalister Mackintosh, a British scientist acting as a special consultant to the U.S. Public Health Service, wrote these lines in 1952: ". . . the mere preparation of a closely defined code of regulations would defeat its own purpose. Human beings are not alike, and a code of regulations obeyed to the letter by one research worker might well result in irretrievable damage of a patient. There is no code that could cover the frailties of an inefficient worker, or the sinister vagaries of a research student who placed his own ambitions above the human needs and rights of the patient."[54] Likewise, Beecher believed that "the problems of human experimentation do not lend themselves to a series of rigid rules. In most cases, these are more likely to do harm than good."[55]

Other physicians of the time also were critical of ethical codes; they believed, however, that some boundaries were essential. That attitude was inherent in the International Code of Medical Ethics adopted by the WMA in 1949. It began as follows:

'As ye would that men should do to you, do ye even so to them,' is a Golden Rule for all men. A Code of Ethics for physicians can only amplify or focus this and other golden rules and precepts to the special relations of practice. As a stream cannot rise above its source, so a code cannot change a low-grade man into a high-grade doctor, but it can help a good man to be a better man and a more enlightened doctor. It can quicken and inform a conscience, but not create one.[56]

Physician, Cure Thyself

The necessity of codified regulations for experiments on humans was underlined especially by physicians who were conversant with both the law and medicine. In a review of "Ethical and Legal Aspects of Medical Research on Human Beings" in 1954, the Associate Director of Research Planning at the National Institutes of Health (NIH), Irving Ladimer of New York City, alerted readers to substantial differences between the legal and the medical professions in the consideration of experiments on humans. The law, deeply protective of human integrity and life, insisted that there be no experimentation with these rights, not recognizing that any medical intervention was, to some extent, experimental. The position of legal writers and of jurists was highly conservative. Although the legal system allowed that it was the duty of a physician to keep up with advancements in his profession, any forging ahead of the perimeter of the field was condemned. In the judicial mind, medical experimentation was equated with disregard or negligence. In Ladimer's view, the untenable gap that existed between the law and the realities of medicine could be narrowed only by considering the experiment objectively as "a legitimate scientific endeavor which can be advanced by the recognized research scientist." Ladimer went on to say that "The legal issue would then become not experimentation versus accepted practice of the art of medicine but an evaluation of the plan and conduct of research in relation to specific fact situations, that is, whether the research was conducted with due regard to the interests of the subject. The law has a duty to comprehend the scope and elements of diverse human activity and their places in society if it is to assist in making individual judgments and setting or recognizing general values."[57] This, however, required effort on the part of the medical profession. Ladimer contended that "... the responsible professions have a duty to delineate for their own members and for a critically vigilant public the nature of medical research and the limits within which it may be properly undertaken."[58]

It was not so much recognition of a duty but fear of litigation that induced physicians to call for clear-cut rules in regard to experiments on humans. Ladimer warned that "the physician experiments at his peril,"[59] even if experiments were undertaken under the authority of the government. A representative of the Army Epidemiological Board, which sponsored studies with healthy subjects on various infectious diseases, noted in 1948 that in case of a lawsuit, responsibility would "devolve entirely upon the individual experimenter." In their own interest, experimenters were advised to protect themselves "by means of the usual waiver," and were informed that in case of injury or death of a test subject, the Army could not provide indemnification in the absence of clear authority of Congress. The Army actually considered engaging "individuals or groups in Congress with the idea of having laws passed relating to payment of compensation for disability or release of the experimenter from liability." No specific action was taken, however, because of the assumption "that this would be a dangerous course, and that it might in fact injure clinical investigations generally. There is a very real possibility that unfavorable publicity would quickly result."[60]

Eventually, under the umbrella of a law that gave the military authority to indemnify contractors for risks undertaken in "research and development situations," some relief for researchers was granted by the U. S. Congress in 1952. The law provided "direct indemnification to the contractor and not to the individual human guinea pig." Because the law also covered risks unrelated to medical research, such as accidents involving test pilots, a comprehensive debate in Congress on experiments in humans had been unnecessary.[61]

The unbridled engagement of the U.S. military in studies involving human test subjects induced the Department of Defense to issue guidelines for experimentation on humans. In 1952, the legal advisor to the Armed Forces Medical Policy Council, Stephen S. Jackson, proposed that the ". . . principles and conditions, which were laid down by the Tribunal in the Nuremberg Trials, be adopted," reminding that these principles already had international judicial sanction. Anything short of this would open the military to criticism along the line of, "see – they use only that which suits them." In February 1953, U.S. Secretary of Defense Charles Wilson (Fig. 417), signed a memorandum for the secretaries of the Army, Navy, and Air Force concerning the "use of volunteers in experimental research" that, in addition to all provisions of the Nuremberg Code, required consent in writing and forbade experiments on prisoners of war. One year later, the Nuremberg Code was restated in a document released by the Army Office of the Surgeon General.[62]

FIG. 417
Charles Wilson
(1890-1961)

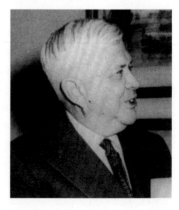

18 · The Aftermath of Nuremberg

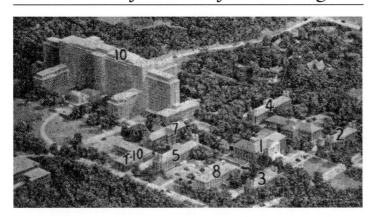

FIG. 418
The Clinical
Center of the
National Insti-
tutes of Health
(building no.
10) at the open-
ing of it in
1953.

The Guidelines of the National Institutes of Health

In 1953, the NIH adopted guidelines for research based on the Nuremberg Code at the time that its Clinical Center opened in Bethesda, Maryland (Fig. 418). That Center was a state-of-the-science research hospital with resources for the care and study of 500 patients. Although devoted entirely to research, the overriding principle governing clinical studies was said to be "that the welfare of individual human beings takes precedence over every other consideration."[63] A pamphlet produced by the NIH explained the role of volunteers in medical research as follows:

The rigid safeguards observed at NIH are based on the so-called 'ten commandments' of human medical research which were adopted at the Nuremberg War Crime Trials after the atrocities performed by Nazi doctors had been exposed. Every volunteer must give his full consent to any test, and he must be told exactly what it involves so that he goes into it with his eyes open. Among other things, the experiment must be designed to yield 'fruitful results for the good of society,' unnecessary 'physical and mental suffering and injury' must be avoided, the test must be conducted by 'scientifically qualified' persons, and the subject must be free to end it at any time he feels unable to go on. And at NIH, a special board of scientists also studies every projected experiment before it is okayed.[64]

The Abuse of Man

The adoption of the principles of the Nuremberg Code by the U.S. Public Health Service through the National Institutes of Health stimulated international interest in developing guidelines for human experimentation that would be acceptable universally. In September 1961, the Committee on Medical Ethics of the World Medical Association submitted a code to its fifteenth General Assembly. The draft code went through a number of revisions, during which several provisions were deleted, including a rule "that children in institutions and not under the care of relatives should not be the subject of human experiments." The code was finalized at a meeting of the Council of the World Medical Association in Luxembourg in March, 1964 (Fig. 419) and was adopted by the eighteenth World Medical Assembly in Helsinki shortly thereafter.[65]

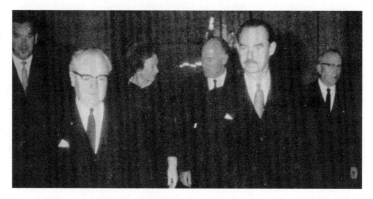

FIG. 419
Fiftieth Meeting of the Council of the World Medical Association in Luxembourg in March 1964: the chairman of the WMA Council, Félix Worré (right), escorts the Grand-Duke of Luxembourg to the Council Session.

The Declaration of Helsinki

In comparison with the WMA's Resolution on Human Experimentation of 1954, the provisions regarding consent were vitiated even further by the Declaration of Helsinki. The basic principles of that Declaration included the following: 1) foundation of human experiments on scientifically established facts, acquired through laboratory and animal experiments; 2) conduction by scientifically qualified persons only; 3) restriction of studies to scientific problems important enough to warrant inherent risks to the subjects; 4) careful assessment of inherent risks in comparison with foreseeable benefits to the subject or to others; and 5) use of special caution in performing clinical research that has the potential to alter the personality of the subject by drugs or experimental procedure. Consent of test subjects was not included in the basic principles. In regard to "Non-Therapeutic Clinical Research," the Declaration of Helsinki maintained that "clinical research on a human subject cannot be undertaken without his free consent, after he has been fully informed; if he is legally incompetent the consent of the legal guardian should be procured." In regard to "Clinical Research Combined With Professional Care," however, informing patients about experimental procedures was required only if "consistent with patient psychology." The independence of physicians was considered more important than the consent of patients.

In the treatment of the sick person the doctor must be free to use a new therapeutic measure if in his judgment it offers hope of saving life, re-establishing health, or alleviating suffering[66] (Fig. 420).

The Helsinki Declaration was praised by physicians as an advance over the Nuremberg Code. Beecher, who had evolved as a leading expert on medical ethics, commented about the matter thus:

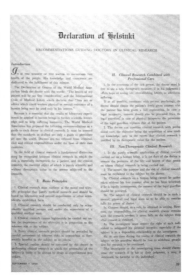

The Nuremberg Code presents a rigid act of legalistic demands ... The Declaration of Helsinki, on the other hand, presents a set of guides. It is an ethical as opposed to a legalistic document and is thus a more broadly useful instrument than the one formulated at Nuremberg . . . Until recently the Western world was threatened with the imposition of the Nuremberg Code as a Western credo. With the Declaration of Helsinki, this danger is apparently now past.[67]

From the perspective of an experimentalist/scientist, Beecher's relief can be understood fully. The Helsinki Declaration made life easier for scientists because it reflected more closely the realities of medical research. The devaluation of the importance of consent also was understandable in that context, based as it was on the consideration that even consent of test subjects could not absolve investigators of taking responsibility for their experiments. By striking consent from the list of basic principles and by stressing the subjective assessment by scientists of importance and risks of experiments as the primary criterion for research on human beings, however, the Helsinki Declaration abetted a cavalier attitude already prevalent toward experiments on humans. Furthermore, the Declaration gave only "recommendations as a guide to each doctor in clinical research;"[68] unlike the Nuremberg Code, it was not a legal document. As a consequence of the continuing debate about guidelines for human experimentation, even the Nuremberg Code, referred to by Beecher derogatorily as a "legalistic document," lost its binding character and came to be viewed as an informal set of recommendations that had no more force than the Declaration of Helsinki.[69]

In short, because of its nonobligatory status and its contents, the Declaration of Helsinki was much more permissive than the Nuremberg Code and by way of that permissiveness encouraged breaches of its own strictures. Michael Shimkin sounded the proper alarm in 1953 when he said that, ". . . science per se is neither moral nor immoral; it becomes moral or immoral only as moral or immoral human beings use its powerful techniques."[70] The denigration of the "rigid act of legalistic demands" embodied in the Nuremberg Code gave immoral activists of medical research a green light.

CHAPTER 19

AN ORGY OF EXPERIMENTS ON HUMANS

O f all the effects of the Nuremberg Code, attraction of
international attention to ethical aspects of experiments on humans probably was the most important.
The discussions that ensued were animated, in part, by profound differences in regard to such experiments between the
professions of medicine and the law. Another impetus to debate
about these matters was the rapid increase in scope of human
experimentation that occurred just after the Second World War
ended.

The new surge to experimentation on humans was especially
impressive in clinical trials of drugs. Between the two world
wars, the pharmaceutical industry had grown dramatically and
had generated an impressive number of synthetic and semi-synthetic products, among them antibiotics, general and local anesthetics, analeptics, analgesics, amphetamines, mercurial diuretics, hypnotics, and sedatives. At first, as was inevitable after they
just had been formulated in laboratories, the effects of most of
these substances on humans were not known fully. Physicians
conversant with clinical trials, therefore, became essential to the
drug companies, just as the pharmaceutical industry became an
indispensable ally of the medical profession. Both sides were

well aware of the advantages to one another of the synergism of their efforts. In the first third of the twentieth century, the leadership, worldwide, of German medicine had been attributed, in large measure, to close cooperation between hospitals and companies of the burgeoning pharmaceutical industry. When, in 1931, German hospitals were criticized for "working in the interest of the chemical industry, and thus for big business," the head of internal medicine at the University of Munich, Friedrich von Müller, answered bluntly in these words: "We have reason to thank the chemical industry for having supplied us in the last decades with a number of effective drugs."[1]

In the postwar period, the pharmaceutical industry, especially that in the United States, continued to expand and, in the process, produced an ever increasing number of drugs that were waiting to be tried on human beings. Between 1955 and 1960, for example, about 370 entirely new substances were introduced every year, compared with less than 45 per year in the early 1980s.[2] Scientists repeated the slogan that despite all the experiments in animals, the ultimate test of a drug could only be done in man, and urged that "some patient, whether for good or ill, must be the first to be exposed to it."[3] They reiterated, too, that what they proposed was no different from what had been practiced in the past. Modern clinical trials may have differed in method from that employed traditionally, but they did not differ in principle. Whereas in former times drugs had been dispensed to patients by individual physicians who recorded the effects of them with a bias inherent in all subjective appraisals, modern trials were carried out on a much broader scale, involved many patients, and were planned more carefully and monitored more closely. Without such trials, researchers argued, the release of a new drug would result in an uncontrolled experiment on masses of people with risks much greater and conclusions much less profound.[4] In order to enhance the significance of clinical trials, new methods were utilized, such as (a) construction of two (or

more) closely similar groups of patients observed at the same time but
whose treatment differed; (b) selection of these groups by some process of
random allocation; and (c) withholding of a form of treatment from one or
other of the groups.[5] The single-blind
method for assessment of drugs had
been introduced in 1930 by Paul Martini of Germany (Fig. 421), who con-

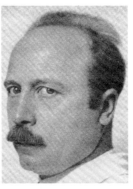

FIG. 421
Paul Martini
(1889-1964)

tended that the purpose of a drug trial could be realized only "if
the different substances to be compared (no matter whether one
of them is fictive or not) cannot be distinguished from one another by the patient."[6] In the 1950s, double-blind trials of drugs
– in which neither the patient nor the investigator knew the
identity of the substances administered – were begun in order to
eliminate bias in the interpretation of data.[7]

Improved methods for study clinically were used not only for
determining the effects of new compounds, but for critical reassessment of old ones. As new modalities of diagnosis and
treatment were validated, some of the time-honored methods
were found to be ineffective. Not uncommonly, studies of established regimens of treatment in conjunction with proper controls using a placebo were criticized at first on ethical grounds
because treatment was withheld from one group of patients and
later were judged unfavorably because treatment was administered to the other group. An example of this criticism involved a
study of the effects of oxygen on premature babies. Suspicion
had arisen that oxygen in high tension was a possible cause of
retrolental fibroplasia and subsequent blindness. When a comparison of two levels of oxygen was undertaken among premature neonates, the attending nurses were indignant because half
of the infants would be denied standard levels of high oxygen. As
the trial continued and it became more apparent that high oxy-

gen likely was a factor in the cause of retrolental fibroplasia, the nurses switched sides and proclaimed that it was "criminal" to place any babies in an atmosphere of high oxygen.[8]

As technology developed more rapidly and became more vast in scope, the notion that "standard diagnostic and therapeutic procedures of to-day [sic] may in five years' time be entirely obsolete"[9] found ever increasing acceptance. The opposite, however, was found to be equally true. As Robert A. McCance, professor of experimental medicine in Cambridge, England, observed in 1951, the physician often "forgets, indeed he may not even know, that what he would have regarded as an 'unjustifiable experiment' five years ago may have become one of his standard diagnostic and therapeutic procedures."[10] An example of that circumstance cited often was cardiac catheterization, introduced in 1929 by Werner Forssmann (Fig. 422). After perfecting his technique on cadavers, the young German surgeon used himself as the first living human subject for passage of a catheter into the right ventricle of the heart; in 1956, he was awarded the Nobel Prize for the work itself and for his courage in performing it. In the years between 1929 and 1956, fatal complications had oc-

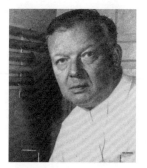

FIG. 422
Werner Forssmann
(1904-1979)

curred in other subjects, but the value of the technique clearly outweighed its risks. Had those complications occurred early in the development of cardiac catheterization, however, investigators might have been accused of risking the life of test subjects in "unjustifiable experiments."[11]

The twin factors of passage of a few years and untimely occurrence of a few rare complications could make the difference between rejection and approval of a new technique; a small controlled study could result in an old method being jettisoned.

19 · An Orgy of Experiments

Everything in medicine appeared to be in flux. From the viewpoint of proponents of medical research, making no effort at diagnosis and treatment of a patient was just as much an experiment as was application of a new procedure whose side effects were yet to be determined. The sophistic argument that no real difference existed between conducting an experiment and abstaining from it was put forward often by physicians in order to justify experiments on humans. For example, Michael Shimkin, then at the University of California's Laboratory of Experimental Oncology, made this argument in 1953: "To do nothing, or to prevent others from doing anything, is itself a type of experiment different from the one proposed. As much knowledge and as weighty reasons are required for one course of action as for the other, and it should be demonstrated that the proposed experiment is more dangerous or more painful than the known results of inaction."[12]

The Conquest of Disease

The inference that any medical decision is an experiment was both an attempt to justify human experimentation and a reflection of the general spirit of the time. Dramatic advances in biomedical research, such as the introduction of effective antibiotics, the elucidation of the structure of DNA, and vaccination against poliomyelitis, had created boundless enthusiasm, a pioneer mentality, and an insatiable wish to conquer the future in regard to disease of all kinds. "World medicine," one editor wrote, "appears to be approaching the threshold of a brilliant new era of discovery in which some of mankind's most dreaded diseases may be wiped out." Proof of this assertion was seen in the "miracle drug," peni-

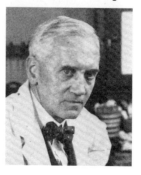

FIG. 423
*Alexander
Fleming
(1881-1955)*

cillin. When Scottish biologist Alexander Fleming (Fig. 423), who shared a Nobel Prize and was knighted for his discovery of antibacterial properties of a penicillin-producing mold, toured the United States in the fall of 1945, he was received as a hero. Fleming's response was exhilarating: "We are only at the beginning of this great study . . . We can certainly expect to do much toward reducing the sum total of human suffering."[13]

The "conquest of infectious disease" was the battle cry in medicine, and no disease was thought to be invincible. This mentality applied to hereditary diseases as well; as in the first decades of the twentieth century, the seeds of eugenics were propagated at medical conferences. In 1960, René Dubos, professor of microbiology at the Rockefeller Institute, identified "prolongation of the life of aged and ailing persons" and the saving of lives of children with genetic defects "the most difficult problems of medical ethics we are likely to encounter within the next decade." That judgment prompted him to ask, ". . . to what extent can we afford to prolong biological life in individuals who cannot derive either profit or pleasure from existence, and whose survival creates painful burdens for the community?" Hermann Joseph Muller of Indiana University (Fig. 424), who in 1946 won the Nobel Prize in medicine and physiology for his work on genetic effects of radiation, proposed "new techniques of reproduction," including a bank for depositing healthy sperm

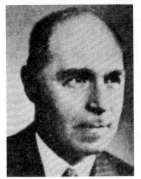

FIG. 424
*Hermann Joseph Muller
(1890-1967)*

for the purpose of preventing what he perceived to be the inevitable degeneration of the race. Physicist William Shockley, another Nobelist, called for serious efforts to improve human intelligence by cloning, artificial insemination, and sterilization. And Sir Julian Huxley (Fig. 425), a British evolutionist and brother of the author of *Brave New World*, Aldous Huxley,

19 · An Orgy of Experiments

proclaimed that ". . . the prospect of radical eugenic improvement could become one of the mainsprings of man's evolutionary advance." As in many other fields, little heed was paid to lessons that should have been learned from the perversion of medicine by the Nazis. The utopia of the "healthy state," a notion fascinating both to physicians and the laity, underwent a revival. At a conference in 1962 titled "Man and His Future," Hungarian Nobel Laureate and biologist, Albert Szent-Györgyi (Fig. 426), made these optimistic remarks:

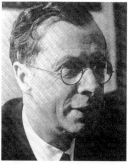

FIG. 425
Julian Sorel Huxley (1887-1975)

You may wish for anything: a cure-all for cancer, a mastery of mutation, an understanding of hormone action, or a cure of any disease you have in mind. None of your wishes need remain unfulfilled, once we have penetrated deep enough into the foundations of life. This is the real promise of medicine.[14]

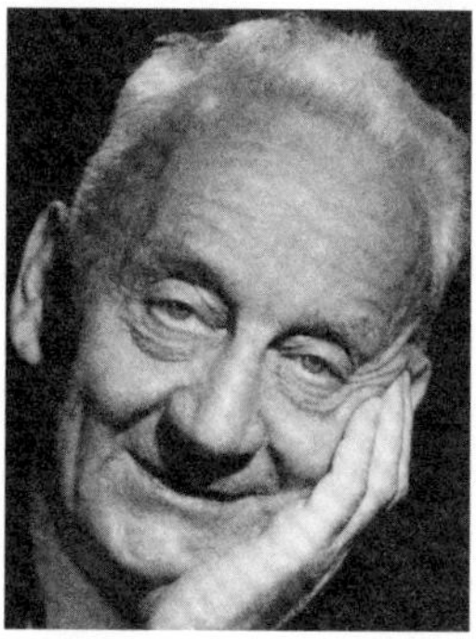

FIG. 426
Albert Szent-Györgyi (1893-1986)

In the United States, enthusiasm for medical research was furthered by a spirit of confidence, optimism, and patriotism that resulted from victory in the war. For Americans, everything seemed to be possible; the daring attitude associated with times of war continued to shape modern research practices in peacetime. Feelings of self-righteousness and self-importance also were running strong. More than ever before, Americans considered themselves to be the chosen people. They had saved the world from the barbarism of the Hitlerite hordes and the kamikaze maniacs of the Japanese Emperor, and were ready and willing to take on a new evil enemy in the form of the Communist Soviet Union. The climate of the Cold War contributed to the conviction that Americans had to be first in everything, even if this meant accepting risks such as those inherent in medical experimentation. "A future aggressor," wrote an editor of *The New York Times*, "will move even more swiftly than Hitler did. Two oceans will not give us time to establish another Office of Scientific Research and Development. Continuous systematic research is an evident necessity. It may be regarded as a kind of military insurance."[15]

Pelted with Money

The need to experiment in medicine was encouraged mightily by the U.S. government, an attitude which fostered a major change in national thinking. Prior to World War II, there had been almost no financial support of research by the federal government. The Committee on Medical Research was a product of the war, and its policy, beginning in 1944, to fund research by making "grants in aid to universities, hospitals, laboratories, and other public or private institutions, and to individuals" had been sanctioned by Congress.[16] As the war drew to a close, President Roosevelt asked the Office of Scientific Research and Development (OSRD) how to sustain the nation's military research efforts in peacetime. The response came in July 1945 in a report captioned, "Science, the Endless Frontier," in which OSRD Director, Vannevar Bush (Fig. 427), made a strong case for continuation of a proactive role for the

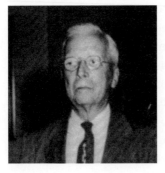

FIG. 427
*Vannevar Bush
(1890-1974)*

federal government in promoting research, arguing that "Scientific progress is one essential key to our security as a nation, to our better health, to more jobs, to higher standard of living, and to our cultural progress."[17] When the Committee on Medical Research ceased operations later

that year, 44 wartime research contracts were transferred to the juris-
diction of the Public Health Service
in order to ensure continuance of
them, thereby providing an impetus
to a program funded by large grants
and administered by what was then
called the National Institute of
Health.[18] In his first message to Con-

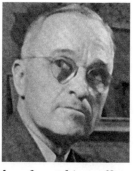

gress in November 1945, seven months after taking office,
Roosevelt's successor, Harry Truman (Fig. 428), proposed
that "Congress adopt a comprehensive and modern health
program for the nation," including the construction of hospitals through federal grants-in-aid to the state, the expansion
of public health services, the expansion of "our compulsory
social security system," and federal support of medical education and medical research.[19]

Truman's message came just at the right time. The results of
coordinated scientific efforts during the war had impressed the
nation. Surgeon General Thomas Parran observed in 1947 that
"never before has there been such keen and widespread interest
in health matters throughout the country."[20] Powerful advocates for medical research, such as activist Mary Lasker (Fig.
429), wife of a prominent and wealthy
New Yorker, used personal money
and personal connections to lobby for
expansion of federal research programs. In December 1944, a committee of the Senate had heard from 16
witnesses, half of whom had been
called to testify at the suggestion of
Mrs. Lasker, that existing sources of
funds for future peacetime medical
research were inadequate.[21] Mary

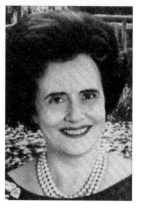

FIG. 429
Mary Lasker

Lasker eventually became the first layperson to serve on an advisory council for national medical research and played an important role in the establishment of the Mental Health Institute, the National Heart Institute, and other branches of the U.S. Public Health Service.[22] Because of the establishment of these new branches, the National Institute of Health pluralized its name in 1948 and became known as the National Institutes of Health (NIH).[23] Influential politicians, such as Senator Lister Hill of Alabama (Fig. 430) and Congressman John Fogarty of Rhode Island (Fig. 431), succeeded in providing the NIH not only with the budget requested by and for it, but with additional funds that might be used to push medical research ahead even more rapidly. Fogarty stated that as long as it helped save lives, he did not care about the cost of research.[24]

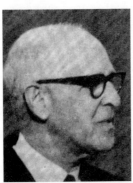

FIG. 430
Lister Hill
(1894-1984)

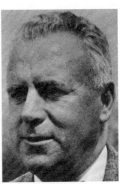

FIG. 431
John Fogarty
(1913-1967)

The magnitude of the increase in funding for medical research was staggering. In 1945, the U.S. government spent approximately $700,000 on medical research. Ten years later, the total had climbed to $36 million, by 1965, to $436 million, and by 1970, the annual appropriations of the NIH reached $1.5 billion.[15] During the first Eisenhower administration, Congress routinely added $8 to $15 million to the annual amount proposed by the administration for the NIH budget.[26] Congress also provided generous funds for the National Science Foundation (NSF), which had been created in 1950 with the specific mission of promoting basic science research, and for the Atomic Energy Commission (AEC), the predecessor of the U. S. Department of Energy, that had been established in 1947.[27] Occasionally, agencies received more money than they could use. In 1947, for example, Congress allocated $175 million to the AEC, with up to $5 million to be reserved for research concerning cancer that did not duplicate the work of other public or private agencies. At first, the AEC had problems finding worthy research projects and, in 1948, actually considered returning cash to the federal treasury. William Bale, who directed wartime studies of radioisotopes at Strong Memorial Hospital in Rochester, New York, recalled that in those days ". . . almost anything could get supported if it had any smattering of sense behind it."[28]

Eventually, the excess of available money created legitimate opportunities to spend it, and the more opportunities arose, the more money was proffered. Any scientist, regardless of affiliation, prominence, or competence, could propose to the NIH a project on almost any subject and have it reviewed for possible funding by a panel of leading scientists from institutions and universities throughout the country. Once the project had been approved and a grant awarded, the scientist was allowed considerable freedom in the design of the research, even changing it to take advantage of new information as the work progressed. A philosophy of academic freedom in the extramural project-grants program of the NIH was thought to be crucial for assuring success in research.[29] President Truman declared proudly in 1952 that the federal government supported one-fourth of all research conducted in medical institutions and, moreover, without exerting any control over scientists or universities.[30] Likewise, Normal H. Topping, Associate Director of the NIH, proclaimed with satisfaction that "those who receive grants [are] free to pursue their own ideas with no federal control or supervision whatever."[31] Stanton Cohn, a veteran of the Manhattan Project, reflected on those times in these words: "It was fantastic – we could buy any piece of machinery or equipment, and you never had to justify it."[32] Another Los Alamos scientist, on returning from Washington, announced gleefully, "I am black and blue from being pelted with money."[33]

The Orgy Begins

In contrast to the lavish provision of funds for medical research, Congress did little to provide financial assistance to medical schools. To be sure, research grants enabled many of those schools to upgrade their educational, as well as their research, programs, but much faculty time and precious space had to be donated to the research effort.[34] As a consequence, more and more graduates of medical schools were attracted by the possibilities of lucrative and prestigious careers in clinical and basic research. Within a few years, a new breed of physicians emerged, one who was interested not in managing individual patients, but in elaborating techniques and finding cures that would benefit mankind and enhance their own careers. Physicians devoted primarily to taking care of patients came to be viewed as second-class and soon were overshadowed professionally by colleagues who spent most of their time doing research. Chairmen of clinical departments no longer were chosen on the basis of clinical skills, but on the basis of the amount of funding they could bring in from the NIH and from other sources such as industry, in particular the pharmaceutical field. Because original studies published in rapid-fire succession were essential to an investigator who sought to acquire such funding, some teaching hospitals were transformed into research centers which soon became an arena for an orgy of human experimentation.

In those years, the development of medicine in the United States resembled that in Germany at the end of the nineteenth century. Because of vigorous research, American medicine seemed to be the best in the world and was a source of great national pride. American researchers became the new "warriors against disease," and test subjects were their "soldiers." The injury and death of soldiers of research were inevitable consequences of the war against disease, and paled in comparison to the dramatic victories on this battlefield. Those victories gave the "warriors" great power that was furthered by their having close ties to the government, such as membership in advisory committees to civilian and military agencies. As a consequence of their power and success, hardly ever were the desires of "warriors against disease" denied. The performance of experiments at will on humans became so widespread that neither physicians nor the laity questioned the justification of it. The maxim of poet Alexander Pope that the "proper study for mankind is man" was translated into practice by scientists who contended that "... the crucial study of new techniques and agents must be carried out in man ... Man as the final test site has come into prominence only in recent decades. The current development of human biochemistry, human physiology, and human pharmacology has made it plain that man is the 'animal of necessity' here."[35]

It had long been recognized by researchers in medicine that experiments on humans, with suitable controls, are indispensable to certain types of research. In the period immediately after the Second World War, however, the situation changed; the necessity of performing experiments on humans became truistic to the laity as well as to physicians. Even Pope Pius XII conceded the importance of experiments on humans. In his comments on medical research in 1952, Pius XII first admonished his international audience that "science is not the highest value," that it has to be "inserted in the order of values," and that some ethical strictures might even be advantageous to science. "The great moral demands," he advised, "force the impetuous flow of human thought and will to flow, like water from the mountains, into certain chan-

nels. They contain the flow to increase its efficiency and useful-
ness. They dam it so that it does not overflow and cause ravages
that can never be compensated for by the special good it seeks. In
appearance, moral demands are a brake. In fact, they contribute
to the best and most beautiful of what man has produced for science . . ." Despite these moralistic claims, Pius XII acknowledged
that ". . . one cannot ask that any danger or any risk be excluded.
That would exceed human possibilities, paralyze all serious scientific research and very frequently would be to the detriment of the
patient."[36] The Pope left no doubt that he was sympathetic toward
"the bold spirit of research" which incites an investigator "to follow newly discovered roads, to extend them, to create new ones
and to renew methods."[37]

Ambiguity in Regard to Ethical Standards for Research

In the 1950s and 60s, the little bell of morality was rung time
and again, but it failed to strike the tympanic membranes of
physicians and the laity, being drowned out as it was by trum-
pets of scientific progress. Even those who rang the bell could
barely hear its sound. They often were ambiguous about their
own orchestration and were desirous of playing in the brass section in concert with others. Henry Beecher, for instance, one of
the most prolific contributors to the establishment of ethical
standards for human experimentation, violated basic principles when it came to research in his own laboratory. Between
1952 and 1954, he conducted for the U.S. Army a secret study at
Harvard University in which hallucinogens were administered
to healthy individuals. According to Louis Lasagna, a research
fellow in Beecher's department who in 1964 would write a
modern version of the Hippocratic Oath, test subjects "weren't
informed about anything."[38]

It was not only individuals who were ambiguous about ethi-

19 · An Orgy of Experiments

cal boundaries for experiments on humans, but also entire agencies. On April 30, 1947, General Manager Carroll Wilson (Fig. 432) of the Atomic Energy Commission prohibited nontherapeutic experiments on humans with radioactive materials and set requirements for fully informed consent of test subjects in therapeutic trials. Wilson set forth those rules to

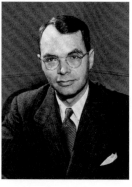

Stafford Warren in a personal letter that was not widely circulated. In the fall of 1947, Wilson informed radiologist Robert Stone that substances "known to be, or suspected of being, poisonous or harmful" should be used on human subjects only under the following circumstances: "(a) that a reasonable hope exists that the administration of such a substance will improve the condition of the patient; (b) that the patient give his complete and informed consent in writing; and (c) that the responsible next of kin give in writing a similarly complete and informed consent, revocable at any time during the course of such treatment."[39] It was in this letter that the term "informed consent" was used for the first time (although the concept of informed consent was very much older). The requirement that not only test subjects but their next of kin had to consent to an experiment was completely new, and it set the bar for human experiments higher than ever, before or since. Wilson's letter to Stone, however, had an even narrower distribution than his earlier letter to Warren.[40] With very few exceptions, institutions that performed research under contract for the AEC never learned of the existence of Wilson's guidelines. Although the prohibition by Wilson of nontherapeutic experiments never was revoked, tracer studies continued to be the mainstay of isotope research sponsored by the AEC. Even when representatives of the Commission were asked specifically about requirements for consent and about "experimental procedures in the human . . . simply for investigational purposes and not for treatment of disease," they declined to give any advice, referring questions to institutions that were subordinate.[41]

When the NIH opened its Clinical Center in 1953, it vowed that "the welfare of the patient takes precedence over every other consideration."[42] Practices of research were to be guided by the "ten commandments" of the Nuremberg Code and every research endeavor projected was to be reviewed by "a special board of scientists."[43] In actuality, the Clinical Center instituted practically no formal procedures or mechanisms to ensure that the goals of research did not take priority over the best interests of patients. According to the Director of what was then called the National Heart Institute, Donald S. Fredrickson, giving an explanation about procedures of research to patients was "by no means universal." The director of clinical investigation for the National Institute of Mental Health admitted that "only a small percentage" of patients signed a specific consent form and, even then, "the negative aspects of therapy" were not usually stipulated and recorded plainly on the form. Moreover, investigators were not obliged by any internal rule to consult with colleagues or to be reviewed prior to initiating a study. Although a Medical Board Committee existed, rarely was it consulted. If an investigator felt that a research protocol was not hazardous, he was given *carte blanche* to proceed with it.[44]

In 1953, the U.S. Department of Defense adopted the principles of the Nuremberg Code for "experimental research in the fields of atomic, biological, and/or chemical warfare," but the memorandum to this effect was classified "top secret." How could a directive issued in secret be implemented?[45] In 1954, the Army Office of the Surgeon General issued an unclassified statement captioned, "Use of Human Volunteers in Medical Research: Principles, Policies and Rules." This document restated the Nuremberg Code and was not limited to atomic, biological, and chemical warfare research. The statement was distributed with this prefatory disclaimer: "To be used as far as applicable as a non-mandatory guide for planning and conducting contract research."[46] It was natural that a "non-mandatory guide" would not be observed strictly. Although officials of the Army sought to apply the policy to all contractors, exceptions were known to be common.

One such dispensation was made in 1962 for Harvard University. When the strictures of the Nuremberg Code appeared suddenly in Army research contracts, members of the Administrative Board of the Harvard Medical School voiced concerns about them. Assistant Dean Joseph W. Gardella (Fig. 433) argued that "the Nuremberg Code was conceived in reference to Nazi atrocities and was written for the specific purpose of preventing brutal excesses from being committed or excused in the name of science. The code, however admirable in its intent, and however suitable for the purpose for which it was conceived, is in our opinion not necessarily pertinent to or adequate for the conduct of medical research in the United States." Henry Beecher, who also belonged to the Administrative Board, warned that "rigid rules will jeopardize the research establishments of this country where experimentation in man is essential." In a meeting with Army Surgeon General Leonard D. Heaton in July 1962, representatives of Harvard Medical School succeeded in extracting a clarification that the principles of the Army were "guidelines" rather than "rigid rules," and thereby were able, as Gardella put it, "to avert the catastrophic impact of the Surgeon General's regulation."[47]

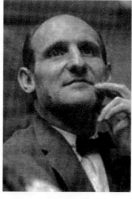

FIG. 433
Joseph Gardella (1915-2001)

Soothing the Concerns of the Public

Years later, in 1975, a review by the U.S. Army Inspector General on the "Use of Volunteers in Critical Agent Research" during the first two decades of the second half of the twentieth century determined that "in spite of clear guidelines concerning the necessity of 'informed consent,' there was a willingness to dilute and in some cases negate the intent of the policy." The report also acknowledged that ". . . this attitude of selective compliance was more the norm than the exception."[48] Failure to implement and control regulations concerning experiments on humans resulted in uncertainty and confusion about the meaning and the stringency of official dictums by the government. The "selective compliance" of government agencies in regard to their own rules may, in actuality, have been more detrimental than having no rules at all. It led, by bad example, to a cavalier attitude among scientists and excused them from having to establish ethical standards themselves. As it turned out, regulations of the government did little to prevent questionable experiments on humans; they served chiefly as a means for calming public concerns. When such experiments were discussed in public forums, scientists were quick to point to the "rigid rules" governing research on human beings, cautioning against exaggeration of the occasional misdemeanors of a few blackguards within the medical community.[49]

In general, the public was entirely uncritical in regard to human experimentation. It failed to recognize that the war on the medical front was associated with severe ethical lapses resulting in harm unnecessarily. The laity was not able to appreciate that some of the greatest successes in medicine – including the development of penicillin and of insulin treatment for diabetes mellitus – had been achieved without extensive experimention on humans.[50] The popular press glorified the warriors of medicine, and magazines such as American Mercury and Reader's Digest ran glowingly complimentary stories of human interest on the "soldiers of research," among them prisoners and conscientious objectors, who were described as "volunteers." *The New York Times* informed readers in 1958 that ". . . among these men and women you will find those who will take shots of the new vaccines, who will swallow radioactive drugs, who will fly higher than anyone else, who will watch malaria infected mosquitos feed on their bare arms." The *Times* contended that test subjects had plausible, often noble, reasons for volunteering for experiments on humans, those motivations being said to be social redemption, religious belief, and service to society – not to mention seeking thrills.[51]

Worries about any aspect of this issue were soothed by trivializing the dangers and side effects associated with such experiments. For example, when dermatologist Albert M. Kligman of the University of Pennsylvania was searching for a substance that would prevent allergic reactions to poison ivy, he gave injections of an immunizing serum to six inmates of Philadelphia's Holmesburg Prison. All developed systemic reactions; four prisoners "went to the hospital in terrible shape;" two others collapsed in the prison and "had no blood pressure." Shortly thereafter, *Life* magazine published a glow-ing article about Kligman's scien-tific quest, portraying him hero-ically "crawling through the bush-es" in search of "bouquets of poi-son ivy," and assuring readers that in 300 trials "only a dozen or so vaccinated volunteers have had more than a brief local rash."[52] This deliberate effort at trivializa-tion was but one example of more to come – and from the very same source (Fig. 434).

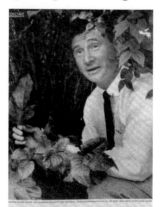

FIG. 434
"Poison Ivy Picker of Pennypack Park" – *an approving article about medical experiments by the dermatologist, Albert M. Kligman, in* Life *magazine in 1955.*

POISON IVY PICKER OF PENNYPACK PARK

Articles in medical journals were somewhat more accurate in regard to methods and results, but the difficulties and distress endured by test subjects, and the risks and complications associated with the experiments rarely were recorded. As in the nineteenth century, when the natural remission of signs of experimentally induced secondary syphilis were carelessly and incorrectly equated with total remission of the disease, dangers that were not apparent immediately were banished from consideration. For example, the effects of sunburn were studied experimentally without any consideration being given to possible implications for carcinogenesis. Test subjects were sensitized to potent allergens without any thought of the possibility of long-term damage that can be caused by reactions to drugs and specific allergic contactants. Countless test subjects were injected with compounds of blood taken from other persons with no reflection having been given to possible transmission of potentially fatal diseases, such as hepatitis.[53] Liver biopsies were performed as part of many experiments, but the mortality of two to three per 1,000 patients associated with the procedure never was mentioned.[54] And whenever reports about severe complications and death appeared in the medical literature, they were accompanied by disclaimers to the effect that such incidents were exceedingly rare.[55] That many fatalities never were made public may be inferred from retrospective studies based on questionnaires sent to heads of departments of medical centers. The responses revealed that instances of severe complications were much greater than was conveyed in the literature. As British physician and champion of subject rights, Maurice H. Pappworth, articulated in 1967, "undoubtedly, and for obvious reasons, the worst experiments go unrecorded."[56]

Sins of Omission

In 1959, Henry Beecher wrote about the problem of falsified reports thus:

19 · An Orgy of Experiments

There have been instances in which certain details and complications have been deleted from published reports to avoid unfavourable criticism. It seems unlikely that such abuses are common, but when they occur it is probable that the study should not have been carried out in the first place. The failure to report serious complications in a final report is inexcusable.[57]

Although Beecher no doubt understated the frequency of that "inexcusable" happening, his conjecture that such studies "should not have been carried out in the first place" was on target exactly. In fact, numerous studies that violated basic principles of medical ethics went unrecorded for fear of hostile reactions. For example, Robert Stone (Fig. 435), chairman of

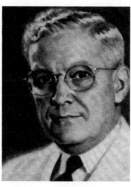

the department of radiology at the University of California in San Francisco and a strong advocate of human experimentation, wanted to release "classified papers containing certain information on human experimentation with radioisotopes conducted within the AEC research program." The AEC, however, warned that "the atmosphere of secrecy and suppression makes one aspect of medical work of the Commission especially vulnerable to criticism" and approved publication of studies only if they corresponded to the rules (mostly uncirculated) laid down by Caroll Wilson.[58] For public consumption, injections of plutonium in unsuspecting human beings simply had never taken place.

Suppression of data that were thought to reflect badly on research was not uncommon. When Los Alamos hematologist Norman Knowlton found "highly significant decreases" in the blood counts of chemists exposed to low amounts of gamma rays, the insurance official of the AEC cautioned against release of his report. He pointed out that there was a "possibility of a

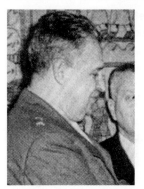

FIG. 436
Leslie Groves
(1896-1970)

shattering effect on the morale of the employees if they become aware that there was substantial reason to question the standards of safety under which they are working. In the hands of labor unions the results of this study would add substance to demands for extra-hazardous pay."[59] This is but one example of the fact that science is no temple of truth. Suppression of data, trivialization of side effects, and exaggeration of successes were part and parcel of the game. Science took place in the real world, where political maneuvers were commonplace and were employed commonly to attain practical goals. That phenomenon was no different for machinations in every other sphere of society. When General Leslie Groves (Fig. 436), the military commander of the Manhattan Project, was summoned to Capitol Hill in November 1945 to testify before a special committee of the Senate about the dangers of radiation, he acknowledged that severe exposure could be fatal. Death through radiation, however, came "without undue suffering," he said, advising that it was "a very pleasant way to die." According to Groves, exposure to low doses of radiation was of little consequence. This is how he stated it: "Anyone who is working with such materials, who accidentally becomes overexposed, just takes a vacation away from the material and in due course of time he is perfectly alright again." Groves made no mention of fatalities that had occurred in the program; he chose to minimize any dangers.[60]

With this kind of behavior being exhibited on the floor of the Senate, how could any researcher as he sat by the bedside of a prospective test subject be expected to adhere strictly to the dicta of truth, full information about all dangers, and abstention from trivialization of side effects? The reality of human experimentation was this: if test subjects were told at all that they were part of a research project, any information given to them was, as a rule, filtered carefully. Leonard Sagan, a physician who worked for the AEC, put it this way:

Doctors who were doing research wanted to be professors, and in order to be a professor, you have to have lots of publications, so your highest priority is to conduct research and publish it. You're the doctor. Here's a patient that you want to experiment on . . . Is it going to contribute to your research if you inform that patient? What can happen is the patient says, 'No, I don't want to do that.' That's not in your interest. Your interest is to have that patient participate, so do you tell him or her? No. Does anybody care? No. So you don't tell them.[61]

Almost nobody did care. Physicians of that time must have been aware of the ethical limits of experiments on humans, discussed as they were repeatedly at medical meetings and in major medical journals. They knew, however, that few cared much about consequences to test subjects and, that being the case, most investigators placed their own interests above those of their charges/subjects. Because there were no sanctions against breaches of rules, scientists sought to outdo one another (in a spirit of competitiveness that is inherent in every step along the way to medical school, during medical school, in securing an internship, a residency, and a fellowship, and for the duration of an entire professional life), thereby leading to an orgy of experiments on human beings. "The impetuous flow of human thought" was not restrained in channels, as Pope Pius XII had demanded it should be, but was allowed to "overflow and cause ravages" that did not enhance the cause of medicine, to say nothing of individual test subjects. As had been the case in the past when human experimentation knew no bounds, countless unnecessary studies were carried out. They were mere repetitions of previous work, attempts to generate data that already were well established; and they were planned and conducted so poorly that their results defied meaningful interpretation. The traditional flaws of experimentation on humans also were maintained in other respects. Experiments were performed chiefly on persons considered to be inferior, unable to defend themselves, and easy to deceive and control – in brief, those in the most vulnerable populations.

CHAPTER 20

THE PRISON
AS TEST SITE

To achieve a particular goal, three conditions must be fulfilled: know where one stands currently, know where one wants to go, and know what steps to take to get there. The most fundamental and important of these conditions is the first – an accurate perception of one's actual position, literally and philosophically. In medicine, the ultimate aim of physicians – health of the patient – is well known to them, and a therapeutic armamentarium may be available to help achieve that desideratum. Without a correct diagnosis, however, treatment cannot be administered in a rational and effective way. The same principle applies to other spheres of endeavor. Without a clear perception of reality – that is, accurate diagnosis of a situation – any effort at achievement is doomed to fail.

In regard to ethics of human experimentation, the aims had been recognized clearly by the mid twentieth century, set forth as they were in the Nuremberg Code and in a variety of other regulations. Measures to achieve those aims also were available. The Nuremberg Code had the status of a legal document that could be used to enforce rules. Several technical procedures and systems, such as review boards for investigations, had been proposed to ensure that ethical limits would not be transgressed in medical research. Appropriate steps to reach these lofty aims, however, were not taken, because the perception of reality in regard to experimentation was blurred. Unethical experiments on humans were not perceived to be a major problem; and, therefore, they continued to be carried out unabated on an ever increasing scale.

The impaired perception of reality was most obvious in medical research done on prisoners. Theoretically, prisons are institutions that serve to rehabilitate inmates of them. When, at the end of the eighteenth century, the Quakers of Pennsylvania instituted a modern system of prisons as places of confinement for ordinary lawbreakers, their intentions were lofty. They sought to make confinement in solitude lend itself to contemplation and an appropriate substitute for forms of punishment common then, such as branding and flogging in public, mutilation, and hanging. By separating individual offenders from other miscreants, shelter would be provided from influences that could be negative mutually. The hope was that lawbreakers, serving their sentences with nothing but the Bible for company, would be brought to repent their sins and achieve, thereby, eternal salvation. The reality was different. Solitary confinement led convicts to become insane rather than penitent and resulted in so many deaths by suicide that by the mid nineteenth century it was abandoned. The regimen of solitary confinement was supplanted by a more "productive" system of "congregate hard labor" by which convicts came once again under the influence of fellow criminals. The corporal punishments that the Quakers had sought to replace with contemplation were exacerbated behind prison walls as wardens and superintendents devised various tortures to maintain discipline and control. Disciplinary measures used in American prisons following World War II ranged from true solitary confinement to brutalization by guards in the form of beatings, whippings, kicking of testicles, and running of gauntlets. At times, prisoners were killed as these punishments were meted out.[1]

Prisons offered inmates the theoretical chance to engage in educational activities, learn a trade, and earn some money by doing productive jobs. In practice, however, there was little opportunity to learn skills that would be useful on the outside. For example, a highly touted program to enable prisoners to learn a trade at San Quentin Penitentiary in California offered only 350 places for a population of over 3,500 prisoners.[2] Good jobs in prisons were rare; jobs with a monthly pay of $5 to $10 were considered to be "money slots." The few dollars allowed for purchases at the prison commissary of cookies, candy, cigarettes, toothbrushes, and other personal items that made the stark, barren life in prison slightly more tolerable. Because prison food was monotonous and often rotten, and items such as writing paper and toilet paper were supplied in very scant quantities, making some money, even a pittance, became a preoccupation of inmates. Those awaiting trial with less severe charges against them could even try to raise enough money to pay their own bail as a first step to freedom.[3] Moreover, money could be used for bribing guards, in a prison system that, in general, was rampant with corruption.[4] Only a few prisoners, however, were given jobs; most simply had to endure a life of unrelieved inactivity and boredom.

When the National Prison Association (NPA) of the United States (later called the American Correctional Association) held its first congress in Cincinnati in 1870, it suggested that prisons be lighted by "way of love." The "thought of inflicting punishment upon prisoners to satisfy so-called justice" was to be replaced by "the real objectives of the system . . . the protection of society by prevention of crime and reformation of criminals." These goals were to be achieved by "men of ability and experience at the head of our penal establishments," that is, persons who had expertise in helping prisoners to become law-abiding citizens.[5] Some enthusiasts of that idealized kind of prison life even went so far as to insist that everyone could profit from a stretch in a penitentiary, that "the world would ultimately be better" if all members of society could be exposed to the "regularity and temperance and sobriety of a good prison."[6] The reality was different. In general, guards were not trained for the high purposes they were meant to serve; most had taken the job because there was no better possibility for them to make a living. Poorly educated and poorly paid, they were considered to be at the bottom of the chain of law enforcement. Any intimacy with prisoners was strictly forbidden. Instead of treating prisoners as individual human beings, guards were expected by their supervisors, as one officer at Raiford State Prison in Florida put it in 1971, "to feel that a convict is the lowest thing on earth."[7]

One of the central ideas of the National Prison Association, voiced first at its congress in 1870 and at numerous meetings thereafter, was that "a criminal is a man who has suffered under a disease evidenced by the perpetration of a crime."[8] The logical conclusion, namely, to "treat the criminal as a patient and the crime as a disease," became particularly popular in the 1950s when prisons instituted programs run by psychiatrists for treatment of the "disease." According to a booklet in 1959 addressed to families of prisoners in California, ". . . the treatment program of the inmate in the prison is planned in terms of an understanding of him as a person . . . human kindness pervades the things that are done." The prison was said to be "like a hospital – only the kinds of troubles treated there are not physical illnesses but personal troubles."[9] In reality, psychiatric treatment was imposed on inmates, whether they wanted it or not. Moreover, prisons were controlled by guards who had total veto power over every detail of every function or operation in every division of them. Psychiatrists who, at the expense of safety rules and prison discipline, tried to establish personal bonds with prisoners, were fired. Consequently, as Harvey Powelson, resident psychiatrist at San Quentin, observed in 1951, ". . . psychiatry in the prison consists primarily in therapeutic practices which have punitive or disciplinary implications: electric shock, insulin shock, fever treatment . . . and so on."[10]

Undermining the Psyche of the Prisoner

When it became evident that psychiatric treatment did not enhance "reformation" of prisoners, behavioral scientists took over and tried out various brainwashing techniques on inmates. Edgar H. Schein, associate professor of psychology at the Massachusetts Institute of Technology, advised prison wardens in 1962 that the best way to change a person's standards of conduct was to "first disorganize the group which supports these standards, then undermine his other emotional supports, then put him in a new and ambiguous situation for which the standards are unclear, and then put pressure on him."[11] Those proposals were then implemented by "spying on the men and reporting back private material" in order to create a sense of widespread distrust among the prisoners, undermining their ties to home by sending inmates to remote prisons, "systematically withholding their mail,"[12] and combining "sensory deprivation with drugs, hypnosis, and astute manipulation of reward and punishment."[13] According to James V. McConnell, controversial professor of psychology at the University of Michigan, the purpose was "to gain almost absolute control over an individual's behavior."[14] Parenthetically, McConnell, because of some of his beliefs, decades later became one of the targets of the Unabomber.

At its first congress, the National Prison Association acknowledged that "granite walls and iron bars, although they deprive the criminal of his liberty and inflict a just physical punishment, do not work that reformation in the soul of the man that will restore him to society regenerated and reformed."[15] To achieve the stated objective of prisons – the "moral regeneration" of the inmate, in contrast to "infliction of vindictive suffering" – it was suggested strongly that sentences be adjusted to fit the character of the prisoner rather than the crime itself for which he was convicted. Hence, the US Congress called for "in-

determinate sentences," under which offenders would be released as soon as "the moral cure" had been effected and "satisfactory proof of reformation" was obtained.[16] Eventually, indeterminate sentences, either directly or indirectly, were introduced throughout the United States, in the form of a parole
system that allowed early release of convicts for good behavior.
The range of indeterminate sentences, that is, the minimum
and maximum time an individual prisoner could be confined,
varied greatly. This was especially true in California where sec-
ond-degree burglary carried a sentence of one to 15 years; rape,
one to 50 years; and robbery or sale of marijuana, five years to
life.[17] The actual time a prisoner had to serve was determined by
parole boards which were said to be "composed of persons who
have demonstrated skills, abilities, and leadership in many
fields."[18] The idea was "to observe a prisoner and release him at
the earliest time within the limits fixed by his sentence."[19]

In reality, the minimum time for an indeterminate sentence
was rarely a realistic consideration, and the average time spent
in prison for a given offense increased progressively and substantially. One reason may have been that parole boards were
not made up of a cross-section of citizens with creditable skills
and accomplishments, but were drawn almost exclusively from
the ranks of law enforcement, such as former policemen, prosecutors, and prison personnel, many of whom were undistin-
guished. Moreover, parole boards took into account not only the
offenses for which a prisoner had been incarcerated, but also
other charges brought against that person, even those based
solely on hearsay. As a result, certain prisoners could be confined
indefinitely, and in that situation they became completely dependent on the correctional authorities who had god-like power
over their lives. The status of prisoners in regard to reformation
of them was assessed once a year on the basis of a brief interview
and on review of their personal files, which were both kept and
updated by the prison staff. Neither prisoners nor their lawyers

were allowed to see those files; if parole were turned down, inmates and their advocates were not entitled to know the reasons why. By keeping prisoners in perpetual suspense, never knowing from year to year what portion of their one-to-20 or five-to-life sentence would have to be served, the authorities in correctional institutions maintained complete control of their body and soul for the entire period of incarceration.[20]

Maximum control also meant that no unfavorable information about the prison could leak to the outside world. All incoming and outgoing mail was censored, and if convicts did succeed in smuggling out information, such as denouncing prison conditions in letters to journalists or editors of newspapers, they ran a serious risk of being punished severely. Access to prisons usually was denied to outsiders, the standard reason given for refusing admittance was that it was "too dangerous." If outsiders were admitted, they had to play by the rules, for example, they were not allowed to speak to prisoners. The rules were determined by the warden, who was the unchallenged ruler of his domain.[21] Behind prison walls, the will of the warden was equivalent to law; in fact, no other laws were in force. Even the courts observed a strict hands-off policy in matters of prison administration, believing that "supervision of inmates . . . rests with the proper administrative authorities, and courts . . . have no power to supervise the management of disciplinary rules of such institutions."[22]

In summary, a vast difference existed between the theory and the reality of life in prison, and it was the distorted perception of the reality that helped legitimize medical experiments on prisoners. Had prisons really been hostels of brotherly love in which individuals with personal problems were treated with respect and decency (as the lofty declarations of correctional authorities indicated they should be), medical research in prisons might not have been so objectionable. In that case, Andrew Ivy's assertion that prisoners were able "to say 'yes' or 'no' without fear of being punished or of being deprived of privileges" would have been plausible.[23] But how could a valid "yes" or "no" be expected from prisoners if correctional authorities believed that "in order to reform a criminal you must first break his spirit"?[24] How could persons who were completely under the control of others "exercise free power of choice"? How could an enlightened decision "without the intervention of any element of force, fraud, deceit, duress, overreaching, or other ulterior form of coercion"[25] be made in an environment so diametric to that called for in the Nuremberg Code? That these questions never were addressed seriously was not by chance or oversight. Reality was disregarded purposely in order to sustain the *status quo*. Just as the idea that prisons were residences for therapy, rather than institutions for punishment, served to assuage the conscience of the public, the fable of a free and independent prisoner volunteering willingly for medical experiments contributed greatly to enhancing even further the preeminence of the United States in medical research. For that reason, the myth was maintained and defended against criticism, both that from within the country and abroad.

A "Sacrifice of Human Dignity"

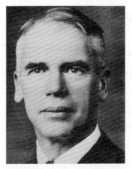

FIG. 437
Shields
Warren

Among the strident critics of medical research on prisoners within the United States were radiologist Joseph Hamilton and radiologist/pathologist Shields Warren, who won the Enrico Fermi Award for his work in atomic energy. When their colleague, Robert Stone, suggested in 1950 that prisoners be utilized for research in projects of the Atomic Energy Commission (AEC), Hamilton dismissed the proposal as having "a little of the Buchenwald touch." Warren

(Fig. 437) asserted that "it's not very long since we got through trying Germans for doing exactly the same thing."[26] To such remarks, proponents of experiments on prisoners reacted with innocence and surprise, claiming that experiments were carried out "on an absolutely voluntary basis."[27]

The more egregious the study, the more vainglorious was the description of the lofty motives of prisoners who participated in it. For example, in 1956, Chester M. Southam of the Sloan-Kettering Cancer Research Institute carried out a study involving subcutaneous injection of live cancer cells into the arms of inmates of Ohio State Penitentiary.[28] According to Southam, all volunteers were informed about possible risks of the experiment, but it is likely that the information provided to them may have been biased because Southam himself "did not regard the experiment as dangerous." Nevertheless, Southam refused to participate as a subject in his own research, arguing thus: "I do not regard myself as dispensable . . . let's face it, there are relatively few skilled cancer researchers, and it seemed stupid to take even the little risk."[28] As it turned out, in healthy test subjects cancer cells were destroyed in but a few days, although "in one normal recipient, a nodule was still growing and contained cancer cells 21 days after inoculation." In prisoners already suffering from another type of cancer, however, "rejection was delayed or did not occur at all during the period of observation . . . in one of these individuals there was metastasis from the inoculation site on the forearm to the axillary nodes."[29] When these experiments were disclosed at a meeting of the New York Academy of Medicine in 1958, Harry S. N. Greene, head of pathology at Yale University, pointed out that Southam had merely confirmed findings that already had been obtained through animal experiments and that "in working with human tumors it is not necessary to use man as an experimental animal." Greene called the use of human subjects a "sacrifice of human dignity." Southam replied thus: "The idea that the participation of volunteers in such work is offensive to their personal dignity is completely foreign to my own thinking. In fact I feel that such altruistic service to mankind is a convincing demonstration of the dignity of man." Southam insisted that prisoners volunteered for the most noble of reasons, their only reward being "the bolstering of their personal sense of dignity."[30] They were not "coming into it for money. Self-satisfaction was the reward . . . altruism was the reason they participated."[31]

Such self-serving responses to criticism or legal impediments to medical experimentation on humans were standard. When Iowa's attorney general ruled in 1967 that "it was not legal to use prison volunteers" in medical research, physicians in Iowa "sought and obtained . . . a specific law permitting the use of prisoners for medical research . . ." Their argument, offered repetitively, was that the "use of prison volunteers for medical research was justified and highly desirable for the investigator, for the subjects, and for society . . . It not only permits the conduct of human investigation under ideal circumstances, but it enables the participants to feel that they are serving a useful function, as indeed they are."[32]

The same arguments were advanced to overcome obstacles internationally. Apart from the United States, the use of prison volunteers for medical experiments was deemed acceptable only in Israel and the Netherlands.[33] A report in 1955 by the Public Health Council of the Netherlands did acknowledge, however, that consent of test subjects "should neither be conditioned by idealistic impulses (nurses and medical students); nor by special conditions (prisoners, etc.)," and stated, unambiguously, that experiments "on prisoners, which involve dangerous risks, inconvenience or pain are not approved."[34] Similar resolutions by international medical societies were frustrated effectively by American experimenters. When the World Medical Association proposed in 1961 that "persons retained in prisons, penitentiaries or reformatories, being captive groups, should not be used as the subjects of experiments," delegates from the United States prevented the adoption of a formal resolution to that effect.[35]

Hiding Behind Prison Walls

The resistance of American researchers to such a stricture was understandable in the context of their having so much to lose. Medical research in the United States depended to a large extent on the exploitation of prisoners as test subjects. According to an estimate in 1960 by R.C. Fox of Columbia University in New York City, as many as 20,000 inmates had participated in medical experiments in federal prisons alone.[36] An unlimited supply of test subjects was the most important advantage of using prisoners for medical research. The hope for a reduction of their sentence and offers of a few dollars almost always seduced "volunteers" enough for any study, no matter how bizarre it might be. Prison research also was cheap. Prisoners were paid much less for their participation in medical experiments than volunteers outside of prison; they could be used as technical assistants for free, and they lived, literally, right next door to the laboratory, thereby eliminating any expense for transportation. Another more insidious advantage for medical investigators was that the conditions of prisoners, that is, living under rigid control in a stark environment, minimized the risk of untoward external influences that might skew results. And, furthermore, there was almost absolute secrecy. The high prison walls prevented unwelcome public scrutiny of any medical research being conducted within their confines.

For many conducting such studies, prevention of scrutiny by the public was considered to be essential. For example, in 1963, renowned endocrinologist, Carl Heller (Fig. 438), proposed "to apply known amounts of ionizing radiation directly to the testes of normal men" for the purpose of studying the effects of

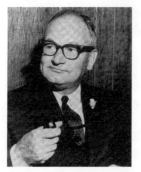

FIG. 438
Carl Heller

it on the secretion of hormones and on male reproductive function, the purpose being to allow him to determine the minimum amount of radiation that would cause "permanent damage" to sperm cells. The Atomic Energy Commission immediately cautioned that "... at some time some 'do-gooder' organization may suddenly realize that we are doing radiation experiments on prisoners and cause such a furor as to bring about a political decision to stop the work." Despite these worries, the Atomic Energy Commission funded Heller's study in which 67 inmates of the Oregon State Prison in Salem had their testicles bombarded with up to 600 rads of radiation, followed by a series of biopsies and a vasectomy at the conclusion of the experiment. A similar study was conducted by a student and colleague of Heller's, C. Alvin Paulsen, at the Washington State Prison in Walla Walla. Heller and Paulsen received hundreds of thousands of dollars for their experiments from the Atomic Energy Commission, being asked only to proceed cautiously and to "minimize publicity."[37]

Both experimenters and prison wardens took great pains to ensure that no information found its way to the outside. A prime example of this was a study by W.J.H. Butterfield, a research fellow at Medical College of Virginia in Richmond. Proposing to study "metabolic aspects of thermal injury" by inducing "16 small shallow burns" on the forearms of prisoners at Virginia State Penitentiary, Butterfield informed prison superintendent W.F. Smith that he faced "these trials with a completely clear conscience" and did not "fear any inquiry." Nevertheless, he advised that "the least said the better." The superintendent initiated appropriate measures, which he summarized in a letter to Butterfield as follows:

I have informed all the inmates and staff members that no publicity should be given to the experiments carried on . . . and the inmates should not have visitors, uncensored mail going in or coming out, and I do not think their name should appear on the daily roster of patients . . . by all means they should not have the privilege of the use of the telephone.[38]

Because of the isolation of the prisons, risks associated with medical experiments could be treated triflingly, and with little fear of consequences. If a prisoner became seriously ill or died in the course of an experiment, it was unlikely that it would ever come to anyone's attention. In the rare instance of an inquiry, medical records that might prove embarrassing conveniently disappeared. In addition, prison volunteers usually were required to sign a waiver releasing anyone and everyone from legal claims that might ensue. Although these waivers were fraudulent and not valid legally, they continued to be used for their effects psychologically. Having signed a waiver, a prisoner – inexperienced, helpless, and unaware of the legal worthlessness of the document – was unlikely in the extreme to bring a lawsuit against medical investigators.[39]

In brief, prisons were ideal sites for medical research and were employed for that purpose accordingly and increasingly. In 1953 the *Federal Prisons Year End Review* recorded a dizzying array of medical experiments in progress, describing in glowing terms their importance to mankind. Among these were malaria experiments on 400 convicts in Atlanta, Georgia, that supposedly contributed to "the discovery of primaquine and chloroquine as impressive agents" in combating the disease. The transmission of viral hepatitis to inmates of federal prisons in Ashland, Kentucky, McNeil Island, Washington, and Lewisburg, Pennsylvania, was claimed to demonstrate that "blood derivative plasma can carry the virus, but that the blood derivatives albumin and gamma globulin apparently do not." A large survey involving federal prisoners at Leavenworth,

Kansas, Atlanta, Georgia, and Terre Haute, Indiana, sought to determine the "relationship between the presence of certain chemical constituents in the blood and the development of heart disease." Transmission of human intestinal protozoan parasites to 175 prisoners at the federal prison in Seagoville, Texas, was responsible for causing diseases such as amebic dysentery, thereby demonstrating that "a very small number of eggs of the parasite . . . can produce infection."[40]

Representatives of all medical specialties in the United States were engaged in prison research. Oncologists injected prisoners with cancer cells and infused them with leukemic blood. Surgeons used prisoners for experimental procedures such as organ transplantations. Internists studied the blood circulation of internal organs by injecting contrast media following catheterization of major arteries.[39] Rheumatologists took "small pieces of muscle tissue and blood samples" for studies of arthritis.[42] Psychiatrists performed secret mind-control experiments for the CIA, subjecting scores of prisoners to lysergic acid diethylamide (LSD) and marijuana in order "to test the effectiveness of certain medications in causing individuals to release guarded information under interrogation."[43] Microbiologists, at different times and in different prisons, disregarded the possiblity of causing serious illness and death in hundreds of convicts when infecting them with "one of the most serious infectious diseases," infectious hepatitis. The defense of the investigators was that it is "necessary to use human volunteers" because "the forms of the virus that produce human hepatitis . . . have no effects on animals."[44]

Immunologists used prisoners as test subjects for new, unproven vaccines against a variety of potentially fatal infectious diseases. For example, a syphilis vaccine was tested in 1954 at New York's Sing Sing prison by inoculating 62 convicts with the spirochete, *Treponema pallidum*.[45] In 1955, the Federal Reformatory in Chillicothe, Ohio, hosted trials of a new vaccine against the common cold. At the same prison, virologist Albert B. Sabin (Fig. 439) studied his oral vaccine against poliomyelitis, which consisted of "highly attenuated strains of live polio virus" and which eventually superseded passive immunization against the disease.[46] In Petersburg, Virginia, John L. Sever of the National Institutes of Health tested vaccines on

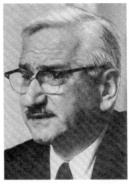

FIG. 439
Albert Bruce
Sabin
(1906-1993)

young prisoners who were willing to expose themselves to a "progressive, uniformly fatal disease which involves a chronic . . . measles infection of the central nervous system."[47] Thirty-one inmates of the Ohio State Penitentiary were put at risk of serious illness by participating in trials of a vaccine against tularemia conducted by the U.S. Army and the Ohio State University Research Foundation.[48] From 1956 to 1975, research concerning tularemia, Q fever, Rift Valley fever, and "other disease-producing agents" was conducted on prisoners at the Maryland House of Corrections by physicians of the University of Maryland under contract with the U.S. Army.[49, 50]

In the first years after the Second World War, dermatologists participated little in the efflorescence of medical experimentation in the United States. In 1950, Donald M. Pillsbury, chairman of the department of dermatology at the University of Pennsylvania School of Medicine, said deploringly that ". . . the skin is the most neglected organ of the human body in terms of lack of support of fundamental studies of it."[51] Although the Society for Investigative Dermatology had been founded in 1937 and launched its *Journal* in 1938 in order to "demonstrate the fact that dermatology has emerged from a state of purely morphologic, static and dead description and classification" to become "a living, integral part of modern medicine,"[52] basic research in the specialty continued to be paltry. Moreover, most experiments on skin diseases were unspectacular. As one example of what seemed banal, a study in 1953 of athlete's foot in Atlanta prisoners revealed "no significant decrease in the incidence of athlete's foot from the use of specially treated shower mats," whereas "treating shoes with formaldehyde fumes" was found to be "an effective procedure."[53] Contrast that result with such breathtaking advances in other fields of medicine, such as the first successful kidney transplant in 1950; the introduction of scintigraphy of the thyroid gland in 1951; the implantation of the first artificial lenses in eyes in 1952; and the first successful use of drugs in the chemotherapy of cancer in 1953. As a consequence of relative absence of basic science research, the profile of dermatology among the specialties of medicine was woefully low. Dermatologists were referred to as "pimple squeezers."[54] In regard to their patients, it was said they "never cure them and never kill them." The practice of dermatology was captured by the maxim, "if it's wet you dry it and if it's dry you wet it!" Because dermatology in the United States was held in such low esteem by both the rest of the profession and the laity, graduates of an American medical school tended not to choose it as a specialty if they had the opportunity to work in a more respected field of medicine. In the ensuing decades, however, the situation would change – and dramatically. One reason for this was the ever increasing effort of dermatologists to participate in experimental research.

"Rules Don't Apply to Genius": Albert Kligman

One of the most important catalyzers of that development was Albert Montgomery Kligman, professor of dermatology at the University of Pennsylvania School of Medicine (Fig. 440). The reasons for Kligman's powerful influence on the maturation of postwar dermatology were manifold. First, he was a fascinating personality, described by contemporaries as "a showman and

entertainer," "a real enigma," "an effer-
vescent man who seems to radiate energy, bombastic opinions, and good
humor," and "a professor who had more
flavor than anyone else in dermatology,
boundless energy, originality, and irreverence." Second, he was a "great teacher"
and "stellar lecturer" who was "very good
at motivating and challenging" his

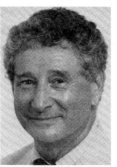

trainees. Third, he was generous to his students, investing his
time and energy in them, making them senior author of scientific articles, the idea for which was his and the work of which
emanated from his laboratory, and trying to further their careers. Many of Kligman's students eventually became chairmen
of university departments of dermatology, both in the United
States and abroad. Among these were John S. Strauss of the
University of Iowa, William L. Epstein of the University of California in San Francisco, Enno Christophers of the University of
Kiel, and Gerd Plewig of the University of Düsseldorf and later
of Munich. Fourth, Kligman had a "facile brain" that was "exploding with ideas." He was thought to be among the few in the
field "who is really creative and original." Last, Kligman seized
any opportunity to bring his ideas to fruition, unconstrained as
he was by scruples, rules, and reservations. As Kligman told his
students, "Rules don't apply to genius; they just get in the way
of creative minds."[55, 56]

The permissiveness generally and utilitarianism ethically of
the postwar period conditioned Kligman's attitude and reflected it. At this same time, young dermatologists, including those
in training, were encouraged by their mentors and peers to
make use of the vast opportunities for experimental research in
penitentiaries. In 1952, Frederick DeForest Weidman (Fig.
441), highly respected professor emeritus of research in dermatology and mycology at the University of Pennsylvania and for-

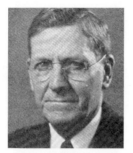

mer president of the prestigious American Dermatological Association (ADA), wrote these lines in the *Journal of Investigative Dermatology*: "We have not been alive enough to the wealth of test material that there is in penitentiaries, and the administrative officers are glad to have doctors work in their institutions. It indicates that special attention is being paid to the welfare of their charges and the inmates really enjoy it."[57]

In 1951, Albert Kligman began a long, industrious, and highly profitable career in prison research after he was called to Holmesburg Prison, just outside of Philadelphia, to treat an outbreak of athlete's foot there (Fig. 442). In an interview in 1966, he recalled that he was amazed on his arrival by what he perceived to be "an anthropoid colony, mainly healthy, under perfect control conditions. All I saw before me were acres of skin. It was like a farmer seeing a fertile field for the first time."[58] The "farmer" soon began to sow seeds for experiments. He met with the top administrator of Holmesburg Prison, Superintendent Frederick S. Baldi, who was a physician himself and,

FIG. 442
*Holmesburg
Prison,
Pennsylvania.*

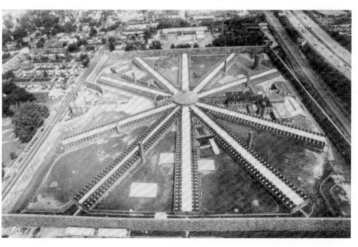

therefore, favorably disposed to Kligman's request to use prisoners for a series of dermatologic experiments. The scope of the experiments soon expanded, a large research unit was created within the prison, and Kligman kept commuting, at least once weekly and episodically several times each week, between the prison and his base at the University of Pennsylvania. He did that for nearly 25 years.

The spectrum of experiments conducted at Holmesburg Prison was extremely broad, ranging from studies on the skin – the anatomy and physiology of normal skin; experimental induction of allergies and acne; effects of x-rays and ultraviolet light; and inoculation with a wide variety of bacteria, fungi, and viruses – to studies on the brain, using a host of psychoactive and hallucinogenic drugs. Among the inoculation experiments were attempts in 1957 by John S. Strauss and Kligman to produce *tinea pedis* and onychomycosis by application of concentrated suspensions of spores of *Trichophyton rubrum*. The impetus of the study was to "gain some fresh appreciation of this disease by studying it experimentally in a prison population. With this group it was possible to do a number of things which would otherwise have been rather difficult. Rigid control over the subjects . . . offered many experimental advantages."[59]

One year later, Kligman and Herbert Goldschmidt (Fig. 443), another professor of dermatology at the University of Pennsylvania, reported on the "experimental inoculation of humans with ectodermotropic viruses." Following dermabrasion or induction of blisters through the application of cantharidin, they performed hundreds of inoculations with matter from *mollusca contagiosa, verrucae vulgares, condylomata acuminata,* and from lesions of herpes simplex, zoster, and vaccinia. The authors em-

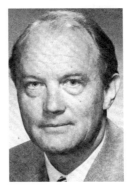

FIG. 443
Herbert
Goldschmidt
(born 1923)

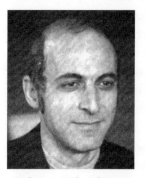

FIG. 444
Howard I.
Maibach (born
1929)

phasized that "students of human infectious diseases have a much greater opportunity to gain an understanding of pathogenesis when the disease can be experimentally produced in man at will."[60]

In 1962, Howard I. Maibach (Fig. 444), while a resident in dermatology at the University of Pennsylvania and working with Kligman at Holmesburg Prison, tried with his mentor to enhance the understanding of pathogenesis of candidal infections by "applying a dense suspension of organisms to the normal skin and covering the site with some form of bandage." On the basis of "about 1,000 inoculations in approximately 150 white and Negro subjects," they followed the course of clinical signs of the infection, starting "with tiny, discrete papules" and "closely spaced small tense pustules" and eventually ending up with "a shallow, continuous lake of pus . . . on a vividly erythematous background." At that stage, "subjects complain bitterly of pain and burning." The further course was characterized by "a violent, inflammatory, exuding, red, swollen dermatitis, accompanied by painful and often incapacitating lymphangitis and regional adenopathy. The subject may be sick and considerably discomforted"[61] (Fig. 445, 446).

From 1959 to 1963, Maibach and Kligman conducted numerous inoculation experiments with cultures of staphylococci. Despite "fear of producing septicemia or generalized furunculosis" in their subjects, more than 1,000 inoculations were performed under a variety of experimental circumstances. For example, prior to inoculation, the test area might be occluded with an adhesive tape or the skin exposed to ultraviolet light, hairs plucked, or the epidermis removed with a scalpel. In many instances, Maibach and Kligman succeeded in producing impetigo, giving them "the opportunity to examine approximately

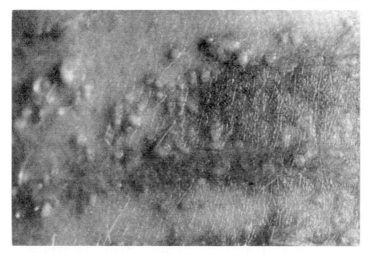

FIG. 445
Pustules that extend beyond the site of inoculation of suspensions of Candida albicans (from the article by Maibach and Kligman).

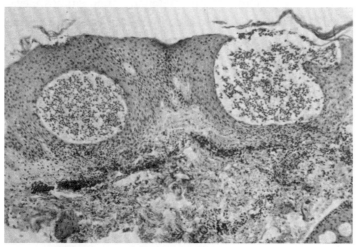

FIG. 446
Intraepithelial pustules following inoculation of suspensions of Candida albicans. (from the article by Maibach and Kligman).

thirty biopsies" of that disease. Following "intradermal injections of staphylococci on his anterior thighs," one test subject developed "marked swelling and local tenderness" as well as fever, for which "blood disseminated organisms must have been responsible."[62] After leaving the University of Pennsylvania, Maibach went on to become a professor of dermatology at the University of California in San Francisco.

A few years later, Kligman resumed the study of "experimental *Staphylococcus aureus* infections in humans" with two dermatologist colleagues, Gurmohan Singh and Richard R. Marples, research trainees of Kligman from abroad. The authors proclaimed that "to induce an infection at will provides an opportunity to study pathogenesis." The two pathogenetic factors essential to enhancing susceptibility to infection were found to be "hydrating the horny layer by sealing the site occlusively" and "elimination of bacterial competitors during the initial phase." With these conditions fulfilled, staphylococci were noted to proliferate rapidly, and in three of 150 prisoners "hot, tender, furunculoid nodules appeared around the infection site a few days after removing the dressings. Two of these had lymphangitis, axillary adenopathy, and modest temperature elevations." Readers were assured that "the discomfort caused by the lesions was cheerfully borne by the volunteers."[63] All inoculation studies were monitored by biopsies of the skin lesions in order to enable the infections to be studied histopathologically.

Biopsies also were performed liberally in other studies. For example, in 1957, Kligman and Walter B. Shelley, then a junior

FIG. 447
"Clinical examples of experimental chloracne" (*from the article by Shelley and Kligman*).

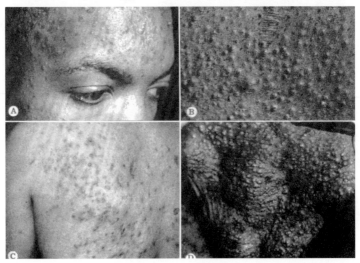

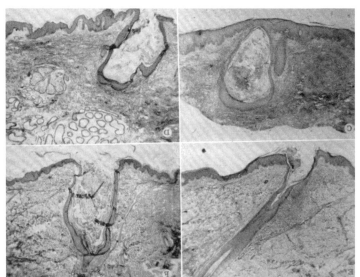

FIG. 448
"*Comparative regional histology of noninflammatory chloracne*" (*from the article by Shelley and Kligman*).

faculty member in the department of dermatology at the University of Pennsylvania, biopsied prisoners following experimental induction of acne through topical administration of penta- and hexachloronaphthalenes.[64] (Fig. 447, 448) Almost 20 years later, Kligman worked with another young dermatologist at the University of Pennsylvania, Kays H. Kaidbey, who performed serial biopsies in prisoners in whom acne had been produced by application of various tars.[65] Strauss and Kligman studied formation of scars after dermabrasion in selected test subjects who had a history of hypertrophic scars and keloids, and found that "hypertrophic scars may definitely follow dermabrasion in predisposed subjects."[66] With Christopher M. Papa, Kligman created an "extremely inflammatory" contact dermatitis by lengthy exposure of the hands and forearms of prisoners to sodium lauryl sulfate, a highly irritating substance, and performed biopsies to assess "the behavior of melanocytes in inflammation."[67] Biopsies also were taken to determine by examination histopathologically the effects of therapeutic compounds, such as the effect of application of aluminum salts on "mechanisms of eccrine anhidrosis"[68] and the "effects of intensive application of retinoic acid on human skin."[69]

Kligman took pride in asking unconventional questions and answering them in ways that were equally unconventional. He asserted that "to raise questions where none existed before, to make mysteries of the obvious . . . is one of the privileges of the scientific outlook." Among those "mysteries of the obvious" was the question, "why do nails grow out instead of up?" In order to resolve that mystery, ". . . 5 mm punch biopsy specimens were removed from the thumb-nail matrices of 2 adult subjects and autografted to the forearm . . ." Kligman acknowledged that this experiment resulted in "slight permanent damage to the nail organ." Once cells of the protective cover of the posterior nail fold had been removed, the matrix produced a cylinder of hard keratin that grew up instead of out.[70]

In the mid 1950s, William L. Epstein and Kligman were curious about what would happen if "elliptical biopsy specimens extending into the subcutis were removed from various parts of the body and were buried completely at some other site."[71] They found that "if the buried autotransplant survived nine months or more, it gradually recovered its normal histologic structure . . . The result was a dermoid-like cyst with functioning hair follicles and sebaceous glands"[72] (Fig. 449). Another study carried out at the same time by Epstein and Kligman concerned the

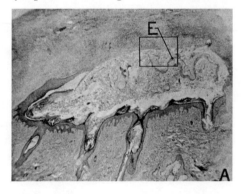

FIG. 449
"Cyst formation seven weeks after burial of scalp skin in the scalp"
(from the article by Epstein and Kligman).

"transfer of allergic contact-type delayed sensitivity in man." In this case, one group of test subjects was "deliberately sensitized" to potent allergens. Then leukocyte suspensions were produced from fluid of artificially produced blisters and from the blood of test subjects. These suspensions were "injected deep intradermally into several sites of the same recipient." All recipients "were Negro males between the ages of 20 and 45 years," none of whom had a history of allergy; "frequently, two or three donors supplied transfer material for the same recipient." When sufficient numbers of leukocytes were used, "transfer resulted in a generalized state of sensitivity."[73] The risk of transferring an unknown infectious disease from donors to test subjects was not a consideration.

Over the course of a quarter of a century, many hundreds, perhaps thousands, of inmates of Holmesburg Prison were sensitized to allergens in a host of experiments. In 1966, for example, Kligman described a method for enhancing sensitization by pretreatment of the exposure sites with sodium lauryl sulfate. A "sequence of alternating 24 hour irritant and 48 hour allergen patches for a total of five exposures of each" was found to be effective in demonstrating "whether specified substances have allergic potentialities and to what degree." Kligman referred to this procedure as the "maximization test," and emphasized that "institutional volunteers are ideal since strict controls can be exerted. Our experimental population was made up of prisoners exclusively. It is not practical to work with children or infants." His reasoning was that "certain discomforts" associated with the test might not be handled well by children. Among the "hazards of maximization testing" were "tachycardia, headache, nausea, vertigo, and altered emotions," as actually developed in some test subjects. According to Kligman, the vast majority of prisoners had "no serious systemic or cutaneous effects . . . even though it was not exceptional for a subject to acquire three or four independent sensitizations."[74]

The induction of allergic contact dermatitis in human test subjects was the starting point of a potpourri of studies by Kligman. In 1955, he and Thomas Kemp reported on "the effect of x-rays on experimentally produced acute contact dermatitis."[75] In 1969, Isaac Willis, then a resident in dermatology at the University of Pennsylvania, along with Kligman, described "photocontact allergic reactions" of "healthy adult male prisoners" who had been presensitized with potent photoallergens. Test subjects were studied "with regard to the quantity of long ultraviolet rays (UV) necessary to elicit reactions."[76] At the same time, Kligman and his pupil from Germany, Reinhard Breit

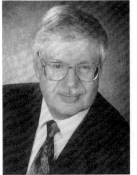

FIG. 450
Reinhard Breit
(born 1936)

(Fig. 450), studied "the identification of phototoxic drugs by human assay." Following oral intake, intradermal injection, or topical application of phototoxic drugs, test areas on the backs of "white, adult prisoner-volunteers" were irradiated with various light sources and intensities, and the resulting inflammatory lesions were studied histopathologically. Kligman and Breit concluded that "these studies indicate the feasibility of using locally treated and irradiated skin as a screening technique for identifying phototoxic agents."[77]

In short, the experiments conducted at Holmesburg Prison were vast both in number and variety. Some were relatively harmless, whereas others were associated with considerable discomfort and, more important, risk of long-term morbidity or even death. It is difficult to estimate how many prisoners were put at serious risk and were seriously harmed because severe complications were concealed and all experimental data were destroyed by Kligman, in highly unscientific fashion, shortly after the research program at the prison was closed down in 1974.[78] As hyposensitization of researchers to the implications of their experiments progressed steadily, even moderately severe side effects of experiments no longer were recorded in scientific publications. For example, when the candidiasis study of Maibach and Kligman, published originally 1962, was repeated and elaborated on 11 years later by Alfredo Rebora, Richard R. Marples, and Kligman, no mention was made of the distress suffered by test subjects.[79] At the same time, the tendency of researchers to flaunt the fact that their experiments had been conducted in a population of prisoners also waned.

In general, prisoners were unaware of possible consequences of the experiments. Although required to sign a waiver releasing Kligman, his coworkers, and prison administrators from responsibility, they were not fully and accurately informed about the nature of the experiments. Most inmates were poorly educated; many could not even read. Later, when the truth began to emerge, the majority of prisoners claimed that they had never heard the words "informed consent,"[80] that they "were never told what was going on," and that they "never had witnesses or a receipt for anything signed."[81] As Kligman's student, Gerd Plewig, later to become chairman of dermatology at the University of Munich, recalled, "during these days uninformed patients were the rule."[82] Kligman himself commented, "We predetermine whether a test is dangerous, and the prisoner has to depend on our judgment."[83]

Experiments also were highly variable in the quality of them scientifically. Although some of them produced data that proved to have value, the vast majority of experiments performed at Holmesburg prison were of questionable scientific worth and the results of many of them were plain wrong. Among these was a study published in 1965 by Papa and Kligman titled, "Stimulation of hair growth by topical application of androgens." The authors claimed that "forty-one institutionalized men with complete frontocentral denudation" had shown "indisputable hair growth" following topical treatment with testosterone.[84] Naturally, the report created great public interest and a feverish clamor by bald and balding men to obtain even ounces of the substance for application to their pelage-poor pates. The data, however, had no validity whatsoever, and many years later Kligman explained, "The prisoners insisted that it grew hair, and I was taken in by their enthusiasm."[85] So much for critical, scientific analysis.

It was not uncommon for Kligman to jump to conclusions without devoting himself to painstaking accumulation of data.[86] Misquoting the father of experimental physiology in France, Claude Bernard, Kligman claimed that the only reason he did the experiments was to please the critics; he already knew the answer ahead of time.[87] If preliminary results supported his expectations, Kligman often stopped experiments well ahead of schedule, assuming an outcome that had not yet been proved, and then proceeded to publish, prematurely, results that often were inaccurate. Accordingly, coworkers criticized his lax methodology and concluded that, despite the firework of ideas, Kligman was "not a good researcher in a pure sense."[88] Even studies without scientific merit, however, did not damage Kligman's reputation as a dermatologic scientist of first rank; the results of these studies were lost in the mountainous verbiage of all the others, and Kligman came to be viewed universally by his colleagues as "one of the greatest of our specialty."[89]

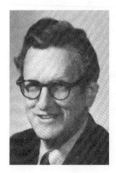

FIG. 451
Walter B.
Shelley (born
1917)

Dermatologic Research at Prisons Throughout the United States

Kligman was not the only dermatologist who utilized the prison as a test site. Independent of Kligman, his contemporary and colleague at the University of Pennsylvania, Walter B. Shelley (Fig. 451), conducted scores of experiments on prisoners. Like

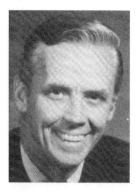

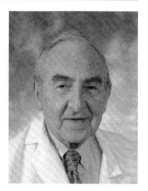

Kligman, Shelley insisted that "the experimental production of disease often permits a clearer view of etiologic factors than can be obtained in regular clinical study."[90] In translating that philosophy into action, he focused mainly on diseases of cutaneous adnexal structures, such as the experimental induction of "apocrine sweat retention in man"[91] and "experimental miliaria in man."[92] With another colleague at the University of Pennsylvania, Harry J. Hurley (Fig. 452), Shelley assessed the effects of testosterone and estrogen on apocrine glands by examining sections of "generous scalpel biopsies" taken from the axillae of "twenty-seven normal healthy adult volunteers" following "long-term subcutaneous implantation of hormone pellets."[93] With his trainee, Milton M. Cahn (Fig. 453), Shelley described "a technique for experimentally producing hidradenitis suppurativa in man." For this study, "the axillae of 12 normal male adult subjects between the ages of 20 and 40 were used as test sites. A perforated belladonna adhesive tape was applied to one axilla, which had been manually epilated. The other axilla served as the control site. One week later, biopsy specimens were secured from each axilla." What came into being were "severe inflammatory changes" that presented themselves clinically as "exquisitely tender deep nodules" in the treated axilla.[94] A similar procedure was used in a study concerning "the experimental production of external otitis in man." The external ear canals of "79 normal adult male volunteers" were either plugged with a rubber or a plastic ear plug or with adhesive tape, or they were treated with chemicals such as a 4 percent solution of formalin. Biopsies from the external ear canal were taken after periods of a few days to several weeks and sections of tissue from the harvested specimens revealed follicular keratoses in association with inflammatory cells around and within the hair follicles.[95]

In the mid 1950s, Cahn established his own research laboratory at Holmesburg Prison. Because Kligman's presence there was so dominant, he later was compelled to transfer his lab to nearby prisons in Bucks and Lancaster counties in Pennsylvania.[96] The spectrum of experiments on prisoners conducted by Cahn ranged from determination of "the effect of a surfactant and of particle size on griseofulvin plasma levels"[97] to the assessment of "normal skin reactions to ultraviolet light." For the latter study, 30 "normal healthy white males," who had been given either placebos or the potent photosensitizer, methoxsalen, were irradiated with ultraviolet light and the skin of them subjected subsequently to biopsy. Cahn noted that "there were no consistent histologic differences in the skin of subjects taking methoxsalen versus placebo, either in sunburned or in pigmented areas."[98]

A similar study was conducted by Thomas B. Fitzpatrick

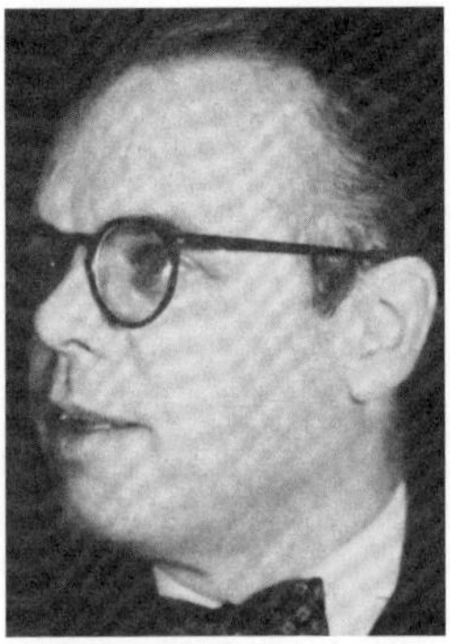

FIG. 454
*Thomas B.
Fitzpatrick
(born 1919)*

(Fig. 454), who later became chairman of dermatology at Harvard University Medical School. With his colleagues, J. Donald Imbrie and Lester L. Bergeron, Fitzpatrick exposed inmates of the Oregon State Prison to ultraviolet light to assess the "erythemal threshold following oral methoxsalen."[99] Robert G. Freeman, a dermatopathologist at the Baylor College of Medicine in Houston,

Texas (Fig. 455), with his colleague, John M. Knox (Fig. 456) and two other coworkers, studied "sunlight as a factor influencing the thickness of epidermis." For that purpose, inmates of the Texas State Department of Correction at Huntsville were subjected to skin biopsies "from three areas which could be reasonably assumed to have received varying amounts of sunlight exposure."[100] Knox also took part in other experiments on humans, such as the "production of infections in humans" by placing cultures of *Staphylococcus aureus, Streptococcus pyogenes, Pseudomonas aeruginosa,* and Corynebacteria on the skin of healthy males and providing the bacteria "with protection plus supplemental nutrients."[101] Israel Zeligman, of Johns Hopkins University School of Medicine in Baltimore (Fig. 457), recruited inmates of the Maryland State Reformatory for Women as test subjects for his studies of the "experimental production of acne by progesterone" by assessment histopathologically of sections of tissue from biopsy specimens taken before and after injections of the hormone.[102]

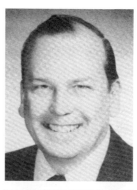

FIG. 455
Robert G.
Freeman
(born 1927)

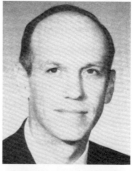

FIG. 456
John M. Knox
(1925-1987)

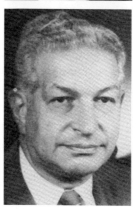

FIG. 457
Israel
Zeligman
(1913-1990)

John Strauss, in collaboration with Peter E. Pochi of Boston University, used inmates of the Massachusetts Correctional Institutions at Walpole and Framingham to study responses of sebaceous glands to a variety of factors, including antibacterial agents,[103] estrogens,[104] and prednisone.[105] In one instance, a highly potent derivative of the female sex hormone, ethinylestradiol, was given to male prisoners for several weeks in order to study its suppressive effect on sebaceous glands. Indeed, "the glands became extremely atrophic." Nevertheless, the authors concluded that female sex hormones play no significant role in the physiology of sebaceous glands because "extremely high unphysiologic amounts of estrogen are necessary to cause the glands to revert to the prepubertal rudimentary state." The authors did note that ". . . the characteristic systemic effects of estrogen were displayed in every subject" who participated in their study.[106]

Among his experiments on inmates of San Quentin Prison, William Epstein attempted "to sensitize previously non-reactive normal human volunteers" to nickel, one of the most ubiquitous of allergens and a common source of severe, incessant allergic contact dermatitis.[107] Other prisoners were injected with zirconium so that the evolution of the resultant granulomatous dermatitis could be studied by examination histopathologically of biopsy sections taken "at intervals ranging from one hour to 8 months after the exposure."[108] A similar experiment had been conducted previously by Shelley and Hurley.[109] For a study about the "mitotic activity of wounded human epidermis," Dennis J. Sullivan and Epstein used a razor blade to produce "seventeen to twenty-five wounds" on the legs of prisoners. From each of these superficial cuts, "biopsy specimens were obtained at precisely six hour intervals" and were studied in regard to the number of mitotic figures found.[110] Epstein and Howard Maibach created research facilities at a prison in Vacaville, California, where they performed many experiments on humans, ranging from devising methods of "poison oak hyposensitization"[111] to the inoculation of pathogenic microorganisms[112] and development of techniques of "screening for drug toxicity" secondary to ultraviolet light.[113] As highly regarded professors, these former trainees of Kligman had students of their own who now learned from their example.

In summary, American dermatology underwent profound transformation during the postwar years. In an effort to keep pace with other specialties of medicine, dermatologists embarked frenetically on basic research in which human experimentation was an integral part. Human skin was appreciated as an organ particularly suitable for scientific study. Walter Shelley described skin for that purpose, vividly, as:

... an incomparable laboratory in which to do experimental work. It is open twenty-four hours a day, seven days a week and provides unlimited bench space. It comes complete with skilled technicians who work constantly, never take vacations or resign. It has servo-controls for temperature, pH, osmotic pressure, chemical composition and a host of unnoticed variables. And it allows the investigator to secure data that will have relevance to clinical disease.[114]

Nowhere in the Western world was it easier to conduct experiments on human beings than in the United States, where prisons were the principal sites for such tests. The promise of an inexhaustible supply of captive human guinea pigs was too tempting for American medical scientists to forsake because of ethical considerations. The exploitation of the skin of prisoners as an "incomparable biology laboratory" enabled dermatology to change its image from that of a relatively unimportant primitive backwater to one of a discipline that was scientifically significant and even avant-garde, and it permitted American dermatologists to present themselves as leaders internationally of that emerging, dynamic field.

CHAPTER 21

THE MENTAL INSTITUTION AS TEST SITE

I t was the abundance of test subjects who were available for long periods of time, lived under close supervision, and could be exploited easily that made prisons so attractive to medical research. These characteristics, however, were not specific for prisons; they were shared equally by other institutions.

The Military in Medical Research

Among the institutions that had attributes in common with prisons was the military. Threatened with court-martial, soldiers could not be disdainful of orders to engage in risky endeavors, and, more than that, disregard them, even outside a combat situation. Between 1951 and 1962, for example, more than 200,000 enlisted men were exposed to radiation during atmospheric tests of atomic bombs in Nevada. In order to simulate battle conditions, many troops were stationed less than a mile from the sites where bombs exploded.[1] Some soldiers, were exposed deliberately in studies aimed at measuring radioisotopes in body fluids or at finding effective methods for decontamination after exposure.[2] In "flash-blindness experiments," soldiers were required to look at an exploding bomb so researchers

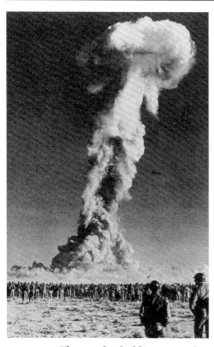

FIG. 458 *Thousands of soldiers exposed to radiation from "Shot Dog," an atomic bomb detonated on November 1, 1951, at the Nevada Test Site.*

could "determine accurately what temporary or permanent effect the flash of an atomic explosion has on the human eye."[3] The experiments on flash-blindness resulted in retinal burns and permanent impairment of vision in some men, and exposure to radiation presumably contributed to a large number of malignancies that developed in these soldiers decades later (Fig. 458).

Experiments on soldiers were numerous and varied. For the study of skin diseases relevant to the military, the Surgeon General of the United States, in 1964, established a dermatologic research program at the Presidio Army base in San Francisco. Among the diseases studied there was *miliaria rubra*, a disorder of sweat ducts induced by the effects of heat and humidity, that had impacted greatly on American forces in Vietnam.[4] In 1967, Tommy B. Griffin, later of the University of North Carolina, Howard Maibach of the University of California in San Francisco, and Marion Baldur Sulzberger (Fig. 459), chairman emeritus of New York University's Skin and Cancer Unit, published the results of a study in which they examined "the relationships between miliaria and anhidrosis in man" by producing miliaria ("heat rash") experimentally in "fifty-one

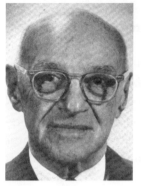

FIG. 459
Marion Bal-
dur Sulzberger
(1895-1983)

apparently healthy Caucasian soldiers on active duty." They applied, for 48 hours, "a double thickness of occlusive plastic wrapping" to "one-half of the entire torso," which was followed by exposure of subjects "to a heat stress of 120ºF and 40 percent relative humidity." Biopsies were taken of the skin lesions so induced and "serial section examination of representative biopsies" was undertaken by a histopathologist.[5] In subsequent experiments, even larger areas of the body were wrapped in plastic. The investigators learned that test subjects suffered from decreased sweating for up to three weeks after all visible signs of miliaria had disappeared. Because the decreased ability to sweat was found to impair the performance physically of test subjects, the conclusion was drawn that *miliaria rubra* could "seriously affect a soldier's ability to perform his duties . . . in hot environments."[6] Another study by Sulzberger, in conjunction with Thomas A. Cortese and W. Mitchell Sams, Jr. (Fig. 460), both of whom were dermatologists newly minted after completing residency training and at that time serving compulsorily in the military, concerned "blisters produced by friction" in "fifty-eight

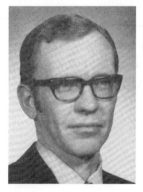

FIG. 460
W. Mitchell
Sams, Jr.
(born 1933)

healthy male volunteers on active military duty." It consisted of examination chemically of fluids aspirated from blisters that had been produced by twisting a pencil eraser, back and forth many times, on the palm of volunteers.[7] Blisters also were brought into being artificially by exposing soldiers to a "linear rubbing machine" that had been designed specifically to induce formation of "friction blisters."[8]

In general, studies concerning skin diseases were relatively harmless. In contrast, some other studies in soldiers were dangerous. Such were a number of experiments with incapacitating substances, like "nerve agents, nerve agent antidotes, psychoactive chemicals, irritants, and vesicant agents."[9] These, unlike an eraser twisted on a palm, twisted the brain, causing permanent emotional, as well as physical damage. In most instances, soldiers "volunteered" for these experiments, but the coercive nature of order and obedience inherent in the military did violence to the concept of true consent. Refusal to volunteer for experiments was perceived by many soldiers as verging on insubordination at best and cowardice at worst.[10] Another coercive factor was the offer of incentives such as extra days off duty. The information provided to the volunteers about risks and inconveniences associated with experiments often was incomplete and even deceptive.

One dupe was James B. Stanley, master sergeant in the U.S. Army, who volunteered in 1958 to be a subject in a study advertised as developing and testing measures for defense against chemical weapons. Stanley became one of thousands of men to be transferred to the Aberdeen, Maryland Proving Grounds for experiments with LSD [lysergic acid diethylamide]. He never was told that he was being given a psychoactive drug. Emotional problems that followed the experiments disrupted his personal life and, in his judgment, contributed to his divorce in 1970, one year after he was discharged from the Army. After learning the truth of the matter in 1975, Stanley filed a suit against the U.S. government that went all the way to the Supreme Court, where it was dismissed in 1987. By a vote of 5 to 4, the justices found that Stanley, like all other former or current members of the Armed Forces, was barred from suing the United States for injuries incurred "incident to service."[11]

Testing in Orphans and the Aged

The advantages of having test subjects living in a controlled environment and exploited easily obtained, too, in homes for the aged and in orphanages. For example, in their study on hair growth in 1965, the results of which proved to be fallacious, Christopher Papa and Albert Kligman recruited not only prisoners as test subjects, but also inmates of the Riverview Home for the Aged in Philadelphia. Papa, then a resident in dermatology at the University of Pennsylvania, served conveniently as medical director at Riverview.[12] Three years later, residents of the same institution were recruited for "an attempt to produce elastosis in aged human skin by means of ultraviolet irradiation." Four different types of UV radiation, combined in part with topical compounds that caused "non specific inflammation" or "an intense phototoxic reaction," were administered to zones on the lower part of the back of the elderly test subjects either daily or every other day for six to twelve months, at the end of which time specimens from "punch biopsies (8 mm) were removed from each of the four sites as well as from an unexposed control area."[13] Yet another experiment on residents of the Riverview Home involved "the effect of autotransplantation on the progression or reversibility of aging in human skin." In that study, "split thickness, 4 cm² sections of skin were reciprocally transplanted from the extensor forearm and abdomen of 18 aged subjects." The coworkers concluded that "the microscopic structural and histochemical hallmarks of the epidermis and dermis . . . convincingly demonstrate that the transplanted skin is not altered by the new dermal milieu onto which it is grafted."[14]

In the 1950s, children in orphanages were used commonly as test subjects; for example, they were given potentially harmful doses of drugs to determine whether such doses were toxic.[15] At that time it was deemed perfectly appropriate to test newly developed vaccines on institutionalized children, especially if the children were retarded mentally.[16] The first provision of the Nuremberg Code – that "the voluntary consent of the human subject is absolutely essential" – played no role at all in the thinking of physicians engaged in such projects. If that code had been observed strictly, any experiment in children and in persons who were incompetent mentally would have been unthinkable. Legally, the right of parents to give consent to actions that were not for the immediate benefit of their child was dubious in itself. Nevertheless, most American physicians subscribed to the position of Andrew Ivy, who, in 1948, wrote that "The ethical principles involved in the use of the mentally incompetent are the same as for mentally competent persons. The only difference involves the matter of consent. Since mental cases are likened to children in an ethical and legal sense, the consent of the guardian is required."[17]

Used Without Being Asked

The main argument in favor of consent by proxy for experiments on children and mentally incompetent persons was the suggestion that stringent adherence to the related clause of the Nuremberg Code was in itself unethical. A total ban on medical experiments on subjects who were incompetent, researchers argued, would have severe adverse effects on the quality of medical care for them. These considerations had prompted Leo Alexander, one of the chief authors of the Nuremberg Code, to propose a special clause in regard to consent for mentally ill patients. In his draft submitted to the Nuremberg tribunal in April 1947, Alexander specified that "In the case of mentally ill patients, for the purpose of experiments concerning the nature and treatment of nervous and mental illness, or related subjects, such consent of the next of kin or legal guardian is required."[18] That provision, however, was deleted by the judges at the Nuremberg Doctors' Trial because they thought it was too permissive. In postwar America, it was ignored by physicians, but because it was too prohibitive! Mentally incompetent persons were considered to be too valuable as test subjects to restrict their use to special arenas of research. Eventually, scores of medical experiments that had nothing to do with "the nature and treatment of nervous and mental illness, or related subjects," were performed on the mentally ill.

Although medical research on incompetent persons was accepted in principal by the vast majority of physicians, concern in regard to the welfare of incompetent test subjects actually was voiced by a few and resistance by them contributed to the establishment of legislation in some states. In Virginia, for example, "legally authorized representatives" of incompetent persons were denied the right to consent to nontherapeutic research associated with a "hazardous risk" to the subject.[19] Some authors called for the prohibition of "all procedures, whether therapeutic in intent or not, which are not designed with the sole intention of improving the lot of the individual upon whom they are performed." They insisted further that "No child must ever be the subject of such an experiment."[20] In California, informed consent given on behalf of an incompetent person was accepted only "for medical experiments related to maintaining or improving the health of the test subject or related to obtaining information about a pathological condition of the human subject."[21] In actuality, many experiments performed on incompetent subjects were unrelated completely to their health and many of them caused major distress and hazards long term.

In the almost total absence of public scrutiny, mental institutions became ideal test sites for those physicians with a blind eye to ethical considerations. Almost anything could be done with the inmates, especially if they were children. As Maurice Pappworth reasoned with biting sarcasm in 1967, "if the test subject of an experiment is incapable of giving or withholding a true consent . . . then he is a very easy subject to get hold of. If it is no use asking for his consent, then he can be used without being asked."[22] Consent of legal guardians usually was obtained with ease, especially if they were not the parents of the subject. The information given to guardians about experiments on those for whom they were responsible often was deceptive. Moreover, guardians were under pressure, knowing that participation of their charges in these experiments was the only way to get those youngsters into certain oversubscribed institutions.[23] In brief, obtaining consent rarely was a problem.

Deviants from God's Great Concept of Man

Another reason researchers resorted to mentally incompetent subjects was that they were not deemed to be full-fledged human beings, but rather to be inferior, deviants from God's great concept of man. The first laws allowing for compulsory sterilization of mentally incompetent persons were not enacted in Nazi Germany, but in the United States. When the Nazis

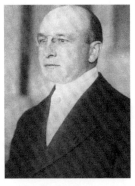

FIG. 461
Alexis Carrel
(1873-1944)

began their "euthanasia" program in 1939, eventually killing more than 70,000 mentally disabled persons, that measure was received sympathetically by many Americans, physicians among them. For example, Nobel laureate Alexis Carrel of the Rockefeller Institute for Medical Research in New York City (Fig. 461) wrote about the matter in 1939 thus:

We have already referred to the vast sums at present spent upon the maintenance of prisons and lunatic asylums in order to protect the public from anti-social and insane persons. Why do we keep all these useless and dangerous creatures alive? . . . In Germany the Government has taken energetic measures against the multiplication of inferior types, the insane and criminals. The ideal solution would be to eliminate all such individuals as soon as they proved dangerous . . . Philosophic theory and sentimental prejudice are not entitled to a hearing in such a matter.[24]

To be sure, only a few of those who experimented in the postwar period with mentally incompetent persons would have subscribed to Carrel's appeal, which literally would deny "inferior types" the right to live. The "inferiority" of mentally disabled test subjects, however, made it easy for researchers to forget boundaries of ethics and measures of safety, and to dismiss scruples disdainfully. Dermatologist Albert Kligman, for example, displayed good humor and an easygoing, if cynical, attitude toward his experiments on mentally disabled children. According to students, he used to say, ". . . these kids want attention so bad, if you hit them over the head with a hammer they would love you for it."[25]

The Vaccine Trials

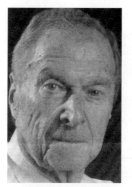

One of the most pressing issues of medical research in the 1940s and early 1950s was the quest for a vaccine against poliomyelitis, a disease that affected thousands of American children every year. President Franklin D. Roosevelt, stricken with the disease himself as a young man, had created the National Foundation for Infantile Paralysis in order to coordinate studies of the disease in different laboratories. In 1950, Hilary Koprowski (Fig. 462), who later became director of the Wistar Institute in Philadelphia, administered the world's first oral polio vaccine to 20 boys and girls at a home for retarded children. At that time, many scientists were wary of giving live polio virus to human beings. When Koprowski presented his data in 1951 at a meeting of the National Foundation in Hershey, Pennsylvania, one of the participants, Thomas Francis of the Rockefeller Institute, asked "what sort of monkeys" had been used as test subjects. According to Koprowski's own recollection, another participant, Jonas E. Salk (Fig. 463), replied, "These are not monkeys, they are children." Francis retorted, "Impossible." But Salk assured him, "Yes, it is possible."[26]

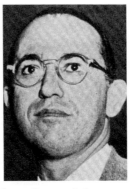

FIG. 463
Jonas E. Salk
(1914-1995)

A few months later, Salk himself conducted one of the most famous and successful of all studies involving the mentally disabled. Having first tried different types of polio vaccine on prisoners, on his laboratory staff, and on himself, Salk, in 1952, tested a noninfectious vaccine on mentally retarded men and boys at a state institution in western Pennsylvania.[27] This was followed, in 1954, by a nationwide field trial on 650,000 children, including 200,000 controls who received a placebo. The vaccine was found to be highly effective and was considered to be completely safe. That, however, was not always to be the case. After the vaccine had become available commercially in 1955, a number of cases of poliomyelitis occurred in vaccinated individuals because some batches of the vaccine inadvertently contained residual living virus.[28] Despite these problems, the vaccination program was overwhelmingly successful. Within three years, the number of cases of paralytic poliomyelitis in the United States dropped from more than 50,000 per year to less than 200.[29] (Fig. 464)

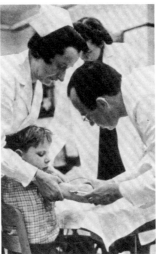

FIG. 464
Jonas E. Salk
administering
a shot during a
mass trial with
a vaccine for
poliomyelitis
in 1954.

Among many other inoculation studies was a trial in England in 1961 of three experimental measles vaccines on 56 institutionalized children who were subnormal mentally. The authors averred that these children "were especially suitable for the study since close medical supervision was possible throughout." The "close medical supervision" did not prevent 48 subjects from getting a rash, 46 from developing fever, and ". . . many of the vaccinated became miserable and fretful during the period of rash and pyrexia." Nine children were recorded to have had a severe reaction to the vaccination, including one who developed bronchopneumonia.[30] Experimental vaccines of measles also were tested throughout the United States. For example, trials took place at a "state school for the mentally deficient operated by the Department of Mental Health of the Commonwealth of Massachusetts;"[31] at the State Home and Training School in Wheatridge, Colorado, which housed "about 800 mentally retarded children and children severely handicapped by congenital abnormalities;"[32] and at the Willowbrook State School for the Retarded on Staten Island, New York, where most inmates suffered from "mongolism, hydrocephaly, microcephaly, brain damage and other causes of mental deficiency."[33]

Between 1956 and 1972, inmates at Willowbrook State School for the Retarded were used for another experiment that could not conceivably benefit them, namely, infection with he-

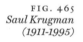
FIG. 465
Saul Krugman
(1911-1995)

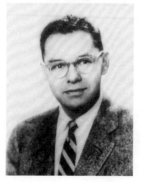

patitis for the purpose of learning whether immunity would develop. The responsible physician, Saul Krugman (Fig. 465), an expert in infectious diseases at New York University, had noted a high incidence of hepatitis among residents of the school, a result of catastrophic conditions hygienically. Krugman hoped that injections of gamma globulins, together with live virus, would induce active immunity against the disease. Some residents of Willowbrook were given both gamma globulin and live hepatitis virus obtained from the feces of patients with the disease, whereas others served as controls and were given the virus without benefit of gamma globulins. Several months later, all residents received another dose of live virus to determine whether immunity was permanent. In the course of his studies, Krugman came to recognize that there were two types of hepatitis, A and B. The same conclusion was reached concurrently by American virologist Baruch Blumberg, who identified the antigen of hepatitis B in his laboratory, without having conducted experiments on humans. Despite Blumberg's more profound, and more humane contribution, for which he was awarded the Nobel Prize in 1976, Krugman was praised for his studies and his "judicious use of human beings."[34]

Critics of Krugman's experiments were silenced by his claim that, inevitably, "most newly admitted children [to Willowbrook] will become infected" anyway. This claim was in stark contrast with a statement made in 1967 by Dr. A. D. Miller, commissioner of the State Department of Mental Hygiene, to the effect that the hepatitis immunization program had resulted in an "80 to 85 percent reduction of this disease at Willowbrook for both patients and employees." Krugman also insisted that the study had been "set up very carefully . . . and in accordance with the World Medical Association's Draft Code of Ethics on Human Experimentation." Interestingly, the Code of the World Medical Association (WMA) was not formulated until eight years after Krugman's study had begun. Moreover, the Code stipulated that "any act or advice which could weaken physical or mental resistance of a human being may be used only in his interest," which surely was not the case at Willowbrook. In addition, it was alleged that the study had been approved by the Committee on Human Experimentation of New York University, but, at the time the study was begun, no such committee existed. Last, the Willowbrook study was justified on the grounds that parents of each of the subjects had been informed about the study and had signed a consent form. That form, however, was deceiving; it indicated that children were to receive a vaccine against the virus, but it made no mention of the virus itself being injected into them. Neither was it clear whether any or all of the parents had been told that hepatitis can progress to cirrhosis, progressive destruction of the liver, and death. Parents did know, however, that the only route for admission of "new" children to Willowbrook School was via the hepatitis unit because in late 1964 they had been informed that gaining entrance to the school was impossible because of its being overcrowded. Shortly after this notice – in some cases as soon as one week later – a second letter was sent out advising parents that there were some vacancies in the hepatitis unit and if the parents would volunteer their children for the study they would be admitted.[35]

Put the Parasites to Use

Some of the experiments carried out on mentally disabled children were designed to investigate physiologic aspects of youth of that age. Pediatricians Richard D. Rowe and L.S. James of the Toronto Hospital for Sick Children and the Columbia Presbyterian Medical Center in New York City, respectively, catheterized the hearts of "fifteen mongoloid infants under one year of age" for the purpose of determining normal pressure in the pulmonary artery during the first few months of life. They found that all subjects were "free from intracardiac defects" and commented that "no sedative was administered" prior to the experiment.[36] In another study, the same authors sought to assess "the pattern of response of pulmonary and systemic arterial pressures in newborn and older infants to short periods of hypoxia." In addition to being subjected to catheterization, "thirteen infants under the age of one year" were fitted with tight face masks and made to breathe a mixture of gases containing 90 percent nitrogen. The authors recorded that ". . . hypoxia with arterial oxygen saturations as low as 50 percent appeared to produce mild somnolence in all infants. However, when the saturation fell to 40 or 30 percent the infants gradually began to move and become restless, finally crying strenuously, sometimes in a gasping fashion. One infant had a period of apnea at the height of anoxia."[37]

At the District of Columbia Training School in Laurel, Maryland, normal iodine metabolism was scrutinized by giving compounds of radioactive iodine to 19 mentally defective children.[38] Seventeen youngsters in the same institution were administered radioactive thyroxine "to further define thyroid hormone metabolism in children."[39] Various aspects of iron and calcium metabolism were studied by the administration, orally and intravenously, of radioactive compounds to mentally retarded children institutionalized at the Walter E. Fernald State School in Waltham, Massachusetts, the first school for the "feeble-minded" in North America.[40] The school was named for psychiatrist Walter E. Fernald, who called "the feeble-minded . . . a parasitic, predatory class, never capable of self-support or of managing their own affairs." To make use of these "parasites," the institute served as a research laboratory for medical schools in nearby Boston. Experiments ranged from use of tracers with radioactive materials to performance of lobotomies and trials of new drugs. Test subjects were not limited to feeble-minded children; healthy orphans and troublesome children who had been dumped at the Fernald school also were utilized as material for research by the scientists. The healthy youngsters worked on the farm, repaired buildings, mowed grass, and gave their bodies to science, but they were not taught to read or write. Despite their lack of formal education, these children could become members of a "science club" formed by investigators in Boston both to repay them for the "inconveniences" suffered during the experiments and to assuage guilt. Members of the science club occasionally were taken to the beach, to ball games, and to Christmas parties, but admittance to the club was dependent wholly on participation in medical experiments.[41]

The range and number of experiments conducted on children and inmates of mental institutions seemed to be without limit, and many experiments concerning diseases of the skin were among them. Some of those experiments consisted of withholding treatment administered routinely for skin lesions. For example, Alan M. Massing and William Epstein of the University of California in San Francisco studied the "natural history of warts" in "one thousand institutionalized, mentally defective children, ranging in age from 4 to 20." The study was undertaken "with the cooperation of the medical staff of the institution," thereby ensuring that "all wart therapy was avoided."[42] In similar fashion, dermatologist Vincent J. Derbes (Fig. 466) and two coworkers of his at Tulane University School of Medicine in New Orleans fol-

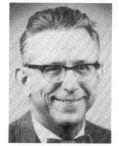

FIG. 466
Vincent J.
Derbes
(1912-1984)

lowed "the course of untreated *tinea capitis* in Negro children." For a period of two to six months, they gave the youngsters a placebo only, never informing either the children or their parents about this deviation from standard practice.[43] In both studies, skin lesions often cleared as they did normally in the absence of treatment; that favorable result, however, does not exonerate the physicians responsible for having exploited particularly vulnerable children for their own purposes.

Sensitizing the Victims

Allergic reactions were one of the chief areas of dermatologic research. Deliberate sensitization of mentally defective persons to potent allergens was a common experimental procedure. The first federally operated mental institution, St. Elizabeths Hospital (a.k.a. Governor Hospital for the Insane and United States Government Hospital for the Insane) in Washington, D.C., was a test site for these experiments. During the 1960s, Naomi M. Kanof, a dermatologist in Washington, D.C. (Fig. 467), editor-in-chief of the *Journal of Investigative Dermatology* for nearly 20 years, and the first woman to receive the Gold Medal of the American Academy of Dermatology, investigated "eczematous sensitizations" at St. Elizabeths along with Adolph Rostenberg (Fig. 468), chairman for many years of the department of dermatology at the

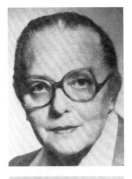

FIG. 467
*Naomi M.
Kanof
(1912-1988)*

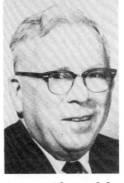

FIG. 468
*Adolph
Rostenberg, Jr.
(1905-1988)*

University of Illinois and at one time a vice-president of the American Academy of Dermatology. Kanof and Rostenberg sought to quantify aspects of sensitization through "comparison between the sensitizing capacities of two allergens and between two different strengths of the same allergen and the effect of repeating the sensitizing dose." To this end, the coworkers decided ". . . to study deliberately induced eczematous sensitizations on a more or less constant population . . . We have had such an opportunity at the St. Elizabeths Hospital, a mental institution, by reason of which the population remains more or less unchanged for many years." The experiments conducted at that infamous institution consisted of applying different dilutions of potent allergens to the skin of test subjects and ". . . these procedures were repeated until each patient had become sensitized or until each patient had had four efforts at sensitization." Rostenberg and Kanof found that "the second attempt at sensitization gave a higher percentage of sensitized individuals than did the first," but "it did not seem that much was to be gained by a third effort at sensitization and still less by a fourth." Another finding was that "Negroes are less readily sensitized than are white persons." The authors expressed, publicly, their "thanks to Dr. W. Overholser, Medical Director of St. Elizabeths Hospital, for his many courtesies." In a discussion of the work presented by Rostenberg and Kanof, Marion Sulzberger, then the dean of American dermatologists and the foremost scientist among them, commented, "We should welcome more and more experimental work of this type."[44]

One of the allergens studied most extensively in the United States was *Rhus radicans*. This was by virtue of the wide distribution of *R. radicans* and *R. diversiloba* in North America and the great sensitizing potential of the allergen housed in their leaves – urushiol, a mixture of catechol derivatives. In an article on "Artificial Sensitization of Infants to Poison Ivy," Henry W. Straus of Brooklyn, New York, declared that a single topical application of a poison ivy paste had sensitized 73 percent of 48 newborn infants.[45] In a discussion of "poison ivy dermatitis" in 1958, Albert Kligman pointed out that "*Rhus* species are by far the Number One cause of allergic dermatitis in the United States, the sufferers from which exceed in number the total of all other forms of allergic disease combined." Kligman also recognized that poison ivy dermatitis "often exists in a severe widespread form" and may be accompanied by kidney disease with "signs of renal tubular damage and the nephrotic syndrome." Although aware of the possibility of serious consequences of sensitization to Rhus antigens, he wrote, with no any attempt at justification, "I sensitized about 85 percent of 34 young children between the ages 2 and 8, who could be presumed not to have been previously exposed."[46]

21 · The Mental Institution as Test Site

A Wealth of Free Biopsy Material

In conjunction with junior coworkers, Kligman carried out a host of experiments on mentally defective children. His test subjects were inmates of a state institution in Pennhurst, Pennsylvania, and two such institutions in southern New Jersey – the Vineland State School, which housed females, and the Woodbine State Colony, which harbored males[47] (Fig. 469, 470). The advantages these institutions offered for purposes of research were praised by Kligman in an article in 1952 about experimental infections with fungi:

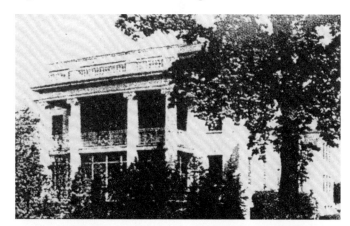

FIG. 469
Vineland Developmental Center, a research laboratory for dermatology.

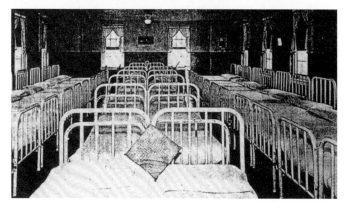

FIG. 470
Dormitory at Vineland Developmental Center.

The work was carried out at a state institution for congenital mental defectives . . . The experimental circumstances were ideal in that a large number of individuals living under confined circumstances could be inoculated at will and the course of the disease minutely studied from its very onset. Biopsy material was freely available.[48]

In the study on fungal infections, the test sites on the skin were either rubbed with a finger or scarified with a blunt knife, followed by inoculation with hairs infected with hyphae or with "a dense water suspension of macroconidia and hyphal fragments." Contact with hairs was found to be more effective in producing infections, and the glabrous skin of the back proved to be more susceptible to that of the occiput. The coauthors noted that "The experimental ringworm lesions reached a maximum size (climax) after 2 to 3 months." Although all of the lesions induced went untreated, "spontaneous resolution of the disease occurred in every case. In most instances this happened within 7 months. In two cases the disease lasted a year, and in one instance 14 months." Different types of fungi were associated with different degrees of inflammation. In the case of *Microsporum canis* (ringworm particularly common in dogs and cats), "an inflammatory reaction ranging from a folliculitis to a mild kerion preceded spontaneous involution in all but one case." Kligman acknowledged that "most of the experimentally infected individuals were subjected to biopsy studies."[49]

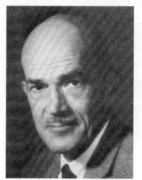

FIG. 471
*J. Walter
Wilson
(1903-1980)*

The biopsies "taken from the scalps of experimental subjects inoculated with *Microsporum audouinii* and *Microsporum canis*" formed the basis of a histopathologic study of *tinea capitis* that was praised enthusiastically at the annual meeting in 1954 of the American Dermatological Association. J. Walter Wilson, a dermatologist/mycologist then at Brown University (Fig. 471) and a future president of the American Academy of Dermatology stated that, "I have long admired Dr. Kligman and his excellent contributions to our knowledge of fungous diseases, and today's presentation is worthy of, and hereby receives, my highest commendation." Francis W. Lynch (Fig. 472), chairman of the department of dermatology at the Mayo Clinic and another future president of the Academy, added this paean:

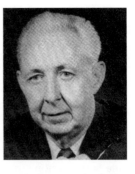

FIG. 472
Francis W. Lynch (1906-1988)

> I congratulate Dr. Kligman on his prize-winning essay. With unusual industry and intelligence he has carried out a unique experimental study . . . Such work cannot be expected from residents, fellows, graduate students, or practitioners of dermatology – it comes only from a dermatologic 'institute' – and only from full-time, at least semi-permanent, scientific workers. Such a paper emphasizes that dermatology sorely needs more such workers and institutions.[50]

Not a single word was wasted on the children who, as unwitting participants in Kligman's study, had been infected and biopsied.

In addition to studying pathogenesis and histopathologic findings, Kligman investigated different treatments of fungal infections in order to compare the results of his investigations. For example, "hairs infected with *Microsporum audouinii* were removed from the scalp of a child experimentally infected 12 days previously" and were "immersed in various types of melted ointments." After more than 30 days of exposure to acidic ointments, fungi could still be grown from the hairs infected. Kligman concluded that "the fungistatic agents are unable to penetrate the hair sufficiently to cause destruction of the hyphae within the hair." He believed that in order to cure an infection, " hyphae growing within the hair must be destroyed." To this end, Kligman and his coworker, W. Ward Anderson, resorted to more drastic measures, which they described as follows:

A tightly fitting rubber bathing cap was placed over the head of the patient and a three inch incision made into the dome of the cap. Through this hole was inserted about six four-inch gauze squares. One hundred milliliters of formalin were poured onto the gauze. The hole was sealed with adhesive. In the beginning 10 percent formalin was used. This was increased to full strength formalin . . . In six cases the individuals were exposed to full strength formalin for one hour. In none of these was a cure effected, nor the hairs rendered culturally negative immediately following treatment. One child in a state mental institution was able to tolerate the formalin treatment for five hours. A failure was recorded in this case also.[51]

Among numerous other inoculation experiments performed by Kligman and his junior associates was one on "the isolation of wart virus in tissue culture and its successful reinoculation into humans." In collaboration with C.G. Mendelson, Kligman removed warts from the soles of men, minced and homogenized them, and then added the homogenate to a culture of monkey kidney cells. After having been grown in fresh cell cultures several times, cell-free fluid of the cultures was "injected intradermally into the palmar aspect of the left thenar eminence of 20 young male patients (age range, 7 to 20) . . . By 3 months, 2 of the 20 subjects inoculated with ultrafiltrates pooled after 6 passages

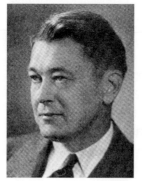

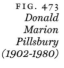

FIG. 473
*Donald
Marion
Pillsbury
(1902-1980)*

developed clinically typical verruca vulgaris . . . The histologic changes of excised experimental lesions were typical for warts." Mendelson and Kligman proclaimed with pride that Koch's postulates had been fulfilled.[52]

At about the same time, Kligman entered into an entirely different field of research – the determination of the effects of ionizing radiation on

human skin. His efforts in that regard were supported vigor-
ously by Donald M. Pillsbury (Fig. 473), chairman of the department of dermatology at the University of Pennsylvania and
one of the leaders in American dermatology. In an attempt to
help secure grants for Kligman's study, Pillsbury wrote a letter
to the chairman of the Armed Forces Epidemiological Board,
Thomas Francis, deploring the "small volume of studies having
to do with the biologic effects of ionizing radiation" and suggesting that "a number of aspects of this problem which were
not the subject of any study" be explored. According to Pillsbury, "the proposed study would be . . . an effort to determine
short- and long-term effects of ionizing radiation on human
skin, under conditions of strict control . . . The subjects to be
used principally would be idiots and feeble-minded children

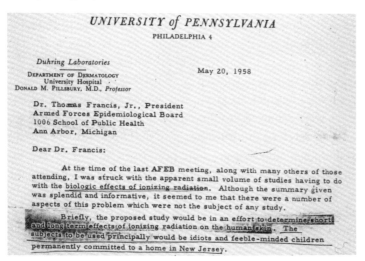

FIG. 474
*Letter of Donald
M. Pillsbury to
Thomas Francis,
Jr., the President
of the Armed
Forces Epidemio-
logical Board,
May 20ᵗʰ, 1958.*

permanently committed to a home in New Jersey." These children offered the advantage of being available "for indefinite periods of time"[53] (Fig. 474). In another letter to the Epidemiological Board, in December 1958, Pillsbury explained the advantages of using inmates of the home in New Jersey for radiation
experiments in these words:

There is no satisfactory study which has dealt with irreversible and long-term changes produced by known varying quantities of gamma rays. The precise doses required to cause permanent damage to such appendages as hair, sweat glands, sebaceous glands, and to blood vessels and connective tissue are merely guesses . . . One may find statements on all these matters in the medical literature, but opinions are at variance, and there is no body of solid experimental evidence. It is the opinion of Dr. Kligman and myself that such experiments could be carried out safely at this institution. There would be no concern about the possible genetic effects; these individuals will never reproduce. No area used would be larger than one which could easily be excised.[54]

The U.S. Army gave its sanction in the form of financial support to the project proposed by Pillsbury on behalf of Kligman; soon radiation experiments on mentally defective children were under way. Among those was a study by John Strauss and Albert Kligman about the "effect of X-rays on sebaceous glands of the human face." In that endeavor, "twenty-three males between the ages of 15 and 30, all but three [of them] inmates at a school for mental defectives, were used as subjects." Different doses of radiation were given, and "biopsy specimens of treated areas were removed at different intervals." For example, "two subjects received 1500r to an area of the cheek two centimeters in diameter," and biopsies were performed "at two weeks, two months, and one year." In addition, "control biopsy specimens of the contralateral cheek were obtained before treatment" in all cases. The radiation resulted in marked, but short-lived, shrinkage of sebaceous glands. In contrast, the effects of the radiation on hair follicles were much more definite and pronounced. One year following application of 1500r in a single dose, "no hair structures were seen although a few undifferentiated epithelial columns, probably follicular remnants, extended down from the epidermis."[55]

21 · The Mental Institution as Test Site

The Effects of Hormones on Sebaceous Glands

Strauss (Fig. 475) and Kligman also collaborated on experiments designed to determine the effects of sex hormones on sebaceous glands. The bulk of the experiments was performed on inmates of three state mental institutions – Vineland, Woodbine, and Fernald. The coworkers centered their attention particularly "on the glands on the face, because the fully developed glands of this region are very large and sebum secretion is high . . . Deep punch biopsy specimens, four to seven millimeters in diameter, have been taken from symmetrical non bearded areas of the cheek before and after hormone administration"[56] (Fig. 476).

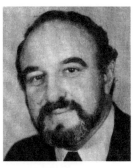

FIG. 475
*John S. Strauss
(born 1926)*

Strauss and Kligman pointed out that "there is general agreement that androgens mediate the enlargement of the sebaceous glands which occurs at puberty."[57] For their studies, they "utilized prepuberal [sic] subjects exclusively because of the high androgenic sensitivity of their glands." For example,

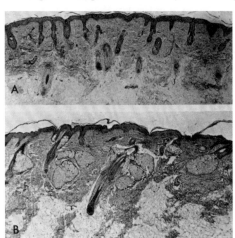

FIG. 476
"Enlargement of the prepuberal sebaceous glands of the cheek of an eleven year old boy given 100 milligrams of methyl testosterone orally daily for twelve weeks" (from the article by Strauss and Kligman).

"fourteen prepuberal children, eight boys and six girls, seven to eleven years of age, were given methyltestosterone orally daily for periods of 7 to 12 weeks ... The glands were studied in cheek biopsy specimens before and after treatment." As expected, the glands were found to enlarge under the influence of testosterone, thereby confirming a fact that already was agreed on generally. This is the conclusion that the authors reached: "We tentatively feel that androgen stimulation can rapidly transform the skin into the postpubertal type, anatomically and functionally."[58]

Following administration of androgens, Strauss and Kligman also noticed "a pronounced growth of coarse black pubic hair, ... a small amount of axillary hair," and a "definite enlargement of the breasts."[59] Boys showed enlargement of the penis. The effects of androgens on sebaceous glands, however, were especially prominent, and the authors were able to advise that "because of their extremely small size, the sebaceous glands of the prepuberal subject are exceedingly useful to measure androgenic effects."[60]

In addition to sex hormones, Strauss and Kligman assessed, too, the effects of other hormones on sebaceous glands. For example, "prepuberal males, post-pubertal females, and post-puberal males," all of whom were "mentally defective inmates of the New Jersey State Colonies at Woodbine and Vineland," were given intramuscular injections of adrenocorticotropic hormone (ACTH) for up to 12 weeks. Other subjects from the same institutions received hydrocortisone by mouth in doses of up to 100 mg per day and "Control biopsy specimens were taken from the cheek before treatment; biopsy specimens were taken from the identical position of the contralateral cheek at varying intervals after therapy." Strauss and Kligman found that "ACTH and hydrocortisone may cause sebaceous gland enlargement in suitable human subjects, namely in prepuberal males and post-puberal females."[61]

21 · The Mental Institution as Test Site

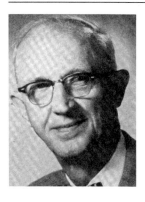

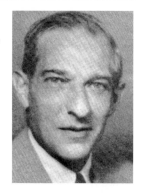

Acceptance of the Unacceptable

Most of the studies just referred to were presented in major forums where participants included leading figures of American dermatology and chairmen of departments of dermatology such as Clarence S. Livingood of the Henry Ford Hospital in Detroit, Michigan; Walter C. Lobitz of Dartmouth University and later the University of Oregon; Eugene Van Scott of the National Cancer Institute in Bethesda, Maryland; Thomas B. Fitzpatrick then of the University of Oregon and later of Harvard University; William S. Becker (Fig. 477) and Stephan Rothman of the University of Chicago (Fig. 478); and Marion Sulzberger and Rudolf L. Baer of New York University School of Medicine (Fig. 479). Although many incisive comments were made in these discussions, not a single utterance was directed at the propriety of using mentally disabled children as test subjects.

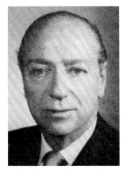

In British medical journals of that same time, the abuse of children as human guinea pigs was denounced repeatedly. For example, in 1953 R.E.W. Fisher of London unambiguously criticized in the *Lancet* nontherapeutic experiments on children. This is what he said:

No medical procedure involving the slightest risk or accompanied by the slightest physical or mental pain may be inflicted on a child for experimental purposes unless there is a reasonable chance, or at least a hope, that the child may benefit thereby.[62]

In a letter to the editor of the *Lancet*, Stephen Goldby of Oxford attacked Saul Krugman for having infected inmates at the Willowbrook State School with hepatitis, calling it "indefensible to give potentially dangerous infected material to children, particularly those who were mentally retarded, with or without parental consent, when no benefit to the child could conceivably result." He also expressed his amazement "that the work was published and that it has been actively supported editorially by the *Journal of the American Medical Association*."[63]

In the United States, questions of ethics were handled differently than in England. When ethics of human experimentation were considered in the United States, it was done mostly in a general and self-promoting way; particular studies were not questioned and specific physicians never were criticized. It is inconceivable that American physicians were unaware of basic principles of human decency that prohibit inflicting harm and pain on innocent children. Those physicians who conducted experiments on humans, however, suppressed considerations that would have interfered with their quest for knowledge, their grasp for grants, and their hope for fame, and, in some instances, fortune. Colleagues who listened to their presentations at scientific meetings and read their articles in medical journals often were not capable of reflection sufficiently critical to enable them to spot infractions ethically; even if they did perceive such violations, they lacked the courage to speak up, to alert others to the misbehavior of fellow medical men, and to dissociate themselves from a pragmatic, insensitive, unempathic mentality that reigned at the time. Those who remained passive also were participants in a conspiracy of silence that furthered exploitation of vulnerable human beings in the name of science.

21 · The Mental Institution as Test Site

It is ironic that in a country proud of its tradition of respect for the individual, mentally disabled children came to be treated like laboratory animals, without any regard for their humanity and individuality, and mental institutions became cages for test subjects who happened to be human beings.

CHAPTER 22

EXPERIMENTS ON
AFRICAN-AMERICANS

O n a risky ride, a prudent person does not use his best
horse because it might be injured. For a risky medical
experiment, physicians, traditionally, have not used
human subjects that they deemed to be crème de la crème. That
role was reserved for those considered to be inferior or dispen-
sible, such as criminals and mentally disabled individuals. To
some medical men, however, the most overt sign of inferiority
was black skin. In the days of slavery, African-Americans were
used commonly as human guinea pigs, sometimes being purchased by researchers for the sole purpose of experimentation.
For example, Dr. T. Stillman of Charleston, South Carolina,
who operated a private infirmary specializing in the treatment
of diseases of the skin, announced in the *Charleston Mercury* in

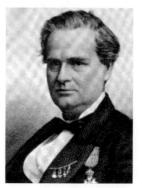

FIG. 480
*James Marion
Sims
(1813-1883)*

1838 that he would purchase from
slave owners any chronically diseased
slaves they might wish to "dispose of."[1]
Other physicians offered experimental treatment for diseased slaves at
low or no cost to their owners. The gynecologist of international renown,
James Marion Sims of Montgomery,
Alabama (Fig. 480), used African-
American female slaves to develop his

surgical technique of closing vesicovaginal fistulae. "If you will give me Anarcha and Betsey for experiment," he proposed to one owner, "I agree to perform no experiment or operation on either of them to endanger their lives, and will not charge a cent for keeping them, but you must pay their taxes and clothe them. I will keep them at my own expense."[2] Between 1845 and 1849, in the days before anesthesia, Sims performed dozens of operations on these hapless women, all the while lauding their "heroism and bravery."[3]

Other American physicians of the nineteenth century placed slaves in pit ovens in order to study heat stroke, poured scalding water over them in an attempt to learn more about typhoid fever, and amputated fingers to assess the efficacy of anesthesia.[4] Slaves often were used as objects in medical demonstrations. Medical schools built their reputations on their ability to procure "clinical material," among which were cadavers for practicing autopsy. At a time when few whites consented to have their bodies investigated post mortem, the presence of a large population of voiceless slaves or "free persons of color" was a distinct advantage in this respect to medical schools in the South. English writer Harriet Martineau commented after a visit to the United States in 1834 that ". . . the bodies of coloured people exclusively are taken for dissection, 'because the whites do not like it, and the coloured people cannot resist.'"[5] Interstate shipments of dead black bodies from the South to medical schools in the North continued well into the twentieth century.[6]

The Inequality of Rights

During the Civil War, Lincoln emancipated all slaves in the United States, and after the war African-Americans, as free persons, were granted, by the thirteenth and fourteenth amendments to the American Constitution, the rights of citizenship. Despite that, however, a Civil Rights Act of 1875 that guaranteed the right of African-Americans to equal accommodations in public facilities was declared unconstitutional by the Supreme Court, which, in 1883, ruled that Congress was to be concerned exclusively with actions by states against the rights of citizens, not with the actions by individuals against other individuals. Thereafter, discriminatory practices against African-Americans went largely unchallenged until World War II. Higher positions in the military, civil service, and private companies simply were unattainable for African-Americans, who had to content themselves with low-level jobs and poor pay. Denied membership in most labor unions, they were assigned to the most menial and hazardous duties, and earned far less than whites doing the same type of work. The unemployment rate among African-Americans was high, and millions living in urban communities required direct relief in terms of food, clothing, fuel, and shelter. When they were in need of medical care, these economically disadvantaged citizens often were perceived as material particularly appropriate for medical experimentation.[7] Typical is a study in 1939 by physicians of the University of Georgia School of Medicine who inoculated four African-Americans with pus from lesions of *granuloma inguinale*, a chronic disabling venereal disease for which no effective treatment was then available. Two test subjects were referred to as "volunteers," one was said to be "a tuberculous patient," and one was "schizophrenic." After about six weeks, fluctuating abscesses and ulcerations developed in three of the four subjects[8] (Fig. 481, 482).

Because of the trying economic circumstances, African-Americans also were the most likely to be seduced by offers of money into participating in medical experiments. In the early 1930s, for example, William Osler Abbott of the University of Pennsylvania utilized "professional guinea pigs" to develop a new technique for intubating rapidly the human intestine,

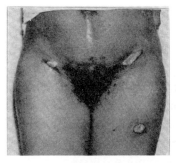

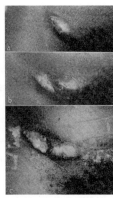

FIG. 482
*Example of
experimental
granuloma
inguinale
(from the
article by
Greenblatt et
al.)*

FIG. 481 *Example of experimental
granuloma inguinale (from the
article by Greenblatt et al.)*

from mouth to rectum. After trying unsuccessfully to recruit unemployed men and beggars as test subjects, he called in his black janitor and promised him 50 cents for every healthy human subject who appeared, in both a sober and a fasting state, at the laboratory door at 8:30 am. Within a short time, Abbott had at his disposal several African-Americans, to whom he referred jokingly as his "animals." Describing his experiences with these subjects, Abbott alluded to the stereotype of their penchant for thievery; nonetheless, he continued to employ them, commenting cynically that "those boys may have been short on morals but they were long in gut."[9]

The high rate of crime among African-Americans was, in large measure, the result of their degrading situation socioeconomically. Denied access to "white" housing areas, most African-Americans lived in the poor quarters of cities, where exposure to crime began in early childhood and continued throughout life. As a consequence, the percentage of African-Americans in populations of prisoners was extremely high, just as it is to this day. Equally important for that disproportionate statistic was the fact that African-Americans were sentenced to prison terms much more readily and for much longer than whites who had committed comparable offenses.[10] As a result, the medical experiments conducted in prisons were chiefly on

African-Americans, even though some investigators tended to "favor" white prisoners when the choice was available. That African-Americans constituted the majority of inmates utilized for research was acknowledged forthrightly in many publications. For example, when Albert Kligman of the department of dermatology of the University of Pennsylvania developed his "maximization test" for screening and rating allergic contact sensitizers, he noted that "the maximization ratings presented in this paper refer to Negroes who comprised 90 percent of our experimental subjects."[11]

Although living conditions and prospects for African-Americans in the North were poor, they were far better than those in the South, where strict segregation of races was still the rule. Separate facilities for Caucasians and African-Americans existed for all aspects of public life, including public transportation, medical facilities, libraries, and schools. Any personal relationship between a white and an African-American was scrutinized closely, and frowned upon; the law of some states prohibited marriage between the races. African-Americans were denied the right to vote, were treated condescendingly by local authorities, and were subjected to arbitrary violence, ranging from minor physical assault to lynching. The organs of law enforcement offered little protection to African-Americans and resort to the courts in conflicts with whites was an exercise in utter futility. In the 1950s, the first steps toward desegregation met with violent resistance on the part of white Southerners. When the Supreme Court of the United States ruled in 1954 that compulsory segregation of African-Americans in public schools was unconstitutional under the fourteenth amendment and directed that public schools must desegregate "with all deliberate speed," the states of Alabama, Georgia, Mississippi, and Virginia threatened to abolish public schools altogether, rather than permit mixing of the races in "hallowed halls." In fact, to avoid desegregation, public schools were closed in one Virginia county from 1959 to 1964. By 1966, only 16.9 percent of African-American students in eleven southern states attended school with white students, and the vast majority of schools were still segregated totally.

The issue of education was crucial because the poor level of schooling of African-Americans helped maintain the strict segregation of the races. Illiteracy being common among African-Americans, they were in no position to claim their rights and challenge their white "superiors." The poor level of education also served to maintain racial prejudice on the part of white Southerners, a prejudice to which physicians, based on their erudition and scientific knowledge, contributed substantially. Differences between races, real or imagined – with respect to such diverse aspects as brain size, facial features, odor, and susceptibility to disease – often were subjects of debate among physicians.[12] Influenced by the ideology of Social Darwinism, physicians had no difficulty in identifying Negroes as the race least likely to triumph in the struggle for survival. They argued that the benevolent side of the institution of slavery, with its elaborate medical care for slaves and its brake consciously on tendencies to self-destructive behavior by them had held in check the decay of the black race. Following the abolition of slavery, however, the Negroid race was thought to be doomed. This is how J. Wellington Byers, a physician in Charlotte, North Carolina, explained it:

The weakest members of the social body...sooner or later succumb to the devitalizing forces of intemperance, disease, and crime and death. The Negro is peculiarly unfortunate ... [because] ... he has not only the inherent frailties of his nature to war against – instincts, passions and appetites; but also those nocuous, seductive, destroying influences that emanate from free institutions in a country of civil liberty.[13]

The Abuse of Man

Syphilis, a Vehicle for Stereotyping

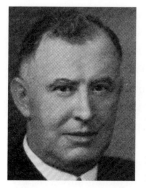

One of the "inherent frailties" of the Negro was said to be his frighteningly strong sex drive. Dermatologist Thomas W. Murrell (Fig. 483) of the University College of Medicine in Richmond, Virginia observed in 1910 that, "... morality among these people is almost a joke, and only assumed as a matter of convenience or when there is a lack of desire and opportunity for indulgence ... I have never seen a negro virgin over 18 years of age ... A negro man will not abstain from sexual intercourse if there is opportunity and no mechanical obstruction ... His sexual powers are those of a specialist in a chosen field."[14]

In the days of slavery, extramarital affairs among slaves, with the exception of those engaged in with their white owners, were prohibited, and visits at night between slave cabins were punished severely. Once that control no longer was exerted, the incidence of venereal diseases among African-Americans increased rapidly; by 1902, more than 50 percent of all African-Americans over the age of 25 were believed to have acquired syphilis.[15] In 1908, Howard Fox (Fig. 484), who later became chairman of dermatology at New York University College of

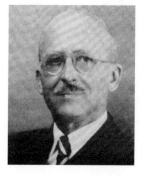

Medicine and the first president of the American Academy of Dermatology (AAD), compared the incidence of skin diseases in more than 4,000 African-Americans and white Americans, and concluded "that syphilis in the Negro is not only very prevalent, but more so than in the white." He agreed "with certain writers who claim that, from a physical standpoint, the negro slaves were infinitely better off than are their descendants of today . . . An utter lack of morality, . . . a strong sexual instinct and lack of cleanliness, seem all that are necessary to have brought about a widespread infection with syphilis."[16]

Statements such as these were heaven-sent for racist Southerners. In general, African-Americans were blamed for their own poor health, the reasons attributed being their wicked lifestyle, their neglect of hygiene on both personal and community basis, and the absence from their homes of proper facilities for the disposal of human waste. It was as if the socioeconomic conditions under which African-Americans suffered were chosen by them. Syphilis, as a disease acquired principally through voluntary sexual intercourse, was an ideal vehicle for furthering the stereotypical representation of the Negro as an inferior human being, incapable of taking responsibility for himself.[17]

This purported lack of responsibility also was emphasized in regard to treatment of syphilis. Because of the long latency period following remission of the initial manifestations of syphilis, it was extremely difficult to convince poorly educated carriers of the disease of the necessity for ongoing treatment of it. A complicating factor was that chemotherapy for syphilis was costly, lengthy, and unpleasant. Intramuscular injections of neoarsphenamine (neosalvarsan), which had to be taken for more than a year, were painful and associated commonly with side effects that were difficult to accept, especially when there were no symptoms or signs of the disease. In the words of a Southern physician, a Negro "thinks where he is taking medicine and can not feel or see anything wrong . . . that the doctor is getting the better of his purse."[18] The consequence, as noted by Thomas Murrell, was this: "They come for treatment at the beginning and at the end. When there are visible manifestations or when harried by pain, they readily come, for as a race they are not averse to physic; but tell them not, though they look well and feel well, that they are still diseased. Here ignorance rates science a fool."[19]

For many Southern physicians, the ignorant state of African-Americans was inherent in their being, and was the root cause of all the problems of that "inferior race." According to Eugene Corson of Atlanta, Georgia, African-Americans did not care whether they caught syphilis or spread it. "This absolute indifference," he wrote, "is a characteristic of the negro, not only as regards syphilis, but of all diseases. He is simply concerned with the present moment, and not always concerned then."[20]

These prejudices, as prejudices always are, were contrary to information then available. Statistics showed that "the occurrence of syphilis among white people of the same social class as the negroes would seem to be about the same . . . "[21] This was true also for compliance with treatment. Some physicians, such as Stewart Welch of Birmingham, Alabama, contended that African-Americans could be "more readily herded in" for treatment than white patients, "not so much through interest in cure but simply due to the fact that they are more readily driven."[22] Henry H. Hazen (Fig.

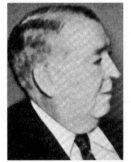

485), professor of dermatology at Georgetown University in Washington, D.C., characterized African-Americans as "very docile patients: while they complain of the pain of intramuscular injections, they will come back for more . . . The secret of treating them is to show them that you are taking an interest in them, and also that you mean just what you say."[23]

A "Ready-Made Situation for Science"

For the United States Public Health Service – so named in 1912 when its mandate became the improvement of all aspects of public health, especially communicable diseases – the high prevalence of syphilis in the rural South presented a major challenge. In 1929, a grant from the Julius Rosenwald Fund was used to explore the prevalence of syphilis among African-Americans and the possibilities of mass treatment of the disease in them in the South. The Rosenwald Study found syphilis to be most prevalent in Macon County, Alabama, an extremely poor region with a mostly illiterate population of blacks. The study found, too, that mass treatment could be implemented successfully among rural blacks for an average of $8.60 per capita, an investment that was expected to pay off handsomely in terms of better efficiency of labor.[24] Although the treatment given was not sufficient to cure all patients, physicians of the Public Health Service were able to render most patients noninfectious.[25] At the same time, however, a worldwide economic crisis erupted and the Rosenwald Fund soon withdrew its financial support for detection and treatment of syphilis. Ironically, it was Taliaferro Clark (Fig. 486), the head of the Venereal Disease Division of Public Health Service and author of the report about the Rosenwald Study, who, in 1932, advocated the very opposite of mass treatment. His suggestion was to assess the natural course of syphilis by deliberately withholding any form of treatment. With the extraordinary prevalence of syphilis and with most blacks remaining untreated anyway, it seemed only natural to Clark to take advantage for the sake of science of that "ready-made situation."[26] Clark's proposal was supported by Surgeon General Hugh Cumming (Fig. 487), who believed

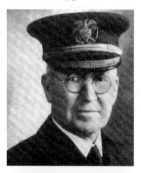

FIG.486
*Taliaferro
Clark
(1867-1948)*

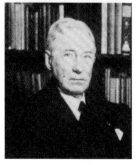

FIG.487
*Hugh Smith
Cumming
(1869-1948)*

that the large concentration of untreated patients with syphilis in Alabama "offers an unparalleled opportunity for carrying on this piece of scientific research which probably cannot be duplicated anywhere else in the world."[27]

A study of untreated syphilis similar to the one proposed by Clark and Cumming actually had been conducted by Caesar Boeck in Norway between 1889 and 1910. Boeck had contended that "the specific therapeutic compounds, potassium iodide and mercury, have a good effect on clinical symptoms, but are unable to eradicate the disease completely and interfere with the inherent regulating effects and healing power of the organism." Boeck had undertaken the study in the hope of realizing a better outcome for his patients. In the 1920s, Boeck's successor as chairman of dermatology at the University of Oslo, Edvin Bruusgaard, conducted a follow-up study of almost 500 of Boeck's patients and found that 70 percent of them went through life without being inconvenienced by the disease. The remaining 30 percent, however, developed severe complications, some of which had not been recognized as being related to syphilis at the time Boeck had begun the study.[28]

More than 30 years later, when Clark suggested that the natural course of syphilis be monitored, complications of the disease already were known well. In his report on the outcome of Boeck's patients, Bruusgaard had called special attention to "affections of vessels and the heart which play a predominant role not only in regard to their frequency but also as causes of death."[29] The Oslo Study had been terminated in 1910 when arsenic compounds became available for treatment of syphilis. By the early 1930s, the therapeutic value of arsenics in primary and secondary syphilis had been established beyond doubt. In regard to latent syphilis, the issue of therapy was undecided. Some dermatovenereologists, such as Paul A. O'Leary, chairman of the department of dermatology of the University of

Minnesota (Fig. 488), recommended no treatment for elderly patients with syphilis in the absence of clinical findings. At Stanford University School of Medicine, patients with serologic evidence of syphilis who were older than 50 years of age and who did not exhibit symptoms or signs of syphilis, positive findings in the cerebrospinal fluid, or signs of aortitis, were left "intentionally untreated" and followed only clinically for many years.[30] On the other hand, Joseph Earl Moore (Fig. 489) of the Venereal Disease Clinic of the Johns Hopkins University School of Medicine and one of the leading American venereologists, wrote these lines in 1933: "Though it imposes a slight though measurable risk of its own, treatment markedly diminishes the risk from syphilis. In latent syphilis, . . . the probability of progression, relapse, or death is reduced from a probable 25-30 percent without treatment to about 5 percent with it; and the gravity of the relapse, if it occurs, is markedly diminished."[31]

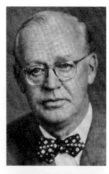

FIG. 488
Paul A.
O'Leary
(1891-1955)

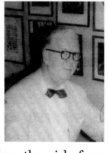

FIG. 489
Joseph Earl
Moore
(1892-1957)

In brief, the risks of untreated syphilis were well known and effective treatment for the disease was available by the early 1930s. In public campaigns, the Public Health Service warned that "uncured syphilis may strike years later" and advised patients who might have the disease to "see your doctor – or local health officer"[32] (Fig. 490). That Clark nevertheless proposed to study the course of untreated syphilis in African-Americans, including young men and those with indubitable clinical evidence of the disease, can be understood only in the context of prejudice racially. By the standards of the 1930s, Clark and other officers of the Public Health Service were veritable liberals in certain aspects in regard to race. They promoted the hir-

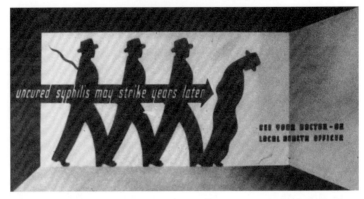

FIG. 490
"Uncured
syphilis may
strike years
later" (health
campaign
poster of the
1930s).

ing of young African-American physicians and used their influence repeatedly to arrange residency training for them.[33] In letters explaining the proposed study, however, Clark emphasized the "rather low intelligence of the Negro population," the "very common promiscuous sex relations of this population group," and the "prevailing indifference with regard to treatment." Joseph Moore, who had called the Oslo Study "a never-to-be-repeated human experiment," endorsed Clark's proposal, arguing that "syphilis in the negro is in many respects almost a different disease from syphilis in the white." Clark's lieutenant, Oliver C. Wenger of the Public Health Service stationed in Hot Springs, Arkansas, advised that ". . . this study will emphasize these differences."[34]

The Tuskegee Syphilis Study Begins

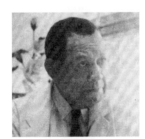

FIG. 491
Eugene H.
Dibble, Jr.
(1893-1968)

With the support of the leading syphilologists of the country, the study of untreated, late-stage syphilis was started at the Tuskegee Institute in Macon County, Alabama, in September 1932. The medical director of the Institute, Eugene H. Dibble, Jr.

(Fig. 491), had offered his cooperation after being assured by Clark that "there would be no cost" to the Institute, that the "hospital and the Tuskegee Institute would get credit for this piece of research work," and that "the results of this study will be sought after the world over."[35]

Originally, the Tuskegee Syphilis Study was scheduled to last for six to twelve months. During that time, black males between the ages of 25 and 60 were to be recruited and screened for late-stage syphilis by means of the Wassermann test. Joseph Moore cautioned that this test was neither specific nor very sensitive in detecting latent syphilis. He acknowledged, however, that for diagnosis of latent syphilis in subjects with a negative test, "a mere history of a penile sore only would not be adequate, inasmuch as the average Negro has had as many penile sores as rabbits have offspring."[36] For that reason, only men with a positive Wassermann reaction were included in the study. They had to undergo a thorough physical examination, laboratory tests, X-rays, and a spinal tap in an effort to determine the incidence of neurosyphilis (Fig. 492).

The recruitment of test subjects proved to be difficult for a variety of reasons. First, the incidence of syphilis was lower

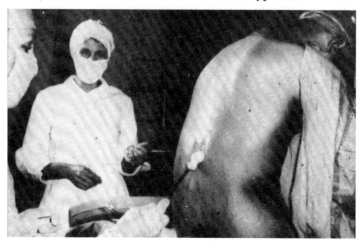

FIG. 492
Spinal tap performed on a subject of the Tuskegee Syphilis Study in 1933.

– 483 –

than anticipated, that is, 20 percent of the population instead of the predicted 35 percent. Second, the number of patients who had sought and received previous treatment exceeded by far the expectations of the Public Health Service. In a letter in March 1933 to his director on site, Raymond H. Vonderlehr, Clark deplored the necessity of testing "such a large number of individuals in order to uncover this relatively limited number of untreated cases."[37] Third, the premise on which the study was based proved to be incorrect, namely, that blacks – promiscuous, lustful, and indifferent to their state of health as they were supposed to be – would not seek treatment for syphilis anyway. On the contrary, subjects with syphilis were quite willing to undergo unpleasant examinations and accept other inconveniences in return for free medical care. The promise of treatment alone elicited cooperation of them. Seizing on this reasonable, but naive, response, investigators told the black men that they would receive treatment for "bad blood," the colloquial expression for syphilis in the rural South. That the examinations actually served no therapeutic purpose was concealed from them carefully. Even spinal taps, which at that time still carried a significant risk of such serious complications as blinding headaches and paralysis, were presented to test subjects as "special free treatment"[38] (Fig. 493, 494).

Some compromise, however, crept into the plan for the study and, at a later time, this would be acknowledged to be a serious impairment to its value scientifically. At the insistence of state health officials in Alabama, some treatment, albeit partial and insufficient, was provided for test subjects.[39] That Clark and his associates at last agreed to administer treatment to test subjects in a study concerning "untreated syphilis" was a consequence of reasons that were less than altruistic. The investigators knew that: (1) the treatment they were to give, usually but a few injections of mercury, had proven to be ineffective; (2) the study was planned initially to last for only six to 12 months, so

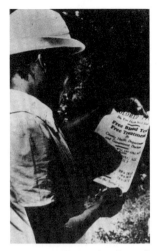

Macon County Health Department

ALABAMA STATE BOARD OF HEALTH AND U. S. PUBLIC HEALTH
SERVICE COOPERATING WITH TUSKEGEE INSTITUTE

Dear Sir:

Some time ago you were given a thorough examination and
since that time we hope you have gotten a great deal of
treatment for bad blood. You will now be given your last
chance to get a second examination. This examination is a
very special one and after it is finished you will be given
a special treatment if it is believed you are in a condition
to stand it.

If you want this special examination and treatment you
must meet the nurse at _____ on
_____at_____ M. She will bring you to
the Tuskegee Institute Hospital for this free treatment. We
will be very busy when these examinations and treatments are
being given, and will have lots of people to wait on. You
will remember that you had to wait for some time when you
had your last good examination, and we wish to let you know
that because we expect to be so busy it may be necessary for
you to remain in the hospital over one night. If this is
necessary you will be furnished your meals and a bed, as well
the examination and treatment without cost.

REMEMBER THIS IS YOUR LAST CHANCE FOR SPECIAL FREE TREAT-
MENT. BE SURE TO MEET THE NURSE.

Macon County Health Department

FIG. 493 *Campaign flyer of the 1930s offering "free treatment" to "colored people" with "bad blood."*

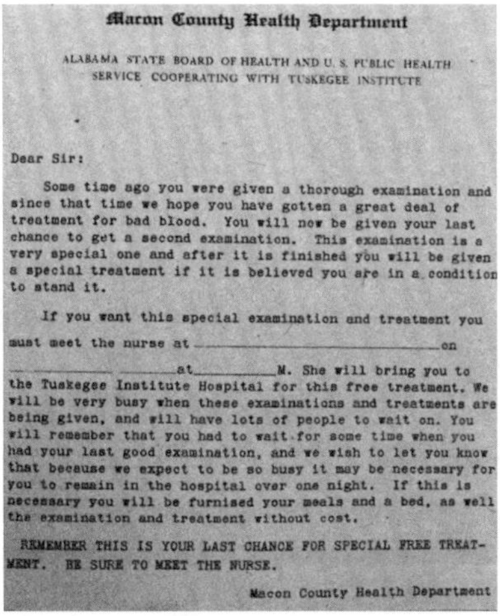

FIG. 494 *Letter to test subjects in 1933 anouncing the "last chance for special free treatment."*

that a few injections near the end of the period were not expected to alter the results; and (3) the injections, whatever they contained, helped to maintain the appearance of a routine medical procedure. In a letter written in 1932, Clark confided that, ". . . in order to secure the cooperation of the planters in this region," for whom the black men were working and who had nearly total control over their lives, "it was necessary to carry on this study under the guise of a demonstration and provide treatment for those cases uncovered found to be in need of treatment."[40] Even though this program of treatment was deficient in the extreme, it came close to exhausting funds that the Public Health Service had allotted to the Tuskegee Study. Raymond Vonderlehr (Fig. 495), who was in charge of the fieldwork, asked Clark repeatedly for more medication, urging thus:

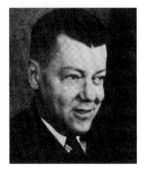

FIG. 495
*Raymond A.
Vonderlehr
(1897-1973)*

Expenditure of several hundred dollars for drugs for these men would be well worthwhile if their interest and cooperation would be maintained in so doing . . . It is my desire to keep the main purpose of the work from the negroes in the county and continue their interest in treatment. That is what the vast majority wants and the examination seems relatively unimportant to them in comparison. It would probably cause the entire experiment to collapse if the clinics were stopped before the work is completed.[41]

The Longest Research Study

The Tuskegee Syphilis Study was rooted in lies and deception. The original study, however, was just the foundation for an even greater deceit that would be fabricated over the next 40 years. Although the Macon County Board of Health had approved the study "with the distinct understanding that treatment be provided for these people," once the data had been accumulated,[42] venereologists of the Public Health Service considered the project to be too intriguing to abandon. Vonderlehr pressed Clark in a letter in April 1933 to keep the experiment going and he said that in these words: "At the end of this project we shall have a considerable number of cases presenting various complications of syphilis who have received only mercury and may still be considered untreated in the modern sense of therapy. Should these cases be followed over a period of from five to ten years, many interesting facts could be learned regarding the course of complications of untreated syphilis."[43] Another argument in favor of continuing the study was the possibility of assessing "the efficacy of present-day antisyphilitic treatment." As Vonderlehr pointed out, "the Public Health Service already has on hand records of a fairly large number of Negroes who have been both adequately and inadequately treated for syphilis and it is our desire to use the untreated group now being examined in Macon County as a comparison to indicate the value of treatment."[44]

22 · Experiments on African-Americans

In a letter to Oliver C. Wenger (Fig. 496), director of the Venereal Disease Clinic of the PHS in Hot Springs, Arkansas, Vonderlehr advised that "the proper procedure is the continuance of the observation of the Negro men used in the study with the idea of eventually bringing them to autopsy."[45] The idea of identifying bodies for dissection in advance – while the individuals under discussion were still alive – was in keeping with medical tradition in the South, where African-Americans had been valued chiefly as vehicles for medical demonstrations and as cadavers for autopsy.[46] Wenger also believed that autopsies were absolutely essential for the subjects of the Tuskegee Syphilis Study, but he advised Vonderlehr of "one danger" in the plan as follows:

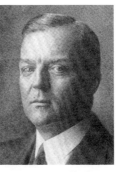

FIG. 496
Oliver Clarence Wenger (1884-1958)

> If the colored population becomes aware that accepting free hospital care means a post-mortem, every darkey will leave Macon County and it will hurt Dr. Dibble's hospital. This can be prevented, however, if the doctors of Macon County are brought into our confidence and requested to be very careful not to let the objective of the plan be known.*

In order to cut costs, Wenger proposed that, except for autopsies, no further examinations be conducted because "we have no further interest in these patients until they die."[47]

The latter suggestion was disregarded by Vonderlehr, who felt that only by supervising patients continuously could they be prevented from being lost to follow-up or going elsewhere for treatment. Compliance of patients was secured by hiring an African-American nurse named Eunice Rivers. According to Vonderlehr's plan, "about once a year some officer of the Service should go to Macon County and spend a few weeks with the idea of checking up on the nurse's work, doing short examinations on the more advanced cases and giving a placebo form of treatment

* Note the pejorative use by physicians of the word "darkey" and the implications of it for treating patients with dark skin as fellow human beings.

FIG. 497
*Nurse Eunice
Rivers dis-
pending "treat-
ment" at a cot-
ton field.*

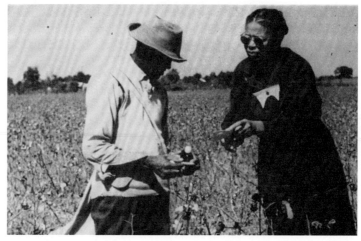

for those desiring it."[48] For the rest of the year, Nurse Rivers was left entirely on her own. She maintained contact with the subjects, picked them up in her own car, took them to the hospital for examinations, organized free hot meals on the days of examinations, provided an opportunity to stop in town on the return trip to shop or visit friends, dispensed noneffective medicines, and procured approval from them for autopsies[49] (Fig. 497). As of 1935, permission for an autopsy was rewarded by an offer of $50 for burial expenses, an amount that increased in 1952 to $100.[50] Rivers had graduated from the Tuskegee Institute School of Nursing and knew the landscape and her charges well. In an article in 1953, coauthored with other members of the Tuskegee team, she explained the

FIG. 498
*Certificate for
twenty-five-
year participa-
tion sent in
1958 to the still
remaining test
subjects of the
Tuskegee
Syphilis Study.*

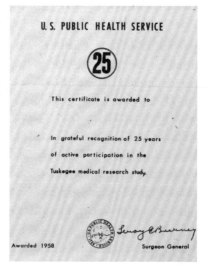

reason for the lures as follows: "Because of the low educational status of the majority of the patients, it was impossible to appeal to them from a purely scientific approach. Therefore, various methods were used to maintain and stimulate their interest ... In our case, free hot meals meant more to the men than $50 worth of free medical examination."[51] Test subjects cherished greatly a certificate given to them in 1958 by the Public Health Service "in grateful recognition of 25 years of active participation in the Tuskegee medical research study." The certificate was especially appreciated because it came with $25 in cash – $1 for each year of participation in the study[52] (Fig. 498).

A Policy of Deceit

From the outset, the Tuskegee Syphilis Study was based on a combination of vague curiosity of the investigators and the availability of men on whom to perform this type of study. There was no methodical, thoughtful, or substantial scientific plan. As a result, numerous changes were made in the design of the study, without in any way their enhancing the scientific quality of it. One such alteration was the recruitment of a control group of healthy, uninfected men. Following approval in 1933 for the continuation of the study by the Public Health Service, Vonderlehr, who had succeeded Clark as chief of the Venereal Disease Division, sent John R. Heller (Fig. 499) to Tuskegee to take charge of the experiment. Heller eventually succeeded Vonderlehr, prior to his becoming Director of the National Cancer Institute in 1948. When recruiting the control group for the Tuskegee Study in 1933, Heller found it necessary to continue the policy of deceit, eliciting cooperation

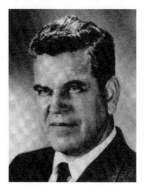

FIG. 499
*John R. Heller
(1905-1989)*

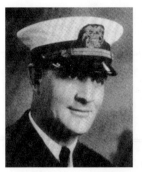

of the healthy subjects by distributing noneffective drugs to them.[53] Control subjects who eventually acquired syphilis themselves simply were transferred to the test group, a shocking violation of standard procedures in research.[54]

In 1938, the study was assessed again by Austin V. Deibert (Fig. 500), a young officer of the Public Health Service, who was "amazed to discover that fully 40 percent of the group had received some treatment, even though inadequate." In a letter to Vonderlehr, Deibert cautioned that "we cannot obtain a true reflection of the course of untreated syphilis in view of 40 percent of the cases having had some treatment."[55] Deibert's comments had a sense of urgency because the incidence of cardiovascular disease among the younger test subjects was lower than he had expected. "The paucity of clinical findings still alarms me," he informed Vonderlehr, "but I feel that the inadequately treated group accounts for this. The majority of this group falls into the 25 to 35 age group, and that none of them have developed aortitis fortifies my belief that even a very little treatment goes a long way in avoiding cardio-vascular complications."[56] Despite these findings, Deibert did not conclude that the benefits of "very little treatment" should be made available to all the subjects. Instead, he suggested supplementation of "the present study with the following plan: . . . 1) Maintain the syphilitic cases who have received some treatment as a study group of inadequately treated cases and on whom subsequent periodic observations can be made. 2) Replace these cases with strictly untreated men of comparable ages and infection dates."[57]

The effort to maintain intact a study group of "strictly untreated men," however, proved to be increasingly difficult. In 1934, Vonderlehr met with physicians in the community to ask for their cooperation in not treating test subjects.[58] In 1937, when the Rosenwald Fund decided to renew its support for programs designed to control syphilis, it sent a physician to Macon County to resume treatment of all patients with syphilis, which could have been a major impediment to the plan of the Tuskegee scientists. Vonderlehr shrewdly arranged to have Nurse Rivers assigned as assistant to the

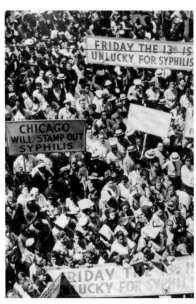

FIG. 501
The campaign to control syphilis launched by Surgeon General Thomas Parran gained wide popular support, as is evident from the size of the crowd gathered in Chicago.

new physician, and as a result, the novice agreed to cooperate fully with the experiment as it was constructed, namely, to prevent subjects in the Tuskegee study from being treated. At the same time, the Surgeon General of the United States, Thomas Parran, launched a nationwide campaign to eradicate venereal diseases, for which he received wide popular attention and sup-

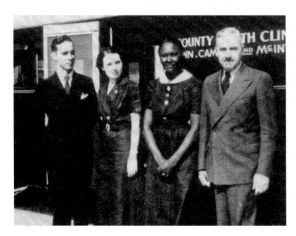

FIG. 502
The mobile clinic of the Public Health Service, called the "Bad Blood Wagon," was staffed by two local nurses and a young PHS officer and future Surgeon General, Leroy Burney (left). Visiting on this occasion was Surgeon General Thomas Parran (right).

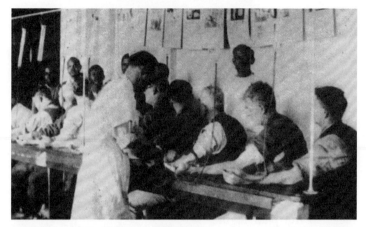

FIG. 503
Rapid Treatment Penicillin Clinic conducted by the U.S. Public Health Service in the late 1940s.

port (Fig. 501). When a mobile treatment unit of the Public Health Service, called the "Bad Blood Wagon," was assigned to Macon County in 1939, Vonderlehr had Nurse Rivers attached to the unit to ensure that test subjects would not be given treatment[59] (Fig. 502). In 1941, several test subjects were drafted by the army and ordered to begin antisyphilitic treatment immediately. When this was brought to the attention of the Health Officer of Macon County, Murray Smith, he "furnished the local board a list containing 256 names of men under 45 years of age and asked that these men be excluded from the list of draftees needing treatment."[60] The chairman of the local draft board, a personal friend of Smith's, complied with that request. Some test subjects, who had already been hospitalized for the purpose of treatment, were released without further explanation,[61] and Vonderlehr boasted in 1942 that "So far, we are keeping the known positive patients from getting treatment."[62] In 1943, the Henderson Act, a new public health law inspired by the realities of the war, required state and local health officials to test everyone between 14 and 50 years of age for tuberculosis and venereal diseases, and to treat those found to be infected. In violation of that law, the subjects in the Tuskegee Study continued to be exempted from treatment.[63]

22 · Experiments on African-Americans

Despite Penicillin, the Study Goes On . . . and On

When penicillin became available in the mid 1940s and "Rapid Treatment Centers" for syphilis were established by the Public Health Service (Fig. 503), the physicians in charge of the Tuskegee Study did their best to withhold penicillin from their test subjects. They were partially successful; although almost 30 percent of the men had received some penicillin by 1952, only 7.5 percent of them had received what could be considered an adequate dose.[64] In a letter to a participating physician, Vonderlehr expressed the hope "that the availability of antibiotics has not interfered too much with this project."[65] Instead of terminating the Tuskegee Study with the advent of penicillin and dispensing that "wonder drug" immediately to those infected systemically with spirochetes, health care officials emphasized the importance of the Study, contending that it could never be duplicated. According to Surgeon General Parran (Fig. 504), the experiment had become "more significant" because it could be used as a "necessary control against which to project not only the results obtained with the rapid schedules of therapy for syphilis but also the costs involved in finding and placing under treatment the infected individuals."[66] Even as late as 1969, officers of the PHS persuaded local physicians of Macon County to abstain from giving antibiotics to subjects of the Tuskegee study, thereby barring them from adequate treatment not only for syphilis, but also for other bacterial infections.[67]

The results of the study were assessed at periodic intervals. In a progress report in 1953, it was mentioned that "each of the patients was followed up with an annual blood test and, whenever the Public Health Service physicians came to Tuskegee,

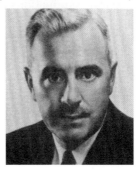

FIG. 504
Thomas Parran (1892-1968)

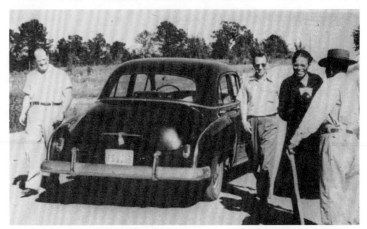

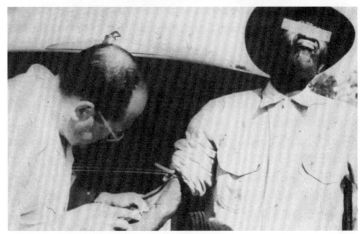

physical examinations were repeated"[68] (Fig. 505, 506). The results of the first assessment of test subjects were published by Vonderlehr in 1936, and they indicated that "only 16 percent of the 399 syphilitic Negroes gave no evidence of morbidity, as compared with 61 percent of the 201 presumably nonsyphilitic Negroes."[69] The second examination was made in the years 1938 and 1939, and the third in 1948. By that time, this is what was known: "First, that untreated syphilis apparently shortens the life expectancy by 20 percent: Second, that there is a greater

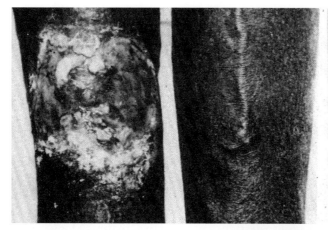

FIG. 507
Ulcerated lesion of syphilis on the leg of a subject of the Tuskegee Study.

involvement of the cardiovascular system, and third, that syphilitics without treatment appear to be subject to a higher rate of other types of morbidity." In 1950, Oliver Wenger admitted some wrongdoing at a seminar in Hot Springs when he said this: "We know now, where we could only surmise before, that we have contributed to their ailments and shortened their lives" (Fig. 507, 508). In spite of these alarming consequences and his own admission of guilt, Wenger did not call for the termination instantly of the study. Instead, he asked for additional funds, exhorting "that we have a high moral obligation to those that have died to make this the best study possible."[70] Likewise, dermatologist Sidney Olansky of Atlanta (Fig. 509), the principal author or coauthor of more publications ema-

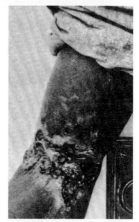

FIG. 508
Ulcerated lesion of syphilis on the arm of a subject of the Tuskegee Study.

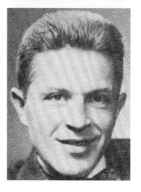

FIG. 509
Sidney Olansky (born 1914)

nating from the Tuskegee Study than anyone else, stressed that the National Health Service had a "responsibility to the survivors, both for their care and really to prove that their willingness to serve, even at risk of shortening of life, as experimental subjects" was rewarded by generating scientific results of merit.[71]

Long Study, Short Results

Of course, survivors had never been asked, and had never expressed their willingness, to serve continuously as experimental subjects. The "care" to which Olansky referred consisted of the administration of noneffective treatment for yet another 20 years. In the end, the scientific results of this long, complex, and behemoth study were meager. From a strictly scientific vantage, the Tuskegee study of untreated syphilis could have led to much better information than that produced by the earlier study of Boeck and Bruusgaard. The Oslo study was retrospective rather than prospective, almost 80 percent of Boeck's original patients being lost to follow-up, and many of the remaining patients being in need of continuous medical care. Thus, the sample examined by Bruusgaard was highly selective and not representative of Boeck's original group. Bruusgaard himself had alerted to the fact that acceptance of his data should be made "with the reservation always required by the nature of the material."[72] The theoretical advantages of a prospective investigation, however, were not utilized in the Tuskegee study. The purpose and the methods of study never were stated clearly; the study groups were not defined precisely, a protocol or procedures for standardization did not exist, and, with the exception of Nurse Rivers, the key personnel changed continually over the years. As a consequence, many examinations remained incomplete. Moreover, insufficient funding prevented sufficient personnel from being employed and made close supervision of test subjects impossible. Originally, Macon County had been chosen as the site for the study not only because of the high incidence of syphilis and the rarity of treatment given there, but also because its poor black population remained in place. In actuality, however, many of the men eventually left the county, if only temporarily, to seek work elsewhere. Outside the county, physicians were not aware of the study and, for that reason, most test subjects received some penicillin, not for syphilis as a rule, but for an unrelated disease. Nevertheless, even a brief course of penicillin diminished greatly the significance of the findings in these subjects.[73]

The physicians responsible for the Tuskegee Study were aware of how poor was the quality of it scientifically. With few exceptions – such as the higher incidence of syphilitic aortitis, lymphadenitis and encephalitis – the findings were not in themselves new. The study merely corroborated what already was known. When Wenger, in 1950, reviewed the findings, such as increased morbidity of test subjects and earlier death of them, he conceded that "this is probably what most people might expect from general knowledge or assumption." Still, he added lamely, ". . . it is important to have the facts documented."[75] Because of flaws inherent in the method, the aspirations for the future of the study were humble. In 1951, Olansky elaborated on plans for a comprehensive workup of test subjects and predicted the following result: "From this type of work-up it is anticipated that data comparable with the Bruusgaard material may be obtained."[76] In spite of the sobering analyses, the study was continued. Its longevity and the costs that had accumulated over the years made it difficult for those responsible to admit that the entire endeavor had been a failure scientifically from the outset. As a senior official of the Public Health Service noted, ". . . we have an investment of almost 20 years of division interest, funds, and personnel."[77] That investment was too high to be written off and, therefore, nothing changed; complete reassessment of test subjects was carried out in 1952, 1954, 1963, and 1970.[78]

On September 10, 1970, James B. Lucas, the assistant chief of the Venereal Disease Branch of the Public Health Service, completed an "analysis of the current status of the Tuskegee Study." This was his view of the matter just as he stated it: "The greatest contribution that the Tuskegee Study has made and can continue to provide has been documented sera for study in our laboratory. Without those sera the problem of evaluating new serologic tests becomes much more difficult and the results less certain. In a great measure the development and our endorsement of the FTA-ABS test rested on Tuskegee sera."[79] The same was true for the VDRL test, another laboratory evaluation employed often for diagnosis of syphilis. The blood samples taken annually from subjects in Tuskegee enabled the Public Health Service to acquire international leadership in serologic aspects of syphilis and thereby dominate a market of considerable commercial value, serologic tests for diagnosis of syphilis being sold throughout the world.[80] In regard to clinical aspects of the Tuskegee Study, Lucas concluded thus:

While some medical knowledge has been gained from this study, its volume and quality has been less than gleaned from the preceding Boeck-Bruusgaard study . . . It must be fully realized that the remaining contribution from this study will be largely of historical interest. Nothing learned will prevent, find, or cure a single case of infectious syphilis or bring us closer to our basic mission of controlling venereal disease in the United States.

Lucas suggested, nevertheless, that "the study may be continued along its present lines."[81]

Beginning To See the Light

Details of the Tuskegee Study were set forth in the medical literature in a series of articles from 1936 through 1973. Although these articles had an estimated readership of up to 100,000 physicians,[82] no comments critical of ethical aspects of the study were voiced until 1965. That year, Irwin J. Schatz of the Henry Ford Hospital in Detroit wrote to Donald H. Rockwell, the author of a progress report about the study, of his own reservations and he did that in these poignant words:

I am utterly astounded by the fact that physicians allow patients with a potentially fatal disease to remain untreated when effective therapy is available. I assume you feel that the information which is extracted from the observation of this untreated group is worth their sacrifice. If this is the case, then I suggest that the United States Public Health Service and those physicians associated with it in this study need to re-evaluate their moral judgments in this regard.[83]

Schatz's letter went unanswered; and for a few years no further criticism of the Tuskegee Study was heard. The times, however, had changed. Discussions about the Declaration of Helsinki, issued in 1964, reminded the medical community of ethical limitations of research, and African-Americans were achieving more strength politically and self-confidence personally and as a group. In the late 1950s and early 1960s, a powerful movement was forged against racial segregation in the South, culminating in 1963 in a demonstration of more than 200,000 persons in Washington, D.C. that ended with an historic speech by Martin Luther King, in which he told fellow Americans of his "dream that one day this nation will rise up and will live out these truths that all men are created equal"[84] (Fig. 510). Largely as a result of these activities, legislation prohibiting racial discrimination was enacted in the ensuing

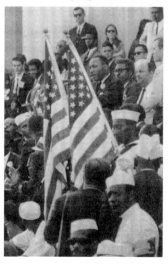

FIG. 510
Martin Luther King speaking at the Lincoln Memorial in 1963.

The Abuse of Man

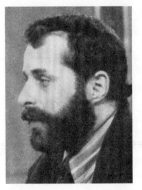

years. In 1964, a Civil Rights Act forbade registrars from applying different standards to white and black citizens who wished to cast a vote, outlawed racial discrimination in public facilities, enjoined private employers and unions from racial discrimination, and authorized the U.S. Attorney General to file a complaint where there was a "pattern or practice" of widespread discrimination. In the context of this sociopolitical background, it was only a matter of time before the emergence of public outrage about a medical experiment in Macon County, Alabama that involved black test subjects exclusively and was conducted in startling violation of accepted ethical principles of research.

The experiment at Tuskegee was brought to public attention widely by Peter J. Buxton (Fig. 511), a young employee of the Public Health Service in San Francisco. One of Buxton's duties was to write a bimonthly narrative about a subject of research related to the work of the Service. In the fall of 1966, he came across the Tuskegee files and compared that study with Nazi medical experiments at Dachau. Ignoring warnings from his superiors that he could be fired, he sent a letter to William J. Brown (Fig. 512), who, as director of the Division of Venereal Diseases, had assumed responsibility for the Tuskegee study in 1957. In it, he explained his "grave moral doubts as to the propriety of this study," especially addressing the following aspects:

1) The group is 100% Negro. This in itself is political dynamite and subject to wide journalistic misinterpretation. It also follows the thinking of Negro militants that Negros have long been used for 'medical experiments' and 'teaching cases' in the emergency wards of county hospitals. 2) The group is not composed of 'volunteers with social motives.' They are largely uneducated, unsophisticated,

and quite ignorant of the effects of un-treated syphilis.

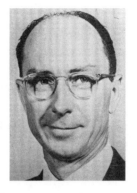

FIG. 512
*William J.
Brown*

Buxton ended his letter by asking Brown to inform him "that the study group has been, or soon will be, treated."[85]

Alarmed by the threat of adverse publicity, Brown, on February 6, 1969, convened a blue-ribbon panel for the purpose of discussing the Tuskegee Study. All participants of the panel were physicians, and only one of them voiced ethical concerns about the study. The other physicians decided, without having stud-ied a single individual case, that treatment at that late stage of syphilis probably would no longer be beneficial and, therefore, saw no point in stopping the study. Instead, they recommended that the study be upgraded scientifically by focusing on findings in syphilis pathologically and by making greater efforts to lo-cate subjects who had been lost to follow-up. When the issues of informing test subjects about the truth of the matter and ob-taining their consent about foregoing treatment were raised, most of the committee assumed the stance that it was impossi-ble to obtain "informed consent" from men of such limited edu-cation and low social status.[86]

Soon after the meeting of the panel, Brown informed Buxton that a "committee of highly competent professionals did not agree nor recommend that the study group be treated. The youngest living member of the study group is 69 years old. The question of treating persons of this age and older, unless it is demonstrated that active disease is present, is a matter of med-ical judgment since the benefits of such therapy must be offset against the risks to the individual . . . You can be assured that competent professionals have studied the point you made and that each person still in the study will be evaluated fully."[87]

In short, nothing changed after Brown's panel had convened, except for the zeal with which the Public Health Service pursued the subjects lost to follow-up. In desperation, Buxton informed a friend in the Associated Press about the study, and, on July 26, 1972, an article about the experiment appeared in the *The New York Times*. The story was picked up by many other news media, instantaneously creating disbelief, furor, and accusations that ranged from "moral astigmatism" to "racial genocide" (Fig. 513, 514). At that time, 74 of the test subjects still were alive. At least 28, but perhaps more than 100, men had died as a direct consequence of advanced syphilis before the study was halted by the Department of Health, Education and Welfare in the summer of 1972.[88] The Tuskegee Syphilis Study, with a duration of 40 years, was the longest nontherapeutic experiment on human beings in medical history.[89]

FIG. 513
"Now can we give him penicillin?" (editorial cartoon by Tony Auth, "Philadelphia Inquirer," July 1972).

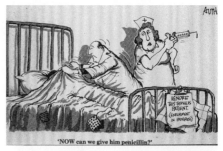

FIG. 514
The "Secret Tuskegee Study" (editorial cartoon by Lou Erikson, "Atlanta Constitution," July 1972).

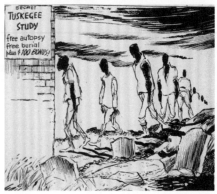

CHAPTER 23

THE "MOST CAPTIVE"
POPULATION

I n the realm of human experimentation, the recruitment of test subjects from vulnerable populations, such as prisoners, orphans, and the mentally incompetent, was an issue of controversy and debate. An American physician with a long history of using prisoners as test subjects, however, averred that "the most coercive element" for volunteers in medical experiments is the patient's "great faith, confidence, and trust in his physician." He acknowledged unflinchingly that "the most captive of the people I have ever used have been patient-subjects."[1]

The Ties That Bind – Patients and Physicians

A patient in the grip of a frightening and possibly fatal disease may, indeed, feel more constrained by his disease than a delinquent collared by a policeman. A patient seeking help for his ailments is more dependent on physicians than, for example, a healthy prisoner. Of course, a patient able physically is free to get up and walk away; such a person has the right to consult freely other physicians. That right, however, rarely has been exercised, and for a variety of reasons. First, most patients cannot afford to be highly selective in their choice of physicians, a reality that is applicable especially to persons who are disadvantaged economically and who, therefore, are most likely to become a victim of medical experiments. Paul Beeson, a specialist in infectious diseases and immunology at Emory University and later chairman of the department of medicine at Yale University, recalled that in regard to patients who were poor, ". . . we were taking care of them, and felt we had a right to get some return from them, since it wouldn't be in professional fees and since our taxes were paying their hospital bills."[2] Before systems of medical insurance were established during the administration of President Lyndon B. Johnson in the mid 1960s, economically impaired citizens of the United States considered themselves fortunate if they were able to obtain advanced medical care at all. That being the case, waiving their doctor's and hospital's fees was a strong incentive for participation in medical experiments. It was standard procedure for the Clinical Center of the National Institutes of Health (NIH) to waive fees in order to recruit test subjects. Because participation in medical research was considered to be "an important contribution for the advancement of knowledge," representatives of the NIH "decided that it would not be proper to require the patient to pay."[3]

Second, patients had no reason to believe that they would be treated by physicians in a manner other than in their own best interests. They had been brought up in a medical system that was based on trust and predicated on a bond with an individual physician. Before World War II, most Americans were cared for by a general practitioner who lived in their neighborhood; many of those physicians had cared for several generations of their family. According to one survey undertaken between 1928 and 1931, in the days when physicians made "house calls," 81 percent of patient visits were to general practitioners,[4] and more than half the patients were seen by a doctor in their own home.[5] In the absence of sophisticated diagnostic techniques, knowing a patient's living conditions and family history was important for management effectively, and physicians relied greatly on exchange of information in direct conversations with their patients.[6] All of this strengthened the personal bond between physician and patient, and the doctor often was perceived as being part of an extended family (Fig. 515).

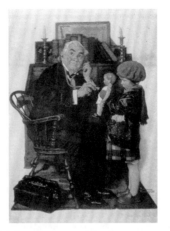

FIG. 515
The physician as friend: "Doctor and Doll" (painting by Norman Rockwell, 1929).

The situation changed with breakthroughs in medical research that resulted in improved medical care, but concurrent with it came progressive alienation of patients from doctors. As new diagnostic techniques became available, conversation between physician and patient seemed to become less necessary and often was sacrificed as pressures of time on doctors mounted. Increasingly, patients came to consult a cadre of "specialists," rather than visiting a general practitioner for their every medical need, thereby exchanging established familiarity for enhanced expertise. By the early 1960s, only 20 percent of physicians identified themselves as general practitioners, and house calls represented less than one percent of all contacts between doctors and patients.[7] Although physicians became strangers to patients, the mentality of trust on the part of the patients nevertheless was sustained. Patients came to hospitals confident that they would receive proper medical care. It never occurred to them that, as they lay ailing in a hospital bed, they could be exposed to unpleasant and often risky procedures that afforded them no benefit whatsoever. Medicine had become so technical and complex that it was impossible for the vast majority of patients to judge whether a given medical procedure was advisable or even necessary. That judgment had to be left to physicians, and patients were not competent enough to challenge the authority of them (Fig. 516).

Third, most patients were not brash enough to challenge

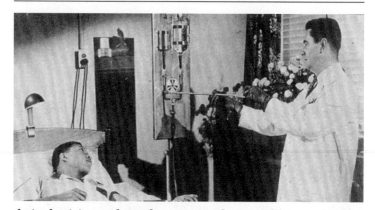

their physicians, who no longer were their neighbors and sometimes even peers socially. To them physicians now seemed like a
caste of priests who in their temples performed miraculous and
frightening procedures. Those temples, with their maze of
buildings, floors, and signs, and their snarl of physicians, nurses, and technicians running to and fro, were impressive and in-
timidating, and they left patients with a distinct sense of pow-
erlessness (Fig. 517). Physicians, too, began to share the feeling
of alienation. More and more they lived in a world apart from
that of their patients, a world of medicine that absorbed most of
their energy, leaving little time for nonmedical activities. In
comparison with prewar medicine, although patients admitted

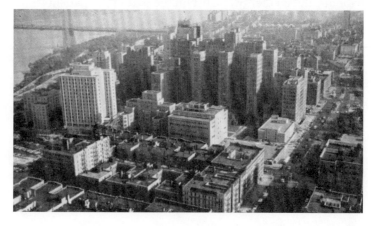

to hospitals in major medical centers were more seriously ill, the length of their stay was shortened. Pressure on physicians to move on to the next "case" made it difficult increasingly for doctors to establish a personal relationship with patients.[8] Moreover, the gap in education, social standing, and economic status between the average patient and the typical doctor was widening. In this regard, Paul Beeson stated that before the advent of Medicare and Medicaid

. . . academics and medical students did their work in charity hospitals. I feel that I am right in saying that we medical students and our teachers looked upon ourselves as belonging to another social class from the patients we were taking care of. That they were lucky to be getting care of the best doctors in the community.[9]

The relationship between physicians and patients no longer was that of partners working together to achieve health for patients, but that of priests and parishioners, kings and subjects. Radiologist Leonard Sagan observed that "in 1945, '50, the doctor . . . was king or queen. It never occurred to a doctor to ask consent for anything . . . They were in charge and nobody questioned their authority."[10] William Silverman, a pediatrician who practiced and did research at the College of Physicians and Surgeons of Columbia University, recalled that

. . . the model was in religion, that is, faith in the priest who will speak to God and get the answer. We were encouraged to behave like priests . . . It was a conscious effort to make patients feel they were in the presence of healers.[11]

The Schizophrenic Nature of the Physician-Scientist

The unquestioned imperial authority of physicians had always been considered to be a rudimentary principle of therapy adjuvant in medicine. The power of suggestion in the restoration of health was well known for centuries; despite the development of increasingly rational regimens of treatment, that power never had lost its potency. What had changed was the way medicine was practiced. Because the relationship between physicians and patients had become more distant and impersonal, patients were viewed increasingly as "cases." This attitude was fostered by a transition in medicine from practice solely to research full-time ideally. As research became more and more the new symbol of status in American medicine, more and more physicians thought of themselves as researchers first, and only secondarily as healers committed singlemindedly to the care of each individual human being in their charge. Although these two modes were not necessarily exclusive mutually, in actuality they had little in common with one another. In his presidential address to the Society of Clinical Research in Chicago in 1952, William B. Bean, then chairman of the department of medicine at the University of Iowa, warned of "the wide cleavage which separates clinicians from investigators in their split personality. As physicians, their prime concern is the intimate personal responsibility in caring for sick people. As investigators, they are goaded by discontent and impelled by curiosity as well as ambition for renown. Such stimuli sometimes suppress the physician altogether."[12] In the same year, Sir William Heneage Ogilvie of Guy's Hospital in London (Fig. 518) made this observation:

In becoming scientists rather than healers, in making the centre of our interest the laboratory rather than the bedside, in organizing ourselves and our work on a nation-wide basis, we are losing that personal contact which has characterized medicine since prehistoric times . . . The science of experimental medicine is something new, and, to those brought up in the Hippocratic tradition, something sinister; for it is capable of destroying in our minds the old faith that we are the servants of the patients whom we have undertaken to care for, and in the minds of the patients the complete trust that they can place their lives, or those of their loved ones, in our care, knowing that we will help them if it is in our power to do so.[13]

23 · The "Most Captive" Population

Philippe Cardon, a psychiatrist at the NIH, said this unambiguously: "If we were more interested in taking care of patients than in research, we wouldn't be here. It is unrealistic to expect most very good investigators also to be very good physicians (and vice versa)."[14] Hungarian Nobel laureate, Albert Szent-Györgyi, commented at an international medical congress in 1961 thus:

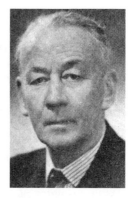

FIG. 518
William Heneage Ogilvie (1887-1971)

The desire to alleviate suffering is of small value in research – such a person should be advised to work for charity. Research wants egoists, damned egoists, who seek their own pleasure and satisfaction, but find it in solving the puzzles of nature.[15]

The difference between the traditional virtue of altruism of physicians and the new virtue of egoism of scientists in pursuit of knowledge prompted Otto Guttentag (Fig. 519) of the School of Medicine of the University of California in San Francisco to propose in 1953 that a distinction be made clearly between the "physician-friend" and the "physician-experimenter."Guttentag explained his thesis in these lines:

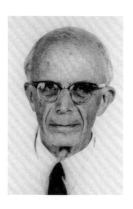

FIG. 519
Otto Guttentag (1900-1992)

The patient-physician relationship is fully understood only when viewed from two aspects. The relationship of the one who performs experiments of no immediate value to the person under observation is impersonal and objective because of the character of the research. Experimentation is the basis on which the two meet, the original bond between them. The fact that the experimenter is a physician is, from this point of view, almost incidental ... Obviously, there exists a second, quite different, relationship between a physician and a sick person. Historically, it is the original and, indeed, the basic justification for our profession. Here one human being is in distress, in need, crying for help; and another fellow human being is concerned and wants to assist him . . . Objective experimentation to confirm or disprove some doubtful or suggested biological generalization is foreign to this relationship. It is not the point of contact between the two partners, for it would involve taking advantage of the patient's cry for help, and of his insecurity.

Guttentag sought to reconcile both aspects of the professional activity of physicians by having strictures of the legal profession adopted by them. "As we all know," he advised, "that profession provides each of the two with a representative of equal stature: there, the prosecuting attorney, and here, the defense attorney. Similar arrangements may have to be developed in the field of human experimentation . . . Research and care would not be pursued by the same doctor for the same person, but would be kept distinct."[16]

In research involving healthy subjects, the dualism between the "physician-friend" and the "physician-experimenter" was irrelevant because the role of the physician as experimenter was evident. In research involving patient-subjects, however, failure to implement Guttentag's suggestion resulted in causing the two aspects of the medical profession to be confused. Physicians who used patients for medical experiments maintained that strict requirements for information and consent would

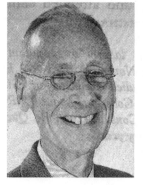

FIG. 520
*Robert
Alexander
McCance
(1898-1993)*

jeopardize the patient's trust in the physician and thus be detrimental to the process of healing. In his president's address to the Royal Society of Medicine in 1950, Robert A. McCance of London (Fig. 520) warned that "the whole atmosphere of trust would be destroyed if patients had to be asked to fill in a printed form of consent for experiment as they are as a rule for an operation."[17] Sir Austin Bradford Hill (Fig. 521), Professor Emeritus of medical statistics at the University of London, in a lecture given to the Royal College of Physicians in 1963, stated that although a patient's consent in regard to participation in therapeutic trials was desirable, it was not always requisite. This is what he said then about consent:

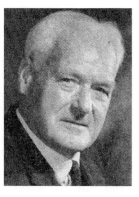

FIG. 521
Austin Bradford Hill (1897-1991)

There are circumstances in which it need not – and even should not – be sought . . . The situation implicit in the controlled trial is that one has two (or more) possible treatments and that one is wholly, or to a very large extent, ignorant of their relative values (and dangers). Can you describe that situation to a patient so that he does not lose confidence in you – the essence of the doctor/patient relationship – and in such a way that he fully understands and can therefore give an understanding consent to his inclusion in a trial? . . . If the patient cannot really grasp the whole situation, or without upsetting his faith in your judgment cannot be made to grasp it, then in my opinion the ethical decision still lies with the doctor, whether or not it is proper to exhibit, or withhold a treatment . . . Having made up your mind that you are not in any way subjecting either patient to a recognized and unjustifiable danger, pain, or discomfort, can anything be gained ethically by endeavouring to explain to them your own state of ignorance and to describe the attempts you are making to remove it?[18]

The comments of Bradford Hill did not go unchallenged. Helen S.U. Hodgson, chairman of a British Patients Association, found it "astonishing to a layman to read a commentary on medical ethics which appears to advocate a doctor/patient relationship based upon deceit."[19] In the discourse that followed, however, most physicians endorsed Hill's view of the matter. One physician posed this question: "In the interests of 'truth' is every patient to be regaled with lists of possible complications and the mortality rate of a recommended operation? Is it deceitful for an honest and ethical doctor to protect his patient from knowledge which he believes to be prejudicial to his welfare?"[20] Another physician merely phrased it differently: "Many patients cannot accept psychologically the full truth about their condition. How then can they make a proper judgment about a trial of treatment?"[21] Similar assertions were made by researchers in the United States. One of the directors of the NIH declared that "the usual patient" wants "to avoid the necessity of grappling with painful facts related to his own welfare. He prefers (and in a real sense he has no other choice) to depend on an overriding faith that the physician and institution will safeguard his interests above any other consideration."[22] Donald Fredrickson of the National Heart Institute contended that providing detailed information to patients about aspects of research would "unduly alarm the patient and hinder his reasonable evaluation of procedures important to his welfare."[23]

In brief, medical researchers, in defending their freedom as "physician-experimenters," advanced arguments on their own behalf as "physician-friends." It was in the best interest of patients, they insisted, that requirements for informed consent had to be curtailed. As a consequence, patients in medical experiments became the least protected of all groups of test subjects. When written consent began to be required in the United States, patient-subjects were excluded. Joseph W. Gardella of Harvard called such a requirement "inappropriate." In a critique of the "Principles, Policies, and Rules of the Surgeon General," Gardella wrote in 1961 that the requirement of written consent is "inappropriate except in connection with healthy volunteers. The legal overtones and implications attendant to such a requirement have no place in a patient-physician relationship based on trust. Here such faith and trust serve as the primary basis of the subject's consent. Moreover, being asked to sign a somewhat formal paper is likely to provoke anxiety in the subject who can but wonder at the need for so much protocol."[24] In response to that criticism, Surgeon General Leonard D. Heaton waived the requirement of written consent of patient-subjects in contracts with Harvard University regarding research on humans. At the Clinical Center of the NIH, formal review and approval of a protocol for experiments on humans was required only for research involving healthy volunteers, not patients.[25] Likewise, the 1964 Declaration of Helsinki created two separate categories in laying out rules for experiments on humans, namely, "Non-therapeutic Clinical Research" and "Clinical Research Combined with Professional Care." In the latter category, physicians were obligated to obtain consent from patient-subjects only when it was "consistent with patient psychology."[26]

Human Lab Rats

In reality, "patient psychology" rarely was considered at all when it came to medical experiments. Patients were conceived to be"clinical material" available readily, which was an expedient solution to the need for human subjects. Louis Lasagna, who was involved in clinical research at Harvard in the 1950s, remembered those days thus:

It was as if, and I'm putting this very crudely purposefully, as if you'd ordered a bunch of rats from a laboratory and you had experimental subjects available for you.[27]

The type of studies carried out on patients varied greatly. Many studies actually were devoted to new therapies and held out possible benefits for those who participated in them. In those instances, informed consent usually was obtained easily. As noted at a conference titled "Concept of Consent in Clinical Research" at Boston University in 1961, informing subjects of potentially beneficial research was "psychologically more comfortable for investigators" because "the expectations of potential subjects coincide with the purpose and expected results of the experiments." When experiments held out no possible benefits for patients, however, the policy in regard to informing them was different. The report of the conference made clear that "it is most often subjects in this category to whom disclosure is not made." The conferees acknowledged that rather than seeking consent from patients to research that offers them no benefit, the "therapeutic illusion is maintained, and the patient is often not even told that he is participating in research. Instead, he is told he is 'just going to have a test.'"[28]

Even if experiments offered no direct benefit to patients, many of those studies were concerned with the disease that itself afflicted the patients. Studies on pregnant women carried out between 1945 and 1947 at Vanderbilt University in Nashville, Tennessee, are illustrative of that phenomenon. To find out how pregnancy and parturition are affected by diet and nutrition, radioactive iron was administered to 829 women under the guise of "a little cocktail" that will "make you feel better." During the time that experiment was being conducted, the physician responsible for the study, Paul Hahn (Fig. 522), informed colleagues that ". . . radioactive iron, regardless of the amount of activity contained, is, to my knowledge, of no value whatsoever in therapy" because the half-life of it is "far too long." Consideration of that knowledge, however, was reserved only for ordinary patients but was neglected completely for subjects of research. In

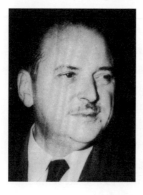

the years that followed, many of the mothers and children exposed *in utero* to radioactive iron in the experiment at Vanderbilt developed effects such as loss of teeth and hair, dermatoses, anemia, and cancer. A follow-up study of the offspring in 1969 revealed that fatal malignancies had developed in four children who had been exposed to radiation *in utero*, whereas no cancers were found in a control group. For the authors, those results suggested "a cause and effect relationship." In their judgment, the findings represented "a small, but statistically significant increase . . . consistent with previous radiobiologic experience."[29]

Pregnant women also were exposed to other types of radiation. For example, a physician in St. Louis, a certain Dr. Hartnett, decided in 1948, "to investigate the possible value of aortography in the diagnosis of placenta praevia." He subjected 66 pregnant women who, at that time, did not have any serious medical condition, to translumbar aortography.[30] The procedure not only was associated with prolonged exposure to X-irradiation, but it also carried the risk of inadvertent puncture of internal organs, such as kidneys, colon, and pancreas. Moreover, injection of the contrast medium into the wall of the aorta was a dreaded complication that could lead to dissection and rupture of the wall of the major blood vessel, with subsequent death.[31] In Hartnett's study, no fatal complications were recorded, although the contrast medium was injected inadvertently outside the aorta in 13 patients.[32] In 1961, physicians of the State University of New York at Brooklyn probed the circulation of the placenta by injecting a contrast medium into the femoral artery of 20 parturients and then taking serial X-rays of the blood vessels of the uterus and placenta. The authors acknowledged that "the consequences of radiation exposure have become a major concern in roentgenology and particularly where pregnant women are concerned." They noted also that "arteriography is not advocated as a routine procedure, but in indicated cases which present difficult diagnostic problems, this procedure may be of considerable diagnostic value." In the particular patients being studied, however, there was no problem in regard to diagnosis. The authors stated unabashedly that "no particular effort was made to select patients either for diagnosis or because they showed abnormalities, but rather to survey the possibilities of the technique as a diagnostic tool and as a research instrument for the study of placental circulation."[33]

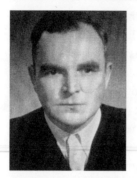

FIG. 523
*Herbert
Gerstner
(born 1910)*

Patients with cancer often were preyed on by physicians and other scientists. For example, the U.S. military, in an effort to enhance its knowledge on the effects of radiation, initiated trials of total-body irradiation in patients with cancer at different medical centers in the United States. One such trial was carried out in the mid 1950s at the M.D. Anderson Cancer Center in Houston, Texas, under the supervision of Herbert Gerstner (Fig. 523), a German physiologist and former Nazi who had been brought to the United States through "Operation Paperclip." Thirty patient-subjects, most of whom were still ambulatory and capable of performing "light tasks," were exposed to a single dose of up to 200 roentgens of total-body irradiation, an amount that was associated with severe side effects such as nausea and vomiting. Following radiation, patients had to perform psychomotor tests – such as operating two crank handles to keep a cursor positioned on a moving target – that were "chosen because of their proven relationship to the skills required in basic pilotry." Within 20 months, all 30 patients who had received 200 roentgens died. Scientists concluded that total body irradiation did not alter significantly the course of the disease. In only three subjects, they claimed, did it seem to have produced a transitory, and clinically unsupported, sense of well-being.[34]

Despite these discouraging results, the wish to learn more about the effects of radiation resulted in several other trials of total-body irradiation. In order to transpose findings in patients with cancer to subjects who were healthy, researchers specifically sought patients with radioresistant tumors, stable blood status, and normal kidney function. These subjects resembled closely healthy soldiers or persons who worked with radioactive material, results of the studies thus being unlikely

to be confused by effects therapeutically. In other respects, studies also were
adjusted to the needs of the military
agencies who paid for them. Eugene
Saenger (Fig. 524), who conducted an
extensive trial of total-body irradiation
at Cincinnati General Hospital in the
1960s and early 1970s, informed the
Defense Department that, "... whenev-

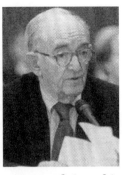

FIG. 524
*Eugene Saenger
(born 1917)*

er possible, unidirectional radiation will be attempted since this
type of exposure is of military interest." Moreover, patient-subjects had to undergo psychological tests that measured depression, hope, denial, and pessimism, while at the same time being
denied medications that would alleviate nausea following total-
body irradiation. This experiment was designed to simulate a
combat situation. In reports to the Defense Atomic Support
Agency, Saenger pointed out that he desired to acquire "a better
understanding of the acute and sub-acute effects of irradiation
in the human" and stressed that "this information is necessary to
provide knowledge of combat effectiveness of troops and to develop additional methods of diagnosis, prognosis, prophylaxis
and treatment of these injuries." Test subjects, who were described in progress reports as "in relatively good health," able to
"perform activities of daily living," and "clinically stable, many of
them working daily," were not informed about the purpose of the
study or of its side effects. Many suffered severe complications,
such as depression of bone marrow, infections, loss of ability to
control body functions, and excruciating pain. In the 1970s, a
faculty committee of the University of Cincinnati reviewed the
study and determined that 19 patients had died within 20 to 60
days after total-body irradiation. They admitted that these patients "could have died from radiation alone."[35]

Patients were used not only for generating data on experimental modalities of treatment that offered them no benefit,

but also for developing new techniques for diagnosis. For example, in 1961, physicians of several New York hospitals described a method called "antethoracic pancardiocentesis" that consisted of transthoracic insertion of needles into the right atrium and the right ventricle of the heart, followed by piercing of the septum to enter the left atrium and the left ventricle. Five of 93 patients, most of whom had valvular disease, developed severe complications, including coronary thrombosis and severe hemorrhage. One of them died secondary to hepatitis brought about by blood transfusions given to combat the hemorrhage. The authors of the study stated that ". . . these undesirable events occurred for the most part in the first dozen examinations. This suggests that we may hope to avoid them with care and experience."[36]

Deliberately Causing More Harm

In many studies undertaken by physicians, effective treatment was withheld from patients. Although it was known that rheumatic fever can be prevented in most instances by treatment of a streptococcal respiratory infection with penicillin, doctors of the U.S. Air Force gave placebos to 109 men suffering from that infection. Two of the men developed acute rheumatic fever and one acute glomerular nephritis, whereas no complications were observed in patients who had been treated with penicillin.[37] The same physician coworkers tried to determine whether complications of acute streptococcal pharyngitis could be prevented by administration of sulfonamides. For that purpose, more than 500 men were denied penicillin, some of them being treated with sulfonamides and others with no antibiotic at all. Rheumatic fever developed in 5.4 and 4.2 percent of the patients, respectively.[38] None of the subjects were informed either of the purpose or the risks, none had consented to the study, and none were aware that they were involved in an experiment.[39] Physicians at Hammersmith Hospital in London with-held insulin from patients with diabetes mellitus in order to investigate the output of sugar by the liver, both before and after injections of insulin: "Aspiration biopsies of the liver were performed in many instances in order that histological changes in the liver might be correlated with the hepatic insulin sensitivity as shown by hepatic vein catheterisation."[40] At the time the study was being conducted, the death rate as a consequence of liver biopsies was estimated to be 2 to 3 per 1,000 cases.[41] In another study, the same English researchers gave patients with diabetes doses of insulin that were high enough to lower the content of blood sugar to a degree that resulted in "sweating, drowsiness, pallor, fainting and fall of blood pressure."[42]

In many experiments that produced no benefit for patients, the diseases from which they suffered were aggravated intentionally. For example, patients with liver disease were given nitrogenous substances of known toxic potential that caused transient, and even persistent, neuropsychological disorders, ranging from tremor of the limbs to disturbances of the brain. The investigators reported that "the first sign noted was usually clouding of the consciousness," and proceeded to declare that the "marked resemblance between this reaction and impending hepatic coma implied that the administration of these substances to patients with cirrhosis may be hazardous."[43] In a project titled "Production of Impending Hepatic Coma by Chlorothiazide and Its Prevention by Antibiotics," the diuretic, chlorothiazide, which was known to be hazardous to patients with liver disease, was given to 20 patients with severe cirrhosis. The authors set out to determine if the mental deterioration that occurred in these patients after administration of the drug was associated with particular changes in levels in serum and urine of ammonia, potassium, and other substances, and whether the mental deterioration could be prevented by administration of antibiotics that were not absorbable.[44] Hundreds of patients with cardiac disease were subjected to catheterization of the heart combined with physical exercise, inhalation of various concentrations of oxygen, and administration of a variety of drugs, the purpose being to elucidate issues such as "the effects of acetylcholine upon respiratory gas exchange in mitral stenosis" and "the relationship of cardiac respiratory effects of exercise and arterial concentrations of lactate and pyruvic acid in patients with rheumatic heart disease." In some patients, acute cardiac failure was induced deliberately by intense physical exercise.[45]

In the remarkable spectrum of diseases that were explored by experimenting on patients who suffered from them, skin diseases were no exception. As but one example, a host of studies with radioactive substances were performed on patients with psoriasis in order to assess the proliferation of epidermal cells and the role of vascular changes. Edward H. Ferguson and William L. Epstein of San Francisco studied "the local hemodynamics of psoriatic plaques" by measuring "skin clearance of radioactive substances" injected into the skin.[46] Gerald D. Weinstein and Eugene J. Van Scott (Fig. 525) of the dermatology branch of the National Cancer Institute at Bethesda, Maryland performed an "autoradiographic analysis of turnover times of normal and psoriatic epidermis" by examining biopsy specimens following intradermal injection of tritiated thymidine. In

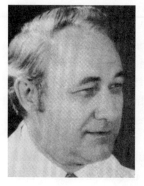

FIG. 525
Eugene J.
Van Scott
(born 1922)

each of their patients, 10 different lesions of psoriasis were selected for the injections and "sequential 4 mm punch biopsy specimens were obtained from injected sites at 1, 12, 24 hours, and at 2, 3, 8, 10, 12, 14, and 16 days." Sequential biopsies from normal appearing skin of patients with psoriasis, mycosis fungoides, and basal-cell carcinoma served as con-

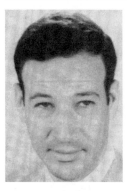

FIG. 526
Phillip Frost
(born 1936)

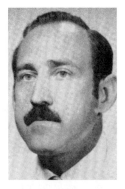

FIG. 527
Gerald D.
Weinstein
(born 1936)

trols.[47] The same protocol was used by Philip Frost (Fig. 526), Gerald D. Weinstein (Fig. 527), and Eugene J. Van Scott in order to assess the proliferation of keratinocytes in ichthyosis vulgaris, lamellar ichthyosis, and epidermolytic hyperkeratosis.[48] Frost, Weinstein, and two other colleagues performed autoradiographic studies with tritiated thymidine to determine the "location of proliferating cells in human epidermis" in patients with psoriasis and different types of ichthyoses, and in healthy controls.[49]

Peter I. Long of Dayton, Ohio, transplanted normal skin of patients with psoriasis into psoriatic plaques and vice versa. He noted that six of 10 transplanted psoriatic lesions "survived and spread into surrounding normal skin," whereas "seven normal skin transplants developed psoriasis when placed into a psoriatic lesion."[50] Long's report prompted William E. Clendenning and Eugene J. Van Scott to perform a more extensive study of "autografts in psoriasis," which included transplantation of split-thickness skin autografts from "normal skin to normal skin . . . normal skin to a plaque of psoriasis . . . psoriatic plaque to psoriatic plaque," and "psoriatic plaque to normal skin"[51] (Fig. 528). R.W. Fardal and Richard K. Winkelmann (Fig. 529) performed autotransplantations of "full thickness cylinders of tissue" in patients with pustular psoriasis of palms and soles.[52] Eugene M. Farber (Fig. 530) and coworkers of the department

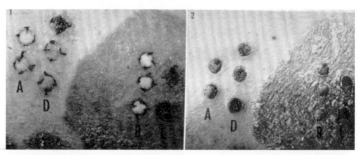

FIG. 528 *Autografts of "normal skin to normal skin" (A), "normal skin to psoriatic plaque" (B), "psoriatic plaque to psoriatic plaque" (C), and "psoriatic plaque to normal skin" (D) on day 2 (Fig. 1) and day 7 (Fig. 2) of the experiment.*

FIG. 529
*Richard K.
Winkelmann
(born 1924)*

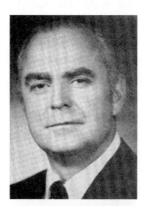

FIG. 530
*Eugene M.
Farber
(1917-2000)*

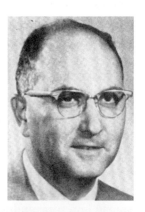

FIG. 531
*Walter C.
Lobitz
(born 1911)*

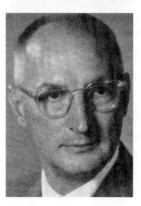

FIG. 532
*Clarence S.
Livingood
(1911-1998)*

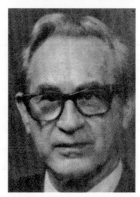

of dermatology of Stanford University School of Medicine in California examined the "cellular response to skin abrasion in psoriasis." In "hospitalized patients with psoriasis" who were "in the eruptive stage of the disease," test sites "were scraped until minute bleeding was evident" and "3 mm punch biopsy specimens were removed immediately after scraping, and at 3, 9, 12, and 24 hours after the initial injury."[53] A similar study was conducted by Yusho Miura and Walter C. Lobitz (Fig. 531) of the University of Oregon Medical School on patients with atopic dermatitis. In order to assess the response to "controlled strip injury" at the cellular level, the cornified layer of the epidermis was removed with an adhesive tape. Two "biopsy specimens were removed from each of these . . . areas before the injury and 4, 18, and 24 hours after the injury."[54] Clarence S. Livingood (Fig. 532) and coworkers of the department of dermatology at the Henry Ford Hospital in Detroit conducted "human skin window studies" on patients with recurrent furunculosis, impetiginized chronic dermatitis, and "various dermatoses of non-bacterial etiology" that consisted of abrading small areas of skin and exposing them to a variety of test substances, such as suspensions of living staphylococci.[55]

These are but a few of many hundreds of examples of experiments on human beings, and no mention of consent of patients was made in any of the publications about them. Although most of these studies were relatively harmless, others were associated with significant risks. For example, in a report in 1958 about poison ivy dermatitis, Albert M. Kligman of the University of Pennsylvania acknowledged that "the administration of an allergen which is the cause of an already existent dermatitis is senseless and contraindicated . . . To bombard sensitive tissue via the hematogeneous route can only add to the patient's woes." Nevertheless, in order "to gain more information on the hazards" of the procedure, Kligman "deliberately administered 0.2 cc. of 10 percent PDC in sesame oil intramuscularly to 11 patients with acute poison ivy dermatitis. The injection of this quantity (20 mg.) in two highly sensitized patients with a generalized dermatitis resulted in their hospitalization with the following findings: temperature to 104 F, leukocytosis (up to 18,000 leukocytes per cubic millimeter), eosinophilia (11 percent and 18 percent respectively), headache, malaise, intense coughing in one case, and menigismus in one case."[56]

Not all experiments on patients were related to the disease the patients bore themselves; patients were thought of as "clinical material" that could be used for all kinds of experimental purposes. For example, the first angiographies of the liver through a catheter inserted into the hepatic vein were performed in the mid 1940s on a group of young men who were "under penicillin therapy for primary or secondary syphilis. Except for syphilis, they appeared to be in good health and, as far as could be judged clinically, had no evidence of hepatic disease."[57] Patients with skin diseases commonly were subjected to biopsies designed to assess problems unrelated to those diseases. Eugene Leibsohn of Boston, for instance, studied the "respiration of human skin" by taking "biopsy specimens of human skin, without anesthesia . . . from dermatological patients not having lesions on or near the biopsy site."[58] Likewise, Van Scott and Thomas M. Ekel of the NIH did scalp biopsies on patients with "either carcinoma of the breast, choriocarcinoma of the uterus, or basal cell carcinoma of the skin" to determine the "geometric relationships between the matrix of the hair bulb and its dermal papilla in normal and alopecic scalp."[59]

In the mid 1960s, William Epstein and Howard Maibach, protégés both of Albert Kligman, studied the "immunologic competence of patients . . . receiving cytotoxic drug therapy" by exposing them to sensitizing doses of potent allergens such as poison ivy, dinitrochlorobenzene, and plague vaccine. For those investigations, they could have used patients with a wide variety of diseases, but they chose patients with psoriasis because they were readily available.[60] At the same time, physicians of Harvard Medical School studied the "effect of thymectomy on skin-homograft survival in children." As noted in the report about the work, "eighteen children of both sexes from three and a half months to eighteen years of age were chosen from among those operated upon at the Children's Hospital Medical Center for congenital heart disease. Eleven of these patients were randomly selected to have a total thymectomy whereas the remaining 7 had only a biopsy of the thymus and served as controls. At the conclusion of each heart operation a full-thickness skin homograft, approximately 1 cm in diameter and obtained from an unrelated adult donor, was sutured in place on the chest wall. The grafts were biopsied when initial gross evidence of rejection, such as edema, loss of pink color or failure to blanch with pressure, was apparent. When indicated serial biopsies were taken." The authors found "no apparent difference in skin homograft survival . . . between the two groups," but announced their "specific plan to repeat the elements of this study" and to "observe closely the growth and development of these children over the years" in order to discover whether thymectomy had adverse effects.[61]

The Most Vulnerable of the Vulnerable

The very young, the very old, and the critically ill, that is, those patients who were defenseless, were at the greatest risk of being abused by physicians as guinea pigs. For example, when physicians of the University of California School of Medicine in San Francisco came across an 18-month-old child with exanthema subitum, they withdrew blood from the child, separated blood cells from the serum, and, within five minutes, injected the serum "intravenously into a 6-month-old susceptible recipient who had had no previous illness." Nine days later, the recipient fell ill and thereby demonstrated what already was well known, namely, "the infectious nature of exanthema subitum."[62] Another example of the exploitation of the most vulnerable patients is a study on "the characteristics of peripheral transport of radioactive palmitic acid," for which physicians of Duke University, North Carolina injected that substance intravenously into 16 hospitalized patients, all but one of whom were "free of serious disease." The one exception, a patient who was speechless and paralysed consequent to a progressive disease of the nervous system, was injected with 10 times the amount of the radioactive substance given to the other patients.[63]

In 1950, physicians of Cincinnati General Hospital set forth a technique for diagnosis called "retrograde cardiac catheterization," for which an incision was made in the main artery of the arm or thigh, followed by passage of a catheter against the blood stream to the main branches of the thoracic aorta. One of the test subjects was an 88-year-old woman who was comatose as a result of a stroke. She died immediately after a series of injections of a contrast medium. Another comatose subject died six hours after the experiment, but the authors contended that "the procedure was probably not at fault." A third subject was a young woman who was semi-conscious following a head injury. The collaborators wrote that "after a second injection of the contrast medium this patient became very excited at this point, but soon quieted. Because the brachial artery had been damaged during the period of excitement it was considered advisable to ligate it . . . The patient was discharged later, completely recovered."[64]

In those days, being unconscious in itself was risky. Not infrequently, advantage was taken of patients under general anesthesia by experimenting on them. For example, studies of the function of the lung, studies of the circulation of the liver by X-rays following injection of a contrast medium into the portal vein, and measurements of circulating adrenalin after catheterization of the heart, the brachial artery, and the pulmonary artery were carried out on patients who were anesthetized in preparation for operations designed for entirely different purposes.[65] In 1957, two anesthesiologists of Harvard Medical School reported on "changes in circulation consequent to manipulation during abdominal surgery." In 68 patients, "a deliberate series of maneuvers was carried out to ascertain the effective stimuli and the areas responsible for development of the expected circulatory changes." In most of the patients, maneuvers such as rubbing "localized areas of the parietal and visceral peritoneum" resulted in "moderate to marked" hypotension and even may have caused a silent myocardial infarction in some of them.[66]

In 1958, patients undergoing "minor surgical procedures" were used to study the effects of elevated tension of carbon dioxide during anesthesia with cyclopropane. Carbon dioxide was injected into the closed respiratory system until a cardiac arrhythmia appeared. One subject developed continuous ventricular extrasystoles for 90 minutes that easily could have led to fatal fibrillation.[67] At about this same time, patients undergoing various head and neck operations at the Presbyterian and Frances Delafield Hospitals in New York City had a small hole made in their skull through which a "trephine button" was inserted that allowed the circulation of the brain to be monitored. The recording was done in order to show the effects of various procedures, such as compression of the carotid arteries, inhalation of carbon dioxide, and intravenous injection of a variety of substances, including nicotinic acid and half a pint of a 10 percent solution of alcohol.[68] This experiment was far more abusive than the biopsies of the brain using a "dental drill" that Udo Wile had carried out and that had aroused public outrage nearly half a century earlier.

"Research by Fraud"

Even being conscious did not prevent patients from being used for medical studies without being informed of them. Most patients did not have the slightest idea of what was being done to them; experiments were disguised as routine components of efforts at diagnosis and treatment. In 1952, William Heneage Ogilvie of London described that ever increasing practice in these words:

Experiment is not new... What is new is research by fraud, the performance on patients who have come to us in good faith for the cure of their ailment of any number of tests and investigations, many of them unpleasant, some of them dangerous, all of them unnecessary for the diagnosis and treatment of their ailment, but performed in a general search for information, or merely as a bit of practice in technique.[69]

Occasionally, patients who came to a hospital "in good faith for the cure of their ailment" had to pay with their lives for their trustfulness. Among them was a former professional tennis player, 42-year-old Harold Blauer, who died at the Psychiatric Institute in New York City in 1952. Blauer had been transferred to the Psychiatric Institute because of depression that seemed to follow on a divorce from his wife. He was given a course of psychotherapy, to which he responded well, and then was told that he was to receive an experimental drug, but he was not made aware that the drug was not intended to help him. Evidence for the wholly experimental purpose of the "treatment" was the wide variation of doses recorded in the medical logs, a finding not consistent with a therapeutic measure. The Psychiatric Institute, which was staffed entirely by psychiatrists of Columbia University, had agreed, in a secret contract with the Army Chemical Corps, to obtain data "which will provide a firmer basis for the utilization of psycho-chemical agents both for offensive use as sabotage weapons and for protection against them." As an unwitting test subject, Blauer received injections of three different derivatives of mescaline. The research physician who gave the injections reported that Blauer was "very apprehensive" and that "considerable persuasion" was required to get him to accept the injections. After the first four injections, Blauer developed tremors and hallucinations, but despite his protests he was given a fifth injection that was 16 times larger than the dose of the same version of mescaline that he had received originally. Blauer sweated profusely, his body stiffened, his teeth clenched, his arms and legs began to jerk randomly, he lapsed into coma, became cyanotic, and died less than 15 hours following the injection.[70]

Another example, one that never was published in a medical journal, happened at a London hospital, where a physician-experimenter wished to practice the technique of lumbar aortography. The subjects chosen for the experiments were eight patients who had been admitted to the hospital with gastric ulcers and who were given the impression that the experiment was merely part of X-ray examination of their stomach. As a direct result of the experiment, three of eight patients died.[71]

Other patients knew that they were being subjected to an experimental procedure and had consented to participate in it, but often they were unaware of the extent and risks of the experiment. All too often, several experiments were carried out in the same patient although the patient had consented to only one of them. Even more often, the explanation given to patients was not accurate and even deceptive deliberately. In the 1960s, for example, Chester M. Southam of the Sloan-Kettering Institute for Cancer Research in New York City injected live cancer cells into 19 patients at the Jewish Chronic Disease Hospital in Brooklyn, New York. The patients, who suffered from chronic debilitating diseases, were informed verbally that they were participating in an experiment, but they were not told that the injections consisted of live cancer cells, because, as a spokesman of the hospital later explained, such knowledge would have effected adversely the emotional and physical condition of the patients. According to the executive director of the hospital, patients "were told that they were to get cells to test their immune reactions to cancer. There was no need to specify the nature of the cells because they were harmless."[72] The assumption that injected cancer cells were incapable of survival in an alien organism and, therefore, harmless, had already been disproven. A few years previously, Southam himself had reported on a metastasis to a lymph node in at least one example of "homotransplantation" of cancer cells.[73]

In principle, the use of patient-subjects for investigating diseases from which they themselves suffered was justifiable because they were the only subjects available. New knowledge derived from those studies could, conceivably, prove to be beneficial to those subjects. Neither of those considerations was applicable, however, to experiments on patient-subjects that were unrelated to the diseases by which they were afflicted. Rather than being the only possible subjects for such research, patients with unrelated diseases actually were less suitable than healthy persons because the diseases from which they suffered could affect the results of the experiments and, more important, risks associated with the experiments were likely to be greater in persons already compromised by a disease than in healthy persons.

In spite of the obvious disadvantages of utilizing for purposes of research patients who suffered from an unrelated disease, such experiments probably were more common than experiments on patients who suffered from the disease under study or than experiments on healthy subjects. The reason was that control subjects who were needed to establish normal values for the phenomena under investigation nearly always were patients sick in a hospital and being treated there for a disease of their own. Using sick patients for the purpose of "normal" controls simply was more convenient than using healthy subjects whose recruitment to a study required an explanation of some kind and consent for it. In regard to patient-subjects, neither explanation nor consent were thought to be necessary. Many experimenters did not even know the subjects personally, but ordered junior physicians to find for them controls on the wards.[74] It was, as Ross G. Mitchell of the University of Aberdeen wrote in 1964, "as though the undertaking of medical care somehow conferred ownership of the patient on the physician."[75]

CHAPTER 24

BIG BUSINESS

I n most human experiments, test subjects had little to gain but a lot to lose. For researchers, the opposite was true. They had little to lose, but a lot to gain in terms of renown, academic advancement, and, not the least, money. With the vast increase in federal spending after World War II, medical research in the United States had become a major enterprise that brought with it handsome financial rewards. In addition to grants awarded for particular projects, researchers now had the opportunity to make contracts on a personal basis with sponsoring agencies, alliances that were even more attractive than grants. One of those who learned this lesson early in his career was Eugene Saenger of the University of Cincinnati. In the 1950s, Saenger discussed grants for research with his friend, John Lawrence of the University of California at Berkeley, known as the "father of nuclear medicine." Saenger later recalled their conversation as follows: "I said to him, 'These grants are really sort of a pain.' He said, 'You mean to tell me that you're still going after grants?' I said, 'John, what should I be doing?' He said, 'Contracts, my boy, contracts.' And it was very interesting because a contract would run forever."[1] Saenger eventually collected almost $700,000 from the Defense Atomic Support Agency for experimental irradiation of the entire body of patients who had tumors that were radioresistent.[2]

The military was not the only big spender for medical research using human subjects. Another was the chemical and pharmaceutical industry. As requirements for experimentation on humans prior to licensing of new compounds became progressively more stringent, the process itself became more difficult and more expensive. An important factor in development of stricter rules was the "Elixir disaster" of 1937. Following the introduction of sulfonamides by Nobel Laureate Gerhard Domagk two years earlier, sulfanilamide became established quickly as an effective and safe drug against streptococci. Then, an obscure pharmaceutical firm in Tennessee placed on the market a solution called "Elixir of Sulfanilamide," hailed at that time as a "wonder drug." Unfortunately, the Elixir had been tested only for "flavor, appearance, and fragrance," and very soon there were alarming reports of toxic reactions to it. Before "Elixir of Sulfanilamide" was withdrawn from the market, it had been responsible, directly, for more than 100 deaths. Investigations showed that the sole cause of death was the solvent, diethylene glycol (akin to antifreeze) in the solution. The nationwide concern aroused by the disaster was described in an editorial in the *Journal of the American Medical Association* in these words:

Seldom has any catastrophe stirred the United States to the extent to which press and public have been aroused by the needless deaths resulting from the Elixir of Sulfanilamide-Massenger.[3]

A Tightening of Regulations in Licensing of Drugs

As a direct consequence of the Elixir disaster, the U.S. Secretary of Agriculture submitted a report to Congress on November 26, 1937, in which he proposed that new drugs be made available only after licensing on the basis of "experimental and clinical tests."

"New drugs" were defined as those that had not been used sufficiently often to become recognized generally as being safe, combinations of chemicals not recognized universally as being safe, drugs not well known, and drugs or combinations of drugs to be prescribed in dosages higher than usual. All drugs found to be dangerous to health would be prohibited, and labels for drugs were to contain a declaration, in full, of their composition and precise directions for the use of them. Against strong opposition by the industry and in rather attenuated form, the proposals of the U.S. Department of Agriculture were incorporated in the Federal Food, Drug, and Cosmetic Act of 1938. Previously, the only restrictions on the marketing of drugs had been that they should not be adulterated, labeled wrongly, or be the subject of false claims in regard to efficacy therapeutically. The new Act brought under the control of the Food and Drug Administration (FDA) any new drug or device for the diagnosis, treatment, or prevention of disease in man or animals, and prohibited traffic in them before they had been proven safe. An exemption was made for drugs intended solely for investigation by qualified scientists.[4]

An event of equal import in motivating a tightening of regulations about licensing of drugs was the thalidomide tragedy. First synthesized in West Germany in 1956, thalidomide was in wide use as a sedative in 1958. Because it usually was well tolerated at doses many times higher than was required for sedation,

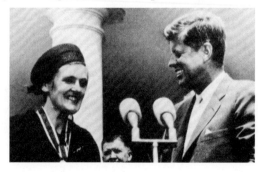

FIG. 533
Frances O. Kelsey of the U.S. Food and Drug Administration being honored by President John F. Kennedy in 1962 for her stubborn scepticism that delayed the approval of Thalidomide in the United States.

it appeared to be ideal for treating women suffering from nausea in the first months of pregnancy. It was not until late 1961 that the first report was published linking the drug to congenital defects of the newborn. In the United States, there were only a few cases of birth defects secondary to thalidomide because the drug had been held up for licensing by Frances O. Kelsey (Fig. 533), an official of the Food and Drug Administration (FDA).

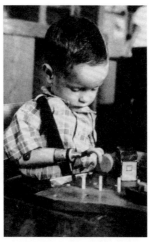

FIG. 534
Intake of Thalidomide by mothers during the first months of pregnancy resulted in severe deformities of limbs called phocomelia.

Nevertheless, photographs of scores of European and Canadian children, perfect in every respect except for a missing or deformed limb, shocked the American public and prompted a reassessment by Congress of the process whereby drugs were approved[5] (Fig. 534).

In 1959, the conduct of pharmaceutical companies was investigated by a Senate Subcommittee on Antitrust and Monopoly. Chaired by Senator Estes Kefauver of Tennessee, the subcommittee found that it was common practice for pharmaceutical companies to provide physicians with samples of experimental drugs, without their having an established record for safety and efficacy. The physicians were then paid to collect data on their patients who, without their knowledge and consent, took the drugs as part of this loosely controlled research. The vivid example of the potential hazards of drugs provided by the thalidomide disaster in 1961 gave Kefauver and other senators new focus and new clout. As a consequence, in 1962, Congress passed the Kefauver-Harris amendments to the Food, Drug, and Cosmetic Act.[6] The amendments required that there be proof of the therapeutic safety and efficacy of drugs, that the labeling of drugs disclose fully contraindications and harmful side effects, and that the FDA impose comprehensive regulations on the testing clinically of new drugs. Moreover, for the first time in the history of the United States, researchers were required to inform subjects of the experimental nature of a drug and receive consent from them before starting an investigation. An exception was made, however, for circumstances in which researchers "deem it not feasible or, in their professional judgment, contrary to the best interests of such human beings."[7]

In February 1963, the FDA issued new regulations that adopted the vague wording of the requirements in the law concerning consent. As a consequence, many investigators eventually interpreted the phrase "not feasible" in the broadest sense possible, that is, not convenient to the design for research they had in mind.[8] The subject-consent provision was the only major aspect in which the FDA did not provide clarification of the amendments. In all other arenas, the provisions of the new law were specified, especially in regard to the design and the procedures of research. Henceforth, the FDA would require pharmaceutical companies to conduct three phases of trials on humans before allowing a drug to be marketed. In the first phase, a new compound that had cleared tests in animals had to be tried on a small group of healthy individuals for possible toxic properties and determination of safe dosages. Phase II trials were then conducted on a slightly larger population to demonstrate further the effectiveness of the compound before application could be made to the FDA to begin large-scale Phase III trials that, if successful, would lead to approval. It was the provisions concerning Phase I studies that especially created problems for pharmaceutical companies who needed large pools of healthy subjects for experiments that had no therapeutic benefit. The problem was solved by the companies when they hit upon the idea of their employing private or university-affiliated physicians with access to the stockpile of human material that lay isolated behind prison walls. The new regulations of the FDA thus created an incredible financial opportunity for physicians who had access to such reserves.[9]

Big Business Behind Bars

From a business vantage, prison research was unparalleled. The customers from the industry were so numerous that even research performed badly did not jeopardize the business, and customers were willing to spend extraordinary sums for the research. The assistants in the research programs were prisoners who were cheap, expendible, and did not complain. Prisoners trained as technicians were paid a smidgen of what counterparts outside confinement secured. For example, an inmate of Holmesburg Prison employed as a photographer by Albert M. Kligman of the University of Pennsylvania was pleased to be paid $25 a month.[10] The supply of "raw material" for experiments on humans was virtually limitless. Prisoners were eager to participate in experiments, hoping for income and early parole. News of fellow inmates who had been released early after participating in medical experiments spread through prisons and captured nationwide attention. One such example was a Sing Sing prisoner named Louis Boy who was serving a life sentence for "complicity in the death of a man in a New York hold up." During the war, Louis Boy volunteered for studies on the treatment of malaria and influenza; in 1949, *The New York Times* reported on his participation in "a perilous medical experiment" on behalf of an 8-year-old girl suffering from leukemia. In an effort to "purify the child's blood of the widely spreading white blood cells characteristic of leukemia," wrote *The Times*, the girl and the prisoner had "their circulatory systems linked together with rubber tubing." The hope was that the "poisoned blood" of the girl would be cleansed as it passed through the body of Louis Boy. The experiment, of course, failed – the girl died within a few days – but six months later, just two days before Christmas, readers of *The Times* were informed on the front page that Louis Boy had been granted his freedom by New York Governor Thomas Dewey because of his "exemplary" prison record and his willingness to participate in "dangerous medical tests and experiments . . . without promise of reward."[11]

Although authorities at correctional institutions and researchers both emphasized repeatedly that there was no "promise of reward," stories such as that of Louis Boy were not lost on other prisoners who hoped for the same sympathetic treatment. In fact, the committee commissioned in 1947 by Governor Dwight Green of Illinois to assess "the ethics governing the service of prisoners as subjects in medical experiments" had stated explicitly that "a reduction of sentence in prison as a recognition for service in a medical experiment is consonant with the statutory 'good time,' 'merit time' and 'industrial credits' provisions of the parole system."[12] Researchers often wrote letters on behalf of test subjects that were included in the prisoners' files. For example, W. J. H. Butterfield of Richmond, who conducted various experiments on humans at the Virginia State Penitentiary, praised the valuable services of inmates in a letter to the State Department of Welfare and Institutions and recommended that "you give to each the maximum commutation of sentence."[13] Robert E. Hodges and William B. Bean of the University of Iowa described practical aspects of "the use of prisoners for medical research" in an article in *JAMA* in 1967, in which they acknowledged that they routinely sent "a letter to the warden at the termination of each experiment expressing our appreciation for the inmate's participation in the study. It is possible that this letter in the prisoner's file may favorably influence the parole board."[14] The vast majority of prisoners, especially those serving time in state or federal institutions, cited early release as an important motivating factor in their participation in experiments.[15]

Other reasons mentioned by inmates for "giving their bodies to science" included altruistic feelings and the expectation of better food, cleaner and more comfortable living quarters, relief from monotony and boredom of prison routine, and a reprieve, no matter how brief, from omnipresent threats of violence on the cell block. For example, the State Prison of Southern Michigan at Jackson was given more than a half million dollars in 1964 by the Upjohn and Parke-Davis drug companies to build a state-of-the-art research laboratory inside the walls. One of the many inmates used as a test subject later told a panel of inquiry that the laboratory was a good place "to hide out a little bit . . . When you are walking around Jackson Prison," he explained, "you have 300 jerks up there that you know have done something wrong. When you look at the guy next to you, he's in maximum security because he's already done something. You know he's capable of tearing your head off at any moment. So, Upjohn and Parke-Davis, far from being something that would be a detriment to me or my colleagues up there, is looked on almost like a chapel. We go to those tests, and it's pure enjoyment. The little bit of irritation that you might be exposed to on Phase I testing is nothing compared to the madness that goes on in the yard."[16]

In short, prisoners had many reasons that had nothing to do with monetary rewards for participating in medical experiments and that ultimately contributed abundantly to the coffers of the investigators. Without question, however, the chief reason for prisoners to participate in medical experiments was money. On a relative scale, prison research was big business, too, for the inmates, who, if they were fortunate enough to get one of the "pay slots" in the echelon of prison employment, normally earned a maximum of $10 to $13 a month[17] (Fig. 535, 536). At Holmesburg, for example, the few jobs available in the shoe shop or the knit-goods mill paid "no more than 50 cents a day."[18] By contrast, a skin biopsy was worth $5 and a deep incision $10.[19] Occasionally, prisoners were successful in bargain-

FIG. 535
*The Holmesburg
Prison's shoe shop
offered long days
and low wages for
the few inmates
lucky enough to win
a job there.*

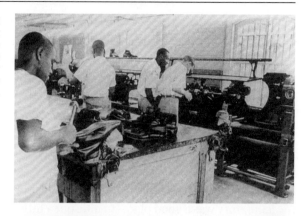

FIG. 536
*The scar on the ab-
domen of a Holmes-
burg prisoner re-
sulted from inci-
sions made for
gauze implants that
paid "$10 for each
cut."*

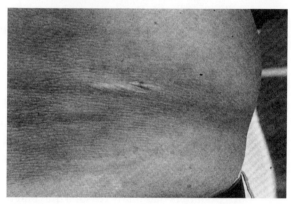

ing with researchers for higher pay. When a physician from the University of Pennsylvania wanted to extract fingernails at $50 each from six inmates, the prisoners refused to cooperate "for fifty bucks." A bargaining session soon yielded a three-fold increase in pay for allowing their fingernails to be ripped out.[20] In other instances, in which the consequences of a procedure were less obvious, prisoners not always were so fortunate. In drug studies, especially, they did not know what to expect because they were not informed about anticipated side effects, and the pay was not as good. Their continued participation in such trials was secured by withholding some, or all, of the pay until a study had been completed. This policy compromised severely the option of test subjects to withdraw from an experiment at any given time. The coercion under which test subjects participated can be appreciated in the description of a trial of drugs directed at obesity and performed by Albert Kligman at Holmesburg Prison. In an article in *The Philadelphia Bulletin* in 1966, Kligman was quoted as follows:

A prison is the right place for such a test . . . How can you do a test like this on the outside – limiting a person to five grams of fat a day? We fed these men a milk-like emulsion. For six long months they had to take this lousy fluid. Now eating is one of the major pleasures of life. Suddenly you take all taste away from the men. They had all kinds of dreams . . . Most of them . . . reached a sensory vacuum. Meals meant nothing to them. But one guy couldn't take it after five months. Somewhere he got an onion and ate it. For him it was a paradisiacal experience after drinking that awful stuff. We discovered it and refused to pay him because the onion ruined the value of his test. Just one lousy onion deprived him of his money. He became violent. But we had to keep discipline.[21]

As is to be expected in business, physicians engaged in prison research tried to keep their expenses down. The income of test subjects, therefore, was very low, and because of the lack of competition and the abundance of prisoner-volunteers, researchers were successful in minimizing costs. In the late 1960s, for example, Robert Hodges (Fig. 537) studied experimentally-induced scurvy by depriving inmates of vitamin C. This resulted in joint pains, swelling of the legs, dental cavities, loss of hair, hemorrhage in the skin, and mental depression. The five inmates of the Iowa State Penitentiary who were recruited for this three-month-long study were paid $1 or $2 per day. Hodges acknowledged that ". . . we had the money, we could have paid much more, of course – but we

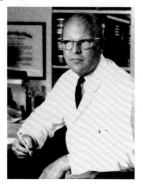

FIG. 537
*Robert Hodges
(1922-1998)*

weren't just being cheap, we were considering the ethics of the situation."[22] Ironically, researchers who seemed to know little about requirements for valid informed consent became very strict about ethics when their own pockets were concerned. While they ignored the Nuremberg Code, researchers in prisons held dear the ethical requirements set forth by Governor Green's Committee that ". . . the prisoners be volunteers, and excessive reward can become undue influence or coercion and would be inconsistent with the principle of voluntary consent."[23] Accordingly, Robert Hodges declared that "it's unethical to pay an amount of money that is too attractive."[24]

Researchers Go Private for Big Bucks

The income derived by researchers from prison work was substantial, the costs were pathetically little, and the profit margins inordinately high. It is no wonder that physicians with access to prisoner-subjects took the opportunity to turn research into big business and to generate windfalls for themselves. An egregious example of such a physician was Austin R. Stough of Oklahoma. A general practitioner with no formal training in pharmacology, Stough, in the mid and late 1960s, is believed to have conducted between 20 and 50 percent of all initial drug tests in the United States. At that time, he, alone, oversaw 130 investigational experiments for 37 pharmaceutical companies, including Bristol-Myers, Merck, Upjohn, and Lederle.[25] The studies were carried out at prisons in Oklahoma, Arkansas, and Alabama, where numerous prison physicians and influential lawyer-legislators were on Stough's "payroll." Many of the studies produced meaningless data because "prisoners failed to swallow pills, failed to report serious reactions to those they did swallow, and failed to receive careful laboratory tests."[26]

Stough also sold blood plasma that was extracted from prisoners solely for that purpose. Plasma was drawn from the whole blood taken from prisoners, and the remaining blood cells were reinjected into donors, enabling them to "donate" blood many times a year. In at least one instance, however, a donor was reinjected with blood cells from another prisoner, with resultant severe serum sickness. In another instance, contamination of equipment led to an outbreak of hepatitis that resulted in many deaths. At Kilby Prison in Alabama, "Joe Willie Tifton, 46, died on March 18. Emzie B. Hasty, 42, died on April 14. Charlie C. Chandler Jr., 31, died on April 16. David McCloud, 27, died on May 22. Each death was attributed to infectious hepatitis . . . 28 percent of the men who participated in Dr. Stough's program came down with the disease. For those who did not take part, the rate was only 1 percent." An official at Cutter Laboratory who visited Stough's operation observed that the plasmapheresis rooms were "sloppy" and that gross contamination with plasma of many donors was evident. Nevertheless, Cutter and other pharmaceutical companies continued to work with Stough, claiming that he had crucial "contacts" and that it was through him that permission was obtained from prison officials to operate the program. By the end of the decade, Stough had retreated from the prison business, but he did not leave empty-handed; in a good year, he grossed in those days close to one million dollars.[27]

Another physician who recognized early on the tremendous commercial opportunities of prison research was Albert M. Kligman. In the early 1960s, Kligman, who was a full Professor, full time, in the department of dermatology at the University of Pennsylvania, situated in a building for research known as Duhring Laboratories, founded a private firm, Ivy Research, for the purpose of performing commercial research at Holmesburg Prison. Calvin Triol, one of the first employees of Kligman in the private sector noted that in his first years at the prison, Kligman's work centered on interests that were purely academic. As the years passed, however, the testing took on a life of its own, attracting scores of major corporate clients and requiring more and more staff and test subjects. The rapidly increasing scope of Kligman's activities is reflected in the annual sums paid out to prisoners: total wages increased from $73,253 in 1959, to $166,000 in 1961, and $272,329 in 1966.[28] It may be inferred that those sums represented less than 10 percent of the income generated by Ivy Research Laboratories. The prison system was paid 20 percent of those amounts, whereas millions of dollars went to the University of Pennsylvania and, the most by far, to Ivy Research.[29] By the end of the decade, Ivy Research employed approximately 30 civilians, in addition to many prisoners who served as research assistants; it was a major player in the business of prison research.[30]

Pursuit of Fame and Fortune

A more sophisticated way of generating money from prisoners was chosen by two former trainees of Kligman, namely, William Epstein and Howard Maibach. In the tradition of their mentor, they conducted research at Vacaville Prison, California, under the aegis of the Solano Institute for Medical and Psychiatric Research. The Institute, which had its headquarters inside the prison, was set up as a nonprofit corporation under California's charitable trust laws. The Institute's administrator, Ralph Urbino, explained that "... we couldn't receive funds from drug companies ... As a nonprofit organization we are barred from receiving money from private business concerns. Our income is derived from the physicians who have been given research grants for the purpose." By turning over their research grants to the Institute, Epstein, Maibach, and several other members of neighboring medical schools in the University of California system served as a conduit for tax-exempt payments from industry. In 1972, an advertisement of the Institute stated proudly that Epstein and Maibach had been "continuously active since the inception of our program here." According to its financial statements, filed with the Registry of Charitable Trusts, the income of the Solano Institute for Medical and Psychiatric Research from "various researchers" rose from $47,000 in 1963, its first year in business, to $266,000 in 1971. Among the "customers" were giant pharmaceutical companies, including Lederle, Wyeth, Dow Chemical, Roche, and Abbott.[31]

The pharmaceutical industry was interested chiefly in Phase I drug studies, which differed from traditional clinical trials in that efficacy of a compound was of no consequence. Phase I studies were trials of how well a drug was tolerated, and were initiated to determine only the margin of safety of a drug. In other words, researchers tried to determine at what dose a drug began to have adverse effects.[32] That circumstance prompted some investigators to look very hard for "positive results," thereby playing a frivolous, but dangerous, game with the health of their subjects. In one study conducted by Epstein (Fig. 538) at Vacaville in 1962, 20 inmates were selected to undergo what Epstein called "pain tolerance studies." The experiment consisted of intramuscular injections of Varidase, a product of Lederle Laboratories composed of fibrinolytic enzymes that still is used for local treatment of skin ulcers and conditions associated with necrosis. Prior to the experiment, little was known about Varidase. According to Dr. William C. Keating, Jr., the Superintendent of Vacaville Prison and a founding member of the Solano Institute, the only information available was "a little brochure that comes with the preparation" and that contained "a list of medical cautions." Epstein explained that he did not know, and was not "expected to know," whether the drug had been "subjected to all the normal procedures required by FDA."

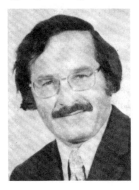

FIG. 538
William L. Epstein (born 1925)

All he knew was that intramuscular injections of Varidase would make people ill and that the *raison d'être* of the study was to find out just how ill test subjects would become. Epstein explained that "The reason we did the experiment was the pain and the fever ... what we were looking for was pain, discomfort, aching in the arm."[33] The experimenters were not disappointed; their test subjects developed those symptoms and more – including "headaches," "cold chills," and "sharp abdominal pains." One prisoner suffered an agonizing, near-fatal disease of the muscles, with his weight dropping from 140 to 75 pounds. Following treatment with corticosteroids for the condition, the prisoner developed gastric ulcers that persisted. When these complications became apparent, Epstein referred to them as an unusually severe but "natural reaction." Instead of terminating the study, he told Lederle that "We are planning this week to try four more men and I am prepared to give them some steroids when the severe symptomatology starts."[34]

Epstein's readiness to continue the experiment was not surprising because Lederle had granted him a "large fund" for the research, from which the share paid to test subjects was "$4; $3 spendable and $1 to retention funds." That test subjects participated in the experiment for only $4 was not surprising either because they had no idea what to expect. According to Dr. Keating, no signed consent was required from prisoner-subjects. He did not believe that "the dangers of any of those possible medical problems were mentioned or explained to any of the potential volunteers for this project." The only surprising aspect was that the story became known at all, a consequence of a lawsuit instituted by one of the prisoners and eventually settled out of court for $6,000. Other experiments with serious sequelae that may have been performed at Vacaville Prison never became public because the Solano Institute for Medical and Psychiatric Research maintained that it was not required under the California Public Records Act to disclose medical data. In its publication addressed to potential customers in 1972, the Institute boasted that its "reservoir of volunteer subjects offers investigational possibilities not found elsewhere" and that "there have been no deaths or serious sequelae resulting from drug research at this institution."[35]

The recklessness demonstrated by Epstein in the pursuit of his "pain tolerance studies" was not an isolated aberration. In 1962, Howard E. Ticktin of Washington, D.C. and Hyman J. Zimmerman of Chicago used "a grant from the Wyeth Laboratories, Radnor, Pennsylvania" to study adverse effects on the liver of the antibiotic, triacetyloleandomycin (TriA), which was to be marketed as a treatment for acne. "In an attempt to determine the incidence and type of hepatic dysfunction relatable to the administration of TriA," the authors recruited 50 "mental defectives or juvenile delinquents" who had "no recognizable organic disease other than the mildly to moderately severe acne for which the drug was given." Eight subjects developed "marked hepatic dysfunction" with symptoms such as abdominal aches and anorexia, and signs such as jaundice. "Liver biopsy was performed at the height of the dysfunction or jaundice, or both, in these 8 patients by the intercostal route with the use of the Menghini needle. In 4 of these patients it was repeated later." Moreover, "four patients were challenged with a 1-gm. dose of the drug after liver function had returned to normal. Within one or two days, hepatic dysfunction again developed in 3 of the 4 . . . In 1 of these, a second challenge after recovery from the effects of the first again led to a rise in the serum glutamic oxalacetic transaminase level." The authors concluded that the development of hepatic dysfunction seemed "reasonably ascribable to the administration of the drug."[36] Of this study a commentator in the *British Medical Journal* said wryly:

Juvenile delinquency in the United States obviously carries hazards which many of us had not previously suspected. The pimpled gangster of today may find himself the bilious guinea pig of tomorrow. It seems a little hard, perhaps, for a boy who has spent his formative years learning how to dodge flick knives to fall victim to intercostal perforation by the Menghini needle.[37]

Another physician who did not hesitate to induce severe adverse reactions in human subjects was Albert M. Kligman, who is credited with many things, including the development of retinoic acid for treatment of acne and for removal of facial wrinkles. Under the names Retin-A® and Renova®, retinoic acid became a gold mine not only for the pharmaceutical company that produced and marketed it, but also for Kligman and the University of Pennsylvania, which received many millions of dollars in revenues, a mere fraction of Kligman's take. Kligman, however, was not the first to recognize the powerful effects of retinoic acid. Long before, Günter Stüttgen (Fig. 539) of the department of dermatology of the University of Düsseldorf had described the keratolytic action of the compound and had warned that irritation of the skin was a common side effect of it.[38] While Stüttgen and others hesitated to pursue experiments with retinoic acid because of those devastating effects, Kligman applied the compound liberally to the backs and faces of scores of inmates of Holmesburg Prison. Kligman was interested not only in the keratolytic effects of retinoic acid, but also in its powers as an irritant. In several publications, he focused on the "extremely inflammatory" reactions produced by the "intensive application of retinoic acid on human skin."[39] Kligman himself admitted in

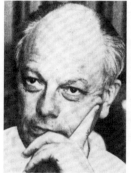

FIG. 539
*Günter
Stüttgen
(born 1919)*

1996 that he experimented at first with "very high doses," so high that "I damn near killed people ... Every one of them got sick."[40]

Kligman's unrestrained efforts to demonstrate adverse effects of drugs is illustrated also by a study in 1965 performed for Dow Chemical Company on the threshold dose for cutaneous changes produced by dioxin, a by-product of the manufacture of herbicides. Dioxin, a powerful carcinogen, was implicated in the cause of acneiform skin eruptions. For $10,000, Kligman agreed to test dioxin on humans and "relieved the Company of any liability" that might be incurred by the experiment. The company acknowledged that dioxin was "highly toxic" and advised, therefore, that "the seriousness of the type of consequences that might develop from testing with this . . . compound require that we approach the matter in a highly conservative manner." This meant beginning the experiment with a very low dose and slow, progressive increasing of it. Kligman initially followed this instruction, but when the cutaneous application of 0.1 to 0.2 micrograms of dioxin produced no results, he deviated from the protocol of Dow Chemical by pushing the dose up much higher. By virtue of a sudden increase in dose, he succeeded in inducing long-standing acneiform lesions in eight of 10 test subjects. Scientists at Dow Chemical were "quite startled" when they learned that Kligman had increased the recommended dose 468 times. They also were dismayed by Kligman's failure to address the purpose of the study, namely, finding the threshold dose for producing acneiform lesions. An official of Dow Chemical stated bluntly that the changes of the protocol initiated by Kligman "caused us to sever the relationship . . . He didn't give us any notice. That was the end of the relationship with Dr. Kligman."[41]

An occasional disappointed customer, however, was no real problem for Kligman and others like him; there were plenty of companies who were satisfied with the methods he used and with the results he provided. For example, Kligman tested a plastic Band-Aid for Johnson & Johnson and reported in the *Archives of Dermatology* in 1957 that the "Band-Aids are simply and quickly applied, but best of all they stick to the skin tenaciously even in the face of sweating and showering." According to Kligman, the Johnson & Johnson product had proven "wonderfully conve-

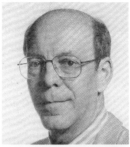

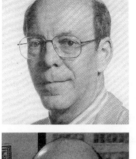

nient and useful" and "superior ... to its rival" from another company.[42] Curiously, the editor of the journal seemed to have no qualms about this patent conflict of interest. This was true also of organizations like the American Academy of Dermatology (AAD), at whose annual meetings Kligman often touted unashamedly the products that he was being paid to test for pharmaceutical and cosmetic companies.

In a study sponsored by the Chocolate Manufacturers Association of the USA, Kligman gave chocolate bars for a month to 35 prisoners at Holmesburg. Along with his trainees, James E. Fulton, Jr. and Gerd Plewig (Fig. 540), he reported in the *Journal of the American Medical Association* that "... ingestion of high amounts of chocolate did not materially affect the course of acne vulgaris."[43] With A. Bernard Ackerman (Fig. 541), who was then a second-year resident in the department of dermatology of the University of Pennsylvania and who would go on to become a dermatopathologist whose contributions were legion and legendary, Kligman studied dandruff in various ways, among them by taking biopsies from the scalp of 65 prisoners at Holmesburg. The DNA synthesis of epidermal cells was studied by injecting tritiated thymidine into the scalp of 11 test subjects and taking biopsies at different intervals.[44] When Ackerman queried Kligman specifically about the propriety of using tritiated thymidine in humans, he was assured that his mentor had full authorization for it from the Atomic Energy Commission. After Ackerman had left the University of Pennsylvania to do his third year of residency at Harvard, which was prior to the completion of the calculation of turnover time for the

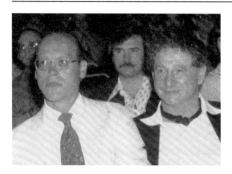

FIG. 542
*Albert M. Kligman (right)
at a symposium together
with his former student,
A. Bernard Ackerman.*

epidermis in "dandruff," Ackerman was surprised to see in the
last draft of the manuscript a series of numbers completely unknown to him that had been supplied by Kligman.[45] (Fig. 542).
The article described dandruff as a disease characterized by "an
increased turnover rate of the epidermis" without "evidence of an
antecedent inflammatory stimulus to power the process."[46] Years
later, with the benefit of decades of experience, Ackerman concluded that, in no small number of instances, he and Kligman
surely had confused dandruff with seborrheic dermatitis and
that dandruff, in fact, was a physiologic phenomenon, to wit,
dander. He pointed out, too, that "such a refrain [of dandruff
being physiologic, not pathologic] would not have been music to
the ears of Proctor & Gamble," manufacturers of the bonanza
treatment for dandruff, *Head and Shoulders*, and a sponsor of
many of Kligman's studies.[47]

Scientific Quest Not for Knowledge, But for Gold

Some bias in the interpretation of findings was unavoidable in
studies conducted chiefly for commercial reasons. In most of
those studies, a true scientific quest for knowledge played a
minor role, if any at all. Accordingly, studies often were performed in careless fashion. For example, prisoners acknowledged that they liked patch tests particularly in their role as test
subjects because they would "hang the patch on the wall" im-

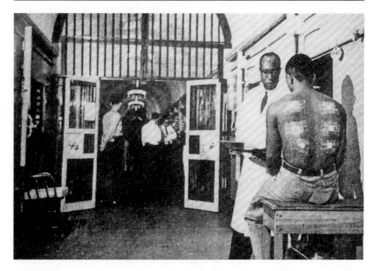

mediately on their return to the cell. Although many experiments were compromised in that way, nobody seemed to care[48] (Fig. 543). The carelessness with which experiments were conducted is illustrated by a study on "the tolerance of the human vagina to daily insertions of medicated and unmedicated suppositories," supervised by Kligman's then wife, Beatrice Troyan, and carried out at the Philadelphia House of Correction. At the outset, Kligman's team made what the contractor, a local paper company, described as an "unfortunate miscarriage of the protocol" consequent to "the misunderstanding of the experimental methods and the dosage regimen." Kligman admitted responsibility saying, "We made a serious error." Then the sponsor requested individual "patient release forms." Kligman wrote back that "Our inmates sign release forms devised by ourselves. I cannot make them available to you." When the sponsor requested data on individual patients, Kligman replied that "The case records were kept as composite notes on the entire group and are not in a form which I feel prepared to submit for inspection." At last, the sponsor apprised Kligman that "our Protocol specifically requires the maintenance and submission of indi-

vidual case reports . . . It is the consensus of our Research Department that this study deviated from the protocol arrange-
ment in so many important respects that not only should no further payments be made, but that a refund of the advance, in so
far as it exceeds out-of-pocket expenses, should be requested."
To this Dr. Kligman responded, "I deeply regret having irreversibly alienated you. Nonetheless, I am truly shocked by your
suggestion that you be relieved of paying the cost of this study . . .
Our costs were substantial and your unwillingness to be even
slightly sympathetic appears to be exceedingly cruel . . . My own
proposal is that you should pay fifty percent (50%) of the original estimate."[49]

Kligman's prison business did not endure great financial hardships. Money kept pouring in, not only from pharmaceutical
companies but also from the U.S. Army. From the 1950s to the
early 1970s, the Army awarded six separate contracts totaling
$650,000 to the University of Pennsylvania. Another $126,000
went directly to Kligman's private company, Ivy Research. The
studies carried out for the Army included attempts to harden the
skin through prolonged exposure to such abrasive and toxic
chemicals as phenol, hydrochloric acid, sodium hydroxide, and
Croton oil. In some of those chemicals, the "systemic toxicity" was
found to be a "severely limiting" factor. After exposure to pure,
undiluted ethylene glycol monomethyl ether, "three of the test
subjects exhibited psychotic reactions (hallucinations, stupor,
etc.) within two weeks and had to be hospitalized." Pure, undiluted dimethylacetamide produced "headaches and febrile reactions." Kligman concluded that solid hardening was "attainable
only if the skin passes through a very intense inflammatory phase
with swelling, redness, scaling, and crusting." Most of the experiments were carried out on the forehead, and it is highly likely that
many black prisoners developed permanent postinflammatory
discoloration.[50]

As a dermatologist, Kligman may have had some scientific

curiosity in regard to the particular aforementioned studies, in addition to his interest commercially. The same cannot be assumed for other studies of his that addressed issues far outside his own region of expertise. Chief among these were experiments with psychoactive drugs on behalf of the Army and the Central Intelligence Agency (CIA). In the mid 1960s, about 200 inmates at Holmesburg were selected for tests with incapacitating agents, for which they were paid several hundred dollars, a fortune for a prisoner in those days. Injections were given in three trailers that the Army had installed at the prison. Each of those trailers housed padded cells and high-tech equipment for monitoring the findings. Following injections, many prisoners went through what they described as horror trips, had all kinds of hallucinations, and became violent. At least one inmate who had been injected with EA 926, a substance known to be "very potent in animals because of its knockdown effect," developed a syncopal reaction and had to be resuscitated. Many others suffered from severe residual symptoms such as "irritability, memory impairment, insomnia, blurred vision, and difficulty in concentrating." After their release from the Army trailers, test subjects were given an identification badge that read: "Please excuse this inmate's behavior. He can't think or act in a coherent manner and is part of the U.S. Army testing program."[51]

One of the reasons that the Army chose to make use of Kligman's services, rather than to perform tests on enlisted men stationed at military facilities near Edgewood Arsenal, Maryland, was that some of the drugs had "unusually prolonged effects" that made long-term follow-up of test subjects mandatory. For that reason, only prisoners who had at least six more months to serve were admitted to the experiments. Unfortunately, Kligman had to inform the Army that some test subjects were "unexpectedly discharged." Representatives of the Chemical Corps of the Army also were unhappy with the psychological reports submitted by Kligman's staff, which they characterized as being "pure gibberish . . . absolutely useless . . . nothing but a list of clichés seemingly pasted together without consideration of coherence in an attempt to provide a facade of competence and ability." Kligman was urged repeatedly to hire a psychopharmacologist; he promised to meet that request, but never did.[52]

Kligman's unwillingness to spend money for qualified personnel also is reflected in his refusal to hire a radiologist to oversee experiments with radioactive substances. To receive a licence from the Atomic Energy Commission (AEC) to store and use radioactive material, appropriate qualifications were required. Kligman received the licence in January 1964 by listing Benjamin Calesnick, professor emeritus of human pharmacology at Hahnemann Medical College and Hospital in Philadelphia, as the "radiation protection officer" and Arthur Wade as the "nucleonics advisor" of the required Isotope Safety Committee. When Calesnick and Wade learned of their ostensible functions from the AEC, they were perplexed, insisting they were "not part of the program," and requested that their names be deleted immediately. Despite this, Kligman had his licence extended after informing the AEC that he had completed a six-month formal course under Dr. Calesnick, in addition to two years of experience in the use of radioisotopes at Hahnemann Hospital and Holmesburg Prison. When, many years later, Benjamin Calesnick heard of that claim by Kligman, he disputed it. "I never taught Kligman anything," he said. "Certainly not about radioactive material and never at Hahnemann. He never took any training program here of any length."[53]

The FDA Grows Suspicious

In 1966, both the scope and laxness of Kligman's research program aroused the suspicion of the FDA, which was being reorganized under new leadership. An administrative review in preparation for testimony to Congress revealed widespread deviations in the industry from required practices of research, including the submission of "wholly fictitious" data. In addition, William W. Goodrich, Assistant General Counsel of the FDA, observed that ". . . patient consent, as required by law, was not being obtained in too many instances."[54] FDA officials were amazed to find that Kligman had conducted 193 studies between 1962 and 1966, and that ". . . used in the studies were 153 experimental drugs, including 26 drugs for which firms were seeking marketing permission and 14 others whose makers wished to market them for new uses." Not surprisingly, Frances Kelsey, the FDA investigator who had prevented thalidomide from being licensed in the United States, "wondered how accurate work could be under such mass production conditions"[55] (Fig. 544, 545, 546).

The interest of the FDA was fostered by a lengthy article Kligman had written about dimethyl sulfoxide (DMSO) and that had appeared in two parts in the *Journal of the American Medical Association* in 1965. Kligman described DMSO as an "organic liquid with exceptional solvent properties" capable of markedly increasing "the penetration of various dyes, steroids, and antiperspirants" through the skin and as "exceptionally nontoxic."[56] Among dozens of experiments performed by Kligman was a study concerning the toxicity of chronic exposure to DMSO, for which "nine milliliters of 90% dimethyl sulfoxide were applied to the entire trunk" of 20 Holmesburg prisoners "once daily for a period of 26 weeks." No systemic symptoms as a consequence of the drug were recorded.[57] The FDA, however, was not so sanguine about DMSO, which had just been banned by it from being tested on humans. When Kligman's operation at Holmesburg was inspected by the FDA, the following irregularities were found:

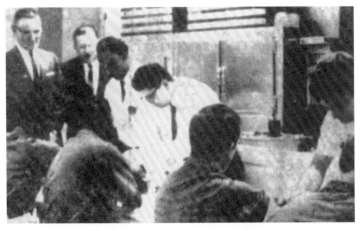

FIG. 544
Technicians performing tests on prisoners in front of Edward Hendrick (far left), the Superintendent of the Philadelphia Prison System.

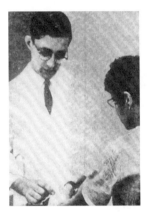

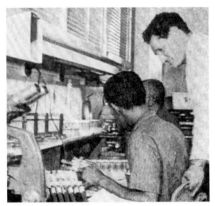

FIG. 545
Medical technician examining the arm of an inmate of Holmesburg Prison for signs of irritation.

FIG. 546
Albert M. Kligman supervising prisoners trained as technicians.

1. A 26-week study ended after 16 weeks, and the number of subjects involved less than what was reported. 2. A test subject who withdrew from the study because of a 'severe adverse reaction' to the test drug was not reported. 3. Questionable blood studies were supposedly drawn from inmates who were not in the prison hospital when the samples were taken. 4. There were no records for a study that was reported.[58]

The study about DMSO was not the only one of Kligman's that the FDA found to be objectionable. It discovered "irregularities or falsification of reports in at least four studies" and "serious discrepancies in the record keeping." Other criticisms included Kligman's involvement "in a number of investigations involving fields other than his specialty." They also complained that it was common practice at Holmesburg Prison to use "an inmate to participate in more than one drug study at a time, e.g., a dermatological and an internal drug at the same time." According to a memorandum of the FDA in May 1966,

Dr. Kligman acknowledged these errors but felt all his work couldn't be condemned . . . He said he thought the least reliable of all his studies were the dermatologic ones since these, until recently, were not done under the medical administrator, but under his own supervision. Dr. Kelsey expressed shock at this since she said we all felt his reputation was chiefly in the field of dermatology.[59]

On July 19, 1966, the FDA notified 33 drug firms who were sponsoring experiments at Holmesburg Prison that Kligman no longer was "eligible to receive investigational drugs." That sanction, and the embarrassing publicity attending it, were thought to be a crucial blow to Kligman's reputation and career. *Time* magazine noted that it was only the second time in its history that "the Food and Drug Administration struck a physician's name from its approved list of researchers who are entitled to test new, investigational drugs on human subjects."[60] In short, the decision was exceptional, but not nearly as remarkable as the events that followed. The ousting of Kligman was

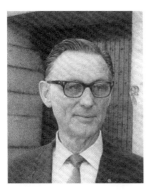

FIG. 547
Edward
Hendrick

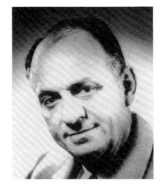

FIG. 548
Luther L. Terry
(1911-1985)

criticized by representatives of the pharmaceutical industry who emphasized that "this facility is badly needed by us" and referred to it as "irreplaceable." Edward Hendrick (Fig. 547), the superintendent of the Philadelphia Prison System, called Kligman's enterprise "a valuable program from our standpoint," one that he "would hate to lose."[61] More importantly, three highly esteemed physicians, Luther L. Terry (Fig. 548), Donald M. Pillsbury, and Aaron B. Lerner, used their good offices on behalf of Kligman. Terry, a former Surgeon General who now was Vice-President for Medical Affairs of the University of Pennsylvania, informed FDA investigators that ". . . while Kligman was eager and an entrepreneur . . . he was thought to be fundamentally honest." Terry claimed that his "chief interest" in the case was "in preserving the good name of the University of Pennsylvania." He did not notify the FDA of the university's financial share in Kligman's enterprise.[62] Lerner (Fig. 549), chairman of the department of dermatology at Yale University School of Medicine and the only dermatologist in the National Academy of Sciences, went to bat for Kligman whom he regarded as an ingeneous medical researcher.[63] Pillsbury, the former chairman of the de-

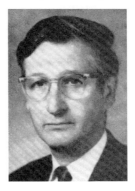

FIG. 549
Aaron B.
Lerner
(born 1920)

partment of dermatology of the University of Pennsylvania, deplored the fact that ". . . the results of this sudden declaration of ineligibility of Dr. Kligman have been absolutely catastrophic." The decision of the FDA had not only "necessitated the sudden dismissal of several very worthy people," but had "removed a highly effective morale-builder at Holmesburg Prison." Pillsbury pledged to "review all protocols" of Kligman's investigative facility, "to expend considerable time and effort to restore it to operation, and to aid in making it as impeccably accurate and reliable as possible."[64]

This three-pronged pressure exerted on the FDA was so strong that Kligman's privilege to investigate new drugs was restored less than a month after the initial action had been taken against him. For Alan Lisook, an FDA investigator, this reversal was a "singular event" in the history of the agency, the "only case" where someone was "disqualified and reinstated in that short a time."[65] All that was demanded of Kligman was the promise to improve his operations and a public correction of his falsified report about the properties of dimethyl sulfoxide. In a letter to the editor of the *Journal of the American Medical Association* in September 1966, Kligman wrote these lines of explanation: "I wish to inform you of a regrettable inaccuracy . . . Owing to inadequate supervision on my part the statements under the section labeled 'Chronic Exposure' . . . are not fully supported by the experimental procedures."[66] Within weeks, Kligman's business was in full swing again and continued to generate huge profits for the University of Pennsylvania and, especially, for himself well into the 1970s.

CHAPTER 25

PUTTING ON
THE BRAKES

S cience is not an endeavor circumscribed by national borders. The desire to acquire new knowledge is a universal human trait. Science, therefore, knows no boundaries, even in its use of available methods, including experiments on humans. In the postwar period, such experiments were not confined to the United States, but were conducted throughout the world. In dermatology, alone, the spectrum of countries in which questionable experiments on humans were performed was as broad as the spectrum of diseases being studied. In 1947, for example, the chairman of the dermatologic clinic of the University of Copenhagen, Holger Haxthausen (Fig. 550), studied vitiligo, morphea, and acrodermatitis chronica atrophicans by transplanting "a piece of tissue from a pathologically altered

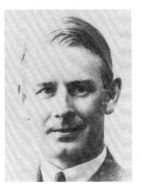

FIG. 550
*Holger
Haxthausen
(1892-1959)*

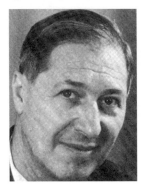

FIG. 551
*Felix Sagher
(1908-1981)*

skin area to normal skin and vice versa."[1] In 1955, Felix Sagher
(Fig. 551) and coworkers at the Hadassah Medical School in
Jerusalem studied reactions of 23 patients suffering from lepromatous leprosy to "the inoculation of living flagellates of
Leishmania tropica . . . Forty-four biopsies of the *L. tropica* inoculation sites were performed at intervals of from 16 days to
20 months after inoculation," sections of tissue from the specimens showing histopathologic changes reminiscent of leprosy[2]
(Fig. 552).

To find out whether the liver was affected in diseases of the
skin, M. Dogliotti, M. Banche, and G. C. Angela of Torino, Italy,
performed liver biopsies in 1954 on patients with eczema, psoriasis, dermatitis herpetiformis, and various other diseases.
Only a few of those patients had abnormal liver function tests.
A similar, but more extensive study was carried out in 1957 by
Claude Huriez and coworkers of the dermatologic department
of the University of Lille, France. Slight changes in the liver
were found in many patients, but a meaningful interpretation
of those findings was impossible because, in the words of the
authors, "such biopsies may reveal antecedent or concomitant
hepatic lesions which may not be responsible for the skin disease." In order "to be prudent," they "attributed to alcohol any
such changes in intemperate patients."[3]

In 1956, the head of the department of dermatology of the

FIG. 552
*"Typical leishma-
niasis lesions, six
to seven months
after the inocula-
tion of L. tropica
in three patients
with lepromatous
leprosy." (from an
article by Liban,
Zuckerman, and
Sagher)*

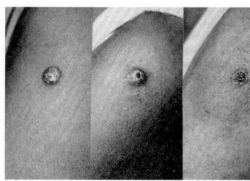

25 · Putting on the Brakes

University of Barcelona, Xavier Vilanova (Fig. 553), reported on the experimental induction of onychomycosis. Although he emphasized the
"prolonged clinical course and resistance to treatment" of onychomycosis, he inoculated fingernails of 14
subjects, including children, with cultures of many different species of
fungi.[4] In 1962, Roberto E. Mancini

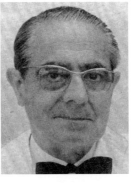

and Jorge V. Quaife of the University of Buenos Aires studied
the "histogenesis of experimentally induced keloids" in nine
"human healthy volunteers" with a previous history of keloids
and in three control subjects. "In all of them an incised wound
15 cm. long reaching the fat layer and an excised wound . . .
about 3/10 mm. thick and 10 to 15 cm. square, were performed
on the abdominal skin under local anesthesia." Biopsy specimens were taken at different intervals, the first one being on the
18th day, and the succeeding biopsies "on the 26th, 33rd, and
42nd day after injury. In the subjects who developed keloids,
new specimens were obtained three, six, nine and 12 months
later."[5] In 1964, physicians of the department of tropical dermatology in Mexico City selected "one hundred male children [in]
years of age from 7 to 11" without "cutaneous lesions or a past
history of dermatophytosis," the purpose being assessment of
the "prophylactic action of griseofulvin." Fifty children were
given that antimycotic drug and 50 others a placebo, followed
by inoculation of the children with strains of *Trichophyton concentricum* and *Trichophyton mentagrophytes*[6] (Fig. 554).

In 1967, David Porter and Sam Shuster of the university department of dermatology in Newcastle-upon-Tyne used "twelve
male and twelve female patients, all schizophrenics" and all
without "evidence of present or past skin disease . . . to measure
the transit time of epidermal cells by incorporation of locally in-

FIG. 554
*Results of in-
oculation of
children
with Tri-
chophyton
concen-
tricum.
(from an ar-
ticle by
González-
Ochoa et al.)*

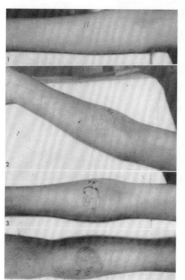

jected C^{14} labeled amino acids into keratin." The authors acknowledged being "grateful to Dr. J. Roy of St. Nicholas Hospital for permission to study patients under his care."[7] In 1969, Kowichi Jimbow, Syozo Sato, and Atsushi Kukita of the department of dermatology at Sapporo Medical College excised "axillary, femoral and inguinal lymph nodes of seven patients with generalized eczematous dermatitis," searching for Langerhans' cells. No purpose diagnostically for the undertaking was stated, and no consent of patients was recorded.[8]

In short, American scientists were not alone in their disregard of ethical boundaries of research on human beings. Nowhere in the world, however, was human experimentation comparable, in terms of scope and zeal, to that in the United States. If any change in the policy of research was to occur, the United States, therefore, was the most likely place for it to happen. The circumstances were comparable to those in Germany at the end of the nineteenth century. At that time, experiments on humans were much more common in Germany than anywhere else, and it was this circumstance that led eventually to the promulgation in 1900 of the first official guidelines for experiments on humans. The Prussian guidelines of 1900, however, were not a consequence of the sheer number of experiments. Other societal factors also played a role, most notably anti-Semitism. Likewise, new currents in American society were needed to change the practice of human experimentation in the United States.

25 · Putting on the Brakes

A Reorientation of Social Thought: Challenge of Authority

In the 1950s, dubious experiments on humans in the United States were very common. The existence of unethical practices of research was acknowledged time and again; no one, however, acted on it. Discussions about the subject remained dispassionate, as if the problems were more conceptual than actual,

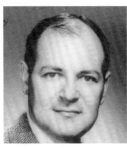

more academically interesting than morally pressing. When, in 1959, the National Society for Medical Research devoted a conference to legal and ethical aspects of clinical research, nary a hint was mentioned of scandal, crisis, or lives at stake. Louis Welt (Fig. 555) of the University of North Carolina School of Medicine addressed the difficulty of obtaining consent that was not coerced, but the group he focused on was medical students, not prisoners or the mentally disabled. One presenter reviewed the matter of human experimentation at the Clinical Center of the National Institutes of Health (NIH) and found the principles guiding it to be adequate; he made no mention, though, of actual practices. In the report of the conference, no doubts were left about the priorities of the National Society for Medical Research, and they were stated thus:

The standards for health research on human subjects should recognize the imperative need for testing new procedures, materials and drugs on human subjects as essential to the public interest. The protection of personal rights of individuals . . . can co-exist with the public necessity to use people – sick or well – as subjects for health research.[9]

Medical circles and society at large still were in awe of research. Any curtailment of the freedom of scientists was thought to be an impediment to progress and, thereby, a threat to the lives of patients who were awaiting the next discovery. Public opinion was guided by visions of wonder drugs, not by nightmare cases; the victory of penicillin had left a more indelible impression than had the disaster of thalidomide. Americans took pride in the achievements of medical research and put their trust in physicians – who they believed would use their discretion in a benevolent way – just as they took pride in their country and put trust in their government.

In the 1960s, however, a progressive reorientation of social thought began. Securing personal rights became more important than obtaining communal goods, and enhancing the prerogatives of the individual was more important than the needs of the community. The civil rights movement sharpened sensibilities in regard to discrimination against minorities, African-American in particular, who began to claim rights instead of accepting humbly whatever sop was handed them. Authority was challenged and paternalism no longer was accepted. In times past, parents and teachers, physicians and politicians had been granted discretion in fulfilling benificent designs, namely, to use their greater knowledge on behalf of their children and students, patients and citizens. In the 1960s, those latter groups came to recognize that that discretion often served self-interest – that parents often furthered their own needs, rather than those of their children; that teachers acted in the best interests of their schools instead of their pupils; that politicians looked to their re-election more than to the needs of their constituents or their country; and that physicians sought to advance careers, often at the expense of test subjects, whose health and lives were treated cavalierly.[10]

For medical researchers, curtailment of the freedom of choice they always had enjoyed was difficult to accept. In general, they adhered to traditional concepts that emphasized the needs of the society rather than those of the individual. William Bean, chair of internal medicine at the University of Iowa (Fig.

556), for example, made this assertion:

In our concern for the rights of the individual we must not forget that society has rights too. Anyone living in a society has a debt to it. Experimental biological science is necessary to advance curative medicine and public health. Exclusive focus on individual and personal rights may accelerate the decline of society down the path of its own self-destruction.[11]

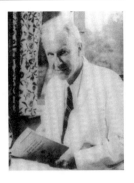

FIG. 556
William B. Bean (1909-1989)

When, in 1965, the NIH assembled an *ad hoc* committee to review procedures of research that had been developed in the past, most members endorsed the hands-off policy that gave investigators sole discretion for determining risk and benefits of experiments, and they did not devise guidelines to govern extramural research. After all, since World War II, this policy had resulted in more than 30 Nobel Prizes in medicine for Americans.[12] Confidence in the ultimate value of research overrode all reservations and was expressed by one director of an institute at the NIH in these words: "Society would be in peril if we did not do clinical research." Nevertheless, there were other scientists who acknowledged that ". . . it is easy to get carried away with the importance of one's own research." One member of the ad hoc committee observed, "We are on the defensive because, whether we like it or not, we have in some senses utilized the concept of the end justifies the means."[13] This was undeniable, and the defense of researchers crumbled as more and more examples of experiments – carried out by investigators who had pursued their own ends by use of questionable means – were publicized. One of the most damaging of those cases was Chester Southam's study on cancer immunology, in which live cancer cells were injected into patients of the Jewish Chronic Disease Hospital. The study and the lawsuit that followed received extensive coverage in the press.

The Abuse of Man

The Finger Points – Reforming Experimental Medicine from Inside

In March 1965, with repercussions of Southam's study still vibrating, Henry Beecher of Harvard Medical School addressed the ethics of research during a medical conference at Brook Lodge Conference Center, Wisconsin. Rather than focusing on general concepts of medical ethics, as he had done before, Beecher spoke about specific studies culled from the literature, the ethics of which disturbed him. He pointed out that "... what seem to be breaches of ethical conduct in experimentation are by no means rare, but are almost, one fears, universal."[14] This statement and its documentation by use of real cases caught the attention of the media, and both *The New York Times* and *The Wall Street Journal* ran lengthy accounts of his presentation. Not surprisingly, the responses of many physicians to Beecher's position were hostile. Two of his colleagues – Thomas Chalmers of the Harvard School of Public Health and David Rutstein, head of preventive medicine at Harvard Medical School – called a press conference to refute Beecher's revelations. Beecher decided to defend his position by turning the Brook Lodge lecture into an article for a professional journal. He accumulated 50 recent examples of what he considered to be investigations of dubious ethical worth and, in August 1965, submitted a

FIG. 557
Beecher's article about "Ethics and Clinical Research" in the New England Journal of Medicine in 1966.

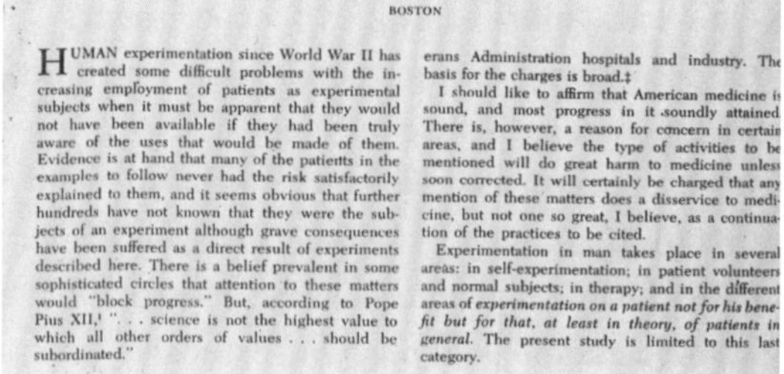

SPECIAL ARTICLE

ETHICS AND CLINICAL RESEARCH*

HENRY K. BEECHER, M.D.†

BOSTON

HUMAN experimentation since World War II has created some difficult problems with the increasing employment of patients as experimental subjects when it must be apparent that they would not have been available if they had been truly aware of the uses that would be made of them. Evidence is at hand that many of the patients in the examples to follow never had the risk satisfactorily explained to them, and it seems obvious that further hundreds have not known that they were the subjects of an experiment although grave consequences have been suffered as a direct result of experiments described here. There is a belief prevalent in some sophisticated circles that attention to these matters would "block progress." But, according to Pope Pius XII,[1] "... science is not the highest value to which all other orders of values ... should be subordinated."

erans Administration hospitals and industry. The basis for the charges is broad.‡

I should like to affirm that American medicine is sound, and most progress in it soundly attained. There is, however, a reason for concern in certain areas, and I believe the type of activities to be mentioned will do great harm to medicine unless soon corrected. It will certainly be charged that any mention of these matters does a disservice to medicine, but not one so great, I believe, as a continuation of the practices to be cited.

Experimentation in man takes place in several areas: in self-experimentation; in patient volunteers and normal subjects; in therapy; and in the different areas of *experimentation on a patient not for his benefit but for that, at least in theory, of patients in general.* The present study is limited to this last category.

long article to the editor of the *Journal of the American Medical Association (JAMA)*, John Talbott, stressing in a cover letter that the message of his article "urgently needs to be disseminated." When Talbott rejected the article, Beecher turned to the *New England Journal of Medicine*, where it was published, in abbreviated form, on June 16, 1966[15] (Fig. 557).

Beecher's article provided brief summaries of 22 experiments on humans that were objectionable ethically, including four conducted at Harvard Medical School and its affiliated hospitals and three at the Clinical Center of the NIH. In almost all 22 studies, the test subjects were institutionalized or were in other situations that compromised their ability to give free consent, such as being newborns, very elderly, terminally ill, mentally disabled children, soldiers, or charity patients in a hospital.[16] Because Beecher wanted to avoid a "condemnation of individuals," he gave neither names nor provided references, but the examples he published were recognizable easily to many readers. Among them were the experimental injection of cancer cells by Chester Southam, the artificial induction of hepatitis in inmates of Willowbrook State School by Saul Krugman, and the study of the effects of thymectomy on the survival of skin homografts by Robert Milton Zollinger and colleagues at Harvard.[17] Perhaps the most bizarre experiment related by Beecher was the transplantation by coworkers at Northwestern University Medical School in 1961 of a cutaneous malignant melanoma from a daughter to her mother. The experiment was conducted "in the hope of gaining a little better understanding of cancer immunity and in the hope that the production of tumor antibodies might be helpful in the treatment of the cancer patient." The mother had volunteered to be a recipient, hoping to help her child recover, but the information given to her probably was inaccurate because her daughter's condition actually was said in the article about the experiment to have been "terminal;" there was no real chance of cure through application of "tumor antibodies" produced by the mother. In fact, the daughter died only one day after the procedure. Nevertheless, the primary implant was allowed to grow for 24 days in the rectus muscle of the mother. When it was excised, together with surrounding "skin, subcutaneous fat and a large piece of rectus fascia and muscle," it already had metastasized. After about two months, the mother "began to complain of constipation and pain in the abdominal wall;" one month later, she developed "high grade partial bowel obstruction." Following treatment with chemotherapeutic agents, "ulcerations of the oral cavity and an almost total alopecia developed. Nausea and distention were marked." The mother died of widespread metastases of melanoma on the 451st day after transplantation.[18]

The study about transplantation of melanoma was one of the few in which consent of a test subject was mentioned. The doubtful ethics of the experiment, itself, corroborated Beecher's reservations about the inherent value of such "consent." According to Beecher, consent "should be emphasized in all cases for obvious moral and legal reasons, but it would be unrealistic to place much dependence on it." Beecher repeated his original view that "consent in any fully informed sense may not be obtainable." Nevertheless, he underscored that ". . . it is absolutely essential to strive for it." In the studies compiled by Beecher, "many of the patients . . . never had the risk satisfactorily explained to them, and it seems obvious that further hundreds have not known that they were the subjects of an experiment although grave consequences have been suffered as a direct result of experiments." Beecher believed that those experiments

. . . will do great harm to medicine unless soon corrected. It will certainly be charged that mention of these matters does a disservice to medicine, but not one so great, I believe, as a continuation of the practices.[19]

Beecher's purpose in having the article published was to reform experimental medicine from the inside. He had compiled examples of unethical experiments because he "hoped that calling attention to them will help to correct abuses present." It was the contention of Beecher "that thoughtlessness and carelessness, not a willful disregard of the patient's rights, accounts for most of the cases encountered." He called on the editors of medical journals to refrain from publishing "data that have been improperly obtained" because "failure to obtain publication would discourage unethical experimentation." Beecher referred to informed consent as one of the two most important components of ethically sound research, but emphasized that "the more reliable safeguard" was the "intelligent, informed, conscientious, compassionate, responsible investigator."[20] Beecher himself, however, must have felt that admonitions alone would not suffice to convert insensitive colleagues into responsible investigators. He must have realized, at least unconsciously, that pressure from the outside was needed if a profound change in medical research were to be effectuated. This was evident in his efforts to create pressure by apprising the media about the forthcoming publication of his article. As a result, the article received wide attention.[21]

At another place or time, Beecher's charges might have created nothing but a mild stir. The place, however, was the United States, and the year was 1966, one that saw the first defeat of the civil rights movement in Congress in regard to the far-reaching issue of "open housing." It also witnessed the transformation of the civil rights movement from one that could dream, in Martin Luther King's words, about "a beautiful symphony of brotherhood" to one that emphasized "black power" as the only way to oppose effectively suppression by the white ruling class. The heightened level of social conflict turned the sensitive issue of experiments on humans into a subject of general significance, especially because scientists represented the establishment and most of their test subjects were disadvantaged.[22]

The Coming of the Review Board

Another factor that heightened the impact of Beecher's article was the way medical research in the United States was organized. Universities and medical schools were dependent on the NIH as their single most important source of funding for research; in turn, the NIH was dependent on Congress that alone allocated its budget and that could embarass leaders of it by requiring them to testify at hearings. The Director of the NIH, James A. Shannon (Fig. 558), conceded that one of his responsibilities was "keeping the Government out of trouble."[23] The centralization of authority in a body that was at the same time subordinate to Congress and superordinate to the research community helped translate public pressure into practical consequences.[24] When a congressman asked officials of the NIH how they intended to respond to Beecher's charges, the associate director for the extramural program assured him that the findings had aroused "considerable interest, alarm, and apprehension" and that "constructive steps have already been taken to prevent such occurrences in research supported by the Public Health Service."[25]

Actually, after grappling with the issue of human experimentation for years, leaders of the NIH had come to understand that, in reality, the clinical investigator "departs from the conventional patient-physician relationship . . .

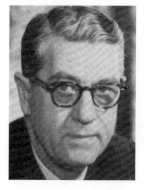

FIG. 558
James A.
Shannon
(1904-1994)

and indeed may not be in a position to develop a purely or a wholly objective assessment of the moral nature or the ethical nature of the act which he proposes to perform."[26] An *ad hoc* group appointed by Shannon to consider policies of the NIH reported to him that if cases of doubtful experiments on humans came to court, the Public

Health Service "would look pretty bad by not having any system or any procedure whereby we could be even aware of whether there was a problem of this kind being created by the use of our funds."[27] The National Advisory Health Council proposed in a resolution on December 3, 1965, ". . . that Public Health Service support of clinical research and investigation involving human beings should be provided only if the judgment of the investigator is subject to prior review by his institutional associates to assure an independent determination of the protection of the rights and welfare of the individual or individuals involved, of the appropriateness of the methods used to secure informed consent, and of the risks and potential medical benefits of the investigation." In February 1966, a few months after Beecher's lecture about the ethics of research but before publication of his article, Surgeon General William Stewart (Fig. 559) issued a Policy Statement that made mandatory "review of the judgment of the investigator by a committee of institutional associates not directly associated with the project" for all federally funded research involving experimentation on humans. Institutions receiving federal research grants were required to furnish information about the review committees and the methods employed to ensure that the advice of the committees would be followed [28] (Fig. 560).

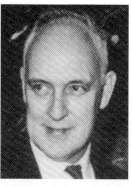

FIG. 559
William H.
Stewart
(born 1921)

A call for independent committees to review experiments on human beings was not novel. Thomas Percival, in his Code of Ethics in 1803, had advised those physicians who were willing to try "new remedies and new methods of chirurgical treatment" that "no such trials should be instituted, without a previous consultation of the physicians or surgeons, according to the nature of the case."[29] In 1902, Albert Moll had suggested in his

FIG. 560
Surgeon General
William Stewart
(middle) and
NIH Director
James A.
Shannon (right)
greeting Lyndon
B. Johnson on a
visit in 1965 to
the campus of the
National Insti-
tutes of Health.

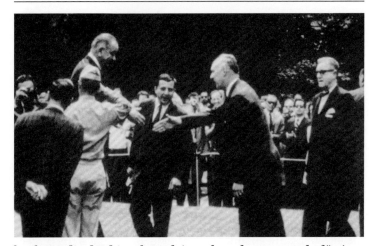

FIG. 560
Surgeon General
William Stewart
(middle) and
NIH Director
James A.
Shannon (right)
greeting Lyndon
B. Johnson on a
visit in 1965 to
the campus of the
National Insti-
tutes of Health.

book, *Medical Ethics*, that advisory boards composed of "scientists, physicians, lawyers, and other learned men" be formed for the purpose of considering the ethical aspects of any planned experiment on human beings.[30] In Germany in the early 1930s, when experiments on humans became the subject of heated debate, members of the Berlin Chamber of Physicians had suggested that bodies of medical men be created for supervision of hospitals and review of proposals of planned experiments. Although the suggestion was taken up by the press, it was repudiated harshly by physicians who were engaged in experiments. Friedrich von Müller, the highly regarded chairman of internal medicine at the University of Munich, wrote in 1930 as follows: "The control of leading hospital physicians through representatives of professional organizations, the state, or local authorities would result in severe conflicts, not to the least because the definition of the term experiment, and therefore of any intervention, is extremely vague. Such a measure would paralyse the creative urge of hospital physicians and would impair scientific work at German hospitals as compared to those of other countries. Furthermore, such control would be impracticable. One should not enact laws that cannot be followed."[31] In the guidelines for experiments on humans circulated by the German Ministry of the Interior in 1931, independent regulatory bodies for medical research were not included.[32]

In the early 1950s, the idea of independent review committees gained momentum in the United States. In September 1950, cardiologist Carl J. Wiggers of Western Reserve University suggested that ". . . the scientific, ethical, and legal considerations pertaining to contemplated studies on human subjects should, whenever possible, be reviewed and approved by a group of colleagues who will not participate in the investigation."[33] At a medical staff conference of the University of California at San Francisco in 1951, Otto Guttentag proposed a model for experiments on humans in which "research and care would not be pursued by the same doctor for the same patient, but would be kept distinct."[34] At the same conference, Michael Shimkin pointed out that ". . . research on human beings is too hazardous and implies too many responsibilities to be undertaken by lone investigators. It should be a group effort supported by a proper consultative body."[35] When the NIH opened its Clinical Center in 1953, a Medical Board Committee was established to ensure that "any nonstandard, potentially hazardous procedure, or any involving normal subjects receives appropriate group consideration before it is undertaken."[36] This was a significant innovation despite the limitation that no "group consideration" was required for experiments on patient-subjects as long as the experimenter did not deem those experiments to be "potentially hazardous." In subsequent years, review committees began to be established at American medical colleges and universities. A survey conducted by Louis Welt in 1960 concerning practices of experimentation on humans, however, revealed that of 66 departments from which came a response, "only eight have a procedural document and only 24 have or favor a committee to review problems in human experimentation."[37] The Policy Statement of the Public Health Service in 1966 that mandated the establishment of institutional review boards (IRBs) as a prerequisite for receiving federal research grants was a landmark in the history of experimentation on human beings.

That Policy Statement established a system of self regulation by research institutions, which were free to decide the composition and the procedures of their own review board. As a result, very few review boards had representatives from outside the world of research, such as lawyers and clergymen. Physicians continued to be monitored by physicians, many of whom knew each another personally and who tended to be sympathetic to each other's aspirations and endeavors. Moreover, the Policy Statement required that informed consent of test subjects was obtained, but it did not spell out definitively the nature of that requirement. The vague wording of the Kefauver-Harris Drug Amendments of 1962, which said that investigators were not required to obtain informed consent when they found it "not feasible or, in their professional judgment, contrary to the best interests of such human beings," was not made more precise or more lucid now. Despite those limitations, experiments on humans moved out of the private sphere of individual investigators into the public domain. The results of that measure soon became apparent. As but one example, the percentage of "problem projects," that is, studies associated with potential hazards to test subjects, submitted to the NIH declined from 7.4 per year in 1966 to 1.7 in 1968.[38]

Like the NIH, the Food and Drug Administration (FDA) also grappled for years with problems raised by experimentation on humans. In contrast with the NIH, the FDA focused on the matter of consent, rather than on the process whereby research was reviewed. In a "Statement of Policy Concerning Consent for Use of Investigational New Drugs on Humans" published on August 30, 1966, the confounding phrases of the old statute – "not feasible" and "contrary to the best interest of such human beings" – were defined. The words "not feasible" were stated to apply to circumstances in which the investigator cannot communicate with the patient or his representative – such as when the patient is comatose or "otherwise incapable" of giving consent and a representative of that patient cannot be reached – and a drug must be administered without delay. The phrase "contrary to the best interest of such human beings" was said to apply "when the communication of information to obtain consent would seriously affect the patient's disease status." In the absence of informed consent, all experiments unrelated to therapy on humans were forbidden. For informed consent to be valid, a person must possess the ability to exercise free choice and be given a "fair explanation" of the procedure, including an understanding of the purpose of the experiment, the nature of it (including the possibility of receiving a placebo in a blind or double-blind study), the duration of it, "all inconveniences and hazards reasonably to be expected," and the availability of any alternative form of therapy.[39]

In summary, regulations issued by the NIH and the FDA in 1966 were important in the development of protection for human subjects of research. Nevertheless, there was a gray zone of considerable breadth in which experiments that were objectionable ethically still could be performed. For example, the NIH continued to sustain the exceptions to the consent requirement laid down in 1962 by the Drug Amendments. The FDA insisted that consent was to be waived only in exceptional cases, but it allowed investigators to determine which cases were exceptional. The IRBs that were being established throughout the country were not supervised by a controlling authority. Free to develop their own policies, they differed greatly in conscientiousness. At Holmesburg Prison, for example, an IRB formed in the early 1970s included an attorney, a clergyman, a sociologist, and two physicians, each of whom received a regular stipend for their participation. One of the physicians, Howard M. Rawnsley of the University of Pennsylvania, explained that ". . . each protocol brought a $5 fee. About 20 to 30 protocols would come in batches and checks would come from Ivy Research," the private company of Albert Kligman. The number of protocols, the fees paid for reviewing them, and the immediate source of those fees provides some insight into the degree of thoroughness, or lack of it, with which the work was conducted. The other physician on the Holmesburg institutional review board, Henry C. Maguire, a student of Kligman and later chairman of the department of dermatology at Hahneman Medical School, recalled that the committee "was not that active a group . . . I can't remember we ever met. There were no formal meetings."[40] With that kind of non-engagement, the committee could not fulfill its obligations, among which was ensuring "the appropriateness of the methods used to secure informed consent." At Holmesburg, test subjects were being told what the tests were about, but they were not informed about possible side effects.[41]

The Gates Shut in Prison Research

It must be noted that the new regulations of the NIH and the FDA applied only to research done under the auspices of those two federal agencies. Outside those arenas, questionable experiments on humans continued unabated and resulted in a staccato of negative publicity. The time when experiments on humans had been praised by the media was over; the public no longer identified with researchers and with triumphs that emanated from their laboratories, but rather with the subjects of the experiments and the harm they sustained. The effects of negative publicity were unleashed on Holmesburg Prison when the police began to investigate the claims of two young inmates that they had been raped in the prison and in sheriff's vans. The investigations revealed that sexual assaults were epidemic in the Philadelphia prison system. Virtually all slightly built young men either were raped repeatedly by gangs of inmates or were forced to seek protection from gang rape "by entering into a homosexual relationship with an individual tormentor." One of those tormentors was Stanley Randle, a prisoner who was employed as a research assistant by Kligman. Furnished with the "power to decide which inmates would serve as subjects on various tests," Randle turned his cell into the left ventricle of a sex-for-money scheme that paid a total in fees to him of between $10,000 and $20,000 a year. In his report about Holmesburg Prison, Alan Davis, an assistant District Attorney in Philadelphia, observed that ". . . the University of Pennsylvania project has had a disastrous effect upon the operations of Holmesburg Prison."[42] In contrast to previous claims that the research program was an important "management tool,"[43] Davis concluded that ". . . the disproportionate wealth and power in the hands of a few inmates leads to favoritism, bribery, and jealousy among the guards, resulting in disrepect for supervisory authority and prison regulations."[44] The Davis report resulted in a series of embarassing newspaper headlines, such as "Lab Testing Program Tied to Prison Sex Corruption," thereby contributing to the growing uneasiness of state authorities about research in prisons. When the Board of Trustees of the Philadelphia prison system decided to abolish prison research in January 1974, many prisoners were dismayed by the loss of income, but the authorities were relieved to have terminated a practice that by then was regarded as "demeaning and dehumanizing."[45]

The censure of research in prisons continued throughout the country until it at last was abandoned entirely in 1983, the only exceptions being studies that dealt with prisons as institutions or prisoners as incarcerated persons, and studies that had the "intent and reasonable probability" of improving the health or well-being of the subjects.[46] Not surprisingly, the curtailment of prison research met with harsh opposition from physicians. When the Director of the Federal Bureau of Prisons, Norman A.

Carlson, embarrassed by questions from lawmakers, announced his intention in 1975 to terminate medical research in federal prisons, he was criticized heatedly by some highly respected scientists. Albert Sabin, the developer of the polio vaccine, underlined the importance of prisons in providing "a stable, long-time permanent study group," and Franz J. Ingelfinger, the editor of the *New England Journal of Medicine*, predicted that a halt in prison research would do severe damage to medical research. By contrast, Carlson's policy was supported by most authorities of correctional institutions and legislators.[47]

Philosophical Resolution of the "Moral Dilemma"

The controversies about termination of prison research reflect the progressive intrusion of "outsiders" into the sphere of medicine. Decisions about ethical aspects of medical research no longer were left exclusively to physicians. There was increasing awareness that traditional maxims, such as "do no harm" and "act only in the interest of the patient," born of a therapeutic context, were not applicable equally to experimental medicine. Hence, the subject of the ethics of medicine became one of concern for other professional groups with expertise in matters ethical, among them philosophers, lawyers, and social scientists. For example, Paul Ramsey, a professor of religion at Princeton University, published a book in 1970 titled, *The Patient as Person*, in which he declared that ethical problems in medicine "are by no means technical problems on which only the expert (in this case the physician) can have an opinion." He warned of the "omnivorous appetite of scientific research ... that has momentum and a life of its own," of any curtailment of the principle of the "inviolability of the individual," and of "a medical and scientific community freed from the shackles of that cultural norm, and proceeding on a basis of an ethos all its own." In Ramsey's view, consent of test subjects was as essential to experimentation on humans as a system of checks and balances was to executive authority, that is, a necessary limitation on the exercise of power. He argued that ". . . man's capacity to become joint adventurers in a common cause makes the consensual relationship possible; man's propensity to overreach his joint adventurer even in a good cause makes consent necessary."[48]

Another philosopher who considered consent to be "a non-negotiable minimum requirement" for experiments on humans was Hans Jonas, professor at the New School for Social Research. Recognizing the importance of consent, Jonas went even further than Ramsey by stating that consent "is not the full answer to the problem." By merely asking for volunteers, Jonas noted in 1969, "some soliciting is necessarily involved." The best way to resolve that moral dilemma was experimentation on oneself: "With self-solicitation, the issue of consent in all its insoluble equivocality is bypassed per se." Jonas was aware "that it would be the ideal, but not a real solution to keep the issue of human experimentation within the research community itself." He believed, nonetheless, that persons who were most capable of giving consent – the best educated with the greatest possibility for choice – should be asked first to volunteer for an experiment. On Jonas' list, research scientists were at the top and prisoners at the bottom in regard to being a test subject. Jonas conceded that this principle of "descending order" might hamper experimentation and slow progress, but he thought that "this should not cause too great dismay." He called for a tempering of the drive to make progress and he did that in these words:

Let us not forget that progress is an optional goal, not an unconditional commitment, and that its tempo in particular, compulsive as it may become, has nothing sacred about it. Let us also remember that a slower progress in the conquest of disease would not threaten society, grievous as it is to those who have to deplore that their particular disease be not yet conquered, but that society would indeed be threatened by the erosion of those moral values whose loss, possibly caused by too ruthless a pursuit of scientific progress, would make its most dazzling triumphs not worth having.[49]

Before long, Jonas's predictions were borne out. When, in 1972, the story about the Tuskegee Syphilis Study broke, revealed not by a single one of the thousands of physicians who knew about it, but by a young law student, Peter J. Buxton, it had a profound and lasting impact on American society. In the eyes of African-Americans, the Tuskegee study was an attempt at genocide, a quintessential symbol of deceit, maltreatment, suppression, and neglect that had shaped Afro-American history for centuries. Confronted with the moral bankruptcy evidenced by the study, many blacks lost faith in their government and no longer had any confidence in health officials who spoke about matters of public concern. When the AIDS epidemic terrified the country some 20 years later, taking an especially high toll on African-Americans living in the inner cities, many black Americans thought, as a lead editorial in *The New York Times* recorded in 1992, "that AIDS and the health measures used against it are part of a conspiracy to wipe out the black race." The editorial cited a survey of black church members in which "an astonishing 35 percent believed AIDS was a form of genocide."[50] Health officials who worked in black communities reported that the Tuskegee study had spawned a legacy of suspicion toward public health authorities and hospitals. According to Mark Smith of the Johns Hopkins University School of Medicine, many African-Americans were "somewhat cynical about the motives of those who arrive in their communities to help them."[51] Many black patients with AIDS refused to take antiretroviral drugs because they were afraid of being used as guinea pigs. Participation of African-Americans in clinical trials was negligible, and prophylactic measures aimed at containing the spread of the disease in African-Americans were crippled by distrust.[52]

25 · Putting on the Brakes

The Birth of Bioethics

When the Tuskegee study became public, the Department of Health, Education, and Welfare (DHEW), as the mother agency of the Public Health Service, tried to soothe criticism by establishing an *ad hoc* advisory panel to review the experiment, as well as the Department's policies and procedures for the protection of human subjects in general. In its final report, issued in April, 1973, the panel observed that "... no uniform Departmental policy for the protection of research subjects exists" and that "... failure to develop a uniform policy has been detrimental to the welfare of research subjects." It warned of "basic defects" in the "existing review committee system," such as low visibility, lack of provision "for the dissemination or publication of review committee decisions," and failure "to conduct continuing review of research projects after their initial approval." The panel advised the following:

Congress should establish a permanent body with the authority to regulate at least all Federally supported research involving human subjects, whether it is conducted in intramural or extramural settings ... This body could be called the National Human Investigation Board ... The members of the Board should be appointed from diverse professional and scientific disciplines, and should include representatives from the public at large.[53]

In Congress, the issue of an independent national commission that would govern experiments on humans had been discussed for years. The reason for this was not so much awareness of practices in experimental research that were objectionable ethically as it was new ethical questions that came to be posed by virtue of the enhanced possibilities of modern medicine. In former times, physicians had used their limited means to preserve the lives of patients, but now they were doubtful whether it was proper, in the words of a pediatrician at Wayne State University, William Zuelzer, to "preserve life against nature's apparent intentions simply because we have the gadgetry that allows us to do so."[54] Was a physician justified, or even obligated, to perform life-saving surgery in a severely handicapped infant against the will of the parents? An instance in which physicians of Johns Hopkins University Hospital had complied with the wishes of parents and had refrained from performing such surgery attracted nationwide attention. It led to the creation in 1971 of the first institute of bioethics at a university, namely, the Kennedy Institute of Ethics at Georgetown University in Washington, D.C., the purpose being to "put theologians next to doctors."[55] Was a physician justified, or even obligated, to turn off equipment for support of life in a comatose individual "whose heart continues to beat but whose brain is irreversibly damaged?" This question induced Harvard Medical School in 1968 to establish a committee to redefine "death." The committee proposed a definition of "brain death" based on two flat EEG readings in a patient who was not on barbiturates and displayed no reflex activity.[56] The definition of death became all the more important with advances in organ transplantation. Kidneys were being transplanted, sometimes involving organs from living relatives and sometimes from cadavers, with gradually increasing frequency and success starting in 1950. The first heart transplantation in December 1967 by Christiaan Barnard of South Africa made the ethical problems more palpable because

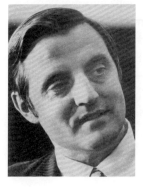

FIG. 561
*Walter
Mondale
(born 1928)*

the heart traditionally had been considered the seat of life and had to be transplanted in a viable state "as close as possible to the moment when death of the donor can be established."[57] Three months after Barnard's transplantation, Senator Walter Mondale (Fig. 561) of Minnesota introduced a bill to establish a Commission on Health Science and Society to assess the ethical, legal, social, and political implications of biomedical advances, warning that those advances had raised

... grave and fundamental ethical and legal questions for our society. Who shall live and who shall die? how long shall life be preserved and how should it be altered? who shall make decisions? how shall society be prepared?[58]

Mondale's initiative met with vocal opposition from the medical profession. In hearings concerning the bill, cardiac transplant surgeon, Adrian Kantrowitz, made this declaration: "We are stepping into areas in the development of medicine where a certain amount of boldness is necessary for success ... I am not sure that committees have established a reputation for courage and boldness." Owen Wangensteen, Professor Emeritus of Surgery at the University of Minnesota, cautioned, "If we are to retain a place of eminence in medicine,

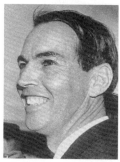

FIG. 562
*Christiaan
Barnard
(1922-2001)*

let us take care not to shackle the investigator with unnecessary strictures, which will dry up untapped resources of creativity." Wangensteen rejected the intrusion of "outsiders" into the sphere of medicine, advising that "the fellow who holds the apple can peel it best." When a senator suggested that the public paid for research and, therefore, should be allowed a role in making decisions about it, Christiaan Barnard (Fig. 562) responded with an echo of the old self-image of physicians as "warriors against disease" thus:

Who pays the costs of war? The public! Who decides where the general should attack? The public? The public is not qualified to make the decision. The general makes the decision. He is qualified to spend the public's money the best way he thinks fit.[59]

Federal Protection for Human Subjects in Research

Formidable opposition by medical researchers quashed Mondale's bill, and when the Senator reintroduced his legislation in 1971, it met the same fate. It took a series of public revelations about disturbing experiments on humans—most importantly the Tuskegee Syphilis Study – to alter attitudes in Congress. In the opening months of 1973, several bills were introduced in Congress to regulate biomedical research, and Senator Edward Kennedy of Massachusetts, who had recently assumed the chair of the Subcommittee on Health of the Committee on Labor and Social Welfare, conducted hearings on the "Quality of Health Care – Human Experimentation." In those hearings, testimony was given not only by physicians but also by victims of questionable experiments, such as subjects of the Tuskegee study and inmates of Holmesburg Prison (Fig. 563). As a consequence, Congress passed the National Research Act in 1974 with a provision creating the National Commission for the Protection of Human Subjects of Biomedical and Behavioral Research.[60]

The National Commission was to be composed of 11 members, only five of whom could be researchers. In negotiations

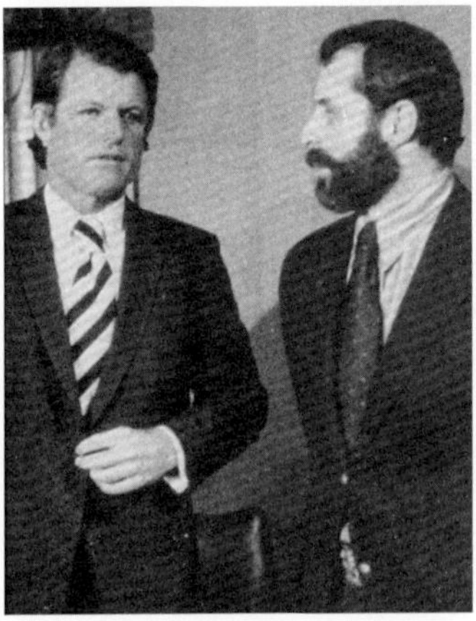

FIG. 563
Senator Edward Kennedy (left) and Peter J. Buxtun in March 1973 at a hearing convened to learn details of the Tuskegee Syphilis Study.

concerning the bill, Kennedy had agreed that the Commission be temporary, rather than permanent, and have no enforcement powers of its own, acting only in an advisory capacity to the secretary of the DHEW. That compromise, however, was based on the condition that the DHEW issue uniform, binding regulations governing research on human subjects. The new regulations were not directed at individual researchers, but at "the institution which receives or is accountable to DHEW for the funds awarded for the support of the activity."[61] They stipulated that "legally effective informed consent" must be obtained by "adequate and appropriate methods" and, ordinarily, should be documented in writing unless subjects are not placed at significant risk. They also closed loopholes that might have offered investigators an opportunity to waive documentation of consent, with the exception of one provision allowing "modified procedures" if "obtaining informed consent would surely invalidate objectives of considerable immediate importance." All research, not only that which placed subjects at risk, was to undergo review.[62]

In the four years of its existence, the National Commission published 17 Reports and Appendices on issues ranging from "Disclosure of Research Information" to "Institutional Review Boards" and "Research Involving Those Institutionalized as Mentally Infirm."[63] Many of the recommendations of the Commission became federal policy with only minor alterations, for example, regulations regarding fetal research and research on children.[64] Other deliberations of the National Commission were more theoretical, but they helped to clarify the significance of guidelines for experiments on humans and the ethical principles that underlay them. This was true especially for the so-called Belmont Report, in which research was defined as "an activity designed to test an hypothesis, permit conclusions to be drawn, and thereby to develop or contribute to generalizable knowledge."[65] The Belmont report also included a scheme according to which guidelines for informed consent should emerge from the principle of respect for persons, guidelines for risk-benefit assessment should emanate from the principle of beneficence, and guidelines for the selection of subjects should issue from the principle of justice.[66] When the statutory limit of the National Commission expired in 1978, Kennedy was able to transform it into the President's Commission for the Study of Ethical Problems in Medicine and provide it the scope that Mondale had urged a decade before.[67]

Tightening Security Around the World

The debate about experiments on humans in the United States soon prompted new activities in that domain internationally. One year after promulgation of the National Research Act, in 1975, the Declaration of Helsinki was revised at the 29th World Medical Assembly (WMA) in Tokyo. In contrast with the original Declaration, the revised version, called "Helsinki II," listed informed consent, either by the subject or by his or her legal guardian, as one of the "Basic Principles":

In any research on human beings, each potential subject must be adequately informed of the aims, methods, anticipated benefits and potential hazards of the study and the discomfort it may entail . . . The doctor should then obtain the subject's freely given informed consent, preferably in writing.

Special consideration was given to obtaining informed consent "if the subject is in a dependent relationship . . . or may consent under duress. In that case the informed consent should be obtained by a doctor who is not engaged in the investigation and who is completely independent of this official relationship." Perhaps the greatest change from Helsinki I to Helsinki II was the inclusion of committees appointed to review ethical issues. In another of the "Basic Principles," the following was stated:

The design and performance of each experimental procedure involving human subjects should be clearly formulated in an experimental protocol which should be transmitted to a specially appointed independent committee for consideration, comment, and guidance.

The Declaration required that research protocols "always contain a statement of the ethical considerations involved and should indicate that the principles enunciated in the present Declaration are complied with." Moreover, it stipulated that "...reports of experimentation not in accordance with the principles laid down in this Declaration should not be accepted for publication."[68]

The revised Declaration of Helsinki came to be recognized as the fundamental guiding principles for the conduct of biomedical research involving human subjects. It was adopted, in modified but similar form, in international texts and national legislation, and by professional medical organizations throughout the world. Further revisions of the Declaration took place in Venice in 1983, in Hong Kong in 1989, and in Somerset West, South Africa in 1996. The latest version was adopted in 2000 at the 52nd General Assembly of the WMA in Edinburgh, Scotland, and included several new provisions. Among them were the obligation of researchers to inform test subjects of sources of funding and "any possible conflicts of interest," and the prohibition of placebos for control groups if effective treatment modalities are available. In regard to the relationship between investigators and review boards, it stated, "The researcher has the obligation to provide monitoring information to the committee, especially any serious adverse events."

In 1982, the principles of the revised Declaration of Helsinki were expanded on by the World Health Organization (WHO) and the Council for International Organizations of Medical Sciences (CIOMS). The resultant guidelines dealt in great detail with problems of informed consent, especially in regard to subjects who lived in developing countries; "vulnerable groups," such as children, pregnant and nursing women, mentally ill and mentally defective persons, and "junior or subordinate members of a hierarchically-structured group;" and community-based research, such as compulsory vaccination programs and the addition of fluoride to a public water supply. The WHO/CIOMS guidelines recognized, in each of these instances, that informed consent might be unobtainable and, therefore, attached even more importance to independent ethical review than was outlined in the Declaration of Helsinki.[69] Although the article of Helsinki II that stipulated "freely given informed consent" was cited, the citation was qualified by the following statement:

Of itself, however, informed consent offers an inadequate safeguard to the subject and it should always be complemented by independent ethical review of research proposals.[70]

The objective of the WHO/CIOMS guidelines was to enable countries to "define a national policy on the ethics of medical and health research and . . . establish adequate mechanisms for ethical review of research activities involving human subjects."[71] Those objectives were reached; institutional review boards were created at research facilities in all developed countries. The fear that having to meet the obligations of ethical guidelines and the complex procedures designed to ensure adherence to them would impair research and retard medical progress was not justified. To be sure, it became more difficult to embark on studies involving experiments on humans, but the quality of those studies improved markedly because they had to be thought through carefully before any investigation was undertaken. The mere necessity of presenting a research proposal to an independent body for review was a strong stimulus to consider every detail that might prove important and that might elicit a negative response. As a consequence, mistakes in the design of studies were avoided from the outset, and, not infrequently, the expertise of members of review boards even helped to improve the studies. One problem created by the establishment of review boards was intrusion into the autonomy of patients. For example, when studies on some retroviral drugs were blocked by institutional review boards (IRBs), desperate patients with acquired immunodeficiency syndrome (AIDS), who had put their hopes for survival on these drugs, could not understand why they should be denied the right to make an autonomous decision about taking them. The advantages offered by IRBs, however, were found to outweigh the problems; review boards have since gained unqualified acceptance.

The debate in the 1960s and 1970s concerning questionable experiments on humans, and regulations that have emerged consequently, have transformed medical research. The impact of that development, however, was even greater because the rules established for medical research were now applied to medicine as a whole. Just as the discretion of physicians was curtailed in laboratories, so, too, was it in hospitals.[72] The days of medical paternalism were over; the autonomy of patients began to be regarded as of prime importance, and written informed consent came to be required even for medical and surgical procedures thought to be banal. These changes in the daily practice of medicine influenced, in turn, the attitudes of researchers, reinforcing respect for autonomy of test subjects and dedication to the welfare of them. After the introduction of regulations by the U.S. Food and Drug Administration and the National Institutes of Health, the establishment of the National Commission for the Protection of Human Subjects of Biomedical and Behavioral Research, the promulgation of the revised version of the Declaration of Helsinki, and the WHO/CIOMS guidelines, medical research on human beings no longer was the same.

CHAPTER 26

THE END OF THE STORY?

When the "Neisser Case" was debated hotly in Germany during the last months of the nineteenth century, leading eventually to the first official regulation governing experiments on humans, the press criticized not only the violation of medical ethics by physicians of that time, but the claim that any ethics were specific for medicine, arguing that "there is only a single, general ethics, and not so and so many ethics in specific professions."[1] This assessment was correct; it did not require ethics specific for medicine to recognize that risky medical experiments on unsuspecting test subjects were unacceptable. Claude Bernard got it right in 1856 when he said, "Christian morals forbid only one thing, doing ill to one's neighbor."[2] Doing ill to test subjects without informing them of hazards of a procedure and obtaining their consent was patently immoral, and it was perceived to be that at the very time the experiments were being performed, as evidenced by harsh reactions of the public whenever dubious experiments on humans became known and by fear of "negative publicity" of investigators and agencies sponsoring them. The "general ethics" were applicable; they allowed right to be distinguished from wrong. This is why claims of investigators that they did not violate ethical standards of their time always rang hollow.

It must be acknowledged, however, that for most of the nineteenth and twentieth centuries unethical experiments on humans were performed with hardly any resistance. How was it possible that studies that violated accepted ethical principles, and were perceived as unacceptable by the public at large, found acceptance in the medical community? The reason was that some principles of "general ethics" were suspended in the context of decisions made by physicians. This phenomenon was not exceptional. Soldiers, for instance, find nothing wrong in killing people as part of their professional duties, and lawyers do not hesitate to help murderers go unpunished and able, therefore, to resume their criminal activities. These examples of "professional ethics" are at odds with "general ethics," but they do not affect the general population on a daily basis and in a personal way. That being the case, they did not elicit as much attention and criticism as particular aspects of the practice of medicine. That doctors used unsuspecting patients for medical experiments was highly alarming to average citizens, who could never be sure that they would not be the next to be experimented on.

The purpose originally of medical ethics was not to suspend, but to reinforce, aspects of "general ethics." In the delicate, unequal relationship between patient and doctor, the one placing his being in the hands of the other and that other engaging the being in order to restore it to health, reinforcement of ethical principles seemed to be necessary for allaying fears and generating trust. The traditional importance attached to ethics in the realm of medicine was supposed to remind physicians and to reassure patients that their relationship served but a single purpose, namely, betterment of the individual seeking medical aid. In the nineteenth and twentieth centuries, that purpose was lost sight of for a variety of reasons, including the advent and increasing importance of experimental medicine, the consideration of advantages for the society and mankind rather than for the individual patient, and the general disregard for ethical issues. Ethics were taught only rarely during the proscribed course of medical education, and the pledge of the Oath of Hippocrates at the time of graduation from medical school was dismissed as antiquated ritual. When traditional ethical boundaries were transgressed time and again by physicians and the trust of patients began to wane, the ethics of medicine had to be rethought, rewritten, and reaffirmed, a process that was long and difficult. The train of unethical experiments on humans has come to a halt time and again, only to pick up momentum anew. As soon as new rules were established in regard to experiments on humans, they were circumvented or ignored. Nevertheless, the efforts have not been in vain. Following the orgy of experimentation on humans in the 1950s and '60s, the practice of medical research has changed, and with it the practice of medicine itself. That change demonstrates convincingly the need for a special ethics of medicine. But has the last word been spoken? Has the train at long last come to its final stop? Is this the end of the story?

Unethical Experiments on Humans Continue to be Performed

It would be naive to think so. In fact, although currently there can be no objection to the vast majority of experiments on humans, dubious experiments continue to be performed. Some of the most egregious examples in the recent past occurred in countries whose government was not a democratic one. Under the Red Khmer government in Cambodia, political prisoners were used routinely for the purpose of demonstrating the anatomy of humans to medical cadres. A notebook recovered near the central prison in Phnom Penh described bizarre experiments, such as bleeding prisoners to death and seeing how long dead bodies take to rise to the surface of a tank of water.[3] In 1990, the World Health Organization investigated claims that an untested treatment for AIDS was being administered to children, mostly orphans, in a hospital in Bucharest, Romania.[4] In 1991, less than one year after the reunification of Germany, it was revealed that East German scientists had used "men, women, and children as human guinea pigs in a state-sponsored research program intended to perfect steroid hormone drugs" in an effort "to develop compounds that would boost the performance of East German athletes." In contrast to clandestine abuse of steroids by athletes in the West, this was "a full-fledged scientific effort – complete with controlled experiments and scientific meetings and seminars." It resulted in several scientific theses that never were published but served as a springboard for an academic career. Test subjects, among them many minors, never were informed about risks associated with taking those substances, among them liver damage, and never were asked for their consent.[5] In Iraq, Saddam Hussein's biological warfare program included field trials on human beings. Although Iraqi officials, in violation of the conditions of a signed peace agreement, placed countless obstacles in the way of UN inspectors seeking to assess Iraq's capability for biological and chemical warfare, the United Nations Special Commission, as the former chairman of it, Scott Ritter, recalled in 1998, found "evidence that 95 political prisoners had been transferred from Abu Gharib Prison to a site in western Iraq, where they had been subjected to lethal testing."[6]

Not only under dictatorships did violations of ethical guidelines governing experiments on humans occur. In Germany in the late 1980s, the psychiatrist, Hans Hippius of Munich, showed frightening pictures and movies to psychiatric patients in order to assess the efficacy on them of drugs designed to alleviate anxiety. The study was sponsored by Germany's *Federal Agency for Civil Defense* (Bundesamt für Zivilschutz).[7] When preparing for the Gulf War, the U.S. Department of Defense received special permission from the Food and Drug Administration to use "unapproved drugs" in "certain battlefield or combat-related" situations without having first obtained informed consent. The regulation noted that the term "combat-related" might mean only the threat of combat. The Department of Defense agreed to give all soldiers asked or ordered to take unapproved drugs an information sheet about what they were taking, but, in reality, hardly ever was that information provided. Among the investigational drugs given to soldiers were a vaccine against botulinum toxin, one of Iraq's biological warfare agents, and pyridostigmine bromide, a drug supposed to protect against attacks with nerve gas but that was known to have neurotoxic effects of its own. On their return from the Gulf, many veterans began to report debilitating illnesses, including fatigue, muscle and joint pain, headaches, and memory loss, which may, conceivably, have been caused by the investigational drugs adminstered without their consent.[8]

In October 1997, the chairman of dermatology of the University of Alabama at Birmingham, W. Mitchell Sams, Jr., was disqualified by the Food and Drug Administration from working with investigational drugs. Sams had conducted a clinical trial with an ointment containing the investigational drug, BCX-34, on patients with cutaneous T-cell lymphoma. At a national dermatology meeting in Chicago in 1995, he had reported on a good response in 14 of 19 patients, including complete remission in seven of them. Three weeks later, the company which had developed the drug and sponsored the study retracted its reports to the Food and Drug Administration and acknowledged that the medication had not been shown to be effective. Further inquiry by the Food and Drug Administration revealed "numerous significant deficiencies in the conduct of the . . . study," including "improper delegations of authority by the principal investigator, failures to follow the protocols, institutional review board deviations," and "serious noncompliance with HHS (Health and Human Services) requirements for the protection of human subjects."[9] Parenthetically, Sams had been president of the American Academy of Dermatology in 1996 and during his tenure had made ethics in medicine his major theme.

In September 1999, an 18-year old man from Tuscon, Arizona (Fig. 564) died as a consequence of a trial of gene therapy conducted by researchers at the University of Pennsylvania School of Medicine. The test subject was suf-

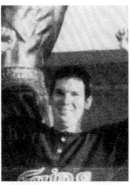

FIG. 564
Jesse Galinger, 18, of Tuscon, Arizona died four days after having received an experimental drug in a gene research study at the University of Pennsylvania on September 17, 1999.

fering from a mild form of deficiency of ornithine transcarbamylase, an enzyme involved in processing ammonia by the liver. He was given an infusion of adenoviruses carrying corrective genes and developed an immune reaction that could not be controlled. The trial was designed to test the safety of that treatment for babies who had a fatal form of ornithine transcarbamylase deficiency. The therapy with genes offered only little benefit to the test subject, whose disease was being controlled through diet and drugs. The test subject had given "informed consent," but the information provided to him had not been comprehesive. For example, the information that monkeys had died after a similar, although stronger, treatment was omitted from the consent form. Moreover, in violation of federal rules, neither the Food and Drug Administration nor the Recombinant DNA Advisory Committee of the National Institutes of Health had been informed when test subjects experienced elevations in liver enzymes significant enough to bring an end to the trial.[10] Four months after the death of the patient, the Food and Drug Administration shut down all experiments about gene therapy at the University of Pennsylvania, citing "numerous deficiencies" in the way the trial was run, including serious lapses in informed consent.[11] A suit against the University of Pennsylvania brought by the family of the deceased young man was settled quickly out of court.

The Abuse of Man

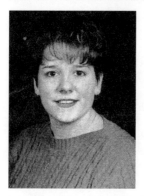

FIG. 565
*Ellen Roche,
24, of Balti-
more died one
month after
having in-
haled an ex-
perimental
drug on June
2, 2001.*

In June 2001, a 24 year-old technician at Johns Hopkins University
(Fig. 565) died after having participated in a study concerning the mechanisms of asthma. In order to determine the role of nerves in the lungs for
the constriction and relaxation of air-
ways, test subjects had to inhale a
drug, hexamethonium, that temporarily blocks nerves from function-
ing normally. One day following the experiment, the test subject developed problems in breathing and she died after having
spent several weeks in an intensive care unit. The subject had
volunteered for the experiment and had signed a consent form
that had been approved by the review board of the university.
The form, however, did not state that hexamethonium had not
been approved by the Food and Drug Administration and that
data on the safety of handling it came from experience with just
20 patients. Moreover, the principal investigator had over-
looked some articles suggesting that the drug might injure the
lungs and had failed to report to the review board side effects in
another test subject, namely, cough and shortness of breath
that lasted for one week after inhalation of hexamethonium. A
few days after recovery of the first subject, the 24-year-old technician took the drug. According to a report by an internal committee of the medical center of Johns Hopkins University, that
drug "was either solely responsible for the subject's illness or
played an important contributory role." In contrast to stonewalling by representatives of the University of Pennsylvania,
the dean and chief executive of Johns Hopkins Medicine, Edward B. Miller, declared immediately after the incident that
"Hopkins takes full resonsibility for what did happen."[12]

These few examples, however, are only the tip of an iceberg.
That the number of cases of unreported dubious experiments

on humans is very high can be concluded from incontrovertible evidence. Chief among them is the fact that many studies involving human beings continue to be performed without their having first been submitted to review boards charged with assessing the ethical aspects of them. Innovative surgical procedures, for example, are not usually subjected to formal review, but are left to the discretion of the surgeon who performs them.[13] The medical literature is replete with articles that house findings obtained during the ordinary management of patients and, in that context, an additional biopsy, an unnecessary blood test, a superfluous gastroscopy, or the choice of a drug whose effectiveness has not been well established for a given disease go unnoticed and unchallenged.

Inherent Flaws in Guidelines Governing Experiments on Humans

But even studies that are subjected to formal review may not always be sound ethically. As is the situation for all guidelines that are general, the revised Declaration of Helsinki has serious flaws in it. Some issues have not been addressed at all, for example, the difficult problem of a selection of test subjects justly. If members of vulnerable groups are to be excluded, and if the term "vulnerable groups" is defined in a broad sense, including not only mentally disabled persons and prisoners, but also children, soldiers, medical students, and poor or poorly educated persons, it becomes extremely difficult, if not impossible, to find volunteers acceptable for a study. And if, for purposes of equality, participation of members of any of those groups had to be restricted to the percentage of them in the general population, it would be practically impossible to conduct any studies on humans.

Another unresolved problem is the powerful influence that a physician exerts on a patient and that may amount to a subtle form of coercion. As pointed out at a recent symposium of the American Dermatologic Association, "investigators, anxious to fulfill their commitment to the drug company and to profit thereby, can easily influence patients who are marginally qualified ... or not particularly enthusiastic" about participating in a study.[14] A recent example is a study concerning an experimental vaccine for treatment of metastases of malignant melanoma. In order to recruit test subjects, the responsible investigator, Michael McGee of the University of Oklahoma, told patients suffering from melanoma that "we have the best vaccine out there" and that he even gave the drug to his father-in-law.[15] But even if an experimenter does his best to explain a study to a patient in a fair and comprehensive way, and to leave the choice of whether or not to take part in it entirely to the patient, that patient may feel obligated to participate.

In several respects, the revised Declaration of Helsinki falls behind the Nuremberg Code. First, it is a non-mandatory set of rules instead of a legal document. Second, the protection of subjects who are incompetent has been weakened. According to the latest version of the Helsinki Declaration that was adopted in Edinburgh in 2000, even non-therapeutic research on incompetent subjects is acceptable "if the physical/mental condition that prevents obtaining informed consent is a necessary characteristic of the research population." Third, provisions regarded formerly as essential were not considered at all. Among them was the participation of investigators themselves as test subjects. According to the fifth paragraph of the Nuremberg Code, experiments in which there was "an a priori reason to believe that death or disabling injury will occur" were permissible when "the experimental physicians also serve as subjects." This statement was susceptible easily to misinterpretation. It was applicable only in the context of all other requirements. As an isolated requirement it would have been unacceptable because willingness of an experimenter to expose himself to serious, and possibly fatal, consequences does not justify recourse to other human subjects. Taken out of context, however, other provisions of the Nuremberg Code also were insufficient safeguards for test subjects, including the one concerning informed consent. In 1949, the president of the Royal Society of Medicine, George Pickering of Oxford (Fig. 566), referred to partici-

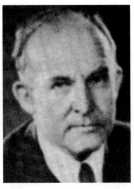

FIG. 566
*George
Pickering
(1904-1980)*

pation of investigators in medical studies as a "golden rule" that helped to decide "whether the experiment is justifiable."[16] In 1959, Henry K. Beecher of Boston made clear that, "whenever doubts exist as to safety, it is advisable for the investigator first to subject himself to the possible hazards involved."[17] In 1969, the philosopher Hans Jonas designated the experimenter the "first natural addressee" in calls for test subjects.[18] In fact, the obligation of experimenters themselves to participate in studies whenever feasible would have prevented the vast majority of unethical experiments that have been performed on humans in the past.

The same may be true for experiments today. One example is a study concerning the industrial pollutant, perchlorate, performed in 2000 by physicians at Loma Linda University Medical Center in San Bernardino, California on behalf of the aerospace giant, Lockheed Martin. In that study, approved by ethical review boards of three medical institutions, test subjects had to swallow, every day for six months, a dose of perchlorate that exceeded the level of safety set by the state health department by 83 times. Perchlorate is a toxic component of rocket fuel that may damage thyroid function and cause cancer. Once used for treatment of thyrotoxicosis, it was discredited in the 1960s as a therapeutic drug because of severe, and sometimes lethal, side effects, such as aplastic anemia and agranulocytosis.

Subjects of the Loma Linda study were not informed comprehensively about those risks, and they did not know that the sponsor of the study, Lockheed Martin, at the very same time, was being sued by a group of San Bernardino residents suffering from thyroid cancer and other disorders that may have been caused by ingestion of perchlorate leaching from a Lockheed Martin plant into water supplies nearby. Lockheed Martin pumped considerable money into the Loma Linda study, hoping that the results would help the company to save millions of dollars in cleanup costs. The offer of $1,000 dollars per subject procured enough volunteers.[19, 20] But would the study have been conducted had the investigators been obligated to participate in it, as demanded in fifth paragraph of the Nuremberg Code? It is startling that what once was perceived as a "golden rule" eventually was struck from consideration.

Fourth, and perhaps most important, responsibility for experiments has shifted from the individual investigator to the institution. Previous codes had emphasized the personal responsibility of investigators. The German "Guidelines for Innovative Therapy and Human Experimentation" of 1931 had identified the chief physician of an institution or service as the person bearing final, non-transferable responsibility for experiments performed in his institution or service. Even though the physician in charge could not be expected to oversee personally every particular experiment, his responsibilty for maintaining standards of professional performance, for establishing an effective system of cooperation and information, and for representing and re-enforcing the ethos of the institution made him responsible directly and liable for matters which, in the conventional division of labor in a typical organization, are included only indirectly and very loosely, if at all, within the realm of personal professional conduct. The German Guidelines made no mention of boards or committees that might share or dilute responsibility.[21] Following the disastrous experiences in Nazi Germany with a medical system organized hierarchically and that allowed investigators to shift responsibility for experiments to their superiors, the Nuremberg Code, at the end of its first paragraph, stated unequivocally that "the duty and responsibility for ascertaining the quality of consent rests upon each individual who initiates, directs or engages in the experiment. It is a personal duty and responsibility which may not be delegated to another with impunity." No such provision is found in the subsequent codes of the U.S. Department of Health, Education, and Welfare, the World Medical Association, and the World Health Organization. Although comments made episodically do convey the idea that investigators still bear responsibility ultimately, the reality is different. In 1980, for example, an American physician was fired by the Ortho Pharmaceutical Corporation because she refused to participate in certain experiments. When she filed suit against the company on the basis of the responsibility imposed personally on each investigator by the Nuremberg Code, the court dismissed her action, arguing that chaos would result if the conscience of individual researchers was allowed to decide whether or not scientific studies should be carried out.[22]

Limitations of Institutional Review Boards

The revised Declaration of Helsinki and other related codes delegated responsibility for the ethical aspects of research to review boards within institutions. Those boards, however, bear no responsibility to test subjects. No member of a review board has ever been convicted of neglect of his or her duties vis-à-vis test subjects. Another problem of review boards is the composition of them. Most members are scientists who usually share the values of fellow investigators. They often are on the faculty of the institution to which the investigators belong, know the investigators personally, and may be disposed inordinately favorably to them and to their wishes. They also know, when sitting in judgment of a research protocol, that their own research projects may be the next to be subjected to scrutiny, and, therefore, they may refrain from insisting on standards of protection for test subjects that would place impediments on the conduct of that particular research or of their own.[23] Moreover, institutional review boards lack the manpower, budget, and time to do much more than review research protocols and check consent forms. The director of the Center for Bioethics at the University of Pennsylvania, Arthur L. Caplan, testified in 1997 that he had "never met an IRB member who has spent any serious amount of time debriefing subjects or visiting with researchers. They almost never talk with researchers or subjects. Thus, they remain uninformed about the extent to which, what they require on paper in the way of informed consent, is actually put into practice."[24] In 1998, an investigation by the Inspector General of the U.S. Department of Health and Human Services found that committees may spend no more than a few minutes reviewing each study.[25] Given that brief amount of time, a thorough review of protocols, including a competent weighing of scientific merit versus risks for test subjects, may be impossible. This is even more true for ongoing review of approved research projects, especially in regard to studies at multiple sites carried out by different investigators at different places.[26] In general, once a study is approved, it is not monitored further by review boards. As a consequence, investigators may deviate from the principles set forth in their application and may fail, too, to reconsider the ethics of a study in the light of new information.

For example, when investigators of the Food and Drug Administration discovered that the dermatologist, W. Mitchell Sams of the University of Alabama, had deviated in a clinical trial in 1995 from decisions of the institutional review board of his university, the review board was criticized for not having fulfilled its obligation to monitor Sam's research and to report any serious noncompliance or unanticipated problems involving risks to subjects or others. Broader scrutiny of the institutional review board prompted the Office for Protection from Research Risks of the National Institutes of Health, in January 2000, to suspend immediately about 550 research projects at the University of Alabama that were funded by the federal government and that utilized human subjects.[27]

In 1999, when officials of the Food and Drug Administration investigated the death of the 18-year old patient in the gene therapy trial conducted at the University of Pennsylvania, they found that the consent form given to patients differed from the one that the agency had approved. They noted also that serious side effects that could have brought a halt to the trial long before the fatal incident occurred had not been called attention to urgently and, moreover, the consent form had not been revised to include them.[28] More extensive scrutiny by the NIH of trials of gene therapy revealed that throughout the country there had been 691 "serious adverse events" in experiments involving the use of adenoviruses, only 39 of which had been recorded formally by scientists.[29]

Despite the existence of institutional review boards, basic research at universities is controlled much less rigorously than research conducted by industry. In order to test an investigational drug on human beings, industry has to apply to the Food and Drug Administration (FDA) for permission, a procedure that takes many months, if not years, of paperwork and sometimes millions of dollars in expense. By contrast, many investigators in academe, who do not have the personnel, time, and money for that procedure, usually turn reflexively to the institutional review board of their university, whose standards for safety tend to be much lower than those of the FDA. For example, when a test subject died in 2001 as a consequence of having inhaled an unapproved drug in a study at Johns Hopkins University, investigations revealed severe shortcomings in preparation for the study. Without having conducted a probing review of the literature concerning side effects of the drug and without having performed experiments on animals, the investigator, with the approval of the institutional review board of the university, went to a chemical supply house, bought the substance, sterilized it, and administered it to human subjects. Because of this laxness of the institutional review board, all federally financed medical research at Johns Hopkins was suspended, a major blow to a university that previously had received more federal research money that any other university in the United States. Although the suspension of federally funded research at Johns Hopkins served as a serious warning to medical schools throughout the country, the real problem remained unresolved. Because of lack of resources, it is difficult for universities to reconcile basic research with strict standards for safety, and, as might be expected, investigators muttered concerns that insistence on approval of studies by the FDA would be "a major disruption to academic research."[30]

Following an investigation of institutional review boards (IRBS) in 1998, the Inspector General of the Department of Health and Human Services asserted that "the effectiveness of IRBS is now in jeopardy." According to his report, the main problems were that 1) IRBS review too much, too quickly, and with too little expertise, 2) IRBS conduct a minimum of continuing review of approved research, 3) IRBS face conflicts that threaten their independence (for example, placing IRBS in the offices where grants and contracts that bring in research dollars are awarded), 4) institutions provide little training for investigators and board members, 5) institutions make little effort to assess the effectiveness of IRBS, and 6) there is an alarming number of violations of informed consent and unethical advertisement for subjects. The report also warned about the potential for self-serving motives in the emergence of for-profit independent IRBS that contract with pharmaceutical firms and hospitals to review research protocols and research itself.[31]

In addition, big pharamaceutical companies, acknowledging the increasing importance of bioethics, have bioethicists on their payroll or give grants to universities or private institutes of bioethics, thereby creating dependency on the part of bioethicists. For example, Stanford University, in 1996, accepted $1 million from the pharmaceutical giant, SmithKline Beecham, to start a program in ethics and genetics. The Hastings Center, a private institute founded in 1969 as the first one devoted specifically to bioethics, received an annual grant of $25,000 from Eli Lilly & Company that was withdrawn after the Center's own journal had published an article critical of a drug produced by that company. Carl Elliott, a bioethicist at the University of Minnesota, alerted to the fact that companies tend to use ethics boards as a kind of corporate window dressing and cautioned that "bioethics boards look like watchdogs, but they are used as show dogs."[32] Curiously, bioethicists at the University of Pennsylvania have avoided scrupulously rendering any opinion in the form of a publication about what might be the responsibilities ethically of that institution to inmates of Holmesburg Prison who, for 25 years, were guinea pigs in experiments carried out there under the aegis of one of the most prominent professors of dermatology of that university. In brief, although the establishment of review boards has been a major advance, various deficiences compromise their functions. As a consequence, review boards cannot be relied on with dependability to prevent certain research projects that should not be done.

Trivialization of Dubious Experiments on Humans

In order to prevent such projects from being done, researchers themselves have to be convinced of the importance of measures to guarantee the safety and autonomy of test subjects. That this is not the case universally can be concluded from how little heed

The Abuse of Man

FIG. 567
*Rudolph
Kampmeier
(1898-1990)*

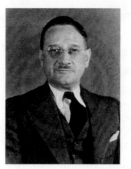

is paid to ethical issues at medical conferences and in medical journals, and from the seemingly irrepressible tendency to trivialize dubious experiments on humans. For example, when the Tuskegee Syphilis Study became public knowledge in 1972, many physicians maintained that nothing had been wrong with it. Among them was Rudolph H. Kampmeier (Fig. 567), a noted syphilologist at Vanderbilt University School of Medicine, who claimed, inaccurately, that "at no time in the 40 year Tuskegee Study is there a hint that treatment desired by a subject was denied him." In an editorial for the Southern Medical Journal, Kampmeier made this statement: "It should be clear that treatment was not withheld, and though no treatment was forced upon men of the Study, they had the freedom of taking what treatment they found convenient or could afford . . . In our free society, anti-syphilitic treatment has never been forced. Since these men did not elect to obtain treatment available to them, the development of aortic disease lay at the subject's door and not in the Study's protocol."[33] Other authors averred that "criticisms of the lack of informed consent are anachronistic,"[34] and defended the decision not to offer penicillin to the test subjects when the drug had become available on the ground that by that time the major damage had already occurred.[35] Almost 30 years later, when experiments on prisoners and mentally disabled children by dermatologists of the University of Pennsylvania were uncovered, reactions were similar. William L. Epstein, chairman emeritus of the department of dermatology of the University of California in San Francisco, and who had worked as a resident with Albert M. Kligman, claimed that "These kids, they don't know what's going on . . . It's not harm." And Kligman, now in his mid-eighties and still active in experimental studies on humans at the

University of Pennsylvania, pointed out that his research "was in keeping with this nation's standard protocol for conducting scientific investigations at that time."[36]*

In 1983, Walter B. Shelley, the former chair of dermatology at the University of Pennsylvania, published a review article titled "Experimental disease in the skin of man." The piece was remarkably comprehensive, except for one aspect, namely, the ethics of experiments on humans. Issues such as the Nuremberg Code and the Declaration of Helsinki, informed consent, and the need for protection of vulnerable members of a population were not just given short shrift; they were not mentioned at all. According to Shelley, all test subjects were volunteers, and in some instances, those "volunteers" were glorified by him in hyperbolic fashion. For example, in regard to the inoculation in 1939 of four subjects with granuloma inguinale, Shelley wrote that "each volunteer should have received a Congressional Medal of Honor for service to their countrymen."[37] The fact that all volunteers had been African-Americans, most likely poorly educated and informed not at all about the consequences of the experiment, and that one of them was said specifically to be "schizophrenic,"[38] was omitted by Shelley. Instead, he praised the blessings brought about by some of the experiments, alerted to the "wondrous feeling of passing from the uneasiness of ignorance into the assurance of knowledge," emphasized that "the ability to produce disease at will is indeed a rich heritage which comes down to us from centuries of work in that incomparable biology laboratory – the human skin," and concluded that "the richest heritage of all is an awareness that there are many more experiments that still may be done in this laboratory."[39] In regard to his own research on humans, including the experimental induction of diseases like acne, hidradenitis suppurativa, miliaria, and external otitis, Shelley declared in 2001 that "I am proud of the experimental work we did and I would repeat it today."[40]

*While this book was in press, Kligman, in an interview with *Dermatology Times* that was published in May 2003, claimed that accusations against him were "preposterous" and denied that any harm had been done by his experiments. He asserted that inmates of Holmesburg Prison were used for studies concerning "dandruff, athlete's foot, and acne," but failed to mention studies performed on them such as those with mind-disabling drugs and with dioxin, and those carried out on disabled children with serious effects. Reminiscent of Udo J. Wile in 1916, Kligman averred that the charge of his having abused human beings in medical experiments "doesn't have the slightest interest for me."

The Abuse of Man

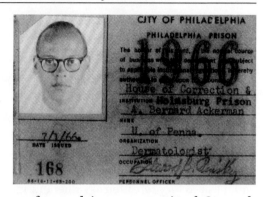

FIG. 568
Card required for admission to Holmesburg Prison, issued on July 1, 1966, to a second-year resident in dermatology at the University of Pennsylvania, A. Bernard Ackerman.

Acknowledgement of wrongdoing was exceptional. One such exception was an "acknowledgement of error and regret," published by the dermatopathologist, A. Bernard Ackerman, who, as a second-year resident in dermatology at the University of Pennsylvania in the mid 1960s, had been involved in experiments on dandruff, devised and orchestrated by Albert Kligman, at Holmesburg Prison.[41] (Fig. 568) That Ackerman's public apology in the year 2000 was a near singular event among physicians is noteworthy in the context of a more general spirit of openness and truthfulness about failure in realms other than medicine. In the same year, Pope John Paul II apologized for atrocities committed by Christians during the Crusades and the Inquisition. In 1998, Japan's Prime Minister, Keizo Obuchi, apologized to the people of Korea for atrocities committed during the Japanese occupation of that country. America's President, William J. Clinton, used a trip to several African countries in 1998 for a belated apology for the injustice and cruelties of slavery.[42] In 1997, Clinton apologized formally to victims of the Tuskegee syphilis study, acknowledging that "the United States government did something that was wrong – deeply, profoundly, morally wrong. It was an outrage to our commitment to integrity and equality for all our citizens."[43] (Fig. 569) With rare exceptions, no similar words have been used by physicians. Instead, a mentality of stonewalling prevailed and prevails, a deliberate effort to hide the facts, to deny, to equivocate, to cover up, to evade, and even to plain lie.[44] The same was done by representatives of universities under whose auspices dubious experiments on humans had been conducted. For example, the University of Pennsylvania, which reaped enormous revenues from Kligman's studies, amounting to tens of millions of dollars, steadfastly denied, and continues to deny, any wrongdoing. In 1998, Richard Tannen, senior vice dean in charge of research and academics at the University of Pennsylvania's School of Medicine, issued this statement: "At that point of time, [human experimention] was widespread and felt to be acceptable practice ... So long as the person gave the appropriate consent, the studies were consistent with the [Hippocratic] Oath.*"[45] Only after persistent public criticism was a formal apology made "to the former inmates who think they may have sustained long-term harm as a result of the experiments at Holmesburg Prison."[46]

* During the second half of the year, 2002, the current dean of the School of Medicine at the University of Pennsylvania, Arthur H. Rubenstein, was sent the chapters in this book that deal with the role of that medical school in regard to dubious medical experimentation and was invited repeatedly, and with *carte blanche*, to respond for publication in this work. He declined to do that.

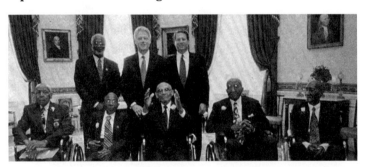

FIG. 569 *Gathering at the White House on May 16, 1997, for the purpose of apology to victims of the Tuskegee Syphilis Study: U.S. Surgeon General David Satcher, President William J. Clinton, and Vice-President Albert Gore together with five survivors of the study.*

Reluctance by the Medical Community to Address Dubious Experiments on Humans

Medical societies are reluctant to address experiments that are objectionable ethically, especially when those experiments have been conducted by their own members. An example is the

American Academy of Dermatology. Following the revelations of the experiments at Holmesburg Prison, the Academy, in 2001, formed an *ad hoc* task force for examining ethical aspects of experiments on human beings. The chairman of the task force, Michael J. Franzblau of San Rafael, California, sent letters to dermatologists who had conducted experiments on humans from the 1950s through the 1970s, asking them to comment on those experiments with the hindsight of up to 50 years. Similar inquiries had been conducted previously by other committees in other fields, for example, by the Advisory Committee on Human Radiation Experiments established by President Clinton. Several recipients of Franzblau's letter, such as Edward H. Ferguson and John H. Epstein, thought that the questions posed had "legitimacy and social value,"[47] and they articulated their own reflections on changes in their perception of the use of vulnerable populations for purposes of research.[48] The officers of the American Academy of Dermatology, however, were furious. They apologized in writing to each physician who had received Franzblau's letter and notified Franzblau that he was not sanctioned "to make inquiries on behalf of the Academy or its Ethics Committee into the research activities of members or other physicians" and, moreover, that his task force had not been authorized by the Academy "to suggest that such experiments may have been in violation of the Nuremberg Code."[49]

In medical journals, contributions alerting readers to ethical flaws in scientific studies continue to be published very uncommonly and only after considerable censorship by editors. In 1967, Maurice H. Pappworth informed that the editor of the *Lancet*, in rejecting a letter in which Pappworth made protests against a study that he deemed to be unethical, had argued that "I know there are times when good comes of speaking strongly and by giving maximum publicity to what appear to be public scandals: but you haven't yet persuaded us here that this is one of those occasions."[50] A similar answer was given when Pappworth criticized a study about catheterizations of the liver and kidney of patients with liver disease that was published in the *Lancet* in 1955. Although 33 of 66 subjects had been delirious and either comatose or stuporous before the experiment was initiated, and 14 were said to be in "the last week of irreversible hepatic coma,"[51] the authors maintained that test subjects "were capable of understanding the nature of the trial."[52] This time, Pappworth's letter was published, but in severely attenuated form, the assistant editor of the *Lancet* explaining his reasons for censoring Pappworth's comments in these words: "I believe there are occasions in medical controversy when the plainest speaking is justified, but I am not convinced that this is one of them."[53]

More than 40 years later, little had changed. When the dubious experiments conducted by Kligman and other dermatologists of the University of Pennsylvania were exposed in 1998 in the book, *Acres of Skin*, by Allen M. Hornblum (Fig. 570), they received wide coverage in the media but only little consideration in journals of dermatology. For example, Ervin Epstein, Sr. (Fig. 571), editor of the *Schoch Letter*, a periodical in the format of a newsletter that purports to be an open forum and vehicle to dermatologists to share ideas with one another, denied publication of a squib about Hornblum's book by contending that "we discussed the matter and reached the conclusion that publishing your item might cause

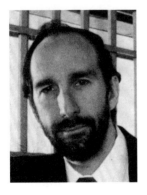

FIG. 570
*Allen M.
Hornblum
(born 1947)*

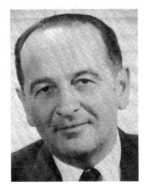

FIG. 571
*Ervin H.
Epstein
(1909-2002)*

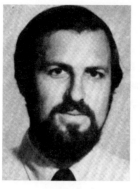

FIG. 572
Kenneth A.
Arndt
(born 1936)

a problem for the Schoch Letter. Therefore, we will be unable to publish your letter."[54]

The only journal that gave substantial consideration to the ethical issues raised by questionable experiments on humans in the realm of dermatology was the *Archives of Dermatology*. Upon urging by the then editor of the "Issues" section of that journal, A. Bernard Ackerman, the editor-in-chief, Kenneth A. Arndt (Fig. 572), agreed to dedicate that section once to the matter of ethics of experiments on humans, including those conducted at Holmesburg Prison. In an article submitted by Allen Hornblum, however, Kligman's name was edited out wherever it appeared – and that was often. The same was done with the name of the University of Pennsylvania, except for a single instance and that being one in which no link was made to the experiments at Holmesburg Prison.[55] Moreover, Hornblum's article was joined by others whose authors tended to trivialize the experiments conducted at Holmesburg Prison, for example, by describing those experiments as "primarily involving dermatologic patch tests" without mentioning studies far more objectionable,[56] by warning that "simply blaming specific people may only have the effect of exonerating everyone else," and even by suggesting vaguely that experiments on prisoners be continued in order to "let them make some money in a reasonable way."[57]

Nevertheless, the articles in the *Archives of Dermatology* generated an angry response by the chairman of the department of dermatology of the University of Pennsylvania, John R. Stanley, who claimed that "outrageous analogies and inflammatory statements" had been made, that "patch testing and skin biopsies" had been described as "horrendous experiments," and that "common sense was lost in exaggerations, misguided analogies, and overly emotional interpretations of what might have happened." Furthermore, Stanley claimed that "it is not clear that any prisoner was harmed by the studies at Holmesburg."[58] In brief, Stanley's letter misrepresented seriously articles critical of what had transpired at Holmesburg Prison and that had appeared in the *Archives of Dermatology*, all of which were devoid of "exaggerations" and "overly emotional interpretations," and it trivialized the objectionable experiments that had been performed by members of the department of dermatology of the University of Pennsylvania before he took charge of it. The editor of the *Archives of Dermatology* sought a response to Stanley's letter, planning to publish the response together with it, but when that response was submitted, it was again subjected to editorial changes that bordered on censorship, such as deletion of the names of Kligman and of the University of Pennsylvania. When those editorial changes were not accepted, Stanley's letter was published, and the response to it was rejected. The explanation given by the editor of the *Archives of Dermatology* was highly reminiscent of arguments used by editors of *The Lancet* in the mid 1950s. This was what Arndt wrote in his letter of rejection: "In my view, the letter would add no light to the discussion of this important topic, but simply a lot more heat. Those manuscripts which I have accepted for publication during my tenure which I have most regretted have been those which in retrospect have been overly provocative." The entire correspondence was later published, unedited, in the journal *Dermatopathology: Practical & Conceptual*.[59]

Breaches of Ethical Rules Continue to be Rewarded

In sum, there is ample evidence that the substantial changes in regulations governing human experiments have not been accompanied by equally profound changes in the mentality of physicians. There also is unimpeachable evidence that most of the reasons that made unethical experiments on humans possible still are operative. Although patients tend to be more critical and better informed than they were in the past, they still depend on physicians to provide them with correct and complete information. Physicians still are caught between the often conflicting requirements of care optimally for individual patients and promotion maximally of their own research. At the universities, the rule of "publish or perish" still obtains. And, perhaps most important, breaches of rules of ethics still are rewarded amply. In 1967, Chester Southam, who injected prisoners and unwitting patients with live cancer cells, was elected vice-president of the American Association for Cancer Research, and in 1968 he became its president. Saul Krugman, who deliberately infected children with hepatitis at the Willowbrook State School for the Retarded, became chairman of the department of pediatrics at New York University School of Medicine. In 1972, on the occasion of being given the John Russell Award of the Markle Foundation, Krugman was praised for demonstrating how clinical research ought to be done. In 1983, he won the Lasker Prize, the highest award given for medical research in the United States.[60] The dermatologist, Albert M. Kligman, has been showered with prizes and honors. In June 1999, for example, the leaders of American dermatology met in Piscataway, New Jersey to discuss "Advances in the Biology and Treatment of the Skin" at "a symposium honoring Albert M. Kligman." The University of Pennsylvania has feted him repeatedly, praised him to the skies in official publications, and even has named a chair for him.

All those honors heaped on Southam, Krugman, Kligman, and others like them, were awarded after unethical experiments by them had become well known. By turning physicians who had violated flagrantly basic rules of human decency into role models for novices in medicine, the universities, especially, forfeited their responsibility as institutions dedicated chiefly to education in the best Socratic sense. One of the pioneers of medical ethics, Albert Moll of Berlin, stated in 1899 that a man who does not shrink from inoculating helpless persons with pathogens "is neither suited to be a physician nor a teacher. More important than all discussions about medical ethics at congresses is the good example."[61] The opposite is also true: nothing could be more detrimental to medical research than a bad example. As a consequence of making miscreants into models, some universities became a breeding ground for scores of experimenters who, in pursuit of their research and advancement of their careers, seemed to pay no heed to ethical scruple. Among them was the University of Pennsylvania, from which came not only Albert Kligman, but also his pupils William Epstein, Howard Maibach, John Strauss, James Fulton, and others. Those students copied Kligman's recipe for success, namely, systematic exploitation of vulnerable human beings for one's own benefit, and, like their teacher, they were feted. The message could not be misread: Violations of ethics in the course of medical research, in the unlikely event that those deviations be uncovered, might cause a tempest in a teapot, but in the long run would pay off handsomely.

And those violations would pay off not only in terms of fame, but also in hard dollars. Kligman, who amassed a fortune from his studies at Holmesburg Prison, was a pioneer in the merger of research and business. Like Kligman, many other scientists have founded private companies in order to shift revenues from research into their own pockets. That development was accelerated by the U.S. Congress which, in 1980, passed the Bayh-Dole Act, a law that encourages universities to patent inventions and then assign the right to those patents to private companies that are able to develop them into products. In an analysis in 1996 of 789 articles in medical journals, Sheldon Krimsky, a professor of urban and environmental policy at Tufts University, found that 34 percent of the authors had a financial interest in the subject matter being studied, and in many of those a patent was pending.[62] That the lure of profit may color scientific integrity cannot be dismissed. In fact, the lesson of numerous studies is that methods and results of research are influenced by financial incentives. According to one study, "articles with drug company support are more likely than articles without drug company support to have outcomes favoring the drug of interest."[63] Another study found "a strong association between authors' published positions on the safety of calcium-channel antagonists and their financial relationships with pharmaceutical manufacturers,"[64] and yet another study came to the conclusion that "pharmaceutical company sponsorship of economic analyses is associated with reduced likelihood of reporting unfavorable events."[65] Likewise, scientists with a financial stake in companies whose fortunes can rise and fall on a single product may be tempted to push for experiments that might not be safe or to withhold information about side effects that might be dangerous.

A recent example of those obstacles is the failure of researchers throughout the United States to fulfill an obligation to report side effects during trials of gene therapy to the Food and Drug Administration and the Recombinant DNA Advisory Committee of the National Institutes of Health. One researcher, Ronald G. Crystal of Weill Medical College of Cornell University, asked the panel not to disclose the fact that a patient had died of an underlying illness during an experiment concerning gene therapy conducted for the company he founded. When the first death secondary to an experiment regarding gene therapy occurred at the University of Pennsylvania in September 1999, investigation of it revealed conflicts of interest. The principal investigator and director of the university's Institute for Human Gene Therapy, James Wilson, also was the founder of a biotechnology company, Genovo, in which both he and the university owned shares of stock. Contributions from Genovo made up one-fifth of the $25 million annual budget of the institute for gene therapy, and in return Genovo had exclusive rights to develop the discoveries of Dr. Wilson into commercial products.[66] Although the fatal outcome of one of the experiments cannot be blamed on that unsettling relationship, the economic prospects of research may enhance the desire for quick results and a disdainful attitude

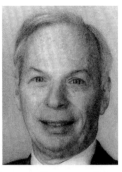

FIG. 573
Richard L. Tannen

toward safety. The Nobel laureate and former director of the National Institutes of Health, Harold Varmus, was one of several critics who asserted that researchers in gene therapy were moving too rapidly into clinical trials.[67]

The gene therapy experiment that met with fatality at the University of Pennsylvania, associated as it was with several violations of federal rules, such as changes of the form for consent approved by the Food and Drug Administration, occurred shortly after Richard L. Tannen (Fig. 573), senior vice dean of the university's medical school, had averred in a letter to the *Archives of Dermatology* that "the ethical issues of the Holmesburg studies have been addressed." According to Tannen, "the matter of the ethics of conducting research on vulnerable populations was settled some 25 years ago."[68] That Tannen's complacent attitude was disproved almost immediately thereafter by the death of a patient in an experiment supervised laxly at his own medical school is a strong reminder of the limitations of regulations that govern medical research and of the necessity to remain vigilant in regard to ethical aspects of research.

The Importance of Knowing the History of Dubious Experiments on Humans

Vigilance in the present and the future, however, is not conceivable or possible without knowledge of history. As Santayana reminded, if failures of the past are forgotten, they are bound to be repeated. That is why the history of experimentation on humans should be known. In order to be illuminating, that history, as any history, has to be told straight, without serpentine maneuvers and selective omission of facts. This includes the omission of names. The attitude of physicians, ranging from Albert Moll through Henry K. Beecher and Kenneth A. Arndt, in regard to protecting colleagues by deleting their names from articles about dubious experiments on human beings, is incompatible with a mindset that enables history to be studied incisively, reflectively, and dispassionately. It also is incompatible with the openness and truthfulness demanded for the relationship between scientists and test subjects. If scientists cannot be frank with one another in public communications, how can they expect their colleagues to be frank with test subjects in the privacy of an examining room? The desire to protect colleagues from becoming targets of criticism because of wrongdoing by them in the past is understandable. So is the desire to protect oneself from harsh reaction and from the possibility of alienating colleagues or disciples of colleagues who still are alive. These personal considerations, however, have no place in the study of history. The same measuring stick has to be applied to Kligman, William Epstein, and Strauss as to Rinecker, von Bärensprung, and Vonkennel. If any shading is to be made it certainly should not be to the advantage of the former who performed experiments on a much larger scale after the ethics of experimentation on humans had been systematized in the Nuremberg Code and in a battery of articles in scientific journals.

After his experiments on mentally disabled children had been uncovered, the dermatologist, John S. Strauss, stated that "To judge something that took place in the 1950s by the standards of the late 1990s is inherently futile and, in many cases, unfair."[69] There is a kernel of truth in that statement. In the past 50 years, progress has been made in regard to morality. The notion of progress morally, however, implies that morality is more than simply a term for habits approved socially. If that ethical relativism is accepted, neither the medieval practice of torturing criminals nor the government-sanctioned institution of slavery nor the suppression and annihilation of "inferior races" by the Nazis would be objectionable morally, and the termination of those practices could not be considered progress, but only change in politics. Progress morally can be invoked only if the validity of qualities independent of a particular time and culture is accepted, qualities such as sensitivity to the pain and suffering of human beings and recognition of the inherent dignity and intrinsic worth of human beings.[70] Those qualities did not originate in the code of William Beaumont, the writings of Claude Bernard, the German guidelines of 1900 and 1931, the Nuremberg Code, or the revised Declaration of Helsinki. Kant's categorical imperative, "People are to be treated as ends, never merely as means to the ends of others," existed long before any of those rules was formulated, and the Nuremberg Code has been referred to rightly as "simply 10 universal standards of human decency."[71] Most of the experiments on humans described in this book were flagrant deviations from human decency.

Study of those experiments is tied inextricably to moral judgment. As the bioethicist, John C. Fletcher, has reminded, "we must make such judgments to be loyal to moral norms and to transmit moral evolution to a new generation . . . If we fail to judge the past, however measured our judgments, we will lose in our collective memory the harm and suffering caused by older practices. We will lose, too, in our moral evolution the ability to change those harmful practices."[72] For those reasons, a judgment has to be made about experiments that are objectionable ethically and about scientists who performed those experiments. That men and women with undeniable qualities and merits become subjects of criticism because of experiments performed several decades ago may be sad and even may induce sympathy for them, but it is essential that it be done. The enforcement of responsibility is one of the strongest factors that maintains the coherence, as well as the integrity, of a society. It is a service to society to demonstrate that one cannot evade responsibility for wrongdoing, that one may be confronted with misdemeanors even after many years, and that neglect of moral imperatives in the conduct of research may not lead to a place in the pantheon of fame, but in the hall of infamy.

Many reasons and excuses have been given for failure to observe basic standards of human decency in the pursuit of knowledge, among them the importance of that knowledge for society, the supposed negligibility of the harm inflicted on test subjects, and the reputed lack of rigid regulations governing certain types of experiments. Because those excuses may at first blush appear compelling, and even persuasive, in a particular context, it is important that the negative consequences of compromising one's conscience and of treating people as means to ends be kept firmly in mind. Despite all procedural safeguards imposed on experiments on humans, the ultimate decision about what to tell a test subject and how to proceed in a particular experimental situation rests with the individual investigator. Study of the behavior of other individuals in similar situations, therefore, should be more illuminating than a theoretical discourse about ethical lapses and requirements. In order to assist individuals in the assessment of their own conduct, the behavior, excuses, and rationalizations of other individuals must be made known. This is especially important for behavior that is not strikingly aberrant and that requires reflection seriously in order to be avoided. The history of dubious experiments on humans is replete with examples of that kind, such as experiments that were associated with negligible harm but were conducted without the consent of subjects, or experiments on subjects who offered themselves as volunteers but, like prisoners, were under duress when they made that offer. A critical assessment of the ethics of those experiments may serve to heighten conscience.

The history of the abuse of man in medical experiments is a history of different societies and their varying ideologies, priorities, and problems, a history of failures and achievements in medicine, a history of the development of ethical guidelines and laws, but most of all a history of specific experiments performed by individual researchers on individual subjects, a history that enables appreciation better of what it means to be treated as a means to the ends of others and to resist the temptation of using others as means to one's own ends. In that respect, the history told in this volume transcends the narrow limits of medical research. Unethical experiments on human beings are not confined to medicine. Attempts to induce a customer to buy a car that is overpriced by far or to induce a jury to neglect facts relevant to an alleged action also are experiments on others that involve deviations from basic principles of decency and fairness. No fundamental difference exists between hiding potential risks from test subjects in medical experiments and hiding facts that allow a customer or a jury to come to an "understanding and enlightened decision." As a "universal standard of human decency," the first provision of the Nuremberg Code is applicable not only to medical research, but to all interactions between human beings. It is in the interaction between experimenter and test subject, however, that the abuse of others for purposes of one's own is expressed most dramatically, distinctively, and poignantly.

Study of that interaction and of the rules that have been developed to govern it, therefore, may be rewarding not only to physicians and bioethicists, but to everyone. That is particularly true in regard to one issue that is at the core of dubious experimentation on humans, although it is never mentioned in ethical codes, namely, the belief that some human beings are inferior, do not deserve respect, and can be used at will. This attitude of stratification of human beings is not entirely alien to any one of us. Depending on the persons with whom we interact, the feeling of superiority cannot always be avoided. It may not always be easy to treat someone else with respect. If one lesson is to be learned from the history of experimentation on humans, however, it is that our own feelings of superiority must be curbed whenever they surface, and that every individual, irrespective of age, sex, race, nationality, religion, or social status, must be treated with the respect that that fellow human being, individual person that he or she is, deserves.

OATH OF HIPPOCRATES

I swear by Apollo the Physician and Aesculapius and Hygieia and Panaceia and all the gods and goddesses, making them my witnesses, that I will fulfill according to my ability and judgment this oath and this covenant:

To hold him who has taught me this art as equal to my parents and to live my life in partnership with him, and if he is in need of money to give him a share of mine, and to regard his offspring as equal to my brothers in male lineage and to teach them this art – if they desire to learn it – without fee and covenant; to give a share of precepts and oral instruction and all the other learning to my sons and to the sons of him who has instructed me and to pupils who have signed the covenant and have taken an oath according to the medical law, but to no one else.

I will apply dietetic measures for the benefit of the sick according to my ability and judgment; I will keep them from harm and injustice.

I will neither give a deadly drug to anybody if asked for it, nor will I make a suggestion to this effect. Similarly I will not give to a woman an abortive remedy. In purity and holiness I will guard my life and my art.

I will not use the knife, not even on sufferers from stone, but will withdraw in favor of such men as are engaged in this work.

Whatever houses I may visit, I will come for the benefit of the sick, remaining free of all intentional injustice, of all mischief and in particular of sexual relations with both female and male persons, be they free or slaves.

What I may see or hear in the course of the treatment or even outside of the treatment in regard to the life of men, which on no account one must spread abroad, I will keep to myself holding such things shameful to be spoken about.

If I fulfill this oath and do not violate it, may it be granted to me to enjoy life and art, being honored with fame among all men for all time to come; if I transgress it and swear falsely, may the opposite of all this be my lot.

CODE OF THOMAS PERCIVAL · 1803

Whenever cases occur, attended with circumstances not heretofore observed, or in which the ordinary modes of practice have been attempted without success, it is for the public good, and in especial degree advantageous to the poor (who, being the most numerous class of society, are the greatest beneficiaries of the healing art) that new remedies and new methods of chirurgical treatment should be devised. But in the accomplishment of the salutary purpose, the gentlemen of the faculty should be scrupulously and conscientiously governed by sound reason, just analogy, or well authenticated facts. And no such trials should be instituted, without a previous consultation of the physicians or surgeons, according to the nature of the case.

CODE OF WILLIAM BEAUMONT · 1833

1. There must be recognition of an area where experimentation in man is needed.

2. Some experimental studies in man are justifiable when the information cannot otherwise be obtained.

3. The investigator must be conscientious and responsible.

4. A well-considered, methodological approach is required so that as much information as possible will be obtained whenever a human subject is used. No random studies are to be made.

5. The voluntary consent of the subject is necessary.

6. The experiment is to be discontinued when it causes distress to the subject.

7. The project must be abandoned when the subject becomes dissatisfied.

INSTRUCTIONS OF THE PRUSSIAN MINISTER OF CULTURE TO THE DIRECTORS OF CLINICS, POLYCLINICS, AND OTHER HEALTH CARE INSTITUTIONS · 1900

I. I wish to point out to the directors of clinics, polyclinics, and similar establishments that medical interventions for purposes other than diagnosis, therapy, and immunization are absolutely prohibited, even though all other legal and ethical requirements for performing such interventions are fulfilled if:

1. The person in question is a minor or is not fully competent on other grounds;

2. The person concerned has not declared unequivocally that he consents to the intervention;

3. The declaration has not been made on the basis of an appropriate explanation of the adverse consequences that may result from the intervention.

II. In addition, I prescribed that:

1. Interventions of this nature may be performed only by the director of the institution himself or with his special authorization;

2. In every intervention of this nature, an entry must be made in the medical case-record book certifying that the requirements laid down in Items 1-3 of section I and Item 1 of Section II have been fulfilled, specifying details of the case.

CIRCULAR OF THE MINISTER OF THE INTERIOR OF THE GERMAN REICH CONCERNING GUIDELINES FOR INNOVATIVE THERAPY AND HUMAN EXPERIMENTATION · 1931

1. Medical science, if it is not to come to a standstill, cannot refrain from introducing in suitable cases New Therapy using agents and methods that have yet to be tested sufficiently. Also, medical science cannot dispense completely with Human Experimentation. Otherwise, progress in diagnosis, therapy, and prevention of disease would be hindered or even rendered impossible.

    The special rights to be granted to the physician under these new Guidelines must be balanced by the special duty of the physician to be aware of the grave responsibility which he bears for the life and health of each individual undergoing innovative therapy or human experimentation.

2. The term *innovative therapy* used in these Guidelines defines therapeutic experimentation and modes of treatment of humans which serve the process of healing, i.e., pursuing in specific individual cases the recognition, healing, or prevention of an illness or suffering, or the removal of a bodily defect, even though the effects and consequences of the therapy cannot yet be adequately determined on the basis of available knowledge.

3. The term *human experimentation*, as defined in the Guidelines, means operations and modes of treatment of humans carried out for research purposes without serving a therapeutic purpose in an individual case, and whose effects and consequences cannot be adequately determined on the basis of available knowledge.

4. Any innovative therapy must be in accord with the principles of medical ethics and the rules of the medical arts and sciences, both in its design and its realization.

    A consideration and calculation of possible harms must be undertaken to determine whether they stand in a suitable relationship to expected benefits. Innovative therapy may only be

– 628 –

initiated after first being tested in animal experimentation, where this is at all possible.

5. Innovative therapy may only be applied if consent or proxy consent has been given in a clear and incontrovertible manner following an expedient instruction provided in advance.

    Innovative therapy may only be introduced without consent if it is urgently required, and cannot be postponed because of a need to save life or prevent severe damage to health, and if prior consent could not be obtained owing to special circumstances.

6. Introduction of innovative therapy in the treatment of children and minors under eighteen requires especially careful consideration.

7. Medical ethics rejects any exploitation of social hardship in order to undertake innovative therapy.

8. Innovative therapy using living micro-organisms requires heightened caution, especially in the case of live pathogens. Such therapy may only be considered permissible if a relative degree of harmlessness in the procedure can be assumed, and if the achievement of equal benefits by other means cannot be expected under any given circumstances.

9. In medical clinics, polyclinics, hospitals, or other health care institutions, innovative therapy may only be conducted by the chief physician himself or, at his specific request and with his full responsibility, by another physician.

10. A written report on any new therapy is required and must contain information about the design, justification, and administration of therapy. Such a report shall state specifically that the subject, or his or her legal representative, has been instructed expediently and has given consent. If innovative therapy is applied without consent, according to 5.2, the report must specify these preconditions clearly.

11. Publication of results of innovative therapy must respect the patient's dignity and the commandments of humanity.

12. Numbers 1 through 11 of these Guidelines are equally applicable to human experimentation (article 3). In addition, the following requirements for such experimentation apply:

(a) Without consent, under no circumstances is nontherapeutic research permissible.

(b) Any human experimentation which could as well be carried out in animal experimentation is not permissible. Only after all basic information has been obtained should human experimentation begin. This information should first be obtained by means of scientific biological or laboratory research and of animal experimentation for reasons of clarification and safety. Given these premises, unfounded or random human experimentation is not permissible.

(c) Experimentation with children or minors is not permissible if it endangers the child or minor in the slightest degree.

(d) Experimentation with dying persons conflicts with the principles of medical ethics and therefore is not permissible.

13. Assuming that, in accordance with these Guidelines, physicians and, in particular, responsible directors in charge of medical institutions will be guided by a strong sense of responsibility toward the patients entrusted to them, it also is to be hoped that they will maintain receptive to their responsibility to seek relief, improvement, protection, or cure for the patient along new paths, when the accepted and actual state of medical science, according to their medical knowledge, no longer seems adequate.

14. In teaching academically, every opportunity should be taken to stress the special duties of a physician in regard to undertaking innovative therapy or human experimentation; these special responsibilities also apply to the publication of the results of innovative therapy and human experimentation.

CODE OF THE AMERICAN MEDICAL ASSOCIATION · 1946

In order to conform to the ethics of the American Medical Association, three requirements must be satisfied: (1) the voluntary consent of the person on whom the experiment is to be performed; (2) the danger of each experiment must be previously investigated by animal experimentation; and (3) the experiment must be performed under proper medical protection and management.

THE NUREMBERG CODE · 1947

1.   The voluntary consent of the human subject is absolutely essential. This means that the person involved should have legal capacity to give consent; should be so situated as to be able to exercise free power of choice, without the intervention of any element of force, fraud, deceit, duress, overreaching, or other ulterior form of constraint or coercion; and should have sufficient knowledge and comprehension of the elements of the subject matter involved as to enable him to make an understanding and enlightened decision. This latter element requires that, before the acceptance of an affirmative decision by the experimental subject, there should be made known to him the nature, duration, and purpose of the experiment; the methods and means by which it is to be conducted; all inconveniences and hazards reasonably to be expected; and the effects upon his health or person which may possibly come from his participation in the experiments.

   The duty and responsibility for ascertaining the quality of the consent rests upon each individual who initiates, directs or engages in the experiment. It is a personal duty and responsibility which may not be delegated to another with impunity.

2.   The experiment should be such as to yield fruitful results for the good of society, unprocurable by other methods or means of study, and not random and unnecessary in nature.

3.   The experiment should be so designed and based on the results of animal experimentation and a knowledge of the natural history of the disease or other problem under study that the

anticipated results will justify the performance of the experiment.

4. The experiment should be so conducted as to avoid all unnecessary physical or mental suffering and injury.

5. No experiment should be conducted where there is an *a priori* reason to believe that death or disabling injury will occur; except, perhaps, in those experiments where the experimental physicians also serve as subjects.

6. The degree of risk to be taken should never exceed that determined by the humanitarian importance of the problem to be solved by the experiment.

7. Proper preparations should be made and adequate facilities provided to protect the experimental subject against even remote possibilities of injury, disability, or death.

8. The experiment should be conducted only by scientifically qualified persons. The highest degree of skill and care should be required through all stages of the experiment of those who conduct or engage in the experiment.

9. During the course of the experiment, the human subject should be at liberty to bring the experiment to an end if he has reached the physical or mental state where continuation of the experiment seems to him to be impossible.

10. During the course of the experiment, the scientist in charge must be prepared to terminate the experiment at any stage, if he has probable cause to believe, in the exercise of the good faith, superior skill and careful judgment required of him, that a continuation of the experiment is likely to result in injury, disability, or death to the experimental subject.

DECLARATION OF GENEVA · 1948

Now being admitted to the profession of medicine, I solemnly pledge to consecrate my life to the service of humanity. I will give respect and gratitude to my deserving teachers. I will practice medicine with conscience and dignity. The health and life of my patient will be my first consideration. I will hold in confidence all that my patient confides in me. I will maintain the honor and the noble traditions of the medical profession. My colleagues will be as my brothers. I will not permit considerations of race, religion, nationality, party politics, or social standing to intervene between my duty and my patient. I will maintain the utmost respect for human life from the time of its conception. Even under threat I will not use my knowledge contrary to the laws of humanity. These promises I make freely and upon my honor.

CODE OF THE WORLD MEDICAL ASSOCIATION · 1954

PRINCIPLES FOR THOSE IN RESEARCH AND EXPERIMENTATION

1. Scientific and Moral Aspects of Experimentation

    The word *experimentation* applies not only to experimentation itself but also to the experimenter. An individual cannot and should not attempt any kind of experimentation. Scientific qualities are indisputable and must always be respected. Likewise, there must be strict adherence to the general rules of respect for the individual.

2. Prudence and Discretion in the Publication of the First Results of Experimentation

    This principle applies primarily to the medical press and we are proud to note that in the majority of cases, this rule has been adhered to by the editors of our journals. Then there is the general press, which does not in every instance have the same rules of prudence and discretion as the medical press. The World Medical Association draws attention to the detrimental effects of premature or unjustified statements. In the interest of the public, each national association should consider methods of avoiding this danger.

3. Experimentation on Healthy Subjects

    Every step must be taken in order to make sure that those who submit themselves to experimentation be fully informed. The paramount factor in experimentation in human beings is the responsibility of the research worker and not the willingness of the person submitting to the experiment.

4. Experimentation on Sick Subjects

    Here it may be that, in the presence of individual and desperate cases, one may attempt an operation or a treatment of a rather daring nature. Such exceptions will be rare and require the approval either of the person or his next of kin. In such a situation it is the doctor's conscience which will make the decision.

5. Necessity of Informing the Person Who Submits to Experimentation of the Nature of the Experimentation, the Reasons for the Experiment, and the Risks Involved

    It should be required that each person who submits to experimentation be informed of the nature of, the reason for, and the risk of the proposed experiment. If the patient is irresponsible, consent should be obtained from the individual who is legally responsible for the individual. In both instances, consent should be obtained in writing.

DECLARATION OF HELSINKI · JUNE 1964

It is the mission of the doctor to safeguard the health of the people. His knowledge and conscience are dedicated to the fulfillment of this mission.

The Declaration of Geneva of the World Medical Association binds the doctor with the words, "The health of my patient will be my first consideration;" and the International Code of Medical Ethics, which declares that "Any act or advice which could weaken physical or mental resistance of a human being may be used only in his interest."

Because it is essential that the results of laboratory experiments be applied to human beings to further scientific knowledge and to help suffering humanity, the World Medical Association has prepared the following recommendations as a guide to each doctor in clinical research. It must be stressed that the standards as drafted are only a guide to physicians all over the world. Doctors are not relieved from criminal, civil, and ethical responsibilities under the laws of their own countries.

In the field of clinical research, a fundamental distinction must be recognized between clinical research, in which the aim is essentially therapeutic for a patient, and clinical research the essential object of which is purely scientific and without therapeutic value to the person subjected to the research.

I · BASIC PRINCIPLES

1. Clinical research must conform to the moral and scientific principles that justify medical research, and should be based on laboratory and animal experiments or other scientifically established facts.

2. Clinical research should be conducted only by scientifically qualified persons and under the supervision of a qualified medical man.

3. Clinical research cannot legitimately be carried out unless the importance of the objective is in proportion to the inherent risk to the subject.

4. Every clinical research project should be preceded by careful assessment of inherent risks in comparison to foreseeable benefits to the subject or to others.

5. Special caution should be exercised by the doctor in performing clinical research in which the personality of the subject is liable to be altered by drugs or experimental procedure.

II · CLINICAL RESEARCH COMBINED WITH PROFESSIONAL CARE

1. In the treatment of the sick person the doctor must be free to use a new therapeutic measure if in his judgment it offers hope of saving life, re-establishing health, or alleviating suffering.

If at all possible, consistent with patient psychology, the doctor should obtain the patient's freely given consent after the patient has been given a full explanation. In case of legal incapacity, consent should also be procured from the legal guardian; in case of physical incapacity, the permission of the legal guardian replaces that of the patient.

2. The doctor can combine clinical research with professional care, the objective being the acquisition of new medical knowledge, only to the extent that clinical research is justified by its therapeutic value for the patient.

III · NON-THERAPEUTIC CLINICAL RESEARCH

1. In the purely scientific application of clinical research carried out on a human being, it is the duty of the doctor to remain the protector of the life and health of that person on whom clinical research is being carried out.

2. The nature, the purpose, and the risk of clinical research must be explained to the subject by the doctor.

3a. Clinical research on a human being cannot be undertaken without his free consent, after he has been fully informed; if he is legally incompetent, the consent of the legal guardian should be procured.

3b. The subject of clinical research should be in such a mental, physical, and legal state as to be able to exercise fully his power of choice.

3c. Consent should as a rule be obtained in writing. However, the responsibility for clinical research always remains with the research worker; it never falls on the subject, even after consent is obtained.

4a. The investigator must respect the right of each individual to safeguard his personal integrity, especially if the subject is in a dependent relationship to the investigator.

4b. At any time during the course of clinical research, the subject or his guardian should be free to withdraw permission for research to be continued. The investigator or the investigating team should discontinue the research if in his or their judgment it may, if continued, be harmful to the individual.

DECLARATION OF HELSINKI

REVISED VERSION, TOKYO, OCTOBER 1975

INTRODUCTION

It is the mission of the medical doctor to safeguard the health of the people. His or her knowledge and conscience are dedicated to the fulfillment of this mission.

The Declaration of Geneva of the World Medical Association binds the doctor with the words, "The health of my patient will be my first consideration;" and the International Code of Medical Ethics declares that, "Any act or advice which could weaken physical or mental resistance of a human being may be used only in his interest."

The purpose of biomedical research involving human subjects must be to improve diagnostic, therapeutic and prophylactic procedures and the understanding of the aetiology and the pathogenesis of disease.

In current medical practice, most diagnostic, therapeutic or prophylactic procedures involve hazards. This applies *a fortiori* to biomedical research.

Medical progress is based on research, which ultimately must rest in part on experimentation involving human subjects.

In the field of biomedical research, a fundamental distinction must be recognized between medical research, in which the aim is essentially diagnostic or therapeutic for a patient, and medical research, the essential object of which is purely scientific and without diagnostic or therapeutic value to the person subjected to the research.

Special caution must be exercised in the conduct of research which may affect the environment, and the welfare of animals used for research must be respected.

Because it is essential that the results of laboratory experiments be applied to human beings to further scientific knowledge and to help suffering humanity, the World Medical Association has prepared the following recommendations as a guide to each doctor in biomedical research involving human subjects. They should be kept under review in the future. It must be stressed that the standards as drafted are only a guide to physicians all over the world. Doctors are not relieved from criminal, civil, and ethical responsibilities under the laws of their own countries.

I. BASIC PRINCIPLES

1. Biomedical research involving human subjects must conform to generally accepted scientific principles and should be based on adequately performed laboratory and animal experimentation and on a thorough knowledge of the scientific literature.

2. The design and performance of each experimental procedure involving human subjects should be clearly formulated in an experimental protocol which should be transmitted to a specifically appointed independent committee for consideration, comment, and guidance.

3. Biomedical research involving human subjects should be conducted only by scientifically qualified persons and under the supervision of a clinically competent medical person. The responsibility for the human subject must always rest with a medically qualified person and never rest on the subject of the research, even though the subject has given his or her consent.

4. Biomedical research involving human subjects cannot legitimately be carried out unless the importance of the objective is in proportion to the inherent risk to the subject.

5. Every biomedical research project involving human subjects should be preceded by careful assessment of predictable risks in comparison with foreseeable benefits to the subject or to others. Concern for the interests of the subject must always prevail over the interest of science and society.

6. The right of the research subject to safeguard his or her integrity must always be respected. Every precaution should be taken to respect the privacy of the subject and to minimize the impact of the study on the subject's physical and mental integrity and on the personality of the subject.

7. Doctors should abstain from engaging in research projects involving human subjects unless they are satisfied that the hazards involved are believed to be predictable. Doctors should cease any investigation if the hazards are found to outweigh the potential benefits.

8. In publication of the results of his or her research, the doctor is obliged to preserve the accuracy of the results. Reports of experimentation not in accordance with the principles laid down

in this Declaration should not be accepted for publication.

9. In any research on human beings, each potential subject must be adequately informed of the aims, methods, and anticipated benefits and potential hazards of the study and the discomfort it may entail. He or she should be informed that he or she is at liberty to abstain from participation in the study and that he or she is free to withdraw his or her consent to participation at any time. The doctor should then obtain the subject's freely given informed consent, preferably in writing.

10. When obtaining informed consent for the research project, the doctor should be particularly cautious if the subject is in a dependent relationship to him or her or may consent under duress. In that case, the informed consent should be obtained by a doctor who is not engaged in the investigation and who is completely independent of this official relationship.

11. In case of legal incompetence, informed consent should be obtained from the legal guardian in accordance with national legislation. Where physical or mental incapacity makes it impossible to obtain informed consent, or when the subject is a minor, permission from the responsible relative replaces that of the subject in accordance with national legislation.

12. The research protocol should always contain a statement of the ethical considerations involved and should indicate that the principles enunciated in the present Declaration are complied with.

II. MEDICAL RESEARCH COMBINED WITH PROFESSIONAL CARE
(Clinical Research)

1. In the treatment of the sick person, the doctor must be free to use a new diagnostic or therapeutic measure, if in his or her judgment it offers hope of saving life, reestablishing health or alleviating suffering.

2. The potential benefits, hazards and discomfort of a new method should be weighed against the advantages of the best current diagnostic and therapeutic methods.

3. In any medical study, every patient – including those of a con-

trol group, if any – should be assured of the best proven diagnostic and therapeutic method.

4. The refusal of the patient to participate in a study must never interfere with the doctor-patient relationship.

5. If the doctor considers it essential not to obtain informed consent, the specific reasons for this proposal should be stated in the experimental protocol for transmission to the independent committee (I,2).

6. The doctor can combine medical research with professional care, the objective being the acquisition of new medical knowledge, only to the extent that medical research is justified by its potential diagnostic or therapeutic value for the patient.

III. NON-THERAPEUTIC BIOMEDICAL RESEARCH INVOLVING HUMAN SUBJECTS

(Non-clinical Biomedical Research)

1. In the purely scientific application of medical research carried out on a human being, it is the duty of the doctor to remain the protector of the life and health of that person on whom biomedical research is being carried out.

2. The subjects should be volunteers – either healthy persons or patients for whom the experimental design is not related to the patient's illness.

3. The investigator or the investigating team should discontinue the research if in his/her or their judgment it may, if continued, be harmful to the individual.

4. In research on man, the interest of science and society should never take precedence over considerations related to the well-being of the subject.

DECLARATION OF HELSINKI

REVISED VERSION, EDINBURGH, OCTOBER 2000

A · INTRODUCTION

1. The World Medical Association has developed the Declaration of Helsinki as a statement of ethical principles to provide guidance to physicians and other participants in medical research involving human subjects. Medical research involving human subjects includes research on identifiable human material or identifiable data.

2. It is the duty of the physician to promote and safeguard the health of the people. The physician's knowledge and conscience are dedicated to the fulfillment of this duty.

3. The Declaration of Geneva of the World Medical Association binds the physician with the words, "The health of my patient will be my first consideration," and the International Code of Medical Ethics declares that, "A physician shall act only in the patient's interest when providing medical care which might have the effect of weakening the physical and mental condition of the patient."

4. Medical progress is based on research which ultimately must rest in part on experimentation involving human subjects.

5. In medical research on human subjects, considerations related to the well-being of the human subject should take precedence over the interests of science and society.

6. The primary purpose of medical research involving human subjects is to improve prophylactic, diagnostic, and therapeutic procedures and the understanding of the aetiology and pathogenesis of disease. Even the best proven prophylactic, diagnostic, and therapeutic methods must continuously be challenged through research for their effectiveness, efficiency, accessibility, and quality.

7. In current medical practice and in medical research, most prophylactic, diagnostic, and therapeutic procedures involve risks and burdens.

8. Medical research is subject to ethical standards that promote respect for all human beings and protect their health and rights. Some research populations are vulnerable and need special protection. The particular needs of the economically and medically disadvantaged must be recognized. Special attention is also required for those who may be subject to giving consent under duress, for those who will not benefit personally from the research and for those for whom the research is combined with care.

9. Research Investigators should be aware of the ethical, legal and regulatory requirements for research on human subjects in their own countries as well as applicable international requirements. No national ethical, legal, or regulatory requirement should be allowed to reduce or eliminate any of the protections for human subjects set forth in this Declaration.

B · BASIC PRINCIPLES FOR ALL MEDICAL RESEARCH

10. It is the duty of the physician in medical research to protect the life, health, privacy, and dignity of the human subject.
11. Medical research involving human subjects must conform to generally accepted scientific principles, be based on a thorough knowledge of the scientific literature, other relevant sources of information, and on adequate laboratory and, where appropriate, animal experimentation.
12. Appropriate caution must be exercised in the conduct of research that may affect the environment, and the welfare of animals used for research must be respected.
13. The design and performance of each experimental procedure involving human subjects should be clearly formulated in an experimental protocol. This protocol should be submitted for consideration, comment, guidance, and where appropriate, approval to a specifically appointed ethical review committee, which must be independent of the investigator, the sponsor, or any other kind of undue influence. This independent committee should be in conformity with the laws and regulations of the country in which the research experiment is performed. The committee has the right to monitor ongoing trials. The re-

searcher has the obligation to provide monitoring information to the committee, especially any serious adverse events. The researcher should also submit to the committee, for review, information regarding funding, sponsors, institutional affiliations, other potential conflicts of interest and incentives for subjects.

14. The research protocol should always contain a statement of the ethical considerations involved and should indicate that there is compliance with the principles enunciated in this Declaration.

15. Medical research involving human subjects should be conducted only by scientifically qualified persons and under the supervision of a clinically competent medical person. The responsibility for the human subject must always rest with a medically qualified person and never rest on the subject of the research, even though the subject has given consent.

16. Every medical research project involving human subjects should be preceded by careful assessment of predictable risks and burdens in comparison with foreseeable benefits to the subject or to others. This does not preclude the participation of healthy volunteers in medical research. The design of all studies should be publicly available.

17. Physicians should abstain from engaging in research projects involving human subjects unless they are confident that the risks involved have been adequately assessed and can be satisfactorily managed. Physicians should cease any investigation if the risks are found to outweigh the potential benefits or if there is conclusive proof of positive and beneficial results.

18. Medical research involving human subjects should only be conducted if the importance of the objective outweighs the inherent risks and burdens to the subject. This is especially important when the human subjects are healthy volunteers.

19. Medical research is only justified if there is a reasonable likelihood that the populations in which the research is carried out stand to benefit from the results of the research.

20. The subjects must be volunteers and informed participants in the research project.

21. The right of research subjects to safeguard their integrity must always be respected. Every precaution should be taken to respect the privacy of the subject, the confidentiality of the patient's information and to minimize the impact of the study on the subject's physical and mental integrity and on the personality of the subject.

22. In any research on human beings, each potential subject must be adequately informed of the aims, methods, sources of funding, any possible conflicts of interest, institutional affiliations of the researcher, the anticipated benefits and potential risks of the study, and the discomfort it may entail. The subject should be informed of the right to abstain from participation in the study or to withdraw consent to participate at any time without reprisal. After ensuring that the subject has understood the information, the physician should then obtain the subject's freely-given informed consent, preferably in writing. If the consent cannot be obtained in writing, the non-written consent must be formally documented and witnessed.

23. When obtaining informed consent for the research project, the physician should be particularly cautious if the subject is in a dependant relationship with the physician or may consent under duress. In that case, the informed consent should be obtained by a well informed physician who is not engaged in the investigation and who is completely independent of this relationship.

24. For a research subject who is legally incompetent, physically or mentally incapable of giving consent, or is a legally incompetent minor, the investigator must obtain informed consent from the legally authorized representative in accordance with applicable law. These groups should not be included in research unless the research is necessary to promote the health of the population represented and this research cannot instead be performed on legally competent persons.

25. When a subject deemed legally incompetent, such as a minor child, is able to give assent to decisions about participation in research, the investigator must obtain that assent in addition to the consent of the legally authorized representative.

26. Research on individuals from whom it is not possible to obtain

consent, including proxy or advance consent, should be done only if the physical/mental condition that prevents obtaining informed consent is a necessary characteristic of the research population. The specific reasons for involving research subjects with a condition that renders them unable to give informed consent should be stated in the experimental protocol for consideration and approval of the review committee. The protocol should state that consent to remain in the research should be obtained as soon as possible from the individual or a legally authorized surrogate.

27. Both authors and publishers have ethical obligations. In publication of the results of research, the investigators are obliged to preserve the accuracy of the results. Negative as well as positive results should be published or otherwise made publicly available. Sources of funding, institutional affiliations and any possible conflicts of interest should be declared in the publication. Reports of experimentation not in accordance with the principles laid down in this Declaration should not be accepted for publication.

C · ADDITIONAL PRINCIPLES FOR MEDICAL RESEARCH COMBINED WITH MEDICAL CARE

28. The physician may combine medical research with medical care, only to the extent that the research is justified by its potential prophylactic, diagnostic, or therapeutic value. When medical research is combined with medical care, additional standards apply to protect the patients who are research subjects.

29. The benefits, risks, burdens and effectiveness of a new method should be tested against those of the best current prophylactic, diagnostic, and therapeutic methods. This does not exclude the use of placebo, or no treatment, in studies where no prophylactic, diagnostic or therapeutic method exists.

30. At the conclusion of the study, every patient entered into the study should be assured of access to the best proven prophylactic, diagnostic, and therapeutic methods identified by the study.

31. The physician should fully inform the patient which aspects of

the care are related to the research. The refusal of a patient to participate in a study must never interfere with the patient-physician relationship.

32. In the treatment of a patient where proven prophylactic, diagnostic, and therapeutic methods do not exist or have been ineffective, the physician, with informed consent from the patient, must be free to use unproven or new prophylactic, diagnostic, and therapeutic measures, if in the physician's judgment it offers hope of saving life, reestablishing health or alleviating suffering. Where possible, these measures should be made the object of research, designed to evaluate their safety and efficacy. In all cases, new information should be recorded and, where appropriate, published. The other relevant guidelines of this Declaration should be followed.

REFERENCES

CHAPTER 1 · INTRODUCTION

1. Tröhler U, Reither-Theil S (ed.). *Ethik und Medizin 1947-1997. Was leistet die Kodifizierung der Ethik?* Göttingen: Wallstein, 1997;19–40.

2. Wolff U. *Abschied von Hippocrates. Ärztliche Ethik zwischen Hippokratischem Eid und Genfer Gelöbnis.* Berlin: Colloquium, 1981;16–25.

3. Tröhler U, Reither-Theil S. *Ethik und Medizin;*19–40.

4. Ackerknecht EH. *Geschichte der Medizin.* Stuttgart: Enke, 1979;65.

5. Toellner R. *Illustrierte Geschichte der Medizin.* Salzburg: Andreas & Andreas, 1986;370.

6. Bean WB. Walter Reed and the ordeal of human experimentation. *Bulletin of the History of Medicine* 1977;51:75–92.

7. Elkeles B. *Der moralische Diskurs über das medizinische Menschenexperiment im 19. Jahrhundert.* Stuttgart, Jena, New York: Gustav Fischer, 1996;154ff.

8. Van Doren V. *A History of Knowledge.* New York: Ballantine Books, 1991.

9. Ackerknecht EH. *Geschichte der Medizin.* Stuttgart: Enke, 1979;82f.

10. Bull JP. The historical development of clinical therapeutic trials. *Journal of Chronic Diseases* 1959;10:218–48.

11. Ibid.

12. Ibid.

13. Ibid.

14. Schott H (ed). *Die Chronik der Medizin.* Gütersloh, München: Chronik, 1993;176.

15. Reiss H (ed.) *Kant. Political Writings.* Cambridge: Cambridge University Press, 1970;54.

16. Ackerknecht EH. *Geschichte der Medizin.* Stuttgart: Enke, 1979;116ff.

17. Schott H (ed). *Die Chronik der Medizin.* Gütersloh, München: Chronik, 1993;222.

18. Faden RF, Beauchamp TL. *A History and Theory of Informed Consent.* New York, Oxford: Oxford University Press, 1986;65.

19. Ibid.;61.

20. Van Doren V. *A History of Knowledge.* New York: Ballantine Books, 1991;224.

21. Ebbinghaus A, Dörner K (eds.). *Vernichten und Heilen. Der Nürnberger Ärzteprozess und seine Folgen.* Berlin: Aufbau-Verlag, 2001;74.

22. Faden RF, Beauchamp TL. *A History and Theory of Informed Consent;*67–69.

CHAPTER 2 · STUDIES BY INOCULATION

1. Tashiro E. *Die Waage der Venus. Venerologische Versuche am Menschen zwischen Fortschritt und Moral.* Husum: Matthiesen, 1991;12f.

2. Elkeles B. *Der moralische Diskurs über das medizinische Menschenexperiment im 19. Jahrhundert.* Stuttgart, Jena, New York: Fischer, 1996;42f.

3. Auspitz H. *Die Lehren vom syphilitischen Contagium und ihre thatsächliche Begründung.* Vienna: Wilhelm Braumüller, 1866;56.

4. Ibid.;56f.

5. Ibid.;14.

6. Ibid.;13f.

7. Crissey JT, Parish LC. *The Dermatology and Syphilology of the Nineteenth Century.* New York: Praeger, 1981;82f.

8. Quétel C. *History of Syphilis.* Translated by Judith Braddock and Brian Pike. Baltimore: The Johns Hopkins University Press, 1992;109.

9. Auspitz H. *Die Lehren vom syphilitischen Contagium*;5.

10. Crissey JT, Parish LC. *The Dermatology and Syphilology of the Nineteenth Century*;86f.

11. Auspitz H. *Die Lehren vom syphilitischen Contagium*;82-4.

12. Wallace W. Lectures on cutaneous and venereal diseases and on surgical cases. *The Lancet* 2: 129-33.

13. Ibid.;615.

14. Auspitz H. *Die Lehren vom syphilitischen Contagium*;144.

15. Waller J. Die Contagiosität der secundären Syphilis. *Vierteljahrsschrift für die praktische Heilkunde* 1851;29:112-32.

16. Ibid.

17. Waller J. Weitere Beiträge betreffend die Contagiosität der secundären Syphilis. Nebst einem Anhange über die Inoculation der Syphilis bei Thieren. *Vierteljahrsschrift für die praktische Heilkunde* 1851;31:51-64.

18. Rinecker F. Über die Ansteckungsfähigkeit der constitutionellen Syphilis. *Verhandlungen der Würzburger Physikalisch-Medicinischen Gesellschaft* 1852;3:375-97.

19. Ibid.

20. Weressajew WW. *Bekenntnisse eines Arztes.* Berlin: Buchverlag Der Morgen, 1960;119-21.

21. Tashiro E. *Die Waage der Venus*;21.

22. Weressajew WW. *Bekenntnisse eines Arztes*;121f.

23. Auspitz H. *Die Lehren vom syphilitischen* Contagium;188-91.

24. Ibid.;171f.

25. Ibid.;101-06.

References

26. Bärensprung FWF. Mittheilungen aus der Abtheilung und Klinik für syphilitisch Kranke. *Annalen des Charité-Krankenhauses* 1860;9:110–208.

27. Auspitz H. Die *Lehren vom syphilitischen Contagium*;225–34.

28. Tashiro E. *Die Waage der Venus*;23f.

29. Ibid.;26f.

30. Ibid.;81.

31. Ibid.;81–3.

32. Ibid.;24–6.

33. Bókai A. Ueber das Contagium der acuten Blenorrhoe. *Allgemeine Medicinische Centralzeitung* 1880;49:901–3.

34. Leistikow L. Ueber Bacterien bei den venerischen Krankheiten. *Charité-Annalen* 1882;7:750–72.

35. Bockhart M. Beitrag zur Aetiologie und Pathologie des Harnröhrentrippers. *Vierteljahresschrift für Dermatologie und Syphilis* 1883;10:3–18.

36. Tashiro E. *Die Waage der Venus*;38f.

37. Bumm E. *Der Micro-Organismus der gonorrhoischen Schleimhauterkrankungen 'Gonococcus Neisser.'* Wiesbaden, 1885.

38. Anfuso G. Il gonococco di Neisser. *La Riforma Medica* 1891;7:328.

39. Wertheim E. Die ascendierende Gonorrhoe beim Weibe. *Archiv für Gynäkologie* 1892;42:1–86.

40. Tashiro E. *Die Waage der Venus*;55f.

41. Åhmann CG. Zur Frage der gonorrhoischen Allgemeininfection. *Archiv für Dermatologie und Syphilis* 1897;39:324–34.

42. Tashiro E. *Die Waage der Venus*;70–73.

43. Ibid.;34–7.

44. Vogelsang TM. A serious sentence passed against the discoverer of the leprosy bacillus (Gerhard Armauer Hansen), in 1880. *Medical History* 1963; 7:182–6.

45. Hebra H. Emile Vidal. *Monatshefte für praktische Dermatologie* 1893;17:161–3.

46. Shelley WB. Experimental disease in the skin of man. A review. *Acta Dermato-venereologica* 1983;Suppl. 108:1–38.

47. Steiner J. Zur Inokulation der Varicellen. *Wiener Medizinische Wochenschrift* 1875;25:305–8.

48. Fehleisen F. *Aetiologie des Erysipels.* Berlin, Leipzig: Thieme, 1883.

49. Garré C. Zur Aetiologie acut eitriger Entzündungen (Osteomyelitis, Furunkel und Panaritium). *Fortschritte der Medicin* 1885;6:165–73.

50. Schimmelbusch C. Ueber die Ursachen der Furunkel. *Archiv für Ohrenheilkunde* 1888;27:252–64.

51. Pick FJ. Untersuchungen über Favus. *Zeitschrift für Heilkunde*

1891;12:153–69.

52. Pick FJ. Ist das Molluscum contagiosum kontagiös? *Archiv für Dermatologie und Syphilis, Ergänzungsheft I* 1892;89–94.

53. Jadassohn J. Sind die Verrucae vulgares übertragbar? *Verhandlungen der Deutschen Dermatologischen Gesellschaft* 1896;5:497–512.

54. Grosz S, Kraus R. Bacteriologische Studien über den Gonococcus. *Archiv für Dermatologie und Syphilis* 1898;45:329–56.

CHAPTER 3 · THE CALL OF CONSCIENCE

1. Weressajew WW. *Bekenntnisse eines Arztes.* Berlin: Buchverlag Der Morgen, 1960;121.

2. Annas GJ, Grodin MA (eds.). *The Nazi Doctors and the Nuremberg Code. Human Rights in Human Experimentation.* New York, Oxford: Oxford University Press, 1992;124.

3. Howard-Jones N. Human experimentation in historical and ethical perspectives. *Social Science and Medicine* 1982;16:1429–48.

4. Beecher HK. *Research and the Individual. Human Studies.* Boston: Little, Brown and Co., 1970;219.

5. Crissey JT, Parish LC. *The Dermatology and Syphilology of the Nineteenth Century.* New York: Praeger, 1981;91.

6. Quidde L. *Arme Leute in Krankenhäusern.* Munich: Staegmeyr, 1900;84f.

7. Elkeles B. *Der moralische Diskurs über das medizinische Menschenexperiment im 19. Jahrhundert.* Stuttgart, Jena, New York: Gustav Fischer, 1996;48.

8. Klusemann GG. Die Syphilisation in wissenschaftlicher und sanitätspolizeilicher Beziehung. Mit einer Nachschrift über die Zurechnung des ärztlichen Heilverfahrens von Casper. *Vierteljahrsschrift für gerichtliche und öffentliche Medicin* 1853;3:92–117.

9. Ibid.

10. Schönfeld W. Die Senatsrüge Rineckers anlässlich der Widerlegung syphilitischer Irrlehren, ein zeitgemässer medizingeschichtlicher Rückblick. *Dermatologische Wochenschrift* 1942;115:877–84.

11. Elkeles B. *Der moralische Diskurs über das medizinische Menschenexperiment;*51–55.

12. Vogelsang TM. A serious sentence passed against the discoverer of the leprosy bacillus (Gerhard Armauer Hansen), in 1880. *Medical History* 1963; 7:182–86.

13. Elkeles B. Der moralische Diskurs über das medizinische Menschenexperiment, p. 56.

14. Ibid.;59.

15. Auspitz H. *Die Lehren vom syphilitischen Contagium und ihre thatsächliche Begründung.* Vienna: Wilhelm Braumüller, 1866;191f.

References

16. Bernard C. *An Introduction to the Study of Experimental Medicine.* Translated by HC Greene. Special edition. The Classics of Medicine Library. Birmingham: Division of Grymon Editions, 1980;99.

17. Ibid.;103.

18. Tröhler U, Reither-Theil S (eds.). Ethik und Medizin 1947–1997. *Was leistet die Kodifizierung von Ethik?* Göttingen: Wallstein, 1997;42.

19. Ibid.;47.

20. Bernard C. *An Introduction to the Study of Experimental Medicine*;101.

21. Elkeles B. *Der moralische Diskurs über das medizinische Menschenexperiment*;60.

22. Auspitz H. *Die Lehren vom syphilitischen Contagium*;192.

23. Ibid.

24. Elkeles B. *Der moralische Diskurs über das medizinische Menschenexperiment*;57–59.

25. Auspitz H. *Die Lehren vom syphilitischen Contagium*;183–87.

26. Elkeles B. *Der moralische Diskurs über das medizinische Menschenexperiment*;183.

27. Auspitz H. *Die Lehren vom syphilitischen Contagium*;184.

28. Weressajew WW. *Bekenntnisse eines Arztes*;121.

29. Åhmann CG. Zur Frage der gonorrhoischen Allgemeininfection. *Archiv für Dermatologie und Syphilis*,1897;39:324–34.

30. Bärensprung F. Mittheilungen aus der Abtheilung und Klinik für syphilitisch Kranke. *Annalen des Charité-Krankenhauses*, 1860;9:110–208.

31. Elkeles B. *Der moralische Diskurs über das medizinische Menschenexperiment im 19. Jahrhundert.* Stuttgart, Jena, New York: Gustav Fischer, 1996;59.

32. Crissey JT, Parish LC. *The Dermatology and Syphilology of the Nineteenth Century.* New York: Praeger, 1981;186f.

33. Tashiro E. *Die Waage der Venus. Venerologische Versuche am Menschen zwischen Fortschritt und Moral.* Husum: Matthiesen, 1991;58–60.

34. Savitt TL. The use of blacks for medical experimentation and demonstration in the Old South. *The Journal of Southern History* 1982;48:331–48.

35. Elkeles B. *Der moralische Diskurs über das medizinische Menschenexperiment*;229f.

36. Weá L. Menschenversuche und Seuchenpolitik – zwei unbekannte Kapitel aus der Geschichte der deutschen Tropenmedizin. 1999: *Zeitschrift für Sozialgeschichte des 20. und 21. Jahrhunderts* 1993;8(2):10–50.

37. Elkeles B. *Der moralische Diskurs über das medizinische Menschenexperiment*;228.

38. Ibid.;231.

39. Tashiro E. *Die Waage der Venus.*;142f.

40. Bean WB. Walter Reed and the ordeal of human experimentation. *Bulletin of the History of Medicine,*1977;51:75–92.

41. Frankenthal K. *Der dreifache Fluch: Jüdin, Intellektuelle, Sozialistin — Lebenserinnerungen einer Ärztin in Deutschland und im Exil.* Frankfurt, New York: K.M. Pearle and S. Leibfried, 1981;35f.

42. Crissey JT, Parish LC. *The Dermatology and Syphilology of the Nineteenth Century.* New York: Praeger, 1981;259.

43. Bull JP. The historical development of clinical therapeutic trials. *Journal of Chronic Diseases* 1959;10:218–48.

44. Leven KH. *Die Geschichte der Infektionskrankheiten. Von der Antike bis ins 20. Jahrhundert.* Landsberg: Ecomed, 1997;47.

45. Howard-Jones N. Human experimentation in historical and ethical perspectives;1429f.

46. Merians LE (ed.). *The Secret Malady. Venereal Disease in Eighteenth-Century Britain and France.* Lexington: University Press of Kentucky, 1995;23.

47. Wiesemann C, Frewer A (ed.). *Medizin und Ethik im Zeichen von Auschwitz. 50 Jahre Nürnberger Ärzteprozess.* Erlangen, Jena: Palm & Enke, 1996;19f.

48. Auspitz H. *Die Lehren vom syphilitischen Contagium und ihre thatsächliche Begründung.* Vienna: Wilhelm Braumüller, 1866;13f.

49. Tröhler U, Reither-Theil S (eds.). *Ethik und Medizin 1947-1997;*63.

50. Lederer SE. *Subjected to Science;*12.

51. St. Maur Moritz AA. The inoculation experiments in Hawaii, including notes on those of Arning and Fitch. *International Journal of Leprosy* 1951;19:203–15.

52. Ebbinghaus A, Dörner K (eds.). *Vernichten und Heilen. Der Nürnberger Ärzteprozess und seine Folgen.* Berlin: Aufbau-Verlag, 2001;96.

53. Bärensprung F. Mittheilungen aus der Abtheilung und Klinik für syphilitisch Kranke. *Annalen des Charité-Krankenhauses* 1860;9:130f.

54. Tashiro E. *Die Waage der Venus;*63f.

55. Elkeles B. *Der moralische Diskurs über das medizinische Menschenexperiment;*110f.

56. Tashiro E. *Die Waage der Venus;*155.

57. Ibid.;56f.

58. Mitchell RG. The child and experimental medicine. *Br Med J* 1964;1:721–27.

59. Jones AR. *The Birth of Bioethics.* New York, Oxford: Oxford University Press, 1998;126.

60. Mitchell RG. The child and experimental medicine.

61. Elkeles B. *Der moralische Diskurs über das medizinische Menschenexperiment;*231.

References

62. Janson C. Über Schutzimpfung und Immunität. *Centralblatt für Bakteriologie und Parasitenkunde* 1891;10:40–5.

63. Schreiber J. Ueber das Koch'sche Heilverfahren. *Deutsche Medizinische Wochenschrift* 1891;17:306–09.

CHAPTER 4 · THE VALUE OF EXPERIMENTS ON HUMANS

1. Elkeles B. *Der moralische Diskurs über das medizinische Menschenexperiment im 19. Jahrhundert.* Stuttgart, Jena, New York: Gustav Fischer, 1996;53.

2. Schott H (ed.). *Chronik der Medizin.* Gütersloh, Munich: Bertelsmann, 1993;267.

3. Crissey JT, Parish LC. *The Dermatology and Syphilology of the Nineteenth Century.* New York: Praeger, 1981;82.

4. Pontoppidan E. Ueber einige Inokulationsresultate von Sklerosen auf den Träger. *Vierteljahresschrift für Dermatologie und Syphilis* 1883;15:566–69.

5. Tashiro E. *Die Waage der Venus. Venerologische Versuche am Menschen zwischen Fortschritt und Moral.* Husum: Matthiesen, 1991;28.

6. Vogelsang TM. A serious sentence passed against the discoverer of the leprosy bacillus (Gerhard Armauer Hansen), in 1880. *Medical History* 1963; 7:182–86.

7. Tashiro E. *Die Waage der Venus;*51f.

8. Klusemann GG. Die Syphilisation in wissenschaftlicher und sanitätspolizeilicher Beziehung. Mit einer Nachschrift über die Zurechnung des ärztlichen Heilverfahrens von Casper. *Vierteljahrsschrift für gerichtliche und öffentliche Medicin* 1853;3:92–117.

9. Crissey JT, Parish LC. *The Dermatology and Syphilology of the Nineteenth Century;*82–8.

10. Ibid.;90.

11. Ibid.;217–30.

12. Ibid.;356.

13. Tashiro E. *Die Waage der Venus;*153.

14. Beecher HK. *Research and the Individual Human Studies.* Boston: Little, Brown and Company, 1970;1.

15. Ibid.;45.

16. Crissey JT, Parish LC. *The Dermatology and Syphilology of the Nineteenth Century;*232.

17. Lederer SE. *Subjected to Science. Human Experimentation in America Before the Second World War.* Baltimore, London: Johns Hopkins University Press, 1997;3.

18. Beecher HK. *Research and the Individual. Human Studies.* Boston: Little,

Brown and Company, 1970;8.

19. Altman LK. Auto-experimentation. An unappreciated tradition in medical science. *N Eng J Med* 1972;286:346–52.

20. Drummond JC, Wilbraham A. William Stark, M.D. An eighteenth century experiment in nutrition. *The Lancet* 1935;2:459–62.

21. Peller S. Walter Reed, C. Finlay, and their predecessors around 1800. *Bulletin of the History of Medicine* 1959;33:195–211.

22. Cáceres UG. Historiografia de la enfermedad de Carrión. Ideas e imágenes en la enfermedad de Carrión. Análisis historiográfico de la iconografia de la Bartonellosis Humana. Parte I. *Folia Dermatologica Peruana* 1998;9:47–56

23. Auspitz H. Franz v. Rinecker in Würzburg. *Archiv für Dermatologie und Syphilis* 1883;10:167–71.

24. Pick FJ. Pietro Pellizzari. *Archiv für Dermatologie und Syphilis* 1893;25:348–49.

25. Weindling P. *Health, Race and German Politics Between National Unification and Nazism. 1870-1945.* Cambridge: Cambridge University Press, 1989;167.

26. Lederer SE. *Subjected to Science*;3.

27. Elkeles B. *Der moralische Diskurs über das medizinische Menschenexperiment im 19. Jahrhundert*;109.

28. Crissey JT, Parish LC. *The Dermatology and Syphilology of the Nineteenth Century*;352f.

29. Ibid.;354.

30. Tashiro E. *Die Waage der Venus*;145.

CHAPTER 5 · THERAPEUTIC TRIALS

1. Allbutt TC. *Greek Medicine in Rome, with Other Historical Essays.* London: Macmillan, 1921;418.

2. Bradford Hill A. Medical ethics and controlled trials. *Br Med J* 1963;1:1043–49.

3. Howard-Jones N. Human experimentation in historical and ethical perspectives. *Social Science and Medicine* 1982;16:1429–48.

4. Ackerknecht EH. *Therapie von den Primitiven bis zum 20. Jahrhundert.* Stuttgart: Enke, 1970;53.

5. Moore C. *The Good, the Bad, and the Homely. Essays of an Old-fashioned Country Plastic Surgeon.* New York: Ardor Scribendi, 2000.

6. Ackerknecht EH. *Therapie von den Primitiven bis zum 20. Jahrhundert*;39.

7. Gillispie GC (ed.). *Dictionary of Scientific Biography*, vol. 3. New York: Charles Scribner's Sons, 1970;37f.

8. Bull JP. The historical development of clinical therapeutic trials. *Journal of Chronic Diseases* 1959;10:218–48.

9. Helmchen H, Winau R. *Versuche mit Menschen.* Berlin, New York: Walter de Gruyter, 1986;9f.

10. Wiesemann C, Frewer A (eds.) *Medizin und Ethik im Zeichen von Auschwitz. 50 Jahre Nürnberger Ärzteprozess.* Erlangen, Jena: Palm & Enke, 1996;17f.

11. Helmchen H, Winau R. *Versuche mit Menschen;*92.

12. Ibid.;95.

13. Ibid.;97.

14. Wiesemann C, Frewer A (eds.) *Medizin und Ethik im Zeichen von Auschwitz;*19.

15. Howard-Jones N. Human experimentation in historical and ethical perspectives.

16. Bull JP. The historical development of clinical therapeutic trials.

17. Elkeles B. *Der moralische Diskurs über das medizinische Menschenexperiment im 19. Jahrhundert.* Stuttgart, Jena, New York: Gustav Fischer, 1996;14f.

18. Sherwood J. Syphilization: Human experimentation in the search for a syphilis vaccine in the nineteenth century. *J Hist Med* 1999;54:364–86.

19. Elkeles B. *Der moralische Diskurs über das medizinische Menschenexperiment;*18.

20. Ibid.;25.

21. Ibid.;30.

22. Helmchen H, Winau R. *Versuche mit Menschen;*99f.

23. Ibid.;125.

24. Ibid.;127–31.

25. Tashiro E. *Die Waage der Venus. Venerologische Versuche am Menschen zwischen Fortschritt und Moral.* Husum: Matthiesen, 1991;61f.

26. Ibid.;111–13.

27. Rothman DJ. *Strangers at the Bedside. A History of How Law and Bioethics Transformed Medical Decision Making.* New York: Basic Books, 1991;20.

28. Bull JP. The historical development of clinical therapeutic trials.

29. Geison GL. Pasteur, Roux, and rabies: scientific versus clinical mentalities. *J Hist Med* 1990;45:341–65.

30. Rothman DJ. *Strangers at the Bedside;*22.

31. Ibid.

32. Burke DS. Joseph-Alexandre Auzias-Turenne, Louis Pasteur, and early concepts of virulence, attenuation, and vaccination. *Perspectives in Biology and Medicine* 1966;39:171–86.

33. Sherwood J. Syphilization: Human experimentation in the search for a syphilis vaccine in the nineteenth century.

34. Burke DS. Joseph-Alexandre Auzias-Turenne, Louis Pasteur, and early concepts of virulence, attenuation, and vaccination.

35. Ibid.

36. Sherwood J. Syphilization: Human experimentation in the search for a syphilis vaccine in the nineteenth century.

37. Ibid.

38. Tashiro E. *Die Waage der Venus*;19.

39. Koch R. Über bacteriologische Forschung. *Deutsche Medizinische Wochenschrift* 1890;16:756–57.

40. Koch R. Weitere Mittheilungen über ein Heilmittel gegen Tuberkulose. *Deutsche Medizinische Wochenschrift* 1890;16:1029–32.

41. Elkeles B. *Der moralische Diskurs über das medizinische Menschenexperiment*;133ff.

42. Ibid.;140.

43. Henoch E. Mittheilungen über das Koch'sche Heilverfahren gegen Tuberkulose. *Berliner klinische Wochenschrift* 1890;27:1169–71.

44. Elkeles B. *Der moralische Diskurs über das medizinische Menschenexperiment*;141.

45. Crissey JT, Parish LC. *The Dermatology and Syphilology of the Nineteenth Century*;208f.

46. Elkeles B. *Der moralische Diskurs über das medizinische Menschenexperiment*;148–50.

47. Langerhans R. Tod durch Heilserum. *Berliner klinische Wochenschrift* 1896;27:602–04.

48. Schadewaldt H. *Geschichte der Allergie*, vol. 3. Munich: Dustri, 1981:227–30.

49. Neisser A. Was wissen wir von einer Serumtherapie bei Syphilis und was haben wir von ihr zu erhoffen? Eine kritische Uebersicht und Materialien-Sammlung. *Archiv für Dermatologie und Syphilis* 1898;44:431–93.

50. Ehrlich P. Chemotherapeutische Trypanosomen-Studien. *Berliner klinische Wochenschrift* 1907:44:233–36, 280–83, 310–14, 341–44.

51. Ehrlich P, Hata S. *Die experimentelle Chemotherapie der Spirillosen (Syphilis, Rückfallfieber, Hühnerspirillose, Frambösie).* Berlin: Julius Springer, 1910;139ff.

52. Howard-Jones N. Human experimentation in historical and ethical perspectives.

53. Tashiro E. *Die Waage der Venus*;115–18.

CHAPTER 6 · WARRIORS AGAINST DISEASE

1. Tashiro E. *Die Waage der Venus. Venerologische Versuche am Menschen zwischen Fortschritt und Moral.* Husum: Matthiesen, 1991;142.

2. Ibid.;145.

References

3. Ibid.;81.

4. Ibid.;143.

5. Weyers W. *Death of Medicine in Nazi Germany. Dermatology and Dermatopathology under the Swastika.* Philadelphia: Ardor Scribendi, 1998;17.

6. Ebbinghaus A, Dörner K. *Heilen und Vernichten. Der Nürnberger Ärzteprozeá und seine Folgen.* Berlin: Aufbau-Verlag, 2001;72f.

7. Ibid.;80.

8. Ibid.;281.

9. Weindling P. *Health, Race and German Politics Between National Unification and Nazism. 1870-1945.* Cambridge: Cambridge University Press, 1989;159.

10. Ebbinghaus A, Dörner K. *Heilen und Vernichten;*76f.

11. Jütte R (ed.) *Geschichte der deutschen Ärzteschaft. Organisierte Berufs- und Gesundheitspolitik im 19. und 20. Jahrhundert.* Köln: Deutscher Ärzte-Verlag, 1997;79f.

12. Weindling P. *Health, Race and German Politics Between National Unification and Nazism;*161f.

13. Crissey JT, Parish LC. *The Dermatology and Syphilology of the Nineteenth Century.* New York: Praeger, 1981;221-24.

14. Fournier A. Die Prophylaxe der Syphilis durch ihre Behandlung. *Dermatologische Zeitschrift* 1900;7:3.

15. Tashiro E. *Die Waage der Venus;*40.

16. Ibid.;43f.

17. Ibid.;45-8.

18. Krause F. Die Mikrokokken der Blenorrhoea neonatorum. *Centralblatt für praktische Augenheilkunde* 1882;6:134–38.

19. Wassermann A. Ueber Gonokokken-Cultur und Gonokokken-Gift. *Berliner Klinische Wochenschrift* 1897;34:685–702.

20. Gläser JA. Noch einmal der "Rheumatismus gonorrhoicus." *Allgemeine Medicinische Central-Zeitung* 1898;67:415-17,429-32.

21. Weindling P. *Health, Race and German Politics Between National Unification and Nazism;*167.

22. Lang E. Einiges über Syphiliscontagium und Syphilistherapie. *Wiener Medizinische Wochenschrift* 1900;50:1114-5.

CHAPTER 7 · THE MERGER OF ANTIVIVISECTIONISM AND ANTI-SEMITISM

1. Bretschneider H. *Der Streit um die Vivisektion im 19. Jahrhundert.* Stuttgart: Gustav Fischer, 1962;12ff.

2. Wertheim G. Experimentelle Studien über Verbrennung und Verbrühung,

angestellt an Hunden. *Wiener Medizinische Presse* 1867;8:1237–39.

3. Bretschneider H. *Der Streit um die Vivisektion im 19. Jahrhundert*;120f.

4. Ibid.;14–6.

5. Ibid.;1.

6. Ludwig C. Die wissenschaftliche Thätigkeit in den physiologischen Instituten. *Im Neuen Reich* 1879;9:513–26.

7. Bretschneider H. *Der Streit um die Vivisektion im 19. Jahrhundert*;16–24.

8. Ibid.;40f.

9. Ibid.;107f.

10. Ibid.;45–9.

11. Ibid.;64ff.

12. Ibid.;89–91.

13. Ibid.;101f.

14. Ibid.;134.

15. Weyers W. *Death of Medicine in Nazi Germany. Dermatology and Dermatopathology under the Swastika.* Philadelphia: Ardor Scribendi, 1998;6ff.

16. Ibid.

17. Dawidowicz LS. *The War Against the Jews,* 10th Anniversary Edition. New York, Toronto, London, Sydney, Auckland: Bantam, 1996;36f.

18. Weyers W. *Death of Medicine in Nazi Germany*;13f.

19. Ibid.;24f.

20. Bretschneider H. *Der Streit um die Vivisektion im 19. Jahrhundert*;36.

21. Ibid.;44.

22. Ibid.;87.

23. Ibid.;99.

24. Elkeles B. *Der moralische Diskurs über das medizinische Menschenexperiment im 19. Jahrhundert.* Stuttgart, Jena, New York: Gustav Fischer, 1996;168.

25. Hamann B. *Hitlers Wien. Lehrjahre eines Diktators.* Munich, Zurich: Piper, 1996;345.

26. Ibid.;412.

27. Dawidowicz LS. *The War Against the Jews*;9.

28. Weyers W. *Death of Medicine in Nazi Germany*;14f.

CHAPTER 8 · ANTI-SEMITISM AS A VEHICLE TO MORALITY

1. Bretschneider H. *Der Streit um die Vivisektion im 19. Jahrhundert.* Stuttgart: Gustav Fischer, 1962;70.

References

2. Ibid.;49.

3. Elkeles B. *Der moralische Diskurs über das medizinische Menschenexperiment im 19. Jahrhundert.* Stuttgart, Jena, New York: Gustav Fischer, 1996;166.

4. Lederer SE. *Subjected to Science. Human Experimentation in America Before the Second World War.* Baltimore, London: Johns Hopkins University Press, 1997;10f.

5. Elkeles B. *Der moralische Diskurs über das medizinische Menschenexperiment;*180.

6. Ibid.;185.

7. Quidde L. *Arme Leute in Krankenhäusern.* Munich: Staegmeyr, 1900;17f.

8. Elkeles B. *Der moralische Diskurs über das medizinische Menschenexperiment;*183f.

9. Ibid.;186f.

10. Hamann B. *Hitlers Wien. Lehrjahre eines Diktators.* Munich, Zurich: Piper, 1996;333f.

11. Elkeles B. *Der moralische Diskurs über das medizinische Menschenexperiment;*170ff.

12. Ibid.;170.

13. Elkeles B. *Der moralische Diskurs über das medizinische Menschenexperiment;*174f.

14. Weyers W. *Death of Medicine in Nazi Germany. Dermatology and Dermatopathology under the Swastika.* Philadelphia: Ardor Scribendi, 1998;1–4.

15. Elkeles B. *Der moralische Diskurs über das medizinische Menschenexperiment;*188–90.

16. Quidde L. *Arme Leute in Krankenhäusern;*32.

17. Ibid.;28.

18. Elkeles B. *Der moralische Diskurs über das medizinische Menschenexperiment;*172–79.

19. Ibid.;175.

20. Grosz S, Kraus R. Bacteriologische Studien über den Gonococcus. *Archiv für Dermatologie und Syphilis* 1898;45:329–56.

21. Elkeles B. *Der moralische Diskurs über das medizinische Menschenexperiment;*187f.

22. Lewy J. Antisemitismus und Medizin. In Deutschen Reich. *Zeitschrift des Centralvereins deutscher Staatsbürger jüdischen Glaubens* 1899;5:1–19.

23. Hamann B. *Hitlers Wien;*428–431.

24. Weyers W. *Death of Medicine in Nazi Germany;*19f.

25. Lewy J. *Antisemitismus und Medizin;*4f.

26. Elkeles B. *Der moralische Diskurs über das medizinische Menschenexperiment;*175f.

27. Neisser A. Was wissen wir von einer Serumtherapie bei Syphilis und was haben wir von ihr zu erhoffen? Eine kritische Uebersicht und Materialien-Sammlung. *Archiv für Dermatologie und Syphilis* 1898;44:431–93.

28. Quidde L. *Arme Leute in Krankenhäusern*;40.

29. Ibid.;41.

30. Elkeles B. *Der moralische Diskurs über das medizinische Menschenexperiment*;192.

31. Tashiro E. *Die Waage der Venus. Venerologische Versuche am Menschen zwischen Fortschritt und Moral.* Husum: Matthiesen, 1991;88.

32. Elkeles B. *Der moralische Diskurs über das medizinische Menschenexperiment im*;192.

33. Quidde L. *Arme Leute in Krankenhäusern*;57.

34. Elkeles B. *Der moralische Diskurs über das medizinische Menschenexperiment*;194.

35. Ibid.;193.

36. Quidde L. *Arme Leute in Krankenhäusern*;96–100.

37. Elkeles B. *Der moralische Diskurs über das medizinische Menschenexperiment*;193.

38. Tashiro E. *Die Waage der Venus*;95.

39. Elkeles B. *Der moralische Diskurs über das medizinische Menschenexperiment*;174f.

40. Lewy J. *Antisemitismus und Medizin*;4.

41. Notter B. *Leben und Werk der Dermatologen Karl Herxheimer (1861–1942) und Salomon Herxheimer (1841–1899). M.D. diss.*, Johann Wolfgang Goethe University, Frankfurt, 1994;101ff.

42. Ibid.;119f.

43. Hollander A. Geschichtliches aus vergangener Zeit: Politische Bekämpfung der Geschlechtskrankheiten? *Fortschritte der Medizin* 1981;99:927–28.

44. Tashiro E. *Die Waage der Venus*;119f.

45. Hollander A. Geschichtliches aus vergangener Zeit: Politische Bekämpfung der Geschlechtskrankheiten?

CHAPTER 9 · THE DAWN OF INFORMED CONSENT

1. Faden RF, Beauchamp TL. *A History and Theory of Informed Consent.* New York, Oxford: Oxford University Press, 1986;61.

2. Ibid.;63f.

3. Ibid.;66.

4. Ibid.;67–9.

References

5. Howard-Jones N. Human experimentation in historical and ethical perspectives. *Social Science and Medicine* 1982;16:1429–48.

6. Annas GJ, Grodin MA (eds.). *The Nazi Doctors and the Nuremberg Code. Human Rights in Human Experimentation*. New York, Oxford: Oxford University Press, 1992;125.

7. Schönfeld W. Die Senatsrüge Rineckers anlässlich der Widerlegung syphilitischer Irrlehren, ein zeitgemässer medizingeschichtlicher Rückblick. *Dermatologische Wochenschrift* 1942;115:877–84.

8. Klusemann GG. Die Syphilisation in wissenschaftlicher und sanitätspolizeilicher Beziehung. Mit einer Nachschrift über die Zurechnung des ärztlichen Heilverfahrens von Casper. *Vierteljahrsschrift für gerichtliche und öffentliche Medicin* 1853;3:92–117.

9. Lederer SE. *Subjected to Science. Human Experimentation in America Before the Second World War*. Baltimore, London: Johns Hopkins University Press, 1997;13.

10. Wiesemann C, Frewer A (eds.). *Medizin und Ethik im Zeichen von Auschwitz. 50 Jahre Nürnberger Ärzteprozess*. Erlangen, Jena: Palm & Enke, 1996;20.

11. Pagel J. Zum Fall Neisser. *Deutsche Medizinalzeitung* 1900;21:296–97.

12. Baer KE. Der Fall Neisser. *Medicinische Woche* 1900;I:89–91.

13. Düring E. Der Fall Neisser. *Münchener Medicinische Wochenschrift* 1899;46:831–33.

14. Quidde L. *Arme Leute in Krankenhäusern*. Munich: Staegmeyr, 1900;83f.

15. Ibid.;93.

16. Ibid.;23.

17. Ibid.;8.

18. Tashiro E. *Die Waage der Venus. Venerologische Versuche am Menschen zwischen Fortschritt und Moral*. Husum: Matthiesen, 1991;93.

19. Ibid.;94.

20. Ibid.

21. Ibid.;90f.

22. Ibid.;96.

23. Elkeles B. *Der moralische Diskurs über das medizinische Menschenexperiment im 19. Jahrhundert*. Stuttgart, Jena, New York: Gustav Fischer, 1996;223.

24. Ibid.;208f.

25. Moll A. Versuche am lebenden Menschen *Die Zukunft* 1899;29:213–18.

26. Elkeles B. *Der moralische Diskurs über das medizinische Menschenexperiment*;211f.

27. Moll A. *Versuche am lebenden Menschen*;216.

28. Annas GJ, Grodin MA (eds.). *The Nazi Doctors and the Nuremberg Code*.

Human Rights in Human experimentation. New York, Oxford: Oxford University Press, 1992;127.

29. Elkeles B. *Der moralische Diskurs über das medizinische Menschenexperiment*;210–14.

30. Tashiro E. *Die Waage der Venus*;103.

31. Ibid.;105f.

32. Ibid.;126f.

33. Elkeles B. *Der moralische Diskurs über das medizinische Menschenexperiment*;215.

34. Forster E, Tomasczewski E. Nachweis von lebenden Spirochäten im Gehirn von Paralytikern. *Deutsche Medizinische Wochenschrift* 1913;39:1237.

35. Noguchi H. Dementia paralytica und Syphilis. *Münchener Medizinische Wochenschrift* 1913;60:2483–84.

36. Forster E, Tomasczewski E. Nachweis von lebenden Spirochäten im Gehirn von Paralytikern.

37. Habermann R. Fieberkurven von Gonorrhoikern und Normalen nach intravenösen Gonokokken-Vakzineinjektionen. *Deutsche Medizinische Wochenschrift* 1915;41:662.

38. Tomasczewski E. Bakteriologische Untersuchungen über den Erreger des Ulcus molle. *Zeitschrift für Hygiene und Infektionskrankheiten* 1903; 42:327–40.

39. Juliusberg M. Zur Kenntnis des Virus des Molluscum contagiosum des Menschen. *Deutsche Medizinische Wochenschrift* 1905;31:1598–99.

40. Tashiro E. *Die Waage der Venus*;161.

41. Klingmüller V, Baermann G. Ist das Syphilisvirus filtrierbar? *Deutsche Medizinische Wochenschrift* 1904;30:766.

42. Tashiro E. *Die Waage der Venus*;114.

43. Ibid.;108f.

CHAPTER 10 · THE AMERICAN APPROACH TO EXPERIMENTATION ON HUMANS

1. Crissey JT, Parish LC. *The Dermatology and Syphilology of the Nineteenth Century.* New York: Praeger, 1981;252,258,278.

2. Shelley WB, Shelley ED. *A Century of International Dermatological Congresses. An Illustrated History, 1889–1992.* Carnforth: Parthenon Publishing Group, 1992;11–22.

3. Morgan JP. The first reported case of electrical stimulation of the human brain. *J Hist Med* 1982;37:51–64.

4. Wentworth AH. Some experimental work on lumbar puncture of the subarachnoid space. *Boston Med Surg J* 1896;85:132–36,151–61.

References

5. Bean WB. Walter Reed and the ordeal of human experimentation. *Bulletin of the History of Medicine* 1977;51:75–92.

6. Altman LK. *Who Goes First? The Story of Self-Experimentation in Medicine.* Berkeley, Los Angeles, London: University of California Press, 1998;136.

7. Bean WB. Walter Reed and the ordeal of human experimentation;81f.

8. Shelley WB. Experimental disease in the skin of man. A review. *Acta Dermato-venereologica* 1983;Suppl.108:1–38.

9. Freund L. Ein mit Röntgen-Strahlen behandelter Fall von Naevus pigmentosus piliferus. *Wiener Medizinische Wochenschrift* 1897;47:428–34.

10. Freund L. Nachtrag zu dem Artikel 'Ein mit Röntgen-Strahlen behandelter Fall von Naevus pigmentosus piliferus.' *Wiener Medizinische Wochenschrift* 1897;47:856–860.

11. Elkeles B. *Der moralische Diskurs über das medizinische Menschenexperiment im 19. Jahrhundert.* Stuttgart, Jena, New York: Gustav Fischer, 1996;187.

12. Lederer SE. *Subjected to Science. Human Experimentation in America Before the Second World War.* Baltimore, London: Johns Hopkins University Press, 1997;18.

13. Moll A. Versuche am lebenden Menschen. *Die Zukunft* 1899;29:213–18.

14. Bruusgaard E. Über das Schicksal der nicht spezifisch behandelten Luetiker. *Archiv für Dermatologie und Syphilis* 1929;157:309–32.

15. Annas GJ, Grodin MA (eds.). *The Nazi Doctors and the Nuremberg Code. Human Rights in Human Experimentation.* New York, Oxford: Oxford University Press, 1992;121–44.

16. Lederer SE. *Subjected to Science*;9.

17. Ibid.;13.

18. Ibid.;7.

19. Jones AR. *The Birth of Bioethics.* New York, Oxford: Oxford University Press, 1998;159.

20. Lederer SE. *Subjected to Science*;10.

21. Bean WB. Walter Reed and the ordeal of human experimentation;82f.

22. Osler W. *The Principles and Practice of Medicine*, 3rd ed. New York: Appleton, 1898;183.

23. Lederer S. The right and wrong of making experiments on human beings: Udo J. Wile and syphilis. *Bulletin of the History of Medicine* 1984;58:380–97.

24. Lederer SE. *Subjected to Science*;7ff.

25. Morgan JP. The first reported case of electrical stimulation of the human brain.

26. Lederer SE. *Subjected to Science*;17.

27. Ibid.

28. Ibid.;16.

29. Faden RF, Beauchamp TL. *A History and Theory of Informed Consent.* New York, Oxford: Oxford University Press, 1986;123.

30. Lederer SE. *Subjected to Science*;28–32.

31. Ibid.;37.

32. Ibid.;27.

33. Ibid.;7.

34. Altman LK. *Who Goes First?*;71f.

35. Ibid.;94ff.

36. Ibid.;73.

37. Bean WB. Walter Reed and the ordeal of human experimentation.

38. Altman LK. *Who Goes First?*;144ff.

39. Numbers RL. William Beaumont and the Ethics of Human Experimentation. *Journal of the History of Biology* 1979;12:117.

40. Jones AR. *The Birth of Bioethics*;128.

41. Lederer SE. *Subjected to Science*;116.

42. Ibid.;46.

43. Ibid.;20f.

44. Ibid.;15.

45. Lederer SE. *Subjected to Science*;21.

46. Bean WB. Walter Reed and the ordeal of human experimentation;86.

47. Heiman H. A clinical and bacteriological study of the gonococcus Neisser in the male urethra and in the vulvovaginal tract of children. *Journal of Cutaneous and Genito-Urinary Diseases* 1895;13:384–87.

48. Sternberg GM, Reed W. Report on immunity against vaccination conferred upon the monkey by the use of the serum of the vaccinated calf and monkey. *Transactions of the Association of American Physicians* 1895;10:57–69.

49. Knowles FC. Molluscum contagiosum. Report of an institutional epidemic of fifty-nine cases. *JAMA* 1909;53:671–73.

50. Rothman DJ. *Strangers at the Bedside*;28.

51. Chernin E. Richard Pearson Strong and the iatrogenic plague disaster in Bilibid Prison, Manila, 1906. *Reviews of Infectious Diseases* 1989;11:996–1004.

52. Lederer SE. *Subjected to Science*;111.

53. Carpenter KJ, Sutherland B. Eijkman's contribution to the discovery of vitamins. *Journal of Nutrition* 1995;125:155–63.

54. Chernin E. Richard Pearson Strong and the Iatrogenic Plague Disaster in Bilibid Prison, Manila, 1906.

55. Hornblum AM. *Acres of Skin. Human Experiments at the Holmesburg Prison.* New York, London: Routledge, 1998;77.

56. Roussel T. *Traité de la Pellagra et des Pseudo-Pellagres.* Paris, 1866;529.

References

57. Funk C. Prophylaxe und Therapie der Pellagra im Lichte der Vitaminlehre. *Münchener Medizinische Wochenschrift* 1914;61:698–99.

58. Goldberger J. Pellagra: Causation and a method of prevention. *JAMA* 1916;66:471–76.

59. Hornblum AM. *Acres of Skin*;77ff.

60. Lederer SE. *Subjected to Science*;111.

CHAPTER 11 · LEGAL INITIATIVES IN THE UNITED STATES

1. Rosenberg CE. *The Care of Strangers: The Rise of America's Hospital System.* New York: Basic Books, 1987;5.

2. Lederer SE. *Subjected to Science. Human Experimentation in America Before the Second World War.* Baltimore, London: Johns Hopkins University Press, 1997;55.

3. Ibid.;57.

4. McGehee Harvey A. *Science at the Bedside: Clinical Research in American Medicine, 1905–1945.* Baltimore: Johns Hopkins University Press, 1981;78–85.

5. Lederer SE. *Subjected to Science*;53.

6. Ibid.;52–57.

7. Ibid.;57–58.

8. Ibid.;61.

9. Berkley HJ. Studies on the lesions induced by the action of certain poisons on the cortical nerve cell. Study VII: Poisoning with praparations of the thyroid gland. *Bull Johns Hopkins Hosp* 1897;8:137–40.

10. Lederer SE. *Subjected to Science*;62.

11. Wentworth AH. Some experimental work on lumbar puncture of the subarachnoic space. *Boston Med Surg J* 1896;135:132–6,156–61.

12. Lederer SE. *Subjected to Science*;61.

13. Fitch GL. The etiology of leprosy. *Med Rec* 1892;42:293–303.

14. Lederer SE. *Subjected to Science*;63–71.

15. Ibid.;143–146.

16. Ibid.;72.

17. Ibid.;74–87.

18. Ibid.;78.

19. Cannon WB. The responsibility of the general practitioner for freedom of medical research. *Boston Med Surg J* 1909;34:696.

20. Lederer SE. *Subjected to Science*;73.

21. Ibid.;74–89.

22. Knowles FC. Molluscum contagiosum: Report of an institutional epidemic

of fifty-nine cases. *JAMA* 1909;53:671–73.

23. Lederer SE. *Subjected to Science*;82–87.

24. Noguchi H. A cutaneous reaction in syphilis. *J Exp Med* 1911;14:557–68.

25. Wile UJ. Experimental syphilis in the rabbit produced by the brain substance of the living paretic. *J Exp Med* 1916;23:199–202.

26. Lederer SE. *Subjected to Science*;95f.

27. Ibid.;96.

28. Bernard C. *An Introduction to the Study of Experimental Medicine.* Translated by HC Greene. Special edition. The Classics of Medicine Library. Birmingham: Division of Grymon Editions, 1980;103.

29. Lederer SE. *Subjected to Science*;97.

30. Cannon WB. The right and wrong of making experiments on human beings. *JAMA* 1916;67:1372–3.

31. Lederer SE. *Subjected to Science*;98f.

32. Jones AR. *The Birth of Bioethics.* New York, Oxford: Oxford University Press, 1998;132f.

33. Lederer SE. *Subjected to Science*;98f.

34. Ibid.;102f.

35. Stanley LL. An analysis of one thousand testicular substance implantations. *Endocrinology* 1922;6:787–94.

36. McIntosh JA. The etiology of granuloma inguinale. *JAMA* 1926;87:996–1002.

37. Sellards AW, Lacy GR, Schöbl O. Superinfection in yaws. *Philippine Journal of Science* 1926;30:463–74.

38. Hornblum AM. *Acres of Skin*;79f.

39. Hess AF, Fish M. Infantile scurvy: The blood, the blood vessels, and the diet. *American Journal of Diseases of Children* 1914;8:386–405.

40. Lederer SE. *Subjected to Science*;106.

41. Ibid.;109.

42. Black WC. The etiology of acute infectious gingivostomatitis (Vincent's stomatitis). *Journal of Pediatrics* 1942;30:153.

43. Lederer SE. *Subjected to Science*;109f.

44. Ibid.;126ff.

45. Lewis S. *Arrowsmith.* New York: New Americn Library, 1980.

46. De Kruif P. *Microbe Hunters.* New York: Pocket Books, 1962.

47. Lederer SE. *Subjected to Science*;133–36.

48. Ibid.;127f.

References

CHAPTER 12 · EXPERIMENTS ON HUMANS IN A TURBULENT TIME

1. Grüter W. Experimentelle und klinische Untersuchungen über den sogenannten Herpes corneae. *Bericht über die Versammlung der Deutschen Ophthalmologischen Gesellschaft* 1920;42:162–65.

2. Lipschütz B. Untersuchungen über die Ätiologie der Krankheiten der Herpesgruppe (Herpes zoster, Herpes genitalis, Herpes febrilis). *Archiv für Dermatologie und Syphilis* 1921;136:428–82.

3. Kundralitz K. Experimentelle Übertragung von Herpes zoster auf den Menschen und die Beziehungen von Herpes zoster zu Varicellen. *Monatsschrift für Kinderheilkunde* 1925;29:516–23.

4. Schönfeld W. Versuche am Lebenden über den Übergang von Farbstoffen aus dem Blut in die Rückenmarksflüssigkeit und über den Übergang von Arzneimitteln aus der Rückenmarksflüssigkeit in das Blut, nebst Bemerkungen über die intralumbale Salvarsanbehandlung. *Archiv für Dermatologie und Syphilis* 1921;132:162–77.

5. Martenstein H. Experimentelle Untersuchungen bei Hydroa vacciniforme. *Archiv für Dermatologie und Syphilis* 1922;140:300–13.

6. Martenstein H. Experimentelle Untersuchungen über Strahlenempfindlichkeit bei Xeroderma pigmentosum. *Archiv für Dermatologie und Syphilis* 1924;147:499–508.

7. Biberstein H. Über Hautreaktionen bei Applikation von verschiedenen Rhusarten. *Klinische Wochenschrift* 1929;8:99–102.

8. Unna PG. In: Grote LR. *Die Wissenschaft der Gegenwart in Selbstdarstellungen (Medizin)*, vol. 8, Leizig: F. Meiner, 1930;194.

9. Lipschütz B. *Untersuchungen über die Ätiologie des Krankheiten der Herpesgruppe (Herpes zoster, Herpes genitalis, Herpes febrilis)*.

10. Steinmann R. *Die Debatte über medizinische Versuche am Menschen in der Weimarer Zeit. M.D.* diss., Eberhard-Karls-University, Tübingen, 1975;12.

11. Deicher H. Ätiologie und Klinik des Scharlachs. *Klinische Wochenschrift* 1927;50:2361–64.

12. Nohlen A. Experimentelle Anthrakosis und Tuberkulose. *Monatsschrift für Kinderheilkunde* 1927;37:415–23.

13. Vollmer H. Beitrag zur Ergosterinbehandlung der Rachitis. *Deutsche medizinische Wochenschrift* 1927;53:1634–5.

14 Vollmer H. Experimentelle und klinische Untersuchungen mit bestrahltem Ergosterin. *Zeitschrift für Kinderheilkunde* 1928;45:265–88.

15. Bessau G. Ernährungsversuche mit kohlehydratangereicherter Vollmilch. *Monatsschrift für Kinderheilkunde* 1929;42:28–32.

16. Weá L. Menschenversuche und Seuchenpolitik –zwei unbekannte Kapitel aus der Geschichte der deutschen Tropenmedizin. 1999: *Zeitschrift für Sozialgeschichte des 20. und 21. Jahrhunderts* 1993;8,2:10–50.

17. Steinmann R. *Die Debatte über medizinische Versuche am Menschen*;20.

18. Thom A, Caregorodcev GI (eds.). *Medizin unterm Hakenkreuz*. Berlin: VEB Verlag Volk und Gesundheit, 1989;252–54.

19. Steinmann R. *Die Debatte über medizinische Versuche am Menschen*;17.

20. Proctor RN. *Racial Hygiene: Medicine Under the Nazis*. Cambridge, MA: Harvard University Press, 1988;156f.

21. Steinmann R. *Die Debatte über medizinische Versuche am Menschen*;64.

22. Jütte R (ed.). *Geschichte der deutschen Ärzteschaft*. Köln: Deutscher Ärzte-Verlag, 1997;84.

23. Ibid.;107–14.

24. Ibid.;114–119.

25. Ibid.;150.

26. Steinmann R. *Die Debatte über medizinische Versuche am Menschen*;36,72.

27. Ibid.;36.

28. Ibid.;25.

29. Kruse F, Stern A. Über den Einfluss der Nahrung auf die Ausscheidung organischer Säuren im Säuglingsharn. *Zeitschrift für Kinderheilkunde* 1928;45:346–55.

30. Steinmann R. *Die Debatte über medizinische Versuche am Menschen*;29.

31. Wolf R. Wie sag' ich's meiner Öffentlichkeit? *Zeitschrift für ärztliche Fortbildung* 1931;28:442.

32. Steinmann R. *Die Debatte über medizinische Versuche am Menschen*;42.

33. Ibid.;38.

34. Ibid.;47.

35. Ibid.;37.

36. Ibid.;38.

37. Ibid.;46.

38. Tagesgeschichte. *Klinische Wochenschrift* 1929;8:1335.

39. Steinmann R. *Die Debatte über medizinische Versuche am Menschen*;98–103.

40. Ibid.;48–50.

41. Ibid.;48–55.

42. Pirquet C. Allergie nach Lebensalter und Geschlecht bei der Tuberkulose. *Wiener klinische Wochenschrift* 1928;41:797.

43. Rosenfeld S. Der statistische Beweis für die Immunisierung Neugeborener mit B.C.G. *Wiener klinische Wochenschrift* 1928;41:800–04.

44. Wolff G. Calmettes Erfolgsstatistik. *Medizinische Welt* 1930;4:917–8.

45. Steinmann R. *Die Debatte über medizinische Versuche am Menschen*;50–5.

References

46. Ibid.

47. Ibid.;59.

48. Ibid.;67–71.

49. Müller F. Die Zulässigkeit ärztlicher Versuche an gesunden und kranken Menschen. *Münchener Medizinische Wochenschrift* 1931;78:104–07.

50. Stauder A. Die Zulässigkeit ärztlicher Versuche an gesunden und kranken Menschen. *Münchener Medizinische Wochenschrift* 1931;78:107–12.

51. Annas GJ, Grodin MA (eds.). *The Nazi Doctors and the Nuremberg Code. Human Rights in Human Experimentation.* New York, Oxford: Oxford University Press, 1992;130f.

52. Sass H. Reichsrundschreiben 1931: Pre-Nuremberg German regulation concerning new therapy and human experimentation. *Journal of Medicine and Philosophy* 1983;8:99–111.

53. Annas GJ, Grodin MA (eds.). *The Nazi Doctors and the Nuremberg Code*;127–32.

54. Steinmann R. *Die Debatte über medizinische Versuche am Menschen*;3.

55. Maio G. Zum Nutzen des Patienten. Ethische Überlegungen zur Differenzierung von therapeutischen und nichttherapeutischen Studien. *Deutsches Ärzteblatt* 2000;97:A 3242–46.

56. Annas GJ, Grodin MA (eds.). *The Nazi Doctors and the Nuremberg Code*;131f.

57. Sass H. Reichsrundschreiben 1931.

58. Ibid.;130.

59. Steinmann R. *Die Debatte über medizinische Versuche am Menschen*;77.

60. Ibid.;117.

CHAPTER 13 · FROM THE BEST TO THE WORST

1. Wiesemann C, Frewer A (ed.). *Medizin und Ethik im Zeichen von Auschwitz. 50 Jahre* Nürnberger Ärzteprozess. Erlangen, Jena: Palm & Enke, 1996;52.

2. Weyers W. *Death of Medicine in Nazi Germany. Dermatology and Dermatopathology Under the Swastika.* Philadelphia: Ardor Scribendi, Ltd.,1998;18f.

3. Ibid.;141.

4. Proctor RN. *Racial Hygiene. Medicine Under the Nazis.* Cambridge: Harvard University Press, 1988;19.

5. Johnson P. *A History of the American People.* New York: Harper Perennial, 1998;617.

6. Ibid.;667.

7. Ibid.

8. Ibid.

9. Ibid.;670.

10. Jones AR. *The Birth of Bioethics*. New York, Oxford: Oxford University Press, 1998;170.

11. Weyers W. *Death of Medicine in Nazi Germany*;143.

12. Ibid.;148.

13. Ibid.;149f.

14. Alexander L. Medical science under dictatorship. *N Eng J Med* 1949;241:39-47.

15. Kater MH. *Doctors under Hitler*. Chapel Hill: University of North Carolina Press, 1989;177ff.

16. Hollingdale RJ (ed.) *A Nietzsche Reader*. London: Penguin Books, 1977;231.

17. Ibid.;115.

18. Ibid.;231.

19. Weyers W. *Death of Medicine in Nazi Germany*;151.

20. Schultze W. Das Vorgehen gegen asoziale Geschlechtskranke. *Dermatologische Wochenschrift* 1936;36:1227-9.

21. Ibid.

22. Weyers W. *Death of Medicine in Nazi Germany*;45.

23. Hanauske-Abel HM. Not a slippery slope or sudden subversion: German medicine and national socialism in 1933. *Br Med Journal* 1996;313:1453-63.

24. Ibid.

25. Weyers W. *Death of Medicine in Nazi Germany*;94. Jütte R (ed.). Geschichte der deutschen Ärzteschaft. Köln: Deutscher Ärzte-Verlag, 1997;150f.

26. Hanauske-Abel HM. Not a slippery slope.

27. Weyers W. *Death of Medicine in Nazi Germany*;99ff.

28. Ibid.;169ff.

29. Bretschneider H. *Der Streit um die Vivisektion im 19. Jahrhundert*. Stuttgart: Gustav Fischer, 1962;140f.

30. Weyers W. *Death of Medicine in Nazi Germany*;99.

31. Klee E. *Auschwitz, die NS-Medizin und ihre Opfer*. Frankfurt: S. Fischer, 1997;150ff.

32. Hilberg R. *Die Vernichtung der europäischen Juden*, vol. 2. Frankfurt: Fischer Taschenbuch Verlag, 1990;1004.

33. Oppitz DU. Medizinverbrechen vor Gericht. In: Frewer A, Wiesemann C (eds.) *Erlanger Studien zur Ethik in der Medizin*, vol. 7. Erlangen, Jena: Palm & Enke, 1999;144f.

34. Weyers W. *Death of Medicine in Nazi Germany*;99.

35. Hilberg R. *Die Vernichtung der europäischen Juden*;1004.

36. Weyers W. *Death of Medicine in Nazi Germany*;179.

References

37. Klee E. *Auschwitz, die NS-Medizin und ihre Opfer*;261.

38. Ibid.;169.

39. Ibid.;239.

40. Ibid.;229f.

CHAPTER 14 · MEDICAL RESEARCH UNDER THE NAZIS

1. Chagoll L. *Im Namen Hitlers. Kinder hinter Stacheldraht.* Cologne: Pahl-Rugenstein Verlag, 1979;134.

2. Weyers W. *Death of Medicine in Nazi Germany. Dermatology and Dermatopathology Under the Swastika.* Philadelphia: Ardor Scribendi, Ltd., 1998;286ff.

3. Klee E. *Auschwitz, die NS-Medizin und ihre Opfer.* Frankfurt: S. Fischer, 1997;15ff.

4. Hilberg R. *Die Vernichtung der europäischen Juden,* vol. 2. Frankfurt: Fischer Taschenbuch Verlag, 1990;967ff.

5. Klee E. *Auschwitz, die NS-Medizin und ihre Opfer*;248.

6. Ibid.;121.

7. Ibid.

8. Ibid.;407ff.

9. Ibid.;435f.

10. Ibid.;40f.

11. Ibid.;168.

12. Brauchle A, Grote RL. *Ergebnisse aus der Gemeinschaftsarbeit von Naturheilkunde und Schulmedizin,* vol. 2, Leipzig: Reclam, 1939;15f.

13. Klee E. *Auschwitz, die NS-Medizin und ihre Opfer*;147.

14. Ibid.;147ff.

15. Annas GJ, Grodin MA (eds.). *The Nazi Doctors and the Nuremberg Code. Human Rights in Human Experimentation.* New York, Oxford: Oxford University Press, 1992;79.

16. Helmchen H, Winau R. *Versuche mit Menschen.* Berlin, New York: Walter de Gruyter, 1986;72.

17. Annas GJ, Grodin MA (eds.). *The Nazi Doctors and the Nuremberg Code*;21.

18. Klee E. *Auschwitz, die NS-Medizin und ihre Opfer*;356ff.

19. Mitscherlich A, Mielke F. *Doctors of Infamy.* New York, Henry Schuman,1949;82f.

20. Ibid.;83.

21. Klee E. *Auschwitz, die NS-Medizin und ihre Opfer*;371ff.

22. Ibid.;478.

23. Ibid.;451ff.

24. Ibid.;97ff.

25. Annas GJ, Grodin MA (eds.). *The Nazi Doctors and the Nuremberg Code*;36f.

26. Weyers W. *Death of Medicine in Nazi Germany*;263f.

27. Klee E. *Auschwitz, die NS-Medizin und ihre Opfer*;198.

28. Panning G. Wirkungsform und Nachweis der sowjetischen Infanteriesprengmunition. *Der Deutsche Militärarzt* 1942;7:20-30.

29. Annas GJ, Grodin MA (eds.). *The Nazi Doctors and the Nuremberg Code*;83.

30. Klee E. *Auschwitz, die NS-Medizin und ihre Opfer*;87ff.

31. Harris SH. *Factories of Death. Japanese Biological Warfare, 1932-45, and the American Cover-up*. New York: Routledge, 1994;x.

32. Weyers W. *Death of Medicine in Nazi Germany*;303.

33. Klee E. *Auschwitz, die NS-Medizin und ihre Opfer*;269ff.

34. Ibid.;378ff.

35. Ibid.;385f.

36. Ebbinghaus A, Dörner K (eds.). *Vernichten und Heilen. Der Nürnberger Ärzteprozess und seine Folgen*. Berlin: Aufbau-Verlag, 2001;115f.

37. Klee E. *Auschwitz, die NS-Medizin und ihre Opfer*;217.

38. Klee E. *Auschwitz, die NS-Medizin und ihre Opfer*;218.

39. Ibid.;220ff.

40. Ebbinghaus A, Dörner K (eds.). *Vernichten und Heilen*;134f.

41. Klee E. *Auschwitz, die NS-Medizin und ihre Opfer*;231ff.

42. Ibid.;243ff.

43. Ibid.;205ff.

44. Ibid.;259.

45. Voegt H. Zur Aetiologie der Hepatitis epidemica. *Münchener Medizinische Wochenschrift* 1942;89:76-9.

46. Pross C, Aly G, *et al.* (eds.). *Der Wert des Menschen, Medizin in Deutschland 1918-1945*;261-93.

47. Klee E. *Auschwitz, die NS-Medizin und ihre Opfer*;117ff.

48. Héran J, Reumaux B (eds.) *Histoire de la Medicine à Strasbourg*. Strasbourg: La Nuée Bleue, 1997;595ff.

49. Klee E. *Auschwitz, die NS-Medizin und ihre Opfer*;368.

50. Ibid.;281ff.

51. Ebbinghaus A, Dörner K. *Heilen und Vernichten*;184ff.

52. Ibid.;194ff.

53. Ibid.;213ff.

References

54. Klee E. *Auschwitz, die NS-Medizin und ihre Opfer*;156.

55. Ebbinghaus A, Dörner K. *Heilen und Vernichten*;208ff.

56. Weyers W. *Death of Medicine in Nazi Germany*;296f.

57. Ibid.;295.

58. Scholz A. Personal communication.

59. Weyers W. *Death of Medicine in Nazi Germany*;295.

60. Ibid.;334.

61. Klee E. *Auschwitz, die NS-Medizin und ihre Opfer*;19.

62. Ibid.;487.

63. Annas GJ, Grodin MA (eds.). *The Nazi Doctors and the Nuremberg Code*;15f.

CHAPTER 15 · RESEARCH BY THE JAPANESE IN OCCUPIED CHINA

1. Langer PF. Japan zwischen den Kriegen. In: Mann G (ed.) *Weltgeschichte: Eine Universalgeschichte*, vol. IX. Gütersloh: Prisma Verlag, 1980;231-78.

2. Ibid.

3. Ibid.

4. Harris SH. *Factories of Death. Japanese Biological Warfare, 1932-45, and the American Cover-up*. New York: Routledge, 1994;10.

5. Chang I. *The rape of Nanking*. New York: Penguin Books, 1998;26.

6. Langer PF. Japan zwischen den Kriegen.

7. Harris SH. *Factories of Death*;21.

8. Ibid.;25ff.

9. Ibid.

10. Chang I. *The Rape of Nanking*;3ff.

11. Ibid.

12. Ibid.;40.

13. Ibid.;218.

14. Harris SH. *Factories of Death*;58.

15. Ibid.;44.

16. Ibid.;52.

17. Ibid.;34f.

18. Ibid.;54f.

19. Ibid.;62f.

20. Ibid.;64.

21. Bärnighausen T. *Medizinische Humanexperimente der japanischen Truppen für Biologische Kriegsführung in China, 1932-1945*. M.D. diss., University

of Heidelberg, 1996;101ff.

22. Ibid.;144.

23. Harris SH. *Factories of death*;62.

24. Ibid.;68f.

25. Ibid.;61.

26. Ibid.;111.

27. Ibid.;95ff.

28. Ibid.;67.

29. Bärnighausen T. *Medizinische Humanexperimente der japanischen Truppen für Biologische Kriegsführung in China*;166ff.

30. Harris SH. *Factories of death*;70f.

31. Tanaka Y. Poison gas. The story Japan would like to forget. *Bulletin of the Atomic Scientists* 1988;10-19.

32. Harris SH. *Factories of death*;62.

33. Bärnighausen T. *Medizinische Humanexperimente der japanischen Truppen für Biologische Kriegsführung in China*;104f.

34. Harris SH. *Factories of death*;63.

35. Ibid.;129.

36. Bärnighausen T. *Medizinische Humanexperimente der japanischen Truppen für Biologische Kriegsführung in China*;104f.

37. Harris SH. *Factories of Death*;222.

38. Ibid.;179ff.

39. Weyers W. *Death of Medicine in Nazi Germany. Dermatology and Dermatopathology Under the Swastika*. Philadelphia: Ardor Scribendi, Ltd., 1998;330ff.

40. Harris SH. *Factories of Death*;179f.

41. Weyers W. *Death of Medicine in Nazi Germany*;335.

42. Harris SH. *Factories of Death*;188.

43. Weyers W. *Death of Medicine in Nazi Germany*;331ff.

44. Bärnighausen T. *Medizinische Humanexperimente der japanischen Truppen für Biologische Kriegsführung in China*;187ff.

CHAPTER 16 · HUMAN EXPERIMENTS BY THE ALLIES

1. Bärnighausen T. *Medizinische Humanexperimente der japanischen Truppen für Biologische Kriegsführung in China, 1932-1945*. M.D. diss., University of Heidelberg, 1996;146.

2. Moreno JD. *Undue Risk. Secret State Experiments on Humans*. New York: W.H. Freeman and Company 1999;285.

References

3. Wiesemann C, Frewer A (ed.). *Medizin und Ethik im Zeichen von Auschwitz. 50 Jahre Nürnberger Ärzteprozess*. Erlangen, Jena: Palm & Enke, 1996;39.

4. Mellanby K. *Human Guinea Pigs*. London: Merlin Press, 1973.81.

5. Ibid.;154.

6. Ibid.;130.

7. Ibid.;171.

8. Ibid.;129.

9. Ibid.;174.

10. Ibid.;133.

11. Swaminath CS, Shortt HE, Anderson LAP. Transmission of Indian kala-azar to man by the bites of Phlebotomus argentipes, ann. and brun. *Indian Journal of Medical Research* 1942;30:473-7.

12. Obituary notices. Sir Neil Hamilton Fairley. *Br Med J* 1966;1:1117.

13. Mellanby K. *Human Guinea Pigs*;175f.

14. Moreno JD. *Undue Risk*;49f.

15. Mellanby K. *Human Guinea Pigs*;175f.

16. Moreno JD. *Undue Risk*;48ff.

17. Loff B, Cordner S. World War II malaria trials revisited. *The Lancet* 1999;353:1597.

18. Goodwin B. *Keen as Mustard. Britain's Horrific Chemical Warfare Experiments in Australia*. St. Lucia: University of Queensland Press 1998;32f.

19. Wells HG. *The Shape of Things to Come*. London: Hutchinson & Co., Ltd., 1933;171.

20. Goodwin B. *Keen as Mustard*;61ff.

21. Ibid.;93ff.

22. Ibid.;163ff.

23. Ibid.;117.

24. Ibid.;157f.

25. Ibid.;119ff.

26. Ibid.;146.

27. Ibid.;134.

28. Ibid.;162ff.

29. Ibid.;143f.

30. Ibid.;48f.

31. Ibid.;144.

32. Ibid.;231ff.

33. Sinclair D. The clinical features of mustard gas poisoning in man. *Br Med J* 1948;2:290-4.

34. Sinclair D. The clinical reactions of the skin to mustard gas vapour. *Br J Dermatol* 1949;61:113-25.

35. Goodwin B. *Keen as Mustard*;353.

36. Veterans at risk. The health effects of mustard gas and lewisite. Washington, D.C.: *National Academy Press*;51ff.

37. Bordley J III, McGehee Harvey A. *Two Centuries of American Medicine. 1776-1976*. Philadelphia: W.B. Saunders 1976;356.

38. Rothman DJ. *Strangers at the Bedside. A History of How Law and Bioethics Transformed Medical Decision Making*. New York: Basic Books, 1991;31.

39. Bordley J III, McGehee Harvey A. *Two Centuries of American Medicine*;356.

40. Moreno JD. *Undue Risk*;21ff.

41. Rothman DJ. *Strangers at the Bedside*;42.

42. Hornblum AM. *Acres of Skin. Human Experiments at the Holmesburg Prison*. New York, London: Routledge 1998;80.

43. Hornblum AM. *Acres of Skin*;82.

44. Ibid.;82f.

45. Ibid.;84.

46. Rothman DJ. *Strangers at the Bedside*;44.

47. Hornblum AM. *Acres of Skin*;80f.

48. Rothman DJ. *Strangers at the Bedside*;36.

49. Hornblum AM. *Acres of Skin*;81ff.

50. Ibid.

51. Rothman DJ. *Strangers at the Bedside*;36f.

52. Ibid.;44.

53. Ibid.;47ff.

54. Ibid.;33f.

55. Rothman DJ. Ethics and human experimentation. Henry Beecher revisited. *N Eng J Med* 1987;317:1195-9.

56. Rothman DJ. *Strangers at the Bedside*;38.

57. Ibid.;36.

58. Welsome E. *The Plutonium Files. America's Secret Medical Experiments in the Cold War*. New York: The Dial Press, 1999;73.

59. Ibid.;79.

60. Ibid.;126.

61. Ibid.;134.

62. Ibid.

63. Ibid.;126.

64. Ibid.;139.

65. Ibid.;148.

66. Ibid.;130.

67. Ibid.;149f.

68. Ibid.;150ff.

69. Ibid.;178f.

70. Faden RR, *et al*. *Final Report of the Advisory Committee on Human Radiation Experiments*. New York, Oxford: Oxford University Press, 1996;47f.

71. Ibid.

CHAPTER 17 · THE NUREMBERG CODE

1. Harris SH. *Factories of Death. Japanese Biological Warfare, 1932-45, and the American Cover-up*. New York: Routledge, 1994;157.

2. Annas GJ, Grodin MA (eds.). *The Nazi Doctors and the Nuremberg Code. Human Rights in Human Experimentation*. New York, Oxford: Oxford University Press, 1992;8.

3. Oppitz DU. Medizinverbrechen vor Gericht. In: Frewer A, Wiesemann C (eds.) *Erlanger Studien zur Ethik in der Medizin*, vol. 7. Erlangen, Jena: Palm & Enke, 1999;64ff.

4. Annas GJ, Grodin MA (eds.). *The Nazi Doctors and the Nuremberg Code*;8.

5. Ibid.;174f.

6. Ibid.;67.

7. Wiesemann C, Frewer A (ed.). *Medizin und Ethik im Zeichen von Auschwitz. 50 Jahre Nürnberger Ärzteprozess*. Erlangen, Jena: Palm & Enke, 1996;33.

8. Ibid.;34ff.

9. Ibid.;36.

10. Weyers W. *Death of Medicine in Nazi Germany. Dermatology and Dermatopathology Under the Swastika*. Philadelphia: Ardor Scribendi, Ltd., 1998;143f.

11. Ibid.;120f.

12. Ibid.;335f.

13. Klee E. *Auschwitz, die NS-Medizin und ihre Opfer*. Frankfurt: S. Fischer, 1997;252.

14. Ibid.;89.

15. Annas GJ, Grodin MA (eds.). *The Nazi Doctors and the Nuremberg Code*;69.

16. Ibid.;94f.

17. Ibid.;91.

18. Katz J. *Experimentation on Human Beings*. New York: Russell Sage Foundation, 1972;299f.

19. Ibid.;299.

20. Annas GJ, Grodin MA (eds.). *The Nazi Doctors and the Nuremberg Code*;92.

21. Katz J. *Experimentation on Human Beings*;298f.

22. Mitscherlich A, Mielke F. *Doctors of Infamy*. New York: Henry Schuman, 1949;157ff.

23. Ibid.;160f.

24. Annas GJ, Grodin MA (eds.). *The Nazi Doctors and the Nuremberg Code*;88.

25. Ibid.;132f.

26. Katz J. *Experimentation on Human Beings*;300.

27. Ebbinghaus A, Dörner K. *Heilen und Vernichten. Der Nürnberger Ärzteprozeß und seine Folgen*. Berlin: Aufbau-Verlag 2001;358ff.

28. Moreno JD. *Undue Risk. Secret State Experiments on Humans*. New York: W.H. Freeman and Company 1999;68.

29. Ibid.;64ff.

30. Faden RR, *et al. Final Report of the Advisory Committee on Human Radiation Experiments*. New York, Oxford: Oxford University Press, 1996;76.

31. Harkness JM. Nuremberg and the issue of wartime experiments on US prisoners. The Green Committee. *JAMA* 1996;276:1672-5.

32. Annas GJ, Grodin MA (eds.). *The Nazi Doctors and the Nuremberg Code*;134.

33. Supplementary report of the Judicial Council. *JAMA* 1946;132:1090.

34. Katz J. *Experimentation on Human Beings*;300.

35. Moreno JD. *Undue Risk*;76.

36. Ibid.;76f.

37. Tröhler U, Reither-Theil S (ed.). *Ethik und Medizin 1947-1997. Was leistet die Kodifizierung der Ethik?* Göttingen: Wallstein, 1997;193f.

38. Moreno JD. *Undue Risk*;69.

39. Ibid.

40. Ibid.;70.

41. Katz J. *Experimentation on Human Beings*;303f.

42. Ibid.;304.

43. Annas GJ, Grodin MA (eds.). *The Nazi Doctors and the Nuremberg Code*;135.

44. Ibid.

45. Ibid.;102.

46. Ibid.

47. Ibid.;103.

48. Moreno JD. *Undue Risk*;53a.

49. Ebbinghaus A, Dörner K. *Heilen und Vernichten*;136.

References

50. Katz J. The Nuremberg Code and the Nuremberg trial. A reappraisal. *JAMA* 1996;276:1662-6.

51. Annas GJ, Grodin MA (eds.). *The Nazi Doctors and the Nuremberg Code*;95f.

52. Ibid.;105ff.

53. Ibid.;197.

CHAPTER 18 · THE AFTERMATH OF NUREMBERG

1. Annas GJ, Grodin MA (eds.). *The Nazi Doctors and the Nuremberg Code. Human Rights in Human Experimentation.* New York, Oxford: Oxford University Press, 1992;201.

2. Ibid.;228.

3. Harris SH. *Factories of Death. Japanese Biological Warfare, 1932-45, and the American Cover-up.* New York: Routledge, 1994;195ff.

4. Ibid.; 222.

5. Ibid.;190.

6. Ibid.;189.

7. Ibid.;207.

8. Ibid.;212.

9. Ibid.;208.

10. Ibid.;133.

11. Annas GJ, Grodin MA (eds.). *The Nazi Doctors and the Nuremberg Code. Human Rights in Human Experimentation.* New York, Oxford: Oxford University Press, 1992;106f.

12. Moreno JD. *Undue Risk. Secret State Experiments on Humans.* New York: W.H. Freeman and Company, 1999;88ff.

13. Wiesemann C, Frewer A (ed.). *Medizin und Ethik im Zeichen von Auschwitz. 50 Jahre Nürnberger Ärzteprozess.* Erlangen, Jena: Palm & Enke, 1996;39f.

14. Mellanby K. *Human Guinea Pigs.* London: Merlin Press, 1973;179ff.

15. Oppitz DU. Medizinverbrechen vor Gericht. In: Frewer A, Wiesemann C (eds.) *Erlanger Studien zur Ethik in der Medizin.* Vol. 7. Erlangen, Jena: Palm & Enke, 1999;79ff.

16. Ivy AC. The history and ethics of the use of human subjects in medical experiments. *Science* 1948;108:1-5.

17. Ethics governing the service of prisoners as subjects in medical experiments. Report of a committee appointed by Governor Dwight H. Green of Illinois. *JAMA* 1948;136:457-8.

18. Rothman DJ. *Strangers at the Bedside. A History of How Law and Bioethics Transformed Medical Decision Making.* New York: Basic Books, 1991;47.

19. Leys D. Ethical standards in clinical research. *The Lancet* 1953;2:1044.

20. Beecher HK. Experimentation in man. *JAMA* 1959;169:461-78.

21. Shimkin MB. The problem of experimentation on human beings. I. The research worker's point of view. *Science* 1953;117:205-7.

22. Guttentag OE. Problem of experimentation on human beings: II. Physician's point of view. *Science* 1953;117:207-10.

23. Beecher HK. Experimentation in man.

24. Ibid.

25. Auspitz H. *Die Lehren vom syphilitischen Contagium und ihre thatsächliche Begründung.* Vienna: Wilhelm Braumüller, 1866;5.

26. Sherwood J. Syphilization: Human experimentation in the search for a syphilis vaccine in the nineteenth century. *Journal of the History of Medicine* 1999;54:364-86.

27. Rinecker F. Über die Ansteckungsfähigkeit der constitutionellen Syphilis. *Verhandlungen der Würzburger Physikalisch-Medicinischen Gesellschaft* 1852;3:375-97.

28. Tashiro E. *Die Waage der Venus. Venerologische Versuche am Menschen zwischen Fortschritt und Moral.* Husum: Matthiesen, 1991;111-3.

29. Beecher HK. Experimentation in man.

30. Shimkin MB. The problem of experimentation on human beings.

31. Beecher HK. *Research and the Individual. Human Studies.* Boston: Little, Brown and Company, 1970;31.

32. Howard-Jones N. Human experimentation in historical and ethical perspectives. *Social Science and Medicine* 1982;16:1429-48.

33. Lasagna L, von Felsinger JM. The volunteer subject in research. *Science* 1954;120:359-61.

34. Esecover H, Malitz D, Wilkens B. Clinical profiles of paid normal subjects volunteering for hallucinogen drug studies. *Am J Psych* 1961;117:910-5.

35. Beecher HK. *Research and the Individual*;61.

36. Beecher HK. Experimentation in man.

37. Howard-Jones N. Human experimentation in historical and ethical perspectives.

38. Annas GJ, Grodin MA (eds.). *The Nazi Doctors and the Nuremberg Code*;204.

39. The dedication of the physician. *World Medical Association Bulletin* 1949;1:4-13.

40. Organizational News. *World Medical Journal* 1955;2:14-5.

41. Beecher HK. Experimentation in man.

42. Ibid.

43. Annas GJ, Grodin MA (eds.). *The Nazi Doctors and the Nuremberg*

References

Code;156.

44. Altman LK. *Who Goes First? The Story of Self-Experimentation in Medicine*. Berkeley, Los Angeles, London: University of California Press, 1998;126ff.

45. Annas GJ, Grodin MA (eds.). *The Nazi Doctors and the Nuremberg Code*;156.

46. Beecher HK. Experimentation in man.

47. Ibid.

48. Ehrlich P, Hata S. *Die experimentelle Chemotherapie der Spirillosen* (Syphilis, Rückfallfieber, Hühnerspirillose, Frambösie). Berlin: Julius Springer, 1910;139ff.

49. Guttentag OE. Problem of Experimentation on Human Beings.

50. Beecher HK. Experimentation in man.

51. Ibid.

52. Ibid.

53. Ibid.

54. Ibid.

55. Ibid.

56. Ibid.

57. Beecher HK. *Research and the Individual*;236.

58. Ladimer I. Ethical and legal aspects of medical research on human beings. *Journal of Public Law* 1954;3:467-511.

59. Ladimer I. Human experimentation: Medicolegal aspects. *N Eng J Med* 1957;257:18-24.

60. Ibid.

61. Faden RR, *et al. Final Report of the Advisory Committee on Human Radiation Experiments*. New York, Oxford: Oxford University Press, 1996;55f.

62. Ibid.;56.

63. Ibid.;56ff.

64. Topping NH. The United States Public Health Service's Clinical Center for medical research. *JAMA* 1952;150:541-5.

65. Annas GJ, Grodin MA (eds.). *The Nazi Doctors and the Nuremberg Code*;185.

66. Ibid.;157f.

67. Ibid.;331ff.

68. Ibid.;205.

69. Ibid.;331.

70. Tröhler U, Reither-Theil S (ed.). *Ethik und Medizin 1947-1997. Was leistet die Kodifizierung der Ethik?* Göttingen: Wallstein, 1997;124.

71. Shimkin MB. The problem of experimentation on human beings.

CHAPTER 19 · AN ORGY OF EXPERIMENTS ON HUMANS

1. Müller F. Die Zulässigkeit ärztlicher Versuche an gesunden und kranken Menschen. *Münchener Medizinische Wochenschrift* 1931;78:104-7.

2. Helmchen H, Winau R. *Versuche mit Menschen*. Berlin, New York: Walter de Gruyter 1986;108.

3. Bradford Hill A. Medical ethics and controlled trials. *Br Med J* 1963;1:1043-9.

4. Ibid.

5. Howard-Jones N. Human experimentation in historical and ethical perspectives. *Social Science and Medicine* 1982;16:1429-48.

6. Helmchen H, Winau R. *Versuche mit Menschen*;100.

7. Faden R, *et al*. *Final Report of the Advisory Committee on Human Radiation Experiments*. New York, Oxford: Oxford University Press 1996;80.

8. Mainland D. The clinical trial – some difficulties and suggestions. *Journal of Chronic Diseases* 1960;11:484-96.

9. Bradford Hill A. Medical ethics and controlled trials.

10. McCance RA. The practice of experimental medicine. *Proceedings of the Royal Society of Medicine* 1951;44:189-94.

11. Beecher HK. Experimentation in man. *JAMA* 1959;169:461-78.

12. Shimkin MB. The problem of experimentation on human beings. I. The research worker's point of view. *Science* 1953;117:205-7.

13. Rothman DJ. *Strangers at the Bedside. A History of How Law and Bioethics Transformed Medical Decision Making*. New York: Basic Books 1991;52.

14. Jones AR. *The Birth of Bioethics*. New York, Oxford: Oxford University Press, 1998;13ff.

15. Ibid.;53.

16. Swain DC. The rise of a research empire: NIH, 1930 to 1950. *Science* 1962;138:1233-7.

17. Faden RR, *et al*. *Final Report of the Advisory Committee on Human Radiation Experiments*;10f.

18. Swain DC. The rise of a research empire: NIH, 1930 to 1950.

19. Bordley J III, McGehee Harvey A. *Two Centuries of American Medicine, 1776-1976*. Philadelphia: W.B. Saunders 1976;417.

20. Swain DC. The rise of a research empire: NIH, 1930 to 1950.

21. Bordley J III, McGehee Harvey A. *Two Centuries of American Medicine*;359.

22. Ibid.;418f.

23. Swain DC. The rise of a research empire: NIH, 1930 to 1950.

24. Bordley J III, McGehee Harvey A. *Two Centuries of American Medicine*;419ff.

25. Rothman DJ. *Strangers at the Bedside*;53f.

26. Bordley J III, McGehee Harvey A. *Two Centuries of American Medicine*;420f.

27. Ibid.;419.

28. Welsome E. *The Plutonium Files. America's Secret Medical Experiments in the Cold War*. New York: The Dial Press 1999;210.

29. Curran WJ. Governmental regulation of the use of human subjects in medical research: The approach of two federal agencies. *Daedalus* 1969;98(2):542-94.

30. Tröhler U, Reither-Theil S (ed.). *Ethik und Medizin* 1947-1997;195.

31. Topping NH. The United States Public Health Service's Clinical Center for medical research. *JAMA* 1952;150:541-5.

32. Welsome E. *The Plutonium Files*;210.

33. Ibid.

34. Bordley J III, McGehee Harvey A. *Two Centuries of American Medicine. 1776-1976*. Philadelphia: W.B. Saunders 1976;425.

35. Beecher HK. Experimentation in man.

36. Ibid.

37. Beecher HK. *Research and the Individual. Human Studies*. Boston: Little, Brown and Company 1970;189.

38. Faden RR, *et al. Final Report of theAdvisory Committee on Human Radiation Experiments*;79.

39. Moreno JD. *Undue Risk. Secret State Experiments on Humans*. New York: W.H. Freeman and Company 1999;141.

40. Ibid.;142.

41. Ibid.;46ff.

42. Rothman DJ. *Strangers at the Bedside*;54.

43. Annas GJ, Grodin MA (eds.). *The Nazi Doctors and the Nuremberg Code. Human Rights in Human Experimentation*. New York, Oxford: Oxford University Press, 1992;185.

44. Rothman DJ. *Strangers at the Bedside*;54ff.

45. Faden RR, *et al. Final Report of the Advisory Committee on Human Radiation Experiments*;56ff.

46. Ibid.;62.

47. Ibid.;90f.

48. Moreno JD. *Undue Risk*;257.

49. Pappworth MH. *Human Guinea Pigs*. London: Routledge & Kegan Paul, 1967;6f.

50. Ibid.;28.

51. Faden RR, *et al. Final Report of the Advisory Committee on Human Radiation Experiments*;86f.

52. Hornblum AM. *Acres of Skin. Human Experiments at the Holmesburg Prison*. New York, London: Routledge, 1998;15f.

53. Shelley WB. Experimental disease in the skin of man. A review. *Acta Dermato-venereologica* 1983;Suppl. 108:1-38.

54. Beecher HK. Ethics and clinical research.

55. Pappworth MH. *Human Guinea Pigs*;13f.

56. Ibid.;25f.

57. Beecher HK. Experimentation in man.

58. Faden RR, *et al. Final Report of the Advisory Committee on Human Radiation Experiments*;49.

59. Welsome E. *The Plutonium Files*;205.

60. Ibid.;118.

61. Ibid.;212.

CHAPTER 20 · THE PRISON AS TEST SITE

1. Mitford J. *Kind and Usual Punishment*. New York: Alfred A. Knopf, 1973;30ff.

2. Ibid.;86f.

3. Hornblum AM. *Acres of Skin. Human Experiments at the Holmesburg Prison*. New York, London: Routledge 1998;23f.

4. Mitford J. *Kind and Usual Punishment*;43.

5. Ibid.;79ff.

6. Rothman DJ. *Discovery of the asylum*. Boston: Little, Brown and Company, 1971;84f.

7. Mitford J. *Kind and Usual Punishment*;7.

8. Ibid.;95.

9. Fenton N. *Treatment in Prison: How the Family Can Help*. Sacramento: State of California, 1959.

10. Powelson H, Bendix R. Psychiatry in prison. *Psychiatry* 1951;14.

11. Mitford J. *Kind and Usual Punishment*;121.

12. Ibid.

13. Ibid.;125.

14. Ibid.

15. Ibid.;33.

16. Ibid.

17. Ibid.;80.

18. Ibid.;86.

19. Clark R. *Crime in America*. New York: Simon and Schuster, 1970;222.

20. Mitford J. *Kind and Usual Punishment*;79ff.

21. Ibid.;11f.

22. Ibid.;249.

23. Ivy AC. The history and ethics of the use of human subjects in medical experiments. *Science* 1948;108:1-5.

24. Mitford J. *Kind and Usual Punishment*;32.

25. Annas GJ, Grodin MA (eds.). *The Nazi Doctors and the Nuremberg Code*;102.

26. Faden RR, *et al*. *Final Report of the Advisory Committee on Human Radiation Experiments*. New York, Oxford: Oxford University Press, 1996;55.

27. Ibid.

28. Altman LK. *Who Goes First? The Story of Self-Experimentation in Medicine*. Berkeley, Los Angeles, London: University of California Press, 1998;297.

29. Southam CM. Homotransplantation of human cell lines. *Bulletin of the New York Academy of Medicine* 1958;34:416-23.

30. Ibid.

31. Hornblum AM. *Acres of Skin*;95.

32. Ibid.;93.

33. Howard-Jones N. Human experimentation in historical and ethical perspectives. *Social Science and Medicine* 1982;16:1429-48.

34. Beecher HK. Experimentation in man. *JAMA* 1959;169:461-78.

35. Pappworth MH. *Human Guinea Pigs*. London: Routledge & Kegan Paul, 1967;64.

36. Ibid.;61.

37. Welsome E. *The Plutonium Files. America's Secret Medical Experiments in the Cold War*. New York: The Dial Press, 1999;365ff.

38. Hornblum AM. *Acres of Skin*;94.

39. Mitford J. *Kind and Usual Punishment*;143f.

40. Hornblum AM. *Acres of Skin*;89f.

41. Pappworth MH. *Human Guinea Pigs*;65f.

42. Hornblum AM. *Acres of Skin*;91.

43. Ibid.;95.

44. Ibid.;100f.

45. Ibid.;91.

46. Ibid.;90.

47. Ibid.;108.

48. Ibid.;95f.

49. Moreno JD. *Undue Risk. Secret State Experiments on Humans.* New York: W.H. Freeman and Company, 1999;258.

50. DuPont HL, Hornick RB, Weiss CF, Snyder MJ, Woodward TE. Evaluation of chloramphenicol acid succinate therapy of induced typhoid fever and Rocky Mountain spotted fever. *N Eng J Med* 1970;282:53-7.

51. Pillsbury DM, Zimmerman MC, Baldridge GD. Experimental controls in clinical dermatologic investigation. *J Invest Dermatol* 1959;15:359-71.

52. Editorial. *J Invest Dermatol* 1938;1:5-7.

53. Hornblum AM. *Acres of Skin*;90.

54. Ibid.;46.

55. Ibid.;40ff.

56. Ackerman AB. Holmesburg Prison, Philadelphia, September 1966 – June 1967: acknowledgement of error and regret. *Dermatopathol: Pract & Conc* 2000;6:212-9.

57. Weidman FD. Discussion of Kligman AM. The pathogenesis of tinea capitis due to Microsporum adouini and Microsporum canis. *J Invest Dermatol* 1952;18:246.

58. Hornblum AM. *Acres of Skin*;37.

59. Strauss JS, Kligman AM. An experimental study of tinea pedis and onychomycosis of the foot. *Arch Dermatol* 1957;76:70-9.

60. Goldschmidt H, Kligman AM. Experimental inoculation of humans with ectodermotropic viruses. *J Invest Dermatol* 1958;31:175-82.

61. Maibach HI, Kligman AM. The biology of experimental human cutaneous moniliasis (Candida albicans). *Arch Dermatol* 1962;85:113-37.

62. Maibach HI, Hildick-Smith G. *Skin Bacteria and Their Role in Infection.* New York: McGraw Hill, 1965;85-94.

63. Singh G, Marples RR, Kligman AM. Experimental Staphylococcus aureus infections in humans. *J Invest Dermatol* 1971;57:149-62.

64. Shelley WB, Kligman AM. The experimental production of acne by penta- and hexachloronaphthalenes. *Arch Dermatol* 1957;75:689-95.

65. Kaidbey KH, Kligman AM. A human model of coal tar acne. *Arch Dermatol* 1974;109:212-5.

66. Strauss JS, Kligman AM. Acne. Observations on dermabrasion and the anatomy of the acne pit. *Arch Dermatol* 1956;74:397-404.

67. Papa CM, Kligman AM. The behavior of melanocytes in inflammation. *J Invest Dermatol* 1965;45:465-74.

68. Papa CM, Kligman AM. Mechanisms of eccrine anidrosis. II. The antiperspirant effect of aluminium salts. *J Invest Dermatol* 1967;49:139-45.

69. Kaidbey KH, Kligman AM, Yoshida H. Effects of intensive application of retinoic acid on human skin. *Br J Dermatol* 1975;92:693-701.

70. Kligman AM. Why do nails grow out instead of up? *Arch Dermatol* 1961;84:181-3.

71. Epstein WL, Kligman AM. The pathogenesis of milia and benign tumors of the skin. *J Invest Dermatol* 1956;26:1-11.

72. Epstein WL, Kligman AM. Epithelial cysts in buried human skin. *Arch Dermatol* 1957;76:437-45.

73. Epstein WL, Kligman AM. Transfer of allergic contact-type delayed sensitivity in man. *J Invest Dermatol* 1957;28:291-304.

74. Kligman AM. The identification of contact allergens by human assay. III. The maximization test: A procedure for screening and rating contact sensitizers. *J Invest Dermatol* 1966;47:393-409.

75. Kemp TS, Kligman AM. The effect of X-rays on experimentally produced acute contact dermatitis. *J Invest Dermatol* 1954;23:423-5.

76. Willis I, Kligman AM. Photocontact allergic reactions. Elicitation by low doses of long ultraviolet rays. *Arch Dermatol* 1969;100:535-9.

77. Kligman AM, Breit R. The identification of phototoxic drugs by human assay. *J Invest Dermatol* 1968;51:90-9.

78. Hornblum AM. *Acres of Skin*;39.

79. Rebora A, Marples RR, Kligman AM. Experimental infection with Candida albicans. *Arch Dermatol* 1973;108:69-73.

80. Hornblum AM. *Acres of Skin*;26.

81. Ibid.;122.

82. Ibid.;241.

83. Ibid.;38.

84. Papa CM, Kligman AM. Stimulation of hair growth by topical application of androgens. *JAMA* 1965;191:521-5.

85. Hornblum AM. *Acres of Skin*;51.

86. Shelley WB. Personal communication, Orlando, February 1998.

87. Ackerman AB. Personal communication, Orlando, February 1998.

88. Hornblum AM. *Acres of Skin*;40.

89. Breit R. Jede Woche ein neues Wunder. *Hautarzt* 1998;49:435-51.

90. Shelley WB, Cahn MM. The pathogenesis of hidradenitis suppurativa in man. *Arch Dermatol* 1955; 72: 562-5.

91. Hurley HJ, Jr., Shelley WB. Apocrine sweat retention in man: I. Experimental production of asymptomatic form. *J Invest Dermatol* 1954;22:397-404.

92. Shelley WB. Experimental miliaria in man. *J Invest Dermatol* 1954;22:267-71.

93. Shelley WB, Hurley HJ. An experimental study of the effects of subcutaneous implantation of androgens and estrogens on human skin. *J Invest Dermatol* 1957;28:155-8.

94. Shelley WB, Cahn MM. The pathogenesis of hidradenitis suppurativa in man.

95. Shelley WB, Perry ET. The experimental production of external otitis in man. *J Invest Dermatol* 1956;27:281-9.

96. Hornblum AM. *Acres of Skin;*44ff.

97. Marvel JR, Schlichting DA, Denton C, Levy EJ, Cahn MM. The effect of a surfactant and of particle size on griseofulvin plasma levels. *J Invest Dermatol* 1964;42:197-203.

98. Cahn MM, Levy EJ, Shaffer B. Normal skin reactions to ultraviolet light. *J Invest Dermatol* 1961;36:193-8.

99. Imbrie JD, Bergeron LL, Fitzpatrick TB. Further studies demonstrating an increased erythemal threshold following oral methoxsalen. *J Invest Dermatol* 1960;35:69-71.

100. Freeman RG, Cockerell EG, Armstrong J, Knox JM. Sunlight as a factor influencing the thickness of epidermis. *J Invest Dermatol* 1962;39:295-8.

101. Duncan WC, McBride ME, Knox JM. Experimental production of infections in humans. *J Invest Dermatol* 1970;54:319-23.

102. Zeligman I, Hubener LF. Experimental production of acne by Progesterone. *Arch Dermatol* 1957;76:652-8.

103. Strauss JS, Pochi PE. Effect of orally administered antibacterial agents on titratable acidity of human sebum. *J Invest Dermatol* 1966;47:577-81.

104. Pochi PE, Strauss JS. Effect of cyclic administration of conjugated equine estrogens on sebum production in women. *J Invest Dermatol* 1966;47:582-5.

105. Pochi PE, Strauss JS. Effect of prednisone on sebaceous gland secretion. *J Invest Dermatol* 1967;49:456-9.

106. Strauss JS, Kligman AM, Pochi PE. The effect of androgens and estrogens on human sebaceous glands. *J Invest Dermatol* 1962;39:139-55.

107. Vandenberg JJ, Epstein WL. Experimental nickel contact sensitization in man. *J Invest Dermatol* 1963;41:413-8.

108. Epstein WL. Contribution to the pathogenesis of zirconium granulomas in man. *J Invest Dermatol* 1969;34:183-8.

109. Shelley WB, Hurley HJ. Experimental evidence for an allergic basis for granuloma formation in man. *Nature* 1957;180:1060-1961.

110. Sullivan DJ, Epstein WL. Mitotic activity of wounded human epidermis. *J Invest Dermatol* 1963;41:39-43.

111. Epstein WL, Baer H, Dawson CR, Khurana RG. Poison oak hyposensitization. *Arch Dermatol* 1974;109:356-60.

112. Aly R, Maibach HI, Shinefield HR, Strauss WG. Survival of pathogenic microorganisms on human skin. *J Invest Dermatol* 1972;58:205-10.

113. Maibach HI, Sams WM, Epstein JH. Screening for drug toxicity by wave lengths greater than 3,100 A. *Arch Dermatol* 1967;95:12-5.

114. Shelley WB. Experimental disease in the skin of man. A review. *Acta Dermato-venereologica* 1983;Suppl. 108:1-38.

References

CHAPTER 21 · THE MENTAL INSTITUTION AS TEST SITE

1. Welsome E. *The Plutonium Files. America's Secret Medical Experiments in the Cold War.* New York: The Dial Press, 1999;263.

2. Ibid.;9.

3. Ibid.;294f.

4. Sulzberger MB, Griffin TB. Induced miliaria, postmilarial hypohidrosis, and some potential sequelae. *Arch Dermatol* 1969;99:145-51.

5. Griffin TB, Maibach HI, Sulzberger MB. Miliaria and anhidrosis. II. The relationships between miliaria and anhidrosis in man. *J Invest Dermatol* 1967;49:379-85.

6. Sulzberger MB, Griffin TB. Induced miliaria, postmilarial hypohidrosis, and some potential sequelae.

7. Cortese TA, Jr., Sams WM Jr., Sulzberger MB. Studies on blisters produced by friction. II. The blister fluid. *J Invest Dermatol* 1968;50:47-53.

8. Sulzberger MB, Cortese TA, Jr., Fishman L, Wiley HS. Studies on blisters produced by friction. I. Results of linear rubbing and twisting technics. *J Invest Dermatol* 1966;47:456-65.

9. Moreno JD. *Undue Risk. Secret State Experiments on Humans.* New York: W.H. Freeman and Company, 1999;251.

10. Howard-Jones N. Human experimentation in historical and ethical perspectives. *Social Science and Medicine* 1982;16:1429-48.

11. Moreno JD. *Undue Risk*;251ff.

12. Hornblum AM. *Acres of Skin. Human Experiments at the Holmesburg Prison.* New York, London: Routledge, 1998;51.

13. Shellow WVR, Kligman AM. An attempt to produce elastosis in aged human skin by means of ultraviolet irradiation. *J Invest Dermatol* 1968;50:225-6.

14. Papa CM, Carter DM, Kligman AM. The effect of autotransplantation on the progression or reversibility of aging in human skin. *J Invest Dermatol* 1970;54:200-12.

15. Leys D. Ethical standards in clinical research. *The Lancet* 1953;2:1044.

16. Annas GJ, Grodin MA (eds.). *The Nazi Doctors and the Nuremberg Code. Human Rights in Human Experimentation.* New York, Oxford: Oxford University Press, 1992;204.

17. Ivy AC. The history and ethics of the use of human subjects in medical experiments. *Science* 1948;108:1-5.

18. Annas GJ, Grodin MA (eds.). *The Nazi Doctors and the Nuremberg Code*;135.

19. Ibid.;196.

20. Leys D. Ethical standards in clinical research.

21. Annas GJ, Grodin MA (eds.). *The Nazi Doctors and the Nuremberg Code*;196.

22. Pappworth MH. *Human Guinea Pigs*. London: Routledge & Kegan Paul, 1967;59.

23. Faden RR, *et al. Final Report of the Advisory Committee on Human Radiation Experiments*. New York, Oxford: Oxford University Press, 1996;102.

24. Pappworth MH. *Human Guinea Pigs*. London: Routledge & Kegan Paul, 1967;59f.

25. Hornblum AM. *Acres of Skin*;35.

26. Collins H. The gulp heard round the world. The Philadelphia Inquirer, November 6th, 2000;D1, D12.

27. Kladko B. Human Guinea Pigs. Ashbury Park Sunday Press, September 13, 1998;1, 12-13.

28. Parish HJ. *A history of immunization*. Edinburgh, London: E. & S. Livingstone, 1965;279.

29. Lyons AS, Petrucelli RJ (eds.) *Medicine. An illustrated history*. Reprint. New York: Harry N. Adams, 1987;580.

30. Aldous IR, Kirman BH, Butler N, Goffe AP, Laurence GD, Pollock TM. Vaccination against measles. Part III. Clinical trial in British children. *Br Med J* 1961;2:1250-3.

31. Katz SL, Enders JF, Holloway A. Studies on an attenuated measles-virus vaccine. II. Clinical, virologic and immunologic effects of vaccine in institutionalized children. *N Eng J Med* 1960;263:159-61.

32. Kempe CH, Ott EW, Vincent LS, Maisel JC. Studies on an attenuated measles-virus vaccine. III. Clinical and antigenic effects of vaccine in institutionalized children. *N Eng J Med* 1960;263:162-5.

33. Krugman S, Giles JP, Jacobs AM. Studies on an attenuated measles-virus vaccine. VI. Clinical, antigenic and prophylactic effects of vaccine in institutionalized children. *N Eng J Med* 1960;263:174-7.

34. Rothman DJ, Rothman SM. *The Willowbrook Wars*. New York: Harper & Row 1984;262ff.

35. Beecher HK. *Research and the Individual. Human Studies*. Boston: Little, Brown and Company 1970;124ff.

36. Rowe RD, James LS. The normal pulmonary arterial pressure during the first year of life. *Journal of Pediatrics* 1957;51:1-4.

37. James LS. Rowe RD. The pattern of response of pulmonary and systemic arterial pressures in newborn and older infants to short periods of hypoxia. *Journal of Pediatrics* 1957;51:5-11.

38. Haddad HM. Studies on thyroid hormone metabolism in children. *Journal of Pediatrics* 1960;57:391-8.

References

39. Haddad HM. Rates of I[131]-labeled thyroxine metabolism in euthyroid children. *J Clin Invest* 1960;39:1590-4.

40. Bronner F, Harris RS, Maletskos CJ, Benda CE. Studies in calcium metabolism. The fate of intravenously injected radiocalcium in human beings. *J Clin Invest* 1956;35:78-88.

41. Welsome E. *The Plutonium Files*;229ff.

42. Massing, AM, Epstein WL. Natural history of warts. *Arch Dermatol* 1963;87:306-10.

43. Friedman L, Derbes VJ, Hodges EP. The course of untreated tinea capitis in Negro children. *J Invest Dermatol* 1964;42:237-42.

44. Rostenberg A, Kanof NM. Studies in eczematous sensitizations. I. A comparison between the sensitizing capacities of two allergens and between two different strenghts of the same allergen and the effect of repeating the sensitizing dose. *J Invest Dermatol* 1941;4:505-16.

45. Straus HW. Artificial sensitization of infants to poison ivy. *J Allergy* 1931;2:137.

46. Kligman AM. Poison ivy (Rhus) dermatitis. An experimental study. *Arch Dermatol* 1958;77:149-80.

47. Weyers W. The abuse of man. Dubious human experiments in dermatology. *Dermatopathol: Pract and Conc* 1999;5:341-55.

48. Kligman AM. The pathogenesis of tinea capitis due to Microsporum audouini and Microsporum canis. *J Invest Dermatol* 1952;18:231-46.

49. Ibid.

50. Kligman AM. Tinea capitis due to M. audouini and M. canis. *Arch Dermatol* 1955;71:313-337.

51. Kligman AM, Anderson WW. Evaluation of current methods for the local treatment of tinea capitis. *J Invest Dermatol* 1951;16:155-68.

52. Mendelson CG, Kligman AM. Isolation of wart virus in tissue culture. *Arch Dermatol* 1961;83:559-62.

53. Pillsbury DM. Letter to the President of the Armed Forces Epidemiological Board, Thomas Francis, Jr., May 20th, 1958.

54. Pillsbury DM. Letter to the Executive Secretary of the Armed Forces Epidemiological Board, Robert W. Babione, December 5th, 1958.

55. Strauss JS, Kligman AM. Effect of X-rays on sebaceous glands of the human face: radiation therapy of acne. *J Invest Dermatol* 1959;33:347-56.

56. Strauss JS, Kligman AM. The effect of androgens and estrogens on human sebaceous glands. *J Invest Dermatol* 1962;39:139-55.

57. Strauss JS, Kligman AM. The effect of progesterone and progesterone-like compounds on the human sebaceous gland. *J Invest Dermatol* 1961;36:309-19.

58. Strauss JS, Kligman AM. The effect of androgens and estrogens on human sebaceous glands.

59. Strauss JS, Kligman AM. Androgenic effects of a progestational compound, 17α-ethynyl-19-nortestosterone (Norlutin), on the human sebaceous gland. *Journal of Clinical Endocrinology* 1961;21:215-19.

60. Strauss JS, Kligman AM. The effect of progesterone and progesterone-like compounds on the human sebaceous gland.

61. Strauss JS, Kligman AM. The effect of ACTH and hydrocortisone on the human sebaceous gland. *J Invest Dermatol* 1959;33:9-14.

62. Fisher REW. Controls. *The Lancet* 1953;2:993.

63. Goldby S. Experiments at the Willowbrook State School. *The Lancet* 1971;1:749.

CHAPTER 22 · EXPERIMENTS ON AFRICAN-AMERICANS

1. Savitt TL. The use of blacks for medical experimentation and demonstration in the Old South. *The Journal of Southern History* 1982;48:331-48.

2. Sims JM. *The Story of My Life*. New York: D. Appleton, 1894;236.

3. Lederer SE. *Subjected to Science. Human Experimentation in America Before the Second World War*. Baltimore, London: Johns Hopkins University Press, 1997;115f.

4. Faden RF, Beauchamp TL. *A History and Theory of Informed Consent*. New York, Oxford: Oxford University Press 1986;191.

5. Savitt TL. The use of blacks for medical experimentation and demonstration in the Old South.

6. Reverby SM (ed.). *Tuskegee's Truths. Rethinking the Tuskegee syphilis study*. Chapel Hill, London: University of North Carolina Press, 2000;268.

7. Faden RR, *et al. Final Report of the Advisory Committee on Human Radiation Experiments*. New York, Oxford: Oxford University Press, 1996;83.

8. Greenblatt RB, Dienst RB, Pund ER, Torpin R. Experimental and clinical granuloma inguinale. *JAMA* 1939;113:1109-16.

9. Reverby SM (ed.). *Tuskegee's Truths*;269f.

10. Mitford J. *Kind and Usual Punishment*. New York: Alfred A. Knopf, 1973;52ff.

11. Kligman AM. The identification of contact allergens by human assay. III. The maximization test: a procedure for screening and rating contact sensitizers. *J Invest Dermatol* 1966;47:393-409.

12. Jones JH. *Bad Blood. The Tuskegee Syphilis Experiment*. New York: The Free Press, 1993;17.

13. Ibid.;21.

14. Murrell TW. Syphilis and the American Negro: A medico-sociologic study.

References

JAMA 1910;54:846-9.

15. Reverby SM (ed.). *Tuskegee's Truths*;17.

16. Fox H. Observations on skin diseases in the negro. *Journal of Cutaneous Diseases* 1908;26:109-121.

17. Jones JH. *Bad Blood*;22ff.

18. Ibid.;26.

19. Murrell TW. Syphilis in the Negro: its bearing on the race problem. *American Journal of Dermatology and Genito-Urinary Diseases* 1906;10:305-6.

20. Corson ER. Syphilis in the Negro. *American Journal of Dermatology and Genito-Urinary Diseases* 1906;10:241,247.

21. McNeil HL. Syphilis in the Southern Negro. *JAMA* 1916;67:1001-1104.

22. Welch S. Congenital syphilis. *Southern Medical Journal* 1923;16:420.

23. Hazen HH. Syphilis in the American Negro. *JAMA* 1914;63:463-6.

24. Reverby SM (ed.). *Tuskegee's Truths*;63ff.

25. White RM. Unraveling the Tuskegee study of untreated syphilis. *Archives of Internal Medicine* 2000;160:585-98.

26. Reverby SM (ed.). *Tuskegee's Truths*;18.

27. Ibid.;77.

28. Bruusgaard E. Über das Schicksal der nicht spezifisch behandelten Luetiker. *Archiv für Dermatologie und Syphilis* 1929;157:309-332.

29. Ibid.

30. White RM. Unraveling the Tuskegee study of untreated syphilis.

31. Moore JE. *The Modern Treatment of Syphilis*. Baltimore: Charles C. Thomas, 1933;237.

32. Reverby SM (ed.). *Tuskegee's Truths*;181a.

33. Jones JH. *Bad Blood*;172.

34. Reverby SM (ed.). *Tuskegee's Truths*;20.

35. Jones JH. *Bad Blood*;101f.

36. Reverby SM (ed.). *Tuskegee's Truths*;78.

37. Ibid.;21.

38. Jones JH. *Bad Blood*;127.

39. Ibid.;112.

40. Ibid.;100.

41. Reverby SM (ed.). *Tuskegee's Truths*;22.

42. Ibid.;74.

43. Ibid.;82f.

44. Ibid.;87.

45. Ibid.;83.

46. Savitt TL. The use of blacks for medical experimentation and demonstration in the Old South.

47. Reverby SM (ed.). *Tuskegee's Truths*;85.

48. Jones JH. *Bad Blood*;135f.

49. Rivers E, Schuman SH, Simpson L, Olansky S. Twenty years of followup experience in a long-range medical study. *Public Health Reports* 1953;68:391-5.

50. Reverby SM (ed.). *Tuskegee's Truths*;221.

51. Rivers E, Schuman SH, Simpson L, Olansky S. Twenty years of followup experience in a long-range medical study.

52. Reverby SM (ed.). *Tuskegee's Truths*;132.

53. Jones JH. *Bad Blood*;141.

54. Diebert AV, Bruyere MC. Untreated syphilis in the male Negro, III. *Veneral Disease Information* 1946;27:301-14.

55. Reverby SM (ed.). *Tuskegee's Truths*;89.

56. Jones JH. *Bad Blood*;174.

57. Reverby SM (ed.). *Tuskegee's Truths*;89f.

58. Ibid.;25.

59. Jones JH. *Bad Blood*;162.

60. Reverby SM (ed.). *Tuskegee's Truths*;95.

61. Ibid.;144.

62. Jones JH. *Bad Blood*;178.

63. Ibid.

64. Schuman SH, Olansky S, Rivers E, Smith CA, Rambo DS. Untreated syphilis in the male Negro: background and current status of patients in the Tuskegee study. *Journal of Chronic Diseases* 1955;2:550-3.

65. Reverby SM (ed.). *Tuskegee's Truths*;26.

66. Jones JH. *Bad Blood*;179.

67. Ibid.;198f.

68. Rivers E, Schuman SH, Simpson L, Olansky S. Twenty years of followup experience in a long-range medical study.

69. Vonderlehr R, *et al.* Untreated syphilis in the male Negro: A comparative study of treated and untreated cases. *Venereal Disease Information* 1936;17:260-5.

70. Reverby SM (ed.). *Tuskegee's Truths*;97f.

71. Ibid.;100.

72. Bruusgaard E. Über das Schicksal der nicht spezifisch behandelten Luetiker.

73. Benedek T. The "Tuskegee Study" of syphilis. Analysis of moral versus methodologic aspects. *Journal of Chronic Diseases* 1978;31:35-50.

References

74. McDonald CJ. The contribution of the Tuskegee study to medical knowledge. *Journal of the National Medical Association* 1974;66:1-7.

75. Reverby SM (ed.). *Tuskegee's Truths*;98.

76. Ibid.;100.

77. Jones JH. *Bad Blood*;182.

78. Reverby SM (ed.). *Tuskegee's Truths*;221.

79. Ibid.;107.

80. Roy B. The Tuskegee syphilis experiment. Biotechnology and the administrative state. *Journal of the National Medical Association* 1995;87:56-67.

81. Reverby SM (ed.). *Tuskegee's Truths*;107ff.

82. Ibid.;254f.

83. Jones JH. *Bad Blood*;190.

84. O'Callaghan B. *An Illustrated History of the USA*. Harlow, England: Longman, 1990;113.

85. Reverby SM (ed.). *Tuskegee's Truths*;105.

86. Jones JH. *Bad Blood*;193ff.

87. Reverby SM (ed.). *Tuskegee's Truths*;153f.

88. Jones JH. *Bad Blood*;2.

89. Ibid.;91.

CHAPTER 23 · THE MOST CAPTIVE POPULATION

1. Howard-Jones N. Human experimentation in historical and ethical perspectives. *Social Science and Medicine* 1982;16:1429-1448.

2. Faden RR, *et al. Final Report of the Advisory Committee on Human Radiation Experiments*. New York, Oxford: Oxford University Press, 1996;83.

3. Topping NH. The United States Public Health Service's Clinical Center for Medical Research. *JAMA* 1952;150:541-5.

4. Rothman DJ. *Strangers at the Bedside. A History of How Law and Bioethics Transformed Medical Decision Making* New York: Basic Books, 1991;114.

5. Ibid.;112.

6. Ibid.;117.

7. Ibid.;128f.

8. Ibid.;131.

9. Welsome E. *The Plutonium Files. America's Secret Medical Experiments in the Cold War*. New York: The Dial Press, 1999;215f.

10. Faden RR, *et al. Final Report of the Advisory Committee on Human Radiation Experiments*;83.

11. Welsome E. *The Plutonium Files*;214.

12. Pappworth MH. *Human Guinea Pigs*. London: Routledge & Kegan Paul, 1967;11f.

13. Ogilvie H. Whither medicine? *The Lancet* 1952;2:820-4.

14. Rothman DJ. *Strangers at the Bedside*;59.

15. Pappworth MH. *Human Guinea Pigs*;11.

16. Guttentag OE. The problem of experimentation on human beings. II. The physician's point of view. *Science* 1953;117:207-210.

17. McCance RA. The practice of experimental medicine. *Proceedings of the Royal Society of Medicine* 1951;44:189-194.

18. Bradford Hill A. Medical ethics and controlled trials. *Br Med J* 1963;1:1043-9.

19. Hodgson HSU. Medical ethics and controlled trials. *Br Med J* 1963;1:1339-40.

20. Murley RS. Medical ethics and controlled trials. *Br Med J* 1963;1:1474-5.

21. Marshall J. Ethics of human experimentation. *Br Med J* 1963;2:114.

22. Rothman DJ. *Strangers at the Bedside*;58.

23. Ibid.;55.

24. Faden RR, *et al. Final Report of the Advisory Committee on Human Radiation Experiments*;91.

25. Rothman DJ. *Strangers at the Bedside*;58.

26. Faden RR, *et al. Final Report of the Advisory Committee on Human Radiation Experiments*;91.

27. Ibid.;82.

28. Ibid.

29. Welsome E. *The Plutonium Files*;219ff.

30. Hartnett LJ. The possible significance of arterial visualization in the diagnosis of placenta previa. *American Journal of Obstetrics and Gynecology* 1948;55:940-52.

31. Pappworth MH. *Human Guinea Pigs*;23f.

32. Hartnett LJ. The possible significance of arterial visualization in the diagnosis of placenta previa.

33. Solish GI, Masterson JG, Hellman LM. Pelvic arteriography in obstetrics. *American Journal of Obstetrics and Gynecology* 1961;81:57-66.

34. Welsome E. *The Plutonium Files*;330ff.

35. Ibid.;337ff.

36. Pappworth MH. *Human Guinea Pigs*;161f.

37. Chamovitz R, Catanzaro FJ, Stetson CA, Rammelkamp CH, Jr. Prevention of rheumatic fever by treatment of previous streptococcal infections. I. Evalua-

References

tion of Benzathine Penicillin G. *N Eng J Med* 1954;251:466-71.

38. Morris AJ, Chamovitz R, Catanzaro FJ, Rammelkamp CH, Jr. Prevention of rheumatic fever by treatment of previous streptococcic infections: effect of Sulfadiazine. *JAMA* 1956;160:114-6.

39. Beecher HK. Ethics and clinical research. *N Eng J Med* 1966;274:1354-1360.

40. Bearn BH, Billing BH, Sherlock S. Hepatic glucose output and hepatic insulin sensitivity in diabetes mellitus. *The Lancet* 1951;2:698-701.

41. Beecher HK. Ethics and clinical research.

42. Pappworth MH. *Human Guinea Pigs*;129.

43. Phillips GB, Schwartz R, Gabuzda GJ, Jr., Davidson CS. The syndrome of impending hepatic coma in patients with cirrhosis of the liver given certain nitrogeneous substances. *N Eng J Med* 1952;247:239-46.

44. Mackie JE. Stormont JM, Hollister RM, Davidson CS. Production of impending hepatic coma by chlorothiazide and its prevention by antibiotics. *The N Eng J Med* 1958;259:1151-6.

45. Pappworth MH. *Human Guinea Pigs*;151ff.

46. Ferguson EH, Epstein WL. Clearance of I^{131} injected intralesionally in patients with psoriasis. *J Invest Dermatol* 1961;37:441-5.

47. Weinstein GD, Van Scott EJ. Autoradiographic analysis of turnover times of normal and psoriatic epidermis. *J Invest Dermatol* 1965;45:257-62.

48. Frost P, Weinstein GD, Van Scott EJ. The ichthyosiform dermatoses. II. Autoradiographic studies of epidermal proliferation. *J Invest Dermatol* 1966;47:561-7.

49. Penneys NS, Fulton JE, Weinstein GD, Frost F. Location of proliferating cells in human epidermis. *Arch Dermatol* 1970;101:323-7.

50. Long PI. Behavior of psoriatic and normal skin transplants. *Arch Dermatol* 1961;84:109-12.

51. Clendenning WE, Van Scott EJ. Autografts in psoriasis. *J Invest Dermatol* 1965;45:46-51.

52. Fardal RW, Winkelmann RK. Autotransplantation in pustular psoriasis. *J Invest Dermatol* 1966;46:488-91.

53. Aschheim E, Chan TG, Farber EM, Cox AJ, Jr. Cellular response to skin abrasion in psoriasis. *J Invest Dermatol* 1966;46:12-5.

54. Miura Y, Lobitz WC. Histochemical studies in atopic dermatitis: responses following controlled strip injury. *J Invest Dermatol* 1964;42:115-7.

55. Hu F, Fosnaugh RP, Livingood CS. Human skin window studies. II. Comparison of cellular response to staphylococcus in controls and in patients with cutaneous bacterial infections. *J Invest Dermatol* 1963;41:325-34.

56. Kligman AM. Poison ivy (Rhus) dermatitis. An experimental study. *Arch Dermatol* 1958;77:149-80.

57. Bradley SE, Ingelfinger FJ, Bradley GP, Curry JJ. The estimation of hepatic blood flow in man. *J Clin Invest* 1945;24:890-7.

58. Leibsohn E, Appel B, Ullrick WC, Tye MJ. Respiration of human skin. *J Invest Dermatol* 1958;30:1-8.

59. Van Scott EJ, Ekel TM. Geometric relationships between the matrix of the hair bulb and its dermal papilla in normal and alopecic scalp. *J Invest Dermatol* 1958;31:281-7.

60. Epstein WL, Maibach HI. Immunologic competence of patients with psoriasis receiving cytotoxic drug therapy. *Arch Dermatol* 1965;91:599-606.

61. Zollinger RM, Lindem MC, Filler RM, Corson JM, Wilson RE. Effect of thymectomy on skin-homograft survival in children. *The N Eng J Med* 1964; 270: 707-710.

62. Kempe CH, Shaw EB, Jackson JR, Silver HK. Studies on the etiology of exanthema subitum (roseola infantum). *Journal of Pediatrics* 1950;37:561-8.

63. Friedberg SJ, Klein RF, Trout DL, Bogdonoff MD, Estes EH, Jr. The characteristics of the peripheral transport of C^{14}-labeled palmitic acid. *J Clin Invest* 1960;39:1511-5.

64. Pappworth MH. *Human Guinea Pigs*;73.

65. Ibid.;89ff.

66. Rocco AG, Vandam LD. Changes in circulation consequent to manipulation during abdominal surgery. *JAMA* 1957;164:14-8.

67. Lurie AA, Jones RE, Linde HW, Price ML, Dripps RD, Price HL. Cyclopropane anesthesia. 1. Cardiac rate and rhythm during steady levels of cyclopropane anesthesia at normal and elevated end-exspiratory carbon dioxide tensions. *Anesthesiology* 1958;19:457-72.

68. Bridges TJ, Clark K, Yahr MD. Plethysmographic studies of the cerebral circulation: Evidence for cranila nerve vasomotor activity. *J Clin Invest* 1958; 37: 763-772.

69. Ogilvie H. Whither medicine?

70. Moreno JD. *Undue Risk. Secret State Experiments on Humans*. New York: W.H. Freeman and Company, 1999;194ff.

71. Pappworth MH. *Human Guinea Pigs*;26.

72. Ibid.;125.

73. Southam CM. Homotransplantation of human cell lines. *Bulletin of the New York Academy of Medicine* 1958;34:416-423.

74. Pappworth MH. *Human Guinea Pigs*;101ff.

75. Mitchell RG. The child and experimental medicine. *Br Med J* 1964;1:721-27.

CHAPTER 24 · BIG BUSINESS

1. Welsome E. *The Plutonium Files. America's Secret Medical Experimentsin the Cold War*. New York: The Dial Press, 1999;339.

References

2. Ibid.;341.

3. Howard-Jones N. Human experimentation in historical and ethical perspectives. *Social Science and Medicine* 1982; 16: 1429-48.

4. Ibid.

5. Ibid.

6. Faden RR, *et al. Final Report of the Advisory Committee on Human Radiation Experiments.* New York, Oxford: Oxford University Press, 1996;98.

7. Curran WJ. Governmental regulation of the use of human subjects in medical research: The approach of two federal agencies. *Daedalus* 1969;98(2):542-94.

8. Ibid.

9. Hornblum AM. *Acres of Skin. Human Experiments at the Holmesburg Prison.* New York, London: Routledge, 1998;96f.

10. Ibid.;24.

11. Ibid.;87ff.

12. Ethics governing the service of prisoners as subjects in medical experiments. Report of a committee appointed by Governor Dwight H. Green of Illinois. *JAMA* 1948;136:457-58.

13. Hornblum AM. *Acres of Skin*;91.

14. Hodges RE, Bean WB. The use of prisoners for medical research. *JAMA* 1967;202:177-79.

15. Hornblum AM. *Acres of Skin*;22.

16. Basson D, Lipson RE, Ganos DL (eds.). *Troubling Problems in Medical Ethics.* New York: Alan R. Liss, 1981;79.

17. Mitford J. *Kind and Usual Punishment.* New York: Alfred A. Knopf, 1973;144.

18. Hornblum AM. *Acres of Skin*;194.

19. Ibid.;9f.

20. Ibid.;15.

21. Katz A. Prisoners volunteer to save lives. Philadelphia Bulletin, February 27, 1966.

22. Mitford J. *Kind and Usual Punishment*;151f.

23. Ethics governing the service of prisoners as subjects in medical experiments. Report of a committee appointed by Governor Dwight H. Green of Illinois.

24. Mitford J. *Kind and Usual Punishment*;151.

25. Hornblum AM. *Acres of Skin*;97.

26. Katz J. *Experimentation on Human Beings.* New York: Russell Sage Foundation, 1972;1046.

27. Ibid.

28. Hornblum AM. *Acres of Skin*;47, 68.

29. Ibid.;191.

30. Ibid.;61f.

31. Mitford J. *Kind and Usual Punishment*;157f.

32. Howard-Jones N. Human experimentation in historical and ethical perspectives.

33. Mitford J. *Kind and Usual Punishment*;158f.

34. Ibid.;160f.

35. Ibid.;158ff.

36. Ticktin HE, Zimmerman HJ. Hepatic dysfunction and jaundice in patients receiving triacetyloleandomycin. *N Eng J Med* 1962;267:964-68.

37. More human guinea-pigs. *Br Med J* 1962;2:1536-637.

38. Stüttgen G. Zur Lokalbehandlung von Keratosen mit Vitamin-A-Säure. *Dermatologica* 1962;124:65-80.

39. Kaidbey KH, Kligman AM, Yoshida H. Effects of intensive application of retinoic acid on human skin. *Br J Dermatol* 1975; 92: 693-701.

40. Hornblum AM. *Acres of Skin*;211ff.

41. Ibid.;163ff.

42. Kligman AM. Plastic band-aids for patch testing. *Arch Dermatol* 1957;75:739.

43. Fulton JE, Jr., Plewig G, Kligman AM. Effect of chocolate on acne vulgaris. *JAMA* 1969;210:2071-74.

44. Ackerman AB, Kligman AM. Some observations on dandruff. *Journal of the Society of Cosmetic Chemists* 1969;20:81-101.

45. Ackerman AB. Personal communication.

46. Ackerman AB, Kligman AM. Some observations on dandruff.

47. Ackerman AB. Holmesburg Prison, Philadelphia, September 1966 – June 1967: Acknowledgement of error and regret. *Dermatopathol: Pract & Conc* 2000;6:212-19.

48. Hornblum AM. *Acres of Skin*;12, 120.

49. Ibid.;47ff.

50. Ibid.;143ff.

51. Ibid.;119ff.

52. Ibid.

53. Ibid.;149ff.

54. Curran WJ. Governmental regulation of the use of human subjects in medical research.

55. Hornblum AM. *Acres of Skin*;54.

56. Kligman AM. Topical pharmacology and toxicology of dimethyl sulfoxide –

References

Part 1. *JAMA* 1965;193:796-804.

57. Kligman AM. Dimethyl sulfoxide – Part 2. JAMA 1965;193:923-28.

58. Hornblum AM. *Acres of Skin*;53.

59. Ibid.;58f.

60. Ibid.;54f.

61. Ibid.

62. Ibid.;59ff.

63. A.B. Ackerman, personal communication.

64. Hornblum AM. *Acres of Skin*;59ff.

65. Ibid.;56.

66. Kligman AM. Dimethyl sulfoxide. A correction. *JAMA* 1966;197:1109.

CHAPTER 25 · PUTTING ON THE BRAKES

1. Haxthausen H. Studies on the pathogenesis of morphea, vitiligo and acrodermatitis atrophicans by means of transplantation experiments. *Acta Dermato-Venereologica* 1947;27:352-68.

2. Liban E, Zuckerman A, Sagher F. Specific tissue alteration in leprous skin. VII. Inoculation of Leishmania tropica into leprous patients. *Arch Dermatol and Syphilology* 1955;71:442-50.

3. Huriez C, Desmons F, Nenoit M, Martin P. Liver biopsy in eczema and other dermatoses. *Br J Dermatol* 1957;69:237-44.

4. Vilanova X. Onychomycosis. An experimental study. *J Invest Dermatol* 1956;27:77-101.

5. Mancini RE, Quaife JV. Histogenesis of experimentally produced keloids. *J Invest Dermatol* 1962;38:143-81.

6. González-Ochoa A, Ricoy E, Bravo-Becherelle MA. Study of prophylactic action of griseofulvin – human experimental infection with Trichophyton concentricum. *J Invest Dermatol* 1964;42:55-9.

7. Porter S, Shuster S. A new method for measuring replacement of epidermis and stratum corneum in human skin. *J Invest Dermatol* 1967;49:251-55.

8. Jimbow K, Sato S, Kukita A. Cells containing Langerhans cell granules in human lymph nodes of dermatopathic lymphadenopathy. *J Invest Dermatol* 1969;53:295-99.

9. Rothman DJ. *Strangers at the Bedside. A History of How Law and Bioethics Transformed Medical Decision Making*. New York: Basic Books, 1991;67f.

10. Ibid.;98ff.

11. Bean WB. Walter Reed and the ordeal of human experimentation. *Bulletin of the History of Medicine* 1977; 51: 75-92.

12. Bordley J III, McGehee Harvey A. *Two Centuries of American Medicine. 1776-1976*. Philadelphia: W.B. Saunders, 1976;429.

13. Rothman DJ. *Strangers at the Bedside*;59.

14. Beecher HK. Ethics and clinical research. *N Eng J Med* 1966;274:1354-60.

15. Rothman DJ. *Strangers at the Bedside*;72ff.

16. Rothman DJ. Ethics and human experimentation. Henry Beecher revisited. *N Eng J Med* 1987;317:1195-99.

17. Beecher HK. Ethics and clinical research.

18. Scanlon EF, Hawkins RA, Fox WW, Smith WS. Fatal homotransplanted melanoma: A case report. *Cancer* 1965;18:782-89.

19. Beecher HK. Ethics and clinical research.

20. Ibid.

21. Rothman DJ. *Strangers at the Bedside*;74.

22. Ibid.;100.

23. Ibid.;88.

24. Ibid.;86.

25. Ibid.;88.

26. Ibid.;89.

27. Ibid.;88.

28. Curran WJ. Governmental regulation of the use of human subjects in medical research: The approach of two federal agencies. *Daedalus* 1969;98(2):542-94.

29. Beecher HK. *Research and the Individual. Human Studies*. Boston: Little, Brown and Company, 1970;218.

30. Elkeles B. *Der moralische Diskurs über das medizinische Menschenexperiment im 19. Jahrhundert*;210-14.

31. Müller F. Die Zulässigkeit ärztlicher Versuche an gesunden und kranken Menschen. *Münchener Medzinische Wochenschrift* 1931;78:104-07.

32. Sass H. Reichsrundschreiben 1931: Pre-Nuremberg German regulation concerning new therapy and human experimentation. *Journal of Medicine and Philosophy* 1983;8:99-111.

33. Wiggers CJ. Human experimentation: As exemplified by career of Dr. William Beaumont. *Alumni Bulletin of Western Reserve University*, September 1950:60-5.

34. Guttentag OE. Problem of Experimentation on Human Beings: II. Physician's point of view. *Science* 1953;117:207-10.

35. Shimkin MB. The problem of experimentation on human beings. I. The research worker's point of view. *Science* 1953;117:205-07.

36. Rothman DJ. *Strangers at the Bedside*;56.

37. Welt LG. Reflections on the problems of human experimentation. *Connecticut Medicine* 1961;25:75-8.

38. Curran WJ. Governmental regulation of the use of human subjects in medical research.

39. Rothman DJ. *Strangers at the Bedside*;93.

40. Hornblum AM. *Acres of Skin. Human Experiments at the Holmesburg Prison.* New York, London: Routledge, 1998;205ff.

41. Ibid.;203.

42. Ibid.;189ff.

43. Ibid.;19.

44. Ibid.;191.

45. Ibid.;187.

46. Annas GJ, Grodin MA (eds.). *The Nazi Doctors and the Nuremberg Code. Human Rights in Human Experimentation.* New York, Oxford: Oxford University Press, 1992; 191f.

47. Hornblum AM. *Acres of Skin*;111ff.

48. Rothman DJ. *Strangers at the Bedside*;95ff.

49. Jonas H. Philosophical reflections on experimenting with human subjects. *Daedalus* 1969;98(2):219-47.

50. Jones JH. *Bad Blood. The Tuskegee Syphilis Experiment.* New York: The Free Press, 1993;221.

51. Ibid.;236.

52. Reverby SM (ed.). *Tuskegee's Truths. Rethinking the Tuskegee Syphilis Study.* Chapel Hill, London: University of North Carolina Press, 2000;424ff.

53. Ibid.;177ff.

54. Rothman DJ. *Strangers at the Bedside*;194f.

55. Ibid.;191ff.

56. Ibid.;160ff.

57. Ibid.;152ff.

58. Jones AR. *The Birth of Bioethics.* New York, Oxford: Oxford University Press, 1998;91.

59. Ibid.;91ff.

60. Rothman DJ. *Strangers at the Bedside*;182ff.

61. Annas GJ, Grodin MA (eds.). *The Nazi Doctors and the Nuremberg Code*;187.

62. Faden RF, Beauchamp TL. *A History and Theory of Informed Consent.* New York, Oxford: Oxford University Press, 1986;214.

63. Ibid.;230.

64. Annas GJ, Grodin MA (eds.). *The Nazi Doctors and the Nuremberg Code*;189ff.

65. Jones AR. *The Birth of Bioethics*;152.

66. Faden RF, Beauchamp TL. *A History and Theory of Informed Consent*;216.

67. Rothman DJ. *Strangers at the Bedside*;189.

68. Annas GJ, Grodin MA (eds.). *The Nazi Doctors and the Nuremberg Code*;333ff.

69. Ibid.;160ff.

70. Howard-Jones N. Human experimentation in historical and ethical perspectives. *Social Science and Medicine* 1982;16:1429-48.

71. Annas GJ, Grodin MA (eds.). *The Nazi Doctors and the Nuremberg Code*;161.

72. Rothman DJ. *Strangers at the Bedside*;107.

CHAPTER 26 · THE END OF THE STORY ?

1. Quidde L. *Arme Leute in Krankenhäusern*. Munich: Staegmeyr, 1900;93.

2. Beecher HK. Experimentation in man. *JAMA* 1959;169:461-78.

3. Chandler D. *Voices from S-21*. Berkeley, Los Angeles, London: University of California Press, 1999.

4. Dickman S, Aldous P. WHO concern over new drug. *Nature* 1990;347:606.

5. Dickman S. East Germany: Science in the disservice for the state. *Science* 1991;254:26-7.

6. Moreno JD. *Undue Risk. Secret State Experiments on Humans.* New York: W.H. Freeman and Company, 1999;3.

7. Ebbinghaus A, Dörner K. *Heilen und Vernichten. Der Nürnberger Ärzteprozess und seine Folgen.* Berlin: Aufbau-Verlag, 2001;476f.

8. Ibid.;267ff.

9. Hansen J. BioCryst trials led to review of UAB board. *The Birmingham News*, Jan 23, 2000.

10. Stolberg SG. Teenager's death is shaking up field of human gene-therapy experiments. *The New York Times*, Jan 27, 2000.

11. Stolberg SG. Senators press for answers on gene trials. *The New York Times*, Feb 3, 2000.

12. Kolata G. Johns Hopkins admits fault in fatal experiment. *The New York Times*, July 17, 2001.

13. Howard-Jones N. Human experimentation in historical and ethical perspectives. *Social Science and Medicine* 1982;16:1429-48.

14. Sams WM, Freedberg IM. The dermatology-industry interface: defining the boundaries. *JAAD* 2000;43:550-54.

15. Lemonick MD, Goldstein A. At your own risk. *Time*, April 22, 2002;46-56.

16. Pappworth MH. *Human Guinea Pigs.* London: Routledge & Kegan Paul, 1967;79.

17. Beecher HK. Experimentation in man. *JAMA* 1959;169:461-78.

18. Jonas H. Philosophical reflections on experimenting with human subjects. *Daedalus* 1969;98(2):219-47.

19. Cone M. Volunteers ingest pollutant in drinking water study. *Los Angeles*

References

Times, Nov 27, 2000.

20. Walker B, Wiles R. Rocket science: Aerospace contractor pays Californians $1,000 to eat thyroid toxin in first large-scale human test of water pollutant. *Environmental Working Group*, Nov 27, 2000.

21. Sass H. Reichsrundschreiben 1931: Pre-Nuremberg German regulation concerning new therapy and human experimentation. *Journal of Medicine and Philosophy* 1983; 8: 99-111.

22. Tröhler U, Reither-Theil S (ed.). *Ethik und Medizin 1947-1997. Was leistet die Kodifizierung der Ethik?* Göttingen: Wallstein, 1997;205.

23. McCuen GE (ed.). *Human Experimentation. When Research is Evil*. Hudson, Wisconsin: Gary E. McCuen Publications, 1998;160f.

24. Ibid.;168ff.

25. Stolberg SG. Fines proposed for violations of human research rules. *The New York Times*, May 23, 2000.

26. McCuen GE (ed.). *Human Experimentation. When Research is Evil*;168.

27. Hansen J. BioCryst trials led to review of UAB board.

28. Stolberg SG. F.D.A. officials fault Penn team in gene therapy death. *The New York Times*, Dec 9, 1999.

29. Stolberg SG. Agency failed to monitor patients in gene research. *The New York Times*, Feb 2, 2000.

30. Kolata G. Johns Hopkins death brings halt to U.S.-financed human studies. *The New York Times*, July 20, 2001.

31. Reverby SM (ed.). *Tuskegee's Truths. Rethinking the Tuskegee Syphilis Study*. Chapel Hill, London: University of North Carolina Press, 2000;294.

32. Stolberg SG. Bioethicists find themselves the ones being scrutinized. The New York Times, Aug 2, 2001.

33. Kampmeier RH. The Tuskegee Study of syphilis. *Southern Medical Journal* 1972;65:1247-51.

34. Benedek T. The "Tuskegee Study" of syphilis. Analysis of moral versus methodologic aspects. *Journal of Chronic Diseases* 1978; 31: 35-50.

35. Kampmeier RH. The Tuskegee Study of syphilis.

36. Weyers W. The abuse of man: dubious human experiments in dermatology. *Dermatopathol: Pract and Conc* 1999;5:341-55.

37. Shelley WB. Experimental disease in the skin of man. A review. *Acta Dermato-venereologica* 1983;Suppl. 108:1-38.

38. Greenblatt RB, Dienst RB, Pund ER, Torpin R. Experimental and clinical granuloma inguinale. *JAMA* 1939;113:1109-16.

39. Shelley WB. Experimental disease in the skin of man. A review.

40. Shelley WB. Letter to the Deputy Executive Director of the American Academy of Dermatology, Cheryl K. Norstedt, July 18th, 2001.

41. Ackerman AB. Holmesburg Prison, Philadelphia, September 1966 – June

1967: acknowledgement of error and regret. *Dermatopathol: Pract and Conc* 1999;6:212-19.

42. Lübbe H. Schuldbekenntnisse international. *Damals* 2001;5:40-2.

43. Reverby SM (ed.). *Tuskegee's Truths*;574ff.

44. Hornblum AM. On the practice of silence in the medical profession. *Dermatopathol: Pract and Conc* 1999;6:220-21.

45. Sarlat R. Prison experiments leave legacy of pain. *Philadelphia Tribune*, October 27th, 1998.

46. Tannen RL. The ethical issues of the Holmesburg studies have been addressed. *Arch Dermatol* 2000;136:268.

47. Ferguson EH. Letter to the chairman of the ad hoc task force concerning human experiments of the Ethics Committee of the American Academy of Dermatology, Michael J. Franzblau, July 3rd, 2001.

48. Epstein JH. Letter to the chairman of the ad hoc task force concerning human experiments of the Ethics Committee of the American Academy of Dermatology, Michael J. Franzblau, July 2001.

49. Norstedt CK. Letter to the chairman of the ad hoc task force concerning human experiments of the Ethics Committee of the American Academy of Dermatology, Michael J. Franzblau, July 11, 2001.

50. Pappworth MH. *Human Guinea Pigs*;3.

51. Phear E, Sherlock S, Summerskill WHJ. *Lancet* 1955;1:836.

52. Phear E, Sherlock S, Summerskill WHJ. *Lancet* 1955;1:1023.

53. Pappworth MH. *Human Guinea Pigs*;133.

54. Ackerman AB. Holmesburg Prison, Philadelphia, September 1966 – June 1967: acknowledgement of error and regret.

55. Hornblum AM. Ethical lapses in dermatologic "research." *Arch Dermatol* 1999;135:383-85.

56. Webster SB. Medical ethics relating to clinical investigations using human subjects. *Arch Dermatol* 1999;135:457-58.

57. Krivo J. Ethics, the prison system, and dermatology. *Arch Dermatol* 1999;135:469.

58. Stanley JR. Ethical Accusations: The loss of common sense. *Arch Dermatol* 2000;136:268-69.

59. Weyers W. Failure to appreciate the validity of accusations about violations of ethics. *Dermatopathol: Pract and Conc* 2000;6:225-30.

60. Rothman DJ. *Strangers at the Bedside. A History of How Law and Bioethics Transformed Medical Decision Making*. New York: Basic Books, 1991;77.

61. Moll A. Versuche am lebenden Menschen. *Die Zukunft* 1899;29:213-18.

62. Stolberg SG. Biomedicine is receiving new scrutiny as scientists become entrepreneurs. *The New York Times*, Feb 20, 2000.

63. Cho MK, Bero LA. The quality of drug studies published in symposium pro-

ceedings. *Ann Intern Med* 1996;124:485-89.

64. Stelfox HAT, Chua G, O'Rourke K, Detsky AS. Conflict of interest in the debate over calcium-channel antagonists. *N Eng J Med* 1998;338:101-06.

65. Friedberg M, Saffran B, Stinson TJ, Nelson W, Bennett CL. Evaluation of conflict of interest in economic analyses of new drugs used in oncology. *JAMA* 1999;282:1453-57.

66. Stolberg SG. Biomedicine is receiving new scrutiny as scientists become entrepreneurs. *The New York Times*, Feb 20, 2000.

67. Stolberg SG. Despite ferment, gene therapy progresses. *The New York Times*, June 6, 2000.

68. Tannen RL. The ethical issues of the Holmesburg studies have been addressed.

69. Bullard CS. Doctor's research from '50s raises ethical concerns. *Metro Iowa*, Oct 19, 1998.

70. Annas GJ, Grodin MA (eds.). *The Nazi Doctors and the Nuremberg Code. Human Rights in Human Experimentation.* New York, Oxford: Oxford University Press, 1992;240ff.

71. Ibid.;197.

72. Reverby SM (ed.). *Tuskegee's Truths*;279.

FIGURE REFERENCES

PREFACE

1. Shelley WB, Crissey JT. *Classics in Clinical Dermatology.* Springfield: Charles C. Thomas, 1953;0.

2. Ehring F. *Skin Diseases. 5 Centuries of Illustration.* Stuttgart, New York: Gustav Fischer, 1989;69.

3. Blum G. Laurent Theodor Biett (1780-1840): Der erste Schweizer Dermatologe. *Hautarzt* 1985;36:170-2.

4. Ehring F. *Skin Diseases. 5 Centuries of Illustration;*88.

5. Lyons AS, Petrucelli RJ (eds.) *Medicine. An Illustrated History;*379.

6. Toellner R (ed.). *Illustrierte Geschichte der Medizin.* Vol. 3. Salzburg: Andreas & Andreas, 1986;1503.

CHAPTER 1 · INTRODUCTION

7. Carmichael AG, Ratzan RM (eds.). *Medicine. A Treasury of Art and Literature.* New York: Hugh Lauter Levin Ass. 1991;37.

8. Lyons AS, Petrucelli RJ (eds.) *Medicine. An Illustrated History;*220.

9. Ibid;221.

10. Carmichael AG, Ratzan RM (eds.). *Medicine. A Treasury of Art and Literature;*24.

11. Sonnabend H. Der König der Giftmischer. *Damals* 2002;34(4):37.

12. Schott H (ed.) *Die Chronic der Medizin.* Gütersloh: Chronik Verlag, 1993;43.

13. Lyons AS, Petrucelli RJ (eds.) *Medicine. An Illustrated History;*245.

14. Ibid;252.

15. Schott H (ed.) *Die Chronic der Medizin;*54.

16. Lyons AS, Petrucelli RJ (eds.) *Medicine. An Illustrated History;*329.

17. Carmichael AG, Ratzan RM (eds.). *Medicine. A Treasury of Art and Literature;*96.

18. Dörfelt H, Heklau H. *Die Geschichte der Mykologie.* Schwäbisch Gmünd: Einhorn-Verlag Eduard Dietenberger, 1998;360.

19. Lyons AS, Petrucelli RJ (eds.) *Medicine. An Illustrated History;*315.

20. Radunskaja I. *Die Legende vom Ruhm. Forscher, Fehler und Erfolge.* Leipzig, Jena, Berlin: Urania.

21. Schott H (ed.) *Die Chronic der Medizin;*93.

22. Toman R (ed.). *Die Kunst der italienischen Renaissance.* Köln: Könemann, 1994;268. 1984;161a.

23. Bram L, Hendelson WH, Morse JL. *Funk & Wagnalls New Encyclopedia,* vol. 15. New York: Funk & Wagnalls, 1971;150.

24. Carmichael AG, Ratzan RM (eds.). *Medicine. A Treasury of Art and Literature;*85.

Figure References

25. Engelhardt D, Hartmann F (eds.). *Klassiker der Medizin*, vol. 1. München: C.H. Beck, 1991;114.

26. Schott H (ed.) *Die Chronic der Medizin*;145.

27. Ibid;145.

28. Lyons AS, Petrucelli RJ (eds.) *Medicine. An Illustrated History*;433.

29. Schott H (ed.) *Die Chronic der Medizin*;172.

30. Carmichael AG, Ratzan RM (eds.). *Medicine. A Treasury of Art and Literature*;101.

31. Radunskaja I. *Die Legende vom Ruhm*;161a.

32. Schott H (ed.) *Die Chronic der Medizin*;176.

33. Ibid;176.

34. Radunskaja I. *Die Legende vom Ruhm*;161a.

35. Berghaus P, Von Diepenbroik-Grüter HD, Murkewn AH (eds). *Porträt 2. Der Arzt. Graphische Bildnisse des 16.-20. Jahrhunderts aus dem Porträtarchiv Diepenbroik*. Münster: Landschaftsverband Westfalen-Lippe, 1979;207.

36. Schott H (ed.) *Die Chronic der Medizin*;222.

37. Bor J, Petersma E (eds.). *Illustrierte Geschichte der Philosophie*. Bern, München, Wien: Scherz, 1997;274.

38. Lyons AS, Petrucelli RJ (eds.) *Medicine. An Illustrated History*;469.

39. Oliver M. *Die Geschichte der Philosophie*. Augsburg: Weltbild, 1998;95.

40. Ricci FM. *Dizionario Biografico della Storia della Medicina e delle Scienze Naturali* (Liber Amicorum), vol. 3. Milano: Franco Maria Ricci, 1988;223.

41. Percival T. *Medical ethics*: or a code of institutes and precepts, adapted to the professional conduct of physicians and surgeons. Manchester: Johnson, 1803.

CHAPTER 2 · STUDIES BY INOCULATION

42. Berghaus P, et al. Porträt 2. Der Arzt;206.

43. Nékám L (ed.). Deliberationes Congressus Dermatologorum Internationalis IX-I. Budapestini 13-21 Sept. 1935. Volumen IV. Commemorativum. Budapest 1935;139.

44. Berghaus P et al. Porträt 2. Der Arzt;250.

45. Crissey JT, Parish LC. *The Dermatology and Syphilology of the Nineteenth Century*. New York: Praeger 1981;89.

46. Wallace W. Lectures on cutaneous and venereal diseases and on surgical cases. *Lancet* 1835/36;2:534-40 u. 615-22.

47. Waller J. Die Contagiosität der secundären Syphilis. *Vierteljahresschrift für die praktische Heilkunde* 1851;29:112-32.

48. Lesser E. *Lehrbuch der Haut- und Geschlechtskrankheiten*, vol. 2., 12th ed. Leipzig: Vogel, 1906;III.

49. Zieler K. *Lehrbuch und Atlas der Haut- und Geschlechtskrankheiten – Atlas*, 2nd edition. Berlin:Urban & Schwarzenberg, 1928;155.

50. Ibid;140.

51. Lesser E. *Lehrbuch der Haut*;V.

52. Nékám L (ed.). Deliberationes Congressus Dermatologorum Internationalis IX-I;408.

53. Schönfeld W. Die Senatsrüge Rineckers anläßlich der Widerlegung syphilitischer Irrlehren, ein zeitgemäßer medizingeschichtlicher Rückblick. *Dermatologische Wochenschrift* 1942;115:880.

54. Nékám L (ed.). Deliberationes Congressus Dermatologorum Internationalis IX-I;22.

55. Stümpke G. Ulcus molle. Symptomatologie, Diagnose, Prognose, Therapie, Epidemiologie. In: Jadassohn J (ed.). *Handbuch der Haut- und Geschlechtskrankheiten*, vol. 21. Berlin: Julius Springer, 1927;94.

56. Nékám L (ed.). Deliberationes Congressus Dermatologorum Internationalis IX-I;409.

57. Toellner R (ed.). *Illustrierte Geschichte der Medizin*, Vol. 6. Salzburg: Andreas & Andreas, 1986;3216.

58. Braun-Falco O. 50 Jahre Dermatologie im Städtischen Krankenhaus Thalkirchnerstraße – Rückblick und Ausblick. *Hautarzt* 1980;31:38.

59. Shelley WB, Crissey JT. *Classics in Clinical Dermatology*. Springfield: Charles C. Thomas, 1953;163.

60. Nékám L (ed.). Deliberationes Congressus Dermatologorum Internationalis IX-I;250.

61. Ibid;359.

62. Ibid;53.

63. Ehring F. *Skin Diseases. 5 Centuries of Illustration*;232.

64. Nékám L (ed.). Deliberationes Congressus Dermatologorum Internationalis IX-I;299.

65. Toellner R (ed.). *Illustrierte Geschichte der Medizin*;3263.

66. Beck L (ed.). *Zur Geschichte der Gynäkologie und Geburtshilfe. Aus Anlaß des 100jährigen Bestehens der Deutschen Gesellschaft für Gynäkologie und Geburtshilfe*. Berlin, Heidelberg: Springer, 1986;44.

67. Pagel J. *Biographisches Lexikon hervorragender Ärzte des neunzehnten Jahrhunderts*. Wien: Urban & Schwarzenberg, 1901;1478.

68. Galerie hervorragender Ärzte und Naturforscher. Beilage zur *Münchener Medizinischen Wochenschrift* 1926;Blatt 372.

69. Burg G. *Dermatologie*. München, Wien, Baltimore: Urban & Schwarzenberg, 1988;162.

70. Weyers W. The abuse of man. Dubious human experiments in dermatology. *Dermatopathol: Prac & Conc* 1999;5:344.

71. Nékám L (ed.). Deliberationes Congressus Dermatologorum Internationalis IX-I;54.

72. Fehleisen F. *Die Aetiologie des Erysipels*. Berlin: Verlag von Theodor Fischer's medicinischer Buchhandlung, 1883.

73. Galerie hervorragender Ärzte und Naturforscher. *Münchener Medizinische Wochenschrift* 1927;397.

74. Dennhöfer H. *Hundert Jahre Lautenschläger im Auf- und Ausbau der Asepsis.* Cologne: Dennhöfer, 1988;23.

75. Schimmelbusch C. Ueber die Ursachen der Furunkel. *Archiv für Ohrenheilkunde* 1888;27:252-64.

76. Ibid.

77. Sebastian G, Scholz A. Zum 150. Geburtstag von Filip Josef Pick. *Dermatologische Monatsschrift* 1985;171:123.

78. Nékám L (ed.). Deliberationes Congressus Dermatologorum Internationalis IX-I;89.

CHAPTER 3 · THE CALL OF CONSCIENCE

79. Lyons AS, Petrucelli RJ (eds.) *Medicine. An Illustrated History;*504.

80. Rutkow IR. *American Surgery. An Illustrated History.* Philadelphia: Lippincott-Raven 1998;70.

81. Crissey JT, Parish LC. *The Dermatology and Syphilology of the Nineteenth Century.* New York: Praeger, 1981;89.

82. Klusemann GG. Die Syphilisation in wissenschaftlicher und sanitätspolizeilicher Beziehung. Mit einer Nachschrift über die Zurechnung des ärztlichen Heilverfahrens von Casper. *Vierteljahrsschrift für gerichtliche und öffentliche Medicin* 1853;3:92-117.

83. Bayerisches Hauptstaatsarchiv (HSTA), Munich, M Inn 62534.

84. Rabe CM. *Lupus, Lepra, Lues und andere Leiden. Deutsch-skandinavischer Wissenstranfer in der Dermato-Venerologie.* Hamburg: Beiersdorf, 1996;143.

85. Wallach D, Tilles G (eds.). *Dermatology in France.* Toulouse: Éditions Privat, Pierre Fabre Dermo-Cosmétique, 2002;235.

86. Engelhardt D, Hartmann F. *Klassiker der Medizin,* vol. 2. München: C.H. Beck, 1991;137.

87. Crissey JT, Parish LC. *The Dermatology and Syphilology of the Nineteenth Century;*255.

88. Auspitz H. *Die Lehren von syphilitischen Contagium.* Wien: Wilhelm Braumüller, 1866.

89. Hoffman E. Einiges aus dem Leben Julius Bettingers, des Pfälzers Anonymous. *Dermatologische Zeitschrift* 1913;20:223.

90. Ricci FM. *Dizionario Biografico della Storia della Medicina e delle Scienze Naturali;*271.

91. Zieler K. *Lehrbuch und Atlas der Haut- und Geschlechtskrankheiten;*156.

92. Ibid;172.

93. Schott H. *Meilensteine der Medizin.* Dortmund: Harenberg, 1996;417.

94. Ibid;449.

95. Pross C, Aly G (eds.) *Der Wert des Menschen. Medizin in Deutschland 1918-1945.* Berlin: Edition Hentrich, 1989;91.

96. Crissey JT, Parish LC. *The Dermatology and Syphilology of the Nineteenth Century*;279.

97. Carmichael AG, Ratzan RM (eds.). *Medicine. A Treasury of Art and Literature*;86.

98. Leven KH. *Die Geschichte der Infektionskrankheiten. Von der Antike bis ins 20. Jahrhundert.* Landsberg: Ecomed, 1997;47.

99. Gottlieb BJ, Berg A. *Das Antlitz des germanischen Arztes in vier Jahrhunderten.* Berlin: Rembrandt, 1942;150.

100. Ricci FM. *Dizionario Biografico della Storia della Medicina e delle Scienze Naturali*;239.

101. Rabe CM. *Lupus, Lepra, Lues und andere Leiden*;163.

102. Beck L (ed.). *Zur Geschichte der Gynäkologie und Geburtshilfe*;40.

103. Beighton P, Beighton G. *The Man Behind the Syndrome.* Berlin, Heidelberg, New York, Tokyo: Springer, 1986;136.

104. Lyons AS, Petrucelli RJ (eds.) *Medicine. An Illustrated History*;512.

CHAPTER 4 · THE VALUE OF PERFORMING EXPERIMENTS ON HUMANS

105. Freund H, Berg A (eds.). *Geschichte der Mikroskopie*, vol. 2. Frankfurt: Umschau, 1964;256a.

106. Ricci FM. *Dizionario Biografico della Storia della Medicina e delle Scienze Naturali*; 85.

107. Nékám L (ed.). *Deliberationes Congressus Dermatologorum Internationalis IX-I*;309.

108. Ibid;125.

109. Pagel J. *Biographisches Lexikon hervorragender Ärzte des neunzehnten Jahrhunderts.* Wien: Urban & Schwarzenberg, 1901;311.

110. Crissey JT, Parish LC. *The Dermatology and Syphilology of the Nineteenth Century*;89.

111. Shelley WB, Crissey JT. *Classics in Clinical Dermatology.* Springfield: Charles C. Thomas, 1953;186.

112. Goldenbogen N, Hahn S, Heidel CP, Scholz A (eds.). *Hygiene und Judentum.* Dresden: Verein für regionale Politik und Geschichte Dresden 1995;79.

113. Scholz A. Zum 150. Geburtstag von Heinrich Köbner. *Dermatologische Monatsschrift* 1989;175:112.

114. Toellner R (ed.). *Illustrierte Geschichte der Medizin*;3301.

115. Freund H, Berg A (eds.). *Geschichte der Mikroskopie*;304a.

116. Cáceres UG. Ideas e imagenes en la enfermedad de Carrión. Análisis historiográfico de la iconiografia de la Bartonellosis Humana. Parte I. *Folia Dermatologica Peruana* 1998;9:56.

117. Schott H (ed.) *Die Chronic der Medizin*;323.

118. Freund H, Berg A (eds.). *Geschichte der Mikroskopie*;296a.

119. Duin N, Sutcliffe J. *Geschichte der Medizin. Von der Antike bis zum Jahr 2020*. Köln: vgs verlagsgesellschaft 1993;56.

120. Engelhardt D, Hartmann F. *Klassiker der Medizin*, vol. 2. München: C.H. Beck, 1991;248.

121. Schott H. *Meilensteine der Medizin*;370.

122. Freund H, Berg A (eds.). *Geschichte der Mikroskopie*;240a.

123. Toellner R (ed.). *Illustrierte Geschichte der Medizin*;3328.

124. Crissey JT, Parish LC. *The Dermatology and Syphilology of the Nineteenth Century*;357.

CHAPTER 5 · THERAPEUTIC TRIALS

125. Ricci FM. *Dizionario Biografico della Storia della Medicina e delle Scienze Naturali*;29.

126. Bordley J III, McGehee Harvey A. *Two Centuries of American Medicine. 1776-1976*. Philadelphia: W.B. Saunders, 1976;38.

127. Ricci FM. *Dizionario Biografico della Storia della Medicina e delle Scienze Naturali*;63.

128. Schott H (ed.) *Die Chronic der Medizin*;219.

129. Gottlieb, BJ, Berg A. *Das Antlitz des germanischen Arztes in vier Jahrhunderten*;113.

130. Ricci FM. *Dizionario Biografico della Storia della Medicina e delle Scienze Naturali*;141.

131. Dörfelt H, Heklau H. *Die Geschichte der Mykologie*. Schwäbisch Gmünd: Einhorn-Verlag Eduard Dietenberger, 1998;348.

132. Gottlieb BJ, Berg A. *Das Antlitz des germanischen Arztes in vier Jahrhunderten*;146.

133. Archives of the Institute of the History of Medicine, University of Leipzig, Germany.

134. Lyons AS, Petrucelli RJ (eds.) *Medicine. An Illustrated History*;513.

135. Ibid;521.

136. Archives of the Institute of the History of Medicine, University of Vienna.

137. Toellner R (ed.). *Illustrierte Geschichte der Medizin*;3247.

138. Benedum J, Giese C. *375 Jahre Medizin in Giessen*. Giessen: Wilhelm Schmitz Verlag, 1983;91.

139. Archives of the Institute of the History of Medicine, University of Greifswald, Germany

140. Toellner R (ed.). *Illustrierte Geschichte der Medizin*;3225.

141. Nékám L (ed.). *Deliberationes Congressus Dermatologorum Internationalis IX-I*;158.

142. Engelhardt D, Hartmann F (eds.). *Klassiker der Medizin*;310.

143. Schott H. *Meilensteine der Medizin*;285.

144. Ibid;286.

145. Ibid;348.

146. Malkin HM. *Out of the Mist. The Foundation of Modern Pathology and Medicine During the Nineteenth Century.* Berkeley: Vesalius, 1995;253.

147. Burke DS. Joseph-Alexandre Auzias-Turenne, Louis Pasteur, and early concepts of virulence, attenuation, and vaccination. *Perspectives in Biology and Medicine* 1996;39:172.

148. Nékám L (ed.). *Deliberationes Congressus Dermatologorum Internationalis IX-I*;132.

149. *Deutsche Medizinische Wochenschrift* 1890;16:1029.

150. Ehring F. *Skin Diseases. 5 Centuries of Illustration*;135.

151. Shelley WB, Crissey JT. *Classics in Clinical Dermatology*;247.

152. Toellner R (ed.). *Illustrierte Geschichte der Medizin*;3127.

153. Ibid;3227.

154. Schott H (ed.). *Die Chronic der Medizin*;333.

155. Schott H. *Meilensteine der Medizin*;377.

156. Hansen BM. *Die Inseln des Paul Langerhans.* Vienna, Berlin: Ueberreuter, 1988;24.

157. Langerhans R. Tod durch Heilseum. *Berliner klinische Wochenschrift* 1896;602-04.

158. Stühmer A. Erinnerungen an Paul Ehrlich. Ein Beitrag zur Kenntnis seiner Persönlichkeit aus Anlaß seines 100. Geburtstages am 14. März 1954. *Hautarzt* 1954;5:127-34.

159. Schott H. *Meilensteine der Medizin*;441.

160. Ibid.

CHAPTER 6 · WARRIORS AGAINST DISEASE

161. Shelley WB, Crissey JT. *Classics in Clinical Dermatology*;169.

162. Ehring F. *Skin Diseases. 5 Centuries of Illustration*;228.

163. Bram LL, Philipps RS, Dickey NH. *Funk & Wagnalls New Encyclopedia*, vol. 12. New York: Funk & Wagnalls, 1971;284.

164. Toellner R (ed.). *Illustrierte Geschichte der Medizin*;3209.

165. Gottlieb BJ, Berg A. *Das Antlitz des germanischen Arztes in vier Jahrhunderten*;140.

166. Jütte R (ed.). *Geschichte der deutschen Ärzteschaft.* Köln: Deutscher Ärzte-Verlag, 1997;80.

167. Leven KH. *Die Geschichte der Infektionskrankheiten. Von der Antike bis ins 20. Jahrhundert.* Landsberg: Ecomed, 1997;122.

168. Zentner C, Bedürftig F. *Das große Lexikon des Dritten Reiches.* Munich:

Südwest Verlag, 1985;662.

169. Kolle K (ed.). *Grosse Nervenärzte*, vol. 3. Stuttgart: Georg Thieme, 1963;200a.

170. Toellner R (ed.). *Illustrierte Geschichte der Medizin*;3390.

171. Nékám L (ed.). *Deliberationes Congressus Dermatologorum Internationalis IX-I*;255.

CHAPTER 7 · THE MERGER OF ANTIVIVISECTIONISM AND ANTI-SEMITISM

172. Archives of the Institute of the History of Medicine, University of Vienna.

173. Ricci FM. *Dizionario Biografico della Storia della Medicina e delle Scienze Naturali*;90.

174. Lyons AS, Petrucelli RJ (eds.). *Medicine. An Illustrated History*;503.

175. Ibid;505.

176. Bretschneider H. *Der Streit um die Vivisektion im 19. Jahrhundert.* Stuttgart: Gustav Fischer, 1962;33.

177. Pagel J. *Biographisches Lexikon hervorragender Ärzte des neunzehnten Jahrhunderts.* Wien: Urban & Schwarzenberg, 1901;1496.

178. Ricci FM. *Dizionario Biografico della Storia della Medicina e delle Scienze Naturali*;66.

179. Genschorek W. *Wegbereiter der Chirurgie. Joseph Lister, Ernst von Bergmann.* Leipzig: S. Hirzel, 1984;96a.

180. Beighton P, Beighton G. *The Man Behind the Syndrome.* Berlin, Heidelberg, New York, Tokyo: Springer, 1986;132.

181. Toellner R (ed.). *Illustrierte Geschichte der Medizin*;3162.

182. Weber E. *Die Folterkammern der Wissenschaft. Eine Sammlung von Thatsachen für das Laienpublikum.* Berlin, Leipzig: Hugo Voigt, 1879.

183. Hamann B. *Hitlers Wien. Lehrjahre eines Diktators.* München, Zurich: Piper 1996;475.

184. Ibid;492.

185. Pahlen K. *Große Meister der Musik.* Zurich: Orell Füssli, 1968;109.

186. Florey H (ed.). *General Pathology.* London: Lloyd-Luke, 1962;17.

CHAPTER 8 · ANTI-SEMITISM AS A VEHICLE TO MORALITY

187. Pagel J. *Biographisches Lexikon hervorragender Ärzte des neunzehnten Jahrhunderts*;374.

188. Ibid;679.

189. Ibid;1899.

190. Zentner C, Bedürftig F. *Das große Lexikon des Dritten Reiches*;100.

191. Schoeps JH, Schlör J. *Antisemitismus. Vorurteile und Mythen.* München, Zürich: Piper, 1995;76.

192. *Arme Leute in Krankenhäusern.* München: Staegmeyr'sche Verlagshandlung, 1900.

193. Nékám L (ed.). *Deliberationes Congressus Dermatologorum Internationalis IX-I*;401.

194. Grosz S, Kraus R. Bacteriologische Studien über den Gonococcus. *Archiv für Dermatologie und Syphilis* 1898;45:329.

195. Hamann B. *Hitlers Wien. Lehrjahre eines Diktators*;441.

196. Ibid;395.

197. Hubenstorf M. Der Wahrheit ins Auge sehen. *Wiener Arzt* 1995;5:26.

198. Stühmer A. Erinnerungen an Paul Ehrlich. Ein Beitrag zur Kenntnis seiner Persönlichkeit aus Anlaß seines 100. Geburtstages am 14. März 1954. *Hautarzt* 1954;5:127-34.

199. Neisser A. Was wissen wir von einer Serumtherapie bei Syphilis und was haben wir von ihr zu erhoffen? *Archiv für Dermatologie und Syphilis* 1898;44:431-539.

200. Schoeps JH, Schlör J. *Antisemitismus. Vorurteile und Mythen.* München, Zürich: Piper, 1995;114.

201. Schott H (ed.) *Die Chronic der Medizin*;374.

202. Shelley WB, Crissey JT. *Classics in Clinical Dermatology*;351.

203. Schmidt-La Baume F. In memoriam Karl Herxheimer. *Hautarzt* 1953;4:444.

CHAPTER 9 · THE DAWN OF INFORMED CONSENT

204. Killian H. *Meister der Chirurgie und die Chirurgenschulen im gesamten deutschen Sprachraum.* 2nd ed. Stuttgart: Georg Thieme, 1980;I.

205. Pagel J. *Biographisches Lexikon hervorragender Ärzte des neunzehnten Jahrhunderts*;1247.

206. Stade KH. Die Bedeutung Ernst v. Dürings für die Dermatologie. In: Kleine-Natrop HE, Wagner G. *Schriftenreihe der Nordwestdeutschen Dermatologischen Gesellschaft, Heft 3.* Kiel: Lipsius & Tischer, 1952.

207. Ehring F. *Skin Diseases. 5 Centuries of Illustration*;177.

208. Müller F. Die Entwicklung der Stoffwechsellehre und die Münchener Schule. *Münchener Medizinische Wochenschrift* 1933;80:1660.

209. Pagel J. *Biographisches Lexikon hervorragender Ärzte des neunzehnten Jahrhunderts*;1230.

210. Gottlieb BJ, Berg A. *Das Antlitz des germanischen Arztes in vier Jahrhunderten*;194.

211. Pagel J. *Biographisches Lexikon hervorragender Ärzte des neunzehnten*

Jahrhunderts;826.

212. Goldenbogen N, Hahn S, Heidel CP, Scholz A (eds.). *Medizinische Wissenschaften und Judentum*. Dresden: Verein für regionale Politik und Geschichte Dresden, 1996;47.

213. Moll A. *Ärztliche Ethik. Die Pflichten des Arztes in allen Beziehungen seiner Thätigkeit*. Stuttgart: Ferdinand Enke, 1902.

214. Jubiläumsbeilage Lehrer der Heilkunde und ihre Wirkungsstätten. *Münchener Medizinische Wochenschrift* 1933;66.

215. Holubar K. Benjamin Lipschütz (1878-1931) und seine Bedeutung für die Dermatologie (Dermatovirologie). *Hautarzt* 1986;37:266.

216. Jakstat K. *Geschichte der Dermatologie in Hamburg. Bibliotheca Diesbach*, vol. 1. Berlin: Diesbach Verlag 1987;86.

217. *Dermatologische Wochenschrift* 1940.

218. Nékám L (ed.). *Deliberationes Congressus Dermatologorum Internationalis IX-I*;337.

219. Ibid;86.

220. Toellner R (ed.). *Illustrierte Geschichte der Medizin*;3227.

221. Nékám L (ed.).*Deliberationes Congressus Dermatologorum Internationalis IX-I*;81.

CHAPTER 10 · THE AMERICAN APPROACH TO HUMAN EXPERIMENTATION

222. Morgan JP. The first reported case of electrical stimulation of the brain. *Journal of the History of Medicine* 1982;37:56a.

223. Ibid.

224. Ricci FM. *Dizionario Biografico della Storia della Medicina e delle Scienze Naturali*;34.

225. Schadewaldt H. *Geschichte der Allergie*, vol. 1. Munich: Dustri, 1980;283.

226. Lesky E. *Meilensteine der Wiener Medizin: Große Ärzte Österreichs in drei Jahrhunderten*. Vienna: Wilhelm Maudrich, 1981;215.

227. Freund L. "Ein mit Röntgen-Strahlen behandelter Fall von Naevus pigmentosus piliferus." *Wiener Medizinische Wochenschrift* 1897;47:430.

228. Freund L. Nachtrag zu dem Artikel "Ein mit Röntgen-Strahlen behandelter Fall von Naevus pigmentosus piliferus." *Wiener Medizinische Wochenschrift* 1897;47:858.

229. Shelley WB, Crissey JT. *Classics in Clinical Dermatology*;297.

230. Rutkow IR. *American Surgery. An Illustrated History*. Philadelphia: Lippincott-Raven, 1998;408.

231. Beighton P, Beighton G. *The Man Behind the Syndrome*;130.

232. Lyons AS, Petrucelli RJ (eds.) *Medicine. An Illustrated History*;570.

233. Lederer S. *Subjected to Science. Human Experimentation in America before the Second World War*. Baltimore, London: The Johns Hopkins University

Press, 1995;41.

234. Ibid;79.

235. Ibid;48.

236. Ricci FM. *Dizionario Biografico della Storia della Medicina e delle Scienze Naturali*;154.

237. Bordley J III, McGehee Harvey A. *Two Centuries of American Medicine*;188.

238. Courtesy of Anjou Dargar.

239. Courtesy of Anjou Dargar.

240. Lyons AS, Petrucelli RJ (eds.) *Medicine. An Illustrated History*;562.

241. Ibid;560.

242. Malkin HM. *Out of the Mist. The Foundation of Modern Pathology and Medicine During the Nineteenth Century*. Berkeley: Vesalius, 1995;397.

243. Szymanski FJ. *Centennial History of American Dermatological Association. 1876-1976*. Chicago: American Dermatological Association, 1976;123.

244. Chernin E. Richard Pearson Strong and the iatrogenic plague disaster in Bilibid Prison, Manila, 1906. *Reviews of Infectious Diseases* 1989;11:997.

245. Ibid.

246. Raju TNK. The Nobel Chronicles. *Lancet* 1998;352:1868.

247. Kiple KF. *Plague, Pox &Ppestilence*. New York: Barnes & Noble, 1997;121.

248. Mullan F. *Plagues and Politics. The Story of the United States Public Health Service*. New York: Basic Books 1989;75.

CHAPTER 11 · LEGAL INITIATIVES IN THE UNITED STATES

249. Lyons AS, Petrucelli RJ (eds.) *Medicine. An Illustrated History*;545.

250. Bordley J III, McGehee Harvey A. *Two Centuries of American Medicine*;150.

251. Ibid;380.

252. Carmichael AG, Ratzan RM (eds.). *Medicine. A Treasury of Art and Literature*;286.

253. Bordley J III, McGehee Harvey A. *Two Centuries of American Medicine*;191.

254. Ibid.

255. Lederer S. *Subjected to Science. Human Experimentation in America before the Second World War*. Baltimore, London: The Johns Hopkins University Press, 1995;81.

256. Ibid;80.

257. Freund H, Berg A (eds.). *Geschichte der Mikroskopie*, vol. 2. Frankfurt: Umschau, 1964;480a.

258. Courtesy of Anjou Dargar

259. Rutkow IR. *American Surgery. An Illustrated History*. Philadelphia: Lip-

pincott-Raven, 1998;271.

260. Ricci FM. *Dizionario Biografico della Storia della Medicina e delle Scienze Naturali*;47.

261. Ibid;230.

262. Lyons AS, Petrucelli RJ (eds.) *Medicine. An Illustrated History*;588.

263. Jubiläumsbeilage Lehrer der Heilkunde und ihre Wirkungsstätten. *Münchener Medizinische Wochenschrift* 1933;80:50.

264. Schadewaldt H. Zur Geschichte der Allergie. In: Fuchs E, Schulz KH. *Manuale Allergologicum*. Deisenhofen: Dustri, 1997;II,15.

265. *Münchener Medizinische Wochenschrift* 1934;81:27.

266. Weyers W. The abuse of man. Dubious human experiments in dermatology. *Dermatopathol: Prac & Conc* 1999;5:348.

267. Noguchi H. A cutaneous reaction in syphilis. *Journal of Experimental Medicine* 1911;14:557-68.

268. Weyers W. The abuse of man. Dubious human experiments in dermatology. *Dermatopathol: Prac & Conc* 1999;5:349.

269. Wile UJ. Experimental syphilis in the rabbit produced by the brain substance of the living paretic. *Journal of Experimental Medicine* 1916;23:199-202.

270. Sellards AW, Lacy GR, Schöbl O. Superinfection in yaws. *Philippine Journal of Science* 1926;30:474a.

271. Lyons AS, Petrucelli RJ (eds.) *Medicine. An Illustrated History*;582.

272. Schott H. *Meilensteine der Medizin*;452.

CHAPTER 12 · EXPERIMENTS ON HUMANS IN A TURBULENT TIME

273. Scholz A. *Geschichte der Dermatologie in Deutschland*. Berlin, Heidelberg: Springer, 1999;78.

274. Scholz A, Büchner L. Hans Martenstein (1892-1945) – Dermatologe in Breslau und Dresden – zum 100. Geburtstag. *Der Deutsche Dermatologe* 1992;40:1777.

275. Sulzberger MB. Hans Biberstein zum 70. Geburtstag. *Hautarzt* 1959;10:561.

276. Ehring F. *Skin Diseases. 5 Centuries of Illustration*;146.

277. Jubiläumsbeilage Lehrer der Heilkunde und ihre Wirkungsstätten. *Münchener Medizinische Wochenschrift* 1933;1.

278. Knolle K (ed.). *Große Nervenärzte: 21 Lebensbilder*, vol. 1, 2nd ed., Stuttgart: Georg Thieme, 1970;256a.

279. Jubiläumsbeilage. Lehrer der Heilkunde und ihre Wirkungsstätten. *Münchener Medizinische Wochenschrift* 1933;80:78.

280. Goldenbogen N, Hahn S, Heidel CP, Scholz A (eds.). *Medizin und Judentum*. Dresden: Verein für regionale Politik und Geschichte Dresden, 1994;21.

281. Jütte R (ed.). *Geschichte der deutschen Ärzteschaft*;201.

282. Killian H. *Meister der Chirurgie und die Chirurgenschulen im gesamten deutschen Sprachraum.* 2nd ed. Stuttgart: Georg Thieme, 1980;XXXI.

283. Proctor RN. *Racial Hygiene. Medicine Under the Nazis.* Cambridge: Harvard University Press, 1988;257.

284. Moses J. *Der Totentanz von Lübeck.* Radebeul: Dresden, 1930.

285. Jütte R (ed.). *Geschichte der deutschen Ärzteschaft*;119.

286. Galerie hervorragender Ärzte und Naturforscher. *Münchener Medizinische Wochenschrift* 1926;379.

287. Jubiläumsbeilage Lehrer der Heilkunde und ihre Wirkungsstätten. *Münchener Medizinische Wochenschrift* 1933;79.

288. Ricci FM. *Dizionario Biografico della Storia della Medicina e delle Scienze Naturali* (Liber Amicorum), vol. 3. Milano: Franco Maria Ricci, 1988;171.

289. Freund H, Berg A. (eds.). *Geschichte der Mikroskopie. Leben und Werk großer Forscher*, vol. 2. Frabkfurt: Umschau-Verlag, 1964;360a.

290. Ricci FM. *Dizionario Biografico della Storia della Medicina e delle Scienze Naturali*;81.

291. Polano MK. H.W. Siemens zum 60. Geburtstage! *Hautarzt* 1951;2:431.

292. Mann G (ed.) *Weltgeschichte: Eine Universalgeschichte*, vol. 9. Gütersloh: Prisma Verlag, 1980;681.

293. Thom A, Caregorodcev GI. *Medizin unterm Hakenkreuz.* Berlin: VEB Verlag Volk und Gesundheit, 1989;67.

294. Proctor RN. *Racial Hygiene: Medicine Under the Nazis.* Cambridge: Harvard University Press, 1988;142a.

295. Lorant S. *Sieg Heil! Eine deutsche Bildergeschichte von Bismarck zu Hitler.* Frankfurt: Zweitausendeins, 1979;234.

296. Oliver M. *Die Geschichte der Philosophie.* Augsburg: Weltbild, 1998;124.

297. Ehring F. *Skin Diseases. 5 Centuries of Illustration.* Stuttgart, New York: Gustav Fischer, 1989;150.

298. Benedum J, Giese C. *375 Jahre Medizin in Giessen.* Giessen: Wilhelm Schmitz Verlag, 1983;215.

299. Jütte R (ed.). *Geschichte der deutschen Ärzteschaft.* Köln: Deutscher Ärzte-Verlag, 1997;144.

300. Ibid.;145.

301. Goldenbogen N, Hahn S, Heidel CP, Scholz A (eds.). *Medizin und Judentum.* Dresden: Verein für regionale Politik und Geschichte Dresden, 1994;23.

302. Proctor RN. *Racial Hygiene: Medicine Under the Nazis*;162a.

303. Hanauske-Abel HM. Not a slippery slope or sudden subversion: German medicine and national socialism in 1933. *Br Med Journal* 1996;313:1458.

304. Zentner C. *Illustrierte Geschichte des Dritten Reiches.* Eltville: Bechtermünz Verlag, 1990;120.

305. Jubiläumsbeilage. *Münchener Medizinische Wochenschrift* 1933;80:2.

306. Jubiläumsbeilage – Lehrer der Heilkunde und ihre Wirkungsstätten. *Münchener Medizinische Wochenschrift* 1933;80:2.

Figure References

307. Schönfeld W. Die Geschichte der Würzburger Hautklinik bis 1939. *Hautarzt* 1956;7:134.

308. *Dermatologische Wochenschrift* 1970;156.

309. Hoffmann E. Alois Memmesheimer zum 60. Geburtstag am 14. Juli 1954. *Dermatologische Wochenschrift* 1954;130:767.

310. Schulze W. Die dermatologische Klinik der Universität Rostock: Ein Rückblick auf ihre Gründung und Entwicklung. *Hautarzt* 1955;6:84.

311. Ebbinghaus A, Dörner K (eds.). *Vernichten und Heilen. Der Nürnberger Ärzteprozeß und seine Folgen*. Berlin: Aufbau-Verlag, 2001;256a.

312. Zentner C. *Illustrierte Geschichte des Zweiten* Weltkriegs. Eltville: Bechtermünz Verlag, 1990;341.

313. Zentner C, Bedürftig F. *Das große Lexikon des Dritten Reiches*. Munich: Südwest Verlag, 1985;271.

314. Chagoll L. *Im Namen Hitlers. Kinder hinter Stacheldraht*. Cologne: Pahl-Rugenstein Verlag, 1979;140.

315. Lorant S. *Sieg Heil!*;331.

316. Dejas-Eckertz P, Ruckhaberle D, Tebbe A, Tebbe K, Ziesecke C. *Faschismus*. Berlin, Hamburg: Elefanten Press Verlag GmbH, 1976;243.

317. Oppitz DU. Medizinverbrechen vor Gericht. In: Frewer A, Wiesemann C (eds.) *Erlanger Studien zur Ethik in der Medizin*, vol. 7. Erlangen, Jena: Palm & Enke, 1999;33.

318. Zentner C, Bedürftig F. Das große Lexikon des Dritten Reiches;255.

319. Beutelspacher M, Brändle HU, Eberhardt A, *et al. Volk und Gesundheit. Heilen und Vernichten im Nationalsozialismus*. Frankfurt: Mabuse-Verlag, 1988;191.

320. Héran J, Reumaux B (eds.) *Histoire de la Medicine à Strasbourg*. Strasbourg: La Nuée Bleue, 1997;594.

321. Mitscherlich A, Mielke F. *Doctors of Infamy*. New York: Henry Schuman, 1949;86a.

322. Héran J, Reumaux B (eds.) *Histoire de la Medicine à Strasbourg*;592.

323. Dejas-Eckertz P, Ruckhaberle D, *et al. Faschismus*;119.

324. Zentner C, Bedürftig F. *Das große Lexikon des Dritten Reiches*;381.

325. Proctor RN. *Racial Hygiene: Medicine Under the Nazis*;257a.

326. Schott H. *Meilensteine der Medizin*. Dortmund: Harenberg, 1996;407.

327. Chagoll L. *Im Namen Hitlers. Kinder hinter Stacheldraht*. Cologne: Pahl-Rugenstein Verlag, 1979;129.

328. Klee E. *Auschwitz, die NS-Medizin und ihre Opfer*. Frankfurt: S. Fischer, 1997;448.

329. Jubiläumsbeilage - Lehrer der Heilkunde und ihre Wirkungsstätten. *Münchener Medizinische Wochenschrift* 1933,80:42.

330. Benedum J, Giese C. *375 Jahre Medizin in Giessen*;138.

331. Panning G. Wirkungsform und Nachweis der sowjetischen Infanteriesprengmunition. *Der Deutsche Militärarzt* 1942;7: 20-30.

332. Ibid.

333. Pross C, Aly G (eds.) *Der Wert des Menschen. Medizin in Deutschland 1918-1945*. Berlin: Edition Hentrich, 1989;175.

334. Kalkoff K. In memoriam Carl Moncorps. *Hautarzt* 1952;3:143.

335. Pross C, Aly G (eds.) Der Wert des Menschen. Medizin in Deutschland 1918-1945;296.

336. Ibid.;297.

337. Héran J, Reumaux B (eds.) *Histoire de la Medicine à Strasbourg*;595.

338. Klee E. *Auschwitz, die NS-Medizin und ihre Opfer*;232.

339. Ibid.;221.

340. Annas GJ, Grodin MA (eds.). *The Nazi Doctors and the Nuremberg Code. Human Rights in Human Experimentation*. New York, Oxford: Oxford University Press, 1992;119.

341. Oppitz DU. Medizinverbrechen vor Gericht;34.

342. Klee E. *Auschwitz, die NS-Medizin und ihre Opfer*;190.

343. Ibid.;208.

344. Funk C. Heinrich Löhe zum 75. Geburtstag. *Hautarzt* 1952;3:382.

345. Klee E. *Auschwitz, die NS-Medizin und ihre Opfer*;112.

346. Héran J, Reumaux B (eds.) *Histoire de la medicine à Strasbourg*;596.

347. Proppe A. Hans Theo Schreus zum 60. Geburtstage. *Hautarzt* 1952;3:431.

348. Ebbinghaus A, Dörner K (eds.). *Vernichten und Heilen*;256a.

349. Brinkschulte E (ed.). *Weibliche Ärzte: Die Durchsetzung des Berufsbildes in Deutschland*. Berlin: Edition Hentrich, 1993;133.

350. Dejas -Eckertz P, Ruckhaberle D, *et al. Faschismus*;118.

351. Scholz A. *Geschichte der Dermatologie in Deutschland*. Berlin, Heidelberg: Springer, 1999;121.

352. Götz H. In memoriam Joseph Kimmig. 1909-1976. *Hautarzt* 1977;28:60.

353. Harris SH. *Factories of Death. Japanese Biological Warfare, 1932-45, and the American Cover-up*. New York: Routledge, 1994;142a.

354. Chang I. *The Rape of Nanking*. New York: Penguin Books, 1998;146a.

355. Ibid.

356. Ibid.

357. Ibid.

358. Ibid.

359. Harris SH. *Factories of Death*;142a.

360. Ibid.

361. Bärnighausen T. *Medizinische Humanexperimente der japanischen Truppen für Biologische Kriegsführung in China, 1932-1945*. M.D. diss., University of Heidelberg, 1996;220.

362. Ibid.

363. Ibid.;227.

364. Ibid.;226.

Figure References

365. Harris SH. *Factories of Death*;142a.

366. Ibid.

367. Ibid.

368. Toellner R (ed.). *Illustrierte Geschichte der Medizin*. Vol. 6. Salzburg: Andreas & Andreas, 1986;3069.

369. Obituary notices. Sir Neil Hamilton Fairley. *Br Med Journal* 1966;1:1117.

370. Goodwin B. *Keen as Mustard. Britain's Horrific Chemical Warfare Experiments in Australia*. St. Lucia: University of Queensland Press, 1998;174a.

371. Ibid.

372. Ibid.

373. Ibid.

374. Ibid.

375. Ibid.

376. Bordley J III, McGehee HA. *Two Centuries of American Medicine, 1776-1976*. Philadelphia: W.B. Saunders, 1976;125.

377. Courtesy of Anjou Dargar.

378. Hornblum A. *Acres of Skin*. New York, London: Routledge, 1998;154a.

379. Ibid.

380. Bordley J III, McGehee HA. *Two Centuries of American Medicine, 1776-1976*;124.

381. Welsome E. *The Plutonium Files. America's Secret Medical Experiments in the Cold War*. New York: The Dial Press, 1999;212a.

382. Ibid.

383. Ibid.

384. Ibid.

385. Ibid.

386. Ibid.

387. Eisenberg RL. *Radiology. An Illustrated history*. St. Louis: Mosby Year Book, 1992;366.

388. Bram L, Phillips RS, Dickey NH. Funk & Wagnalls New Encyclopedia, vol. 20. New York: Funk & Wagnalls, 1970;176.

389. Mann G (ed.) *Weltgeschichte: Eine Universalgeschichte*, vol. 8. Gütersloh: Prisma Verlag, 1980;855.

390. Danz K, Mitte W. *Bilder und Dokumente zur Weltgeschichte*. Gütersloh: Prisma Verlag, 1980;505.

391. Bram L, Hendelson WH, Morse JL. *Funk & Wagnalls New Encyclopedia*, vol. 21. New York: Funk & Wagnalls, 1971;176.

392. Lovell R. *Churchill's Doctor. A Biography of Lord Moran*. London, New York: Royal Society of Medicine Services Limited, 1992;310.

393. Mitscherlich A, Mielke F. *Doctors of Infamy*;86a.

394. Oppitz DU. Medizinverbrechen vor Gericht;35.

395. Ibid.

396. Mitscherlich A, Mielke F. *Doctors of Infamy*;86a.

397. Galerie hervorragender Ärzte und Naturforscher. *Münchener Medizinische Wochenschrift* 1940;87:559.

398. Jubiläumsbeilage – Lehrer der Heilkunde und ihre Wirkungsstätten. *Münchener Medizinische Wochenschrift* 1934;1.

399. Bleker J, Jachertz N (eds.) *Medizin im "Dritten Reich."* Cologne: Deutscher Ärzte-Verlag, 1989;193.

400. Mitscherlich A, Mielke F. *Doctors of Infamy*;86a.

401. Ebbinghaus A, Dörner K (eds.). *Vernichten und Heilen*;256a.

402. Mitscherlich A, Mielke F. *Doctors of Infamy*;86a.

403. Oppitz DU. Medizinverbrechen vor Gericht;35.

404. Ibid.

405. Benedum J, Giese C. *375 Jahre Medizin in Giessen.* Giessen: Wilhelm Schmitz, 1983;208.

406. Annas GJ, Grodin MA (eds.). *The Nazi doctors and the Nuremberg Code*;117.

407. Mitscherlich A, Mielke F. *Doctors of Infamy*;86a.

408. Schott H (ed.) *Die Chronic der Medizin.* Gütersloh: Chronik Verlag, 1993;483.

409. Courtesy of the Institute of the History of Medicine, Ludwig-Maximilians University, Munich.

410. Mitscherlich A, Mielke F. *Doctors of Infamy*;86a.

411. Ibid.

412. Ibid.

413. Bram L, Philipps RS, Dickey NH. *Funk & Wagnalls New Encyclopedia*, vol. 24. New York: Funk & Wagnalls, 1971;414.

414. Greene NM. Henry Knowles Beecher 1904-1976. *Anesthesiology* 1976;45:377.

415. *World Med J* 1955;2:74.

416. Riedmiller J. Kirche in totalitären Systemen. *Damals* 2001;6:53.

417. Courtesy of Anjou Dargar.

418. New Clinical Research Center. *JAMA* 1953;152:623.

419. Editorial. *World Med J* 1964;12:210.

420. Declaration of Helsinki. Recommendations guiding doctors in clinical research. *World Med J* 1964;12:281.

451. Jubiläumsbeilage - Lehrer der Heilkunde und ihre Wirkungsstätten. *Münchener Medizinische Wochenschrift* 1933;80:6.

422. Schott H (ed.) *Die Chronic der Medizin*;423.

423. Ibid.;421.

424. Sourkes TL. *Nobel Prize Winners in Medicine and Physiology, 1901-1965.* London, New York, Toronto: Abelard-Schuman, 1967;244.

425. Ricci FM. *Dizionario Biografico della Storia della Medicina e delle Scienze Naturali* (Liber Amicorum), vol. 2. Milano: Franco Maria Ricci, 1987;219.

Figure References

426. Courtesy of Anjou Dargar.

427. Szent-Györgyi A. Lost in the twentieth century. *Annual Review of Biochemistry* 1963;32:1a.

428. Heeb C. *USA*. Munich: C.J. Bucher, 1998;118.

429. Bordley J III, McGehee HA. *Two Centuries of American Medicine. 1776-1976*;359.

430. Ibid.;421.

431. Ibid.;420.

432. Courtesy of Anjou Dargar.

433. Courtesy of Anjou Dargar.

434. Hornblum AM. *Acres of Skin*;154a.

435. Brown RF. In memoriam Robert S. Stone, M.D. (1895-1966). *Radiology* 1967;88:807-8.

436. Welsome E. *The Plutonium Files*;212a.

437. Long ER. History of the American Association of Pathologists and Bacteriologists. *Am J Pathol* 1974;77:128S.

438. Welsome E. *The Plutonium Files*;356a.

439. Lyons AS, Petrucelli RJ (eds.) *Medicine. An Illustrated History*. New York: Harry N. Adams, 1987;580.

440. Plewig G. Albert Montgomery Kligman zum 65. Geburtstag. *Hautarzt* 1981;32:392.

441. Abele DC. Presidential messages. *JAAD* 1988;18:813.

442. Hornblum AM. *Acres of Skin*;154a.

443. Nasemann T. Herbert Goldschmidt zum 60. Geburtstag. *Hautarzt* 1983;34:249-50.

444. Weyers W. The abuse of man. Dubious human experiments in dermatology. *Dermatopathol: Prac & Conc* 1999;5:351.

445. Maibach HI, Kligman AM. The biology of experimental human cutaneous moniliasis (Candida albicans). *Archiv Dermatol* 1962;85:114.

446. Ibid.;116.

447. Shelley WB, Kligman AM. The experimental production of acne by penta- and hexachloronaphthalenes. *Archiv Dermatol* 1957;75:690.

448. Ibid.;691.

449. Epstein WL, Kligman AM. Epithelial cysts in buried human skin. *Archiv Dermatol* 1957;76:439.

450. Nasemann T. Reinhard Breit zum 60. Geburtstag. *Hautarzt* 1996;47:559.

451. Abele DC. Presidential messages. *JAAD* 1988;18:838.

452. Szymanski FJ. *Centennial History of American Dermatological Association. 1876-1976*. Chicago: American Dermatological Association, 1976;418.

453. Courtesy of Anjou Dargar.

454. Szymanski FJ. *Centennial History of American Dermatological Association. 1876-1976*. Chicago: American Dermatological Association, 1976;378.

455. Ibid.;460.

456. Ibid.;408.

457. Ibid.;414.

458. Welsome E. *The Plutonium Files*;356a.

459. Stewart WD. Marion B. Sulzberger. *JAAD* 1988;18:878.

460. Szymanski FJ. *Centennial History of American Dermatological Association. 1876-1976*;463.

461. Schott H. *Die Chronik der Medizin.* Gütersloh, München: Chronik-Verlag, 2000;1903.

462. Collins H. The gulp heard round the world. *The Philadelphia Inquirer*, November 20th, 2000;D1.

463. Parish HJ. *A History of Immunization.* Edinburgh, London: E.&S. Livingstone, 1965;272a.

464. Lyons AS, Petrucelli RJ (eds.) *Medicine. An Illustrated History*;580.

465. Courtesy of Anjou Dargar.

466. Szymanski FJ. *Centennial History of American Dermatological Association. 1876-1976*;399.

467. Kestenbaum T. Naomi M. Kanof, M.D. *JAAD* 1988;18:882.

468. Szymanski FJ. *Centennial History of American Dermatological Association. 1876-1976*;414.

469. Kladko B. *Human Guinea Pigs.* Ashbury Park Sunday Press, September 13, 1998.

470. Ibid.

471. Abele DC. Presidential messages. *JAAD* 1988;18:824.

472. Ibid.;821.

473. Shelley ED. Donald M. Pillsbury, M.D. *JAAD* 1988;18:877.

774. Weyers W. The abuse of man. Dubious human experiments in dermatology. *Dermatopathol: Prac & Conc* 1999;5:352.

475. Ibid.;351.

476. Strauss JS, Kligman AM. The effect of androgens and estrogens on human sebaceous glands. *J Investig Dermatol* 1962;39:141.

477. Obermayer ME. Obituary. Samuel William Becker. 1894-1964. *Archiv Dermatol* 1965;91:97.

478. Burnett JW. Stephen Rothman, M.D. *JAAD* 1988;18:876.

479. Hubler WR, Jr. Rudolf L, Baer, M.D. *JAAD* 1988;18:881.

480. Lyons AS, Petrucelli RJ (eds.) *Medicine. An Illustrated History*;523.

481. Greenblatt RB, Dienst RB, Pund ER, Torpin R. Experimental and clinical granuloma inguinale. *JAMA* 1939;113:1111.

482. Ibid.

483. Szymanski FJ. *Centennial History of American Dermatological Association. 1876-1976*;265.

484. Canizares O. Howard Fox: Founding father of the American Academy of Dermatology – a personal reminiscence. *JAAD* 1988;18:793-6.

Figure References

485. Szymanski FJ. *Centennial History of American Dermatological Association. 1876-1976*;137.

486. Jones JH. *Bad Blood. The Tuskegee Syphilis Experiment*. New York: The Free Press, 1993;48a.

487. Mullan F. *Plagues and Politics. The Story of the United States Public Health Service*. New York: Basic Books, 1989;87.

488. Abele DC. Presidential messages. *JAAD* 1988;18:803.

489. Courtesy of Anjou Dargar.

490. Reverby SM (ed.). *Tuskegee's Truths. Rethinking the Tuskegee Syphilis Study*. Chapel Hill, London: University of North Carolina Press, 2000;181a.

491. Ibid.

492. Jones JH. *Bad Blood*;176a.

493. Reverby SM (ed.). *Tuskegee's Tuths*;181a.

494. Ibid.

495. Jones JH. *Bad Blood*;48a.

496. Reverby SM (ed.). *Tuskegee's Truths*;181a.

497. Jones JH. *Bad Blood*;176a.

498. Reverby SM (ed.). *Tuskegee's Truths*;181a.

499. Ibid.

500. Ibid.

501. Mullan F. *Plagues and Politics*;101.

502. Ibid.;100.

503. Reverby SM (ed.). *Tuskegee's Truths*;181a.

504. Mullan F. *Plagues and Politics*;109.

505. Jones JH. *Bad Blood*;176a.

506. Ibid.

507. Ibid.

508. Ibid.

509. Szymanski FJ. *Centennial History of American Dermatological Association. 1876-1976*;387.

510. O'Callaghan B. *An Illustrated History of the USA*. Harlow, England: Longman, 1990;113.

511. Jones JH. *Bad Blood*;176a.

512. Ibid.;48a.

513. Ibid.

514. Ibid.

515. Carmichael AG, Ratzan RM (eds.). *Medicine. A Treasury of Art and Literature*. New York: Hugh Lauter Levin Assoc., 1991;355.

516. Welsome E. *The Plutonium Files*;356a.

517. Bordley J III, McGehee HA. *Two Centuries of American medicine. 1776-1976*;238.

518. Obituary notices. *Br Med J* 1971;2:282.

519. Courtesy of Anjou Dargar.

520. Widdowson EW. R.A. McCance. *Br Med J* 1993;306:851.

521. Obituary notices. *Br Med J* 1991;302:1017.

522. Courtesy of Anjou Dargar.

523. Welsome E. *The Plutonium Files*;356a.

524. Ibid.

525. Szymanski FJ. *Centennial History of American Dermatological Association.* 1876-1976;397.

526. Ibid.;509.

527. Ibid.;505.

528. Clendenning WE, Van Scott EJ. Autografts in psoriasis. *J Investig Dermatol* 1965;45:47.

529. Szymanski FJ. *Centennial History of American Dermatological Association.* 1876-1976;403.

530. Ibid.;377.

531. Daily AD. Walter C. Lobitz, M.D. *JAAD* 1988;18:882.

532. Hubler WR, Jr. Clarence S. Livingood. *JAAD* 1988;18:880.

533. Mullan F. *Plagues and Politics*;166.

534. Ibid.;167.

535. Hornblum AM. *Acres of Skin*;154a.

536. Ibid.

537. Courtesy of Anjou Dargar.

538. Szymanski FJ. *Centennial History of American Dermatological Association.* 1876-1976;416.

539. Stüttgen G (ed.). *Standort und Ausblick der deutschsprachigen Dermatologie. Zum 100jährigen Bestehen der Deutschen Dermatologischen Gesellschaft.* Berlin, Grosse, 1989;3.

540. Küster W. *Geschichte der Düsseldorfer Hautklinik von 1896 bis 1996.* Düsseldorf, Marburg: Küster, Neuse, 1996;90.

541. Courtesy of Lou Manna.

542. Courtesy of A. B. Ackerman.

543. Hornblum AM. *Acres of Skin*;154a.

544. Ibid.

545. Ibid.

546. Ibid.

547. Ibid.

548. Courtesy of University of Iowa Library.

549. Szymanski FJ. *Centennial History of American Dermatological Association, 1876-1976*;379.

550. Burg G (ed.). *Dermatologie. Entwicklungen und Beziehungen zu anderen Fachgebieten.* Munich, Vienna, Baltimore: Urban & Schwarzenberg, 1998:162.

551. Feuerman EH. Im memoriam Felix Sagher. *Hautarzt* 1983;34:101.

552. Liban E, Zuckerman A, Sagher F. Specific tissue alteration in leprous skin. VII. Inoculation of Leishmania tropica into leprous patients. *Arch Dermatol Syphilol* 1955;71:445.

553. Cabré J. Zum Gedenken an Xavier Vilanova. *Dermatol Wochenschr* 1965; 151:1207.

554. González-Ochoa A, Ricoy E, Bravo-Becherelle MA. Study of prophylactic action of griseofulvin – human experimental infection with Trichophyton concentricum. *J Investig Dermatol* 1964;42:56.

555. Courtesy of Anjou Dargar.

556. Courtesy of Anjou Dargar.

557. Beecher HK. Ethics and clinical research. *N Eng J Med* 1966;274:1354.

558. Bordley J III, McGehee HA. *Two Centuries of American Medicine, 1776-1976*;422.

559. Mullan F. *Plagues and Politics*;75.

560. Ibid.;151.

561. Courtesy of Anjou Dargar.

562. Gehrig OM. Ein Herz kann man doch reparieren. *Badische Zeitung*, September 3, 2001;3.

563. Jones JH. *Bad Blood*;176a.

564. Collins H. Penn, family settle suit in gene-therapy death. *The Philadelphia Inquirer*, November 4, 2000;A15.

565. Kolata G. Johns Hopkins admits fault in fatal experiment. *The New York Times*, July 17, 2001.

566. *Br Med J* 1980;281:752.

567. Courtesy of Anjou Dargar.

568. Ackerman AB. Holmesburg Prison, Philadelphia, September 1966 – June 1967: acknowledgement of error and regret. *Dermatopathol: Prac & Conc* 1999;6:213.

569. Reverby SM (ed.). *Tuskegee's Truths*;181a.

570. Courtesy of Allen M. Hornblum.

571. Szymanski FJ. *Centennial History of American Dermatological Association. 1876-1976*;349.

572. Ibid.;506.

573. Courtesy of Anjou Dargar.

INDEX

Index

beriberi, prison inmate study on, 190–191
Berkley, Henry J., 199–200
Berlin Chamber of Physicians, 227–228, 233, 574
Berlin-Spandau gas chamber, poison gas studies, 274–275
Bernard, Claude
  on Christian morals and informed consent, 592, 621
  defense of experiments on humans, 49–52, 208
  effects of heat on animals, 122, 123
  on prisoners as medical test subjects, 62
Besnier, Ernest, 103
Bessau, Georg, 220
Bettinger, Julius, 53, 54
Biberstein, Hans, 217–218
Bible, as early knowledge source, 7
Bicêtre, Paris (prison and hospice), venereal disease tests in, 61–62
Bickenbach, Otto, 275, 337
Bier, August, 182, 227–228
Biggs, Hermann M., 197
Bignami, Amico, 173
Bilibid Prison, Manila
  beriberi study by U.S. in, 190–191
  vaccination testing by U.S. in, 189–190
bioethics
  birth of, 583–585
  pharmaceutical industry and, 607
biological warfare studies
  Geneva Convention and, 336
  Iraqi, 595
  Japanese, 294–295
    destructive aspects of, 303–304
    at Pingfan Research facility, 301–302
    post WWII use of, 363–365
  Nazi, 274–275
Bismarck, Otto von, 130
Black, William C., 212–213
Blackwell, Elizabeth, 179
Blauer, Harold, 528–529
blind adults, gonorrhea experiments on, 35
Blome, Kurt, 274, 342, 359, 365
blood circulation experiments, 11–12, 13
  transfusions, 83–84
  U.S. prison inmates as test subjects, 422
blood components, heart disease and, U.S. prison studies on, 421–422
bloodletting, 83
Blumberg, Baruch, 453
Bockhart, Max, 32–33, 37, 111
Boeck, Caesar
  course of syphilis study, 173–174, 480
  Tuskegee Syphilis Study *versus* study by, 496
Boeck, Carl Wilhelm
  syphilization by, 100–101
Bókai, Arpad, 31–32
Boston University, "Concept of Consent in Clinical Research" conference (1961), 513–514

botulinum toxin vaccine, U.S. Defense Dept. use of, 596
Boylston, Zabdiel, 65
Brack, Viktor, 342, 359
brain
  biopsies on live patients, 163–164
  research from euthanasia program, 271
  skull hole drilling during head and neck surgery for monitoring, 527
Brandt, Karl, 341, 342, 348–349, 353, 359
Brandt, Rudolf, 342, 359
Braun, Wernher von, 365
Breit, Reinhard, 434
Brewer, Earl, 192, 193
Bristol-Meyers, drug testing in prisons and, 542
British Advisory Committee for Medical War Crimes, 340
British Journal of Dermatology (Morris and Brooke), 169
British Medical Journal
  on liver dysfunction from triacetyloleandomycin for acne, 547–548
  on patient consent in Germany, 154
British Medical Research Council
  on patient consent, 375
Brooke, Henry Ambrose Grundy
  British Journal of Dermatology and, 169
Broussais, FranRois-Joseph-Victor, 20–21, 369
Brown, James M., 201
Brown, William J., 500–501
Bruck, Carl, 119
Bruusgaard, Edvin, 173–174, 480, 496
Buchenwald concentration camp, 260, 272, 283, 347
Buchheim, Rudolf, 90–91
Bumm, Ernst, 31, 33–34, 70, 111
Burney, Leroy, 491–492
Buschke, Abraham, 30, 31
Bush, Vannevar, 392–393
business of medical research, U.S.
  drug licensing and, 533–537
  FDA review of, 556–560
  grants *versus* contracts, 532–533
  Kligman model of, 617
  prison inmate recruitment and pay, 537–542
  profit margins for researchers, 542–544
  recklessness of, 544–551
  scientific method and, 552–555
Butterfield, W.J.H., 420–421, 538
Buxton, Peter J., 500–501, 502, 582, 586
Byers, J. Wellington, 475

Cahn, Milton, 428–429
Calesnick, Benjamin, 555
California, experiments on incompetent persons law in, 448
Calmette, Albert Léon Charles, 204, 229–230
calomen, clinical trials of, 93, 369
Cambodia, Red Khmer government procedures on political prisoners, 594

Index

Index

Index

Index

Index

Index

TYPESET IN MILLER, MANTINIA, AND GALLIARD
TYPES DESIGNED BY MATTHEW CARTER.
PRINTED ON ACCENT OPAQUE
PAPER. BOOK DESIGN BY
JERRY KELLY.

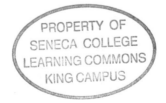